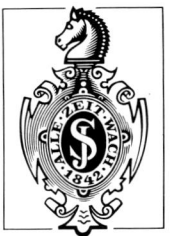

René Louis

Surgery of the Spine

Surgical Anatomy and Operative Approaches

Foreword by Leon L. Wiltse

With 140 Figures in 655 Separate Illustrations

Springer-Verlag
Berlin Heidelberg New York 1983

René Louis
Professor of Anatomy and of Surgery, Chief, Vertebral Surgery Service
Hôpital Hôtel-Dieu; 6, Place Daviel, F-13224 Marseille Cedex 1, France

The original illustrations have been prepared by the author with the
technical assistance of Wahed Ghafar.

Translator: Dr. Elliot Goldstein
1, Square des Feuillants, Parly II, F-78150 Le Chesnay, France

Title of the original French edition: *Chirurgie du rachis*
© Springer-Verlag Berlin Heidelberg New York 1982
ISBN 3-540-11363-0
ISBN 0-387-11363-0

ISBN 3-540-11412-2 Springer-Verlag Berlin Heidelberg New York
ISBN 0-387-11412-2 Springer-Verlag New York Heidelberg Berlin

Library of Congress Cataloging in Publication Data
Louis, René, 1933 –. Surgery of the spine. Translation of: Chirurgie du rachis. Bibliogra-
phy: p. Includes index. 1. Spine-Surgery. 2. Surgery, Operative. 3. Spine-Anatomy. 4. Anatomy, Surgical and topographical.
[DNLM: 1. Spine-Surgery. WE 725 L 888 c] I. Title. RD 533. L 6713 1983 617′.56059 82-16805

© Springer-Verlag Berlin Heidelberg 1983
Printed in Germany

Typesetting and bookbinding: G. Appl, Wemding. Printing: aprinta, Wemding
2124/3140-543210

Foreword

In this comprehensive and original monograph, Professor René Louis presents in minute detail in one volume the gross anatomy, nerve supply, biomechanics, and microcirculation of the spine. He also presents the surgical approaches to the vertebral bodies and their contents. Professor Louis is a great anatomist and this book has been prepared from his personal observations, both anatomical and surgical. His studies have been meticulously conducted and contain much original research, for instance his work on the motion of the neural elements within the lumbar vertebral canal.

The illustrations are nearly all original and very often a photograph of the neural or vascular elements is presented alongside a drawing of a given important anatomical area.

For all these reasons, this inspiring treatise makes a valuable contribution to our knowledge of the spine and forms a basis for an understanding of the intricacies of surgical anatomy and approaches. It will be especially valuable to the spinal surgeon, but the medical student, the orthopedic resident (or registrar), and the anatomist will also find it extremely useful.

Long Beach, July 1982

Leon L. Wiltse, M.D.
Professor of University
of California

Preface

Surgery of the spine, with its twin osteoarticular and neural structure, comes under two specialties, orthopedics and neurosurgery. Because of its axial position in the body, the spine passes through such varied regions as the neck, thorax, and abdomen; to gain access by the anterior approach most surgeons require the collaboration of a specialist in otorhinolaryngology or thoracic, general, or even vascular surgery.

Can this state of affairs be considered the best possible solution to the problems of spinal surgery? The answer is certainly yes if surgical education retains its classical teaching subdivisions. However, the answer would probably be no if the development of surgeons could instead be oriented more toward spinal surgery, leading to it becoming a *full-fledged specialty*. The theoretical and practical teaching of this specialty would have to include the fundamentals of orthopedics, neurosurgery, vascular surgery, and especially general surgery, all applied to the cervical, thoracic and lumbosacral approaches to the spine. During internship and assistant professorship from 1956–1965 my development as a spinal surgeon was accomplished by a self-imposed education of this type, which is at the moment the only way in which the *technical independence* of spinal surgery can be obtained. However, it should be possible to reduce the period of training by offering a consolidated teaching programme. Indeed, the major aim of this book is to bring together the classical, modern, and some personal notions of *anatomy* applied to the surgery of the spine.

The book has been divided into two parts. The first part deals with the fundamental aspects of development, morphology, dynamics, vascularization, and neural systematization of the spine as a whole, and aims to give an understanding of the *main functions* of the spine: statics, stability, dynamics, neural protection, vascular support, and radiculomedullary transmission. Investigation of these functions is necessary in the evaluation of spinal lesions, and their reestablishment should be the primary goal of therapy. The second part of the book deals with the topographical features and surgical approaches in the different regions of the spine. Emphasis is placed on full discussion of regional topography, as this element is basic to safety and efficacy in spinal surgery. Topographical varieties are described in detail, along with the main vasculoneural and visceral anomalies or malformations, which are a potential source of risk if not recognized during surgery. The surgical approaches described represent the outcome of my long experience of constant application and refinement. An effort has been made to identify the possible mishaps and complications of each technique clearly and to present the means of avoiding or treating them. The various anterior and posterior approaches allow access to every part of the spine with full security. Indeed, it is my opinion that the failure to recognize the technical possibilities of these approaches "à la carte" to the spinal regions prevents many surgeons to operating more directly and effectively. For example, fracture of L1 with marked angulation of the vertebral body and anterior compression of the spinal cord would be treated by laminectomy and posterior osteosynthesis if the surgeon were unfamiliar with the anterior approach. However, left thoracophrenolumbotomy would allow full reduction of the angulation, anterior decompression of the spinal cord at the actual site of compression, and stabilization by reconstitution of the anterior column of the spine with intercorporeal grafting and osteosynthesis. The reliability of such direct techniques and the quality of the results obtained should enable the reader to *broaden his technical capability* regarding the approaches to the spine.

A second book, now in the planning stage, will treat the "technical aspects" of surgery of the spine as a function of the etiology of the lesions to be treated.

Thus in any specific clinical situation, this book should allow selection of the surgical approach while the second will help to identify the treatment procedure based on etiology.

The material on which these books are based has been collected patiently since 1956 from my anatomical studies of radiculomedullary topography, the vascular topography of the spine, and vertebral and radiculospinal biodynamics. My experience in surgery of the spine began in Marseilles in 1964, was pursued in Dakar (Senegal) from 1966–1971, and has continued from 1971 onward in the hospital service back in Marseilles, specializing in all aspects of spinal surgery. As a result of this work, all the anatomical and surgical illustrations were personally conceived and drawn, down to their finest details. The final shading of the illustrations was done by my talented collaborator Wahed Ghafar, a visiting fellow from Afghanistan to whom I wish to express my sincere gratitude.

I would also like to thank all those who made this work possible, above all my teachers and friends at the *Marseille School of Anatomy:* Professors M. Salmon, J. Grisoli, J. Gambarelli, P. Bourret, and G. Guerinel. I am indebted to my collaborators and the friends who contributed to my research: Professors A. Manbrini, Y. Baille, D. Obounou-Akong, R. Ouminga, G. Salamon, J. Laffont, and C. Argenson, and Doctors S. Henry, C. Maresca, and P. Auteroche. I express my gratitude to Mrs. V. Azria and Miss A. Orhan for their expert secretarial assistance. Finally, my sincere thanks go to Doctor Götze and his brilliant colleagues from Springer-Verlag for their interest in my work and the perfection they have brought to the publication of this book.

Marseille, July 1982   René Louis

Contents

Part 1

Descriptive and Functional Anatomy

1 Normal and Pathological Development of the Spine

I. Introduction

The appearance of the vertebral column in the animal kingdom is of such great importance that the phylum Vertebrata, in which *Homo sapiens* is the most evolved species, is defined by the presence of this structure. At first simply represented by the notochord, the axial skeleton is associated with the vertebrae in the higher species, solidity thus being added to the flexibility of the primitive spine. The vertebrate animals are also characterized by the formation of a neural tube, developed on the posterior aspect of the notochord and enveloped by the vertebrae. Finally the phenomenon of metamerization, beginning in the higher invertebrates, represents a characteristic evolutionary trait of the vertebrates. The development of the spine is a perfect illustration of metamerization.

Normal embryonic development occurs under the control of *chromosomal genes* followed by a succession of *chemical inductors* determining cellular differentiation and then cellular organization. The chorda-mesoderm represents the primary inductor of the vertebral column. Development of the corporeal form or *morphogenesis* precedes constitution of the organs or *organogenesis,* the final step being *histogenesis.* Because of the successive nature of embryogenesis, the effect of teratogenic agents is all the more severe during early embryonic development. Errors of morphogenesis lead to *monstrosity,* whereas abnormal organogenesis or histogenesis results in *malformation.* Accordingly, after each main stage of vertebral development we shall describe the teratologic series extending from monstrosity to malformation which arises from the more or less precocious and intense alteration of normal embryonic phenomena. Full development of the spine is not restricted to the prenatal period but continues into the first years of postnatal life.

II. Prenatal Development

This period consists of four main stages.

A. Formation of the Primitive Streak

At the end of the second week of intrauterine life the embryonic disc is a bilaminar structure composed of ectoderm and endoderm. The cells in the caudal region of the embryonic disc migrate toward the midline to form the *primitive streak* appearing as a narrow groove flanked by small bulgings with a thickening at the cephalic end known as Hensen's node.

The prochordal plate visible as a thickening in the cephalic region of the endoderm along the axis of the primitive streak is the inductor of the cephalic formations. The embryo thus displays its axial orientation with the future situation of the spine already determined.

Embryonic anomalies arising prior to this stage may lead to symmetrical (gemellary) or asymmetrical (twin monsters) division of the embryo with two spines, either separate or joined by a common region.

B. Formation of the Notochord

Beginning on the 15th day modified ectodermal cells move toward the primitive streak, invaginate, and migrate between the ectodermal and endodermal layers to form the third embryonic layer or *chorda-mesoderm.* The invagination of cells cranially from Hensen's node along the midline forms the *notochord,* which grows until it reaches the prochordal plate. An orifice on the primitive streak, *the primitive pit (blastopore),* extends into the notochordal process to form a lumen known as the *neurenteric canal.* The floor of the notochord fuses with the endoderm and by degeneration allows the neurenteric canal temporarily to connect the yolk sac and amniotic cavity. What remains of the notochord groups together to form a solid midline rod separated from the endoderm, thus obliterating the neurenteric communication. On either side of the notochord the lateral cells of the primitive streak give rise to the *paraxial mesoderm.*

Abnormal development during this phase leads to a teratological series known as notochordal dysraphia (Duhamel 1966) where the common denominator is a local defect in fusion of the notochord. Major forms of dysraphia include esophageal or colic *hernia* through a spinal fissure. A *dorsal enteric fistula* arises when a digestive diverticulum passes through the spine to open on the posterior wall of the trunk. In most cases the fistula regresses before birth, leaving behind only a *dorsal remnant of the enteric fistula,* i.e., pre- or intraspinal cyst, dermal sinus, and duplication of the digestive tube. Anterior rachischisis due to sagittal fissuration of the vertebral bodies and segmental duplication of the spinal cord or diastematomyelia are also related to this series of malformations.

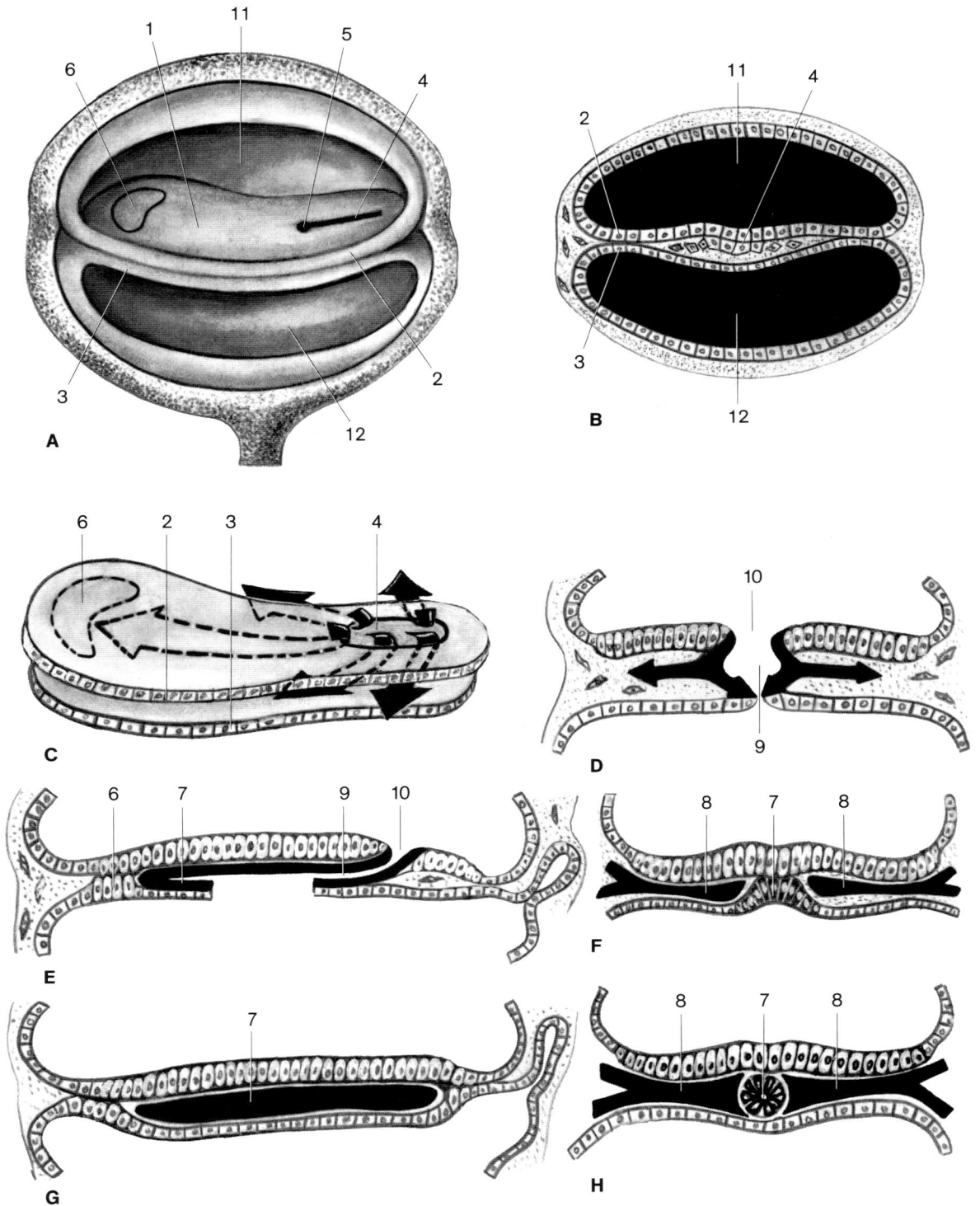

Figure 1 A–H

Sagittal *(left)* and frontal *(right)* sections through the human embryo during the third week of development

1 embryonic disc *2* ectoderm *3* endoderm *4* primitive streak
5 Hensen's node *6* prochordal plate *7* notochord

8 paraxial mesoderm *9* neurenteric canal *10* primitive pit
(blastopore) *11* amniotic cavity *12* yolk sac

C. Formation of the Neuraxis

At the beginning of the third week the ectoderm over the notochord thickens from Hensen's node up to the cephalic end of the embryo to form the *neural plate* of the neurectoderm. A few days later the lateral margins of the neural plate lift up while the midline region depresses thus forming the *neural groove*. The lateral folds of the neural groove continue toward each other and fuse on the midline to create the *neural tube*. Fusion begins in the region of the fourth somite and continues cranially and caudally with persistence of an orifice at either end called the *anterior and posterior neuropores*. These orifices allow communication between the neural tube and the amniotic cavity up to the 23rd day (anterior neuropore) and 25th day (posterior neuropore). During the process of neural tube closure some ectodermal cells on the lateral edges of the neural groove differentiate to form the *neural crests*. Prior to dorsal fusion of the neural tube, the neural crests migrate laterally, later giving rise to the spinal ganglions and latero- and prevertebral vegetative ganglions.

The enlarged cranial end of the neural tube dilates to form three primitive cerebral vesicles and evolves toward the formation of the encephalon. The neural tube caudal to the fourth somite gives rise to the future spinal cord. The inductor of the neural plate and thus of the spinal cord would be Hensen's node or the primordial notochord. Similarly, the closure of the neural tube constitutes an induction for the formation and closure of the posterior envelopes of the spine. Posterior to the neural tube the mesenchyme grows from the embryonic mesoderm giving rise to the endomeninges (pia mater and arachnoid membrane), ectomeninges (dura mater and posterior arches of the vertebrae), and derm, which induces the transformation of the ectoderm into epiblast and then epiderm with exoskeleton.

About the middle of the fourth week the cells of the neurectoderm differentiate to form three layers: the inner *ependymal layer,* surrounding the lumen of the ependymal canal; the middle *mantle layer,* formed of neuroblasts, which gives rise to the gray matter of the spinal cord; and the outer *marginal layer,* containing the nerve fibers, which gives rise to the white matter of the spinal cord.

Up to the third month the spinal cord occupies the entire length of the vertebral canal. However, thereafter the spine grows more rapidly than the neural tube so that the caudal end of the spinal cord apparently ascends within the vertebral canal. According to Barson (1970) the caudal end of the spinal cord lies near L4 at the ninth week and near the lower margin of L2 at term.

As proposed by Duhamel (1966), errors of posterior closure of the neuraxis can be termed encephalomyelodysraphia. The most severe form is complete encephalomyeloaraphia or *anencephaly,* featuring arrested morphological development at the neural groove stage but normal histological development and nerves. This malformation involves the entire spine and cranium. Less advanced forms include *myelodysraphia* or *spina bifida. Spina bifida aperta* or myeloaraphia, most often located in the lower lumbar region, is an exteriorization of the neural plate or neural tube without overlying meninges, bone, or skin. *Meningocele* is characterized by the protrusion of the membranes of the spinal cord through a defect in the posterior vertebral arch. A hernia also containing the spinal cord is termed meningomyelocele. Minor forms of malformation include *spina bifida occulta,* featuring only the defective closure of the posterior arch sometimes accompanied by a tuft of hair on the skin overlying the defect, *circumscribed cutaneous aplasia* with a thin smooth integument, and dermal sinus, which may be either a blind fistula or cystic cavity with an epidermoid lining. Other anomalies can be likened to these malformations of the neuraxis: *diastematomyelia,* where a portion of the spinal cord is divided into two hemicords separated by a bony septum; *hydromyelia* and *syringomyelia,* featuring endomedullary cavities; and finally *myelodysplasia,* associating histological abnormalities of the spinal cord with talipes cavus, spina bifida occulta, and minor neurological disturbances.

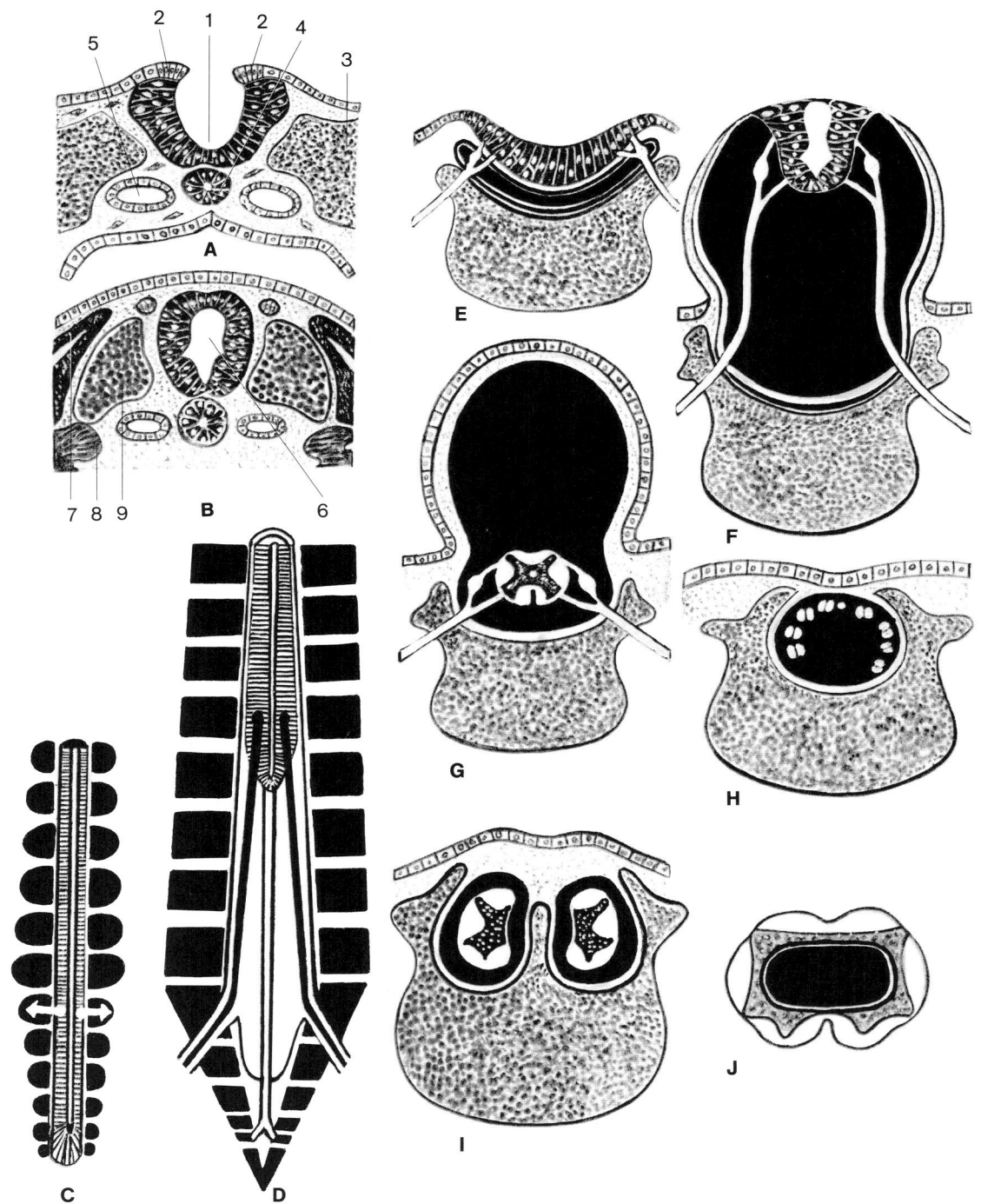

Figure 2 A–J

A Neural groove
B Neural tube
C Caudal end of spinal cord flush with end of vertebral canal before the third month
D Spinal cord terminates at L2 at birth
E Myeloaraphia at the neural groove stage
F Myeloaraphia at the neural tube stage
G Meningocele

H Spina bifida occulta
I Diastematomyelia
J Syringomyelia

1 neural groove 2 neural crest 3 paraxial mesoderm 4 spinal cord
5 dorsal aorta 6 neural tube 7 somite 8 intermediate mesoderm
9 sclerotome

D. Formation of the Sclerotome

On about the 18th day during the formation of the neuraxis, the paraxial mesoderm begins to divide into symmetrical paired cuboidal bodies, called *somites*, lying on either side of the neural groove. The first pair of somites develops a short distance caudal to the cranial end of the notochord and subsequent pairs develop in a craniocaudal sequence yielding eventually 42–44 pairs, i.e., 4 occipital, 8 cervical, 12 thoracic, 5 lumbar, 5 sacral, and 8–10 coccygeal pairs. The first occipital and final coccygeal somites eventually disappear. At the end of the fourth week the somites divide into three cell colonies: the *dermatome*, which migrates under the epiblast to form the dermis and subcutaneous tissue; the *myotome*, giving rise to the musculature; and the *sclerotome*, which takes on the histological aspect of mesenchyme and develops on the right and left of the axial structures (notochord and neural tube). Degeneration of the notochord is the inductor of sclerotome formation. The sclerotome is the initial tissue giving rise to the future vertebral model. It is probable that the sclerotome is segmented like the somites, although Baur (1969) observed at this stage only a homogeneous blastema without metamerization. The developing vertebra is thus paired and symmetrical, the two halves rapidly fusing around the cord and neuraxis. This is the sclerotome stage with a *precartilaginous or membranous vertebra*. Each sclerotome contains a loosely packed cranial zone and a densely packed caudal zone. The densely packed cells migrate opposite the center of the myotome and give rise to the anulus fibrosus of the intervertebral disc and the intervertebral ligaments. The loosely packed cells spread out to occupy the spaces left by the migrating densely packed cells, straddling two myotomes, where they give rise to the precartilaginous vertebral bodies. The notochord degenerates within the vertebral bodies but persists in the intervertebral disc to form the nucleus pulposus. The sclerotome contains two other cell colonies, one of which migrates dorsally to form the model of the future posterior arch. The other colony migrates ventrolaterally to constitute the costal process. Although all the vertebrae present a budding costal process, only those of the thoracic vertebrae develop to form ribs. In the other spinal regions, costal buds take part in the formation of the transverse processes.

During the sixth week three pairs of chondrification centers appear in each mesenchymal vertebra. One pair of centers forms the cartilaginous *centrum* which gives rise to the vertebral body, one pair leads to formation of the posterior arch, and the third gives rise to the costal or transverse processes. This is the stage of the *cartilaginous vertebra*.

From the third month three primary ossification centers appear, thus announcing formation of the *bony vertebra*. There is one ossification center in the centrum and one in each half of the vertebral arch. The lateral primary centers in the vertebral arch are located in the zone of future attachment of the transverse and articular processes. The ossification centers do not appear simultaneously over the entire spine. The ossification centers of the centrum first appear in the thoracolumbar junction, whereas those of the vertebral arch are first seen in the cervical region. The development of the primary ossification centers allows rapid growth of the vertebrae by typical enchondral ossification of the cranial and caudal surfaces and of the dorsal junction with the posterior arch. The cranial and caudal surfaces are the superior and inferior surfaces of the vertebral body on which are inserted the fibers of the anulus fibrosus. A cartilaginous zone known as *Schmorl's intermediate cartilage* is located between the primary centers of the vertebral arch and centrum. The scheme of ossification is slightly different at the two ends of the spine. The atlas presents only two primary ossification centers located in the posterior arch, the third center in the anterior arch appearing as a secondary center near birth. Conversely, in addition to the standard three pairs of primary ossification centers, the axis presents a supplementary pair of centers for the odontoid process which thus appears as the centrum of the atlas attached to the axis. The cartilage between the odontoid process and the body of the axis is homologous to an intervertebral disc. The sacrum is constituted by the grouping together of five vertebrae each having the standard ossification centers. The costal processes of the first three sacral vertebrae fuse together to form the ala sacralis. The coccyx is limited to the median primary centers of the centrum of a few vertebrae.

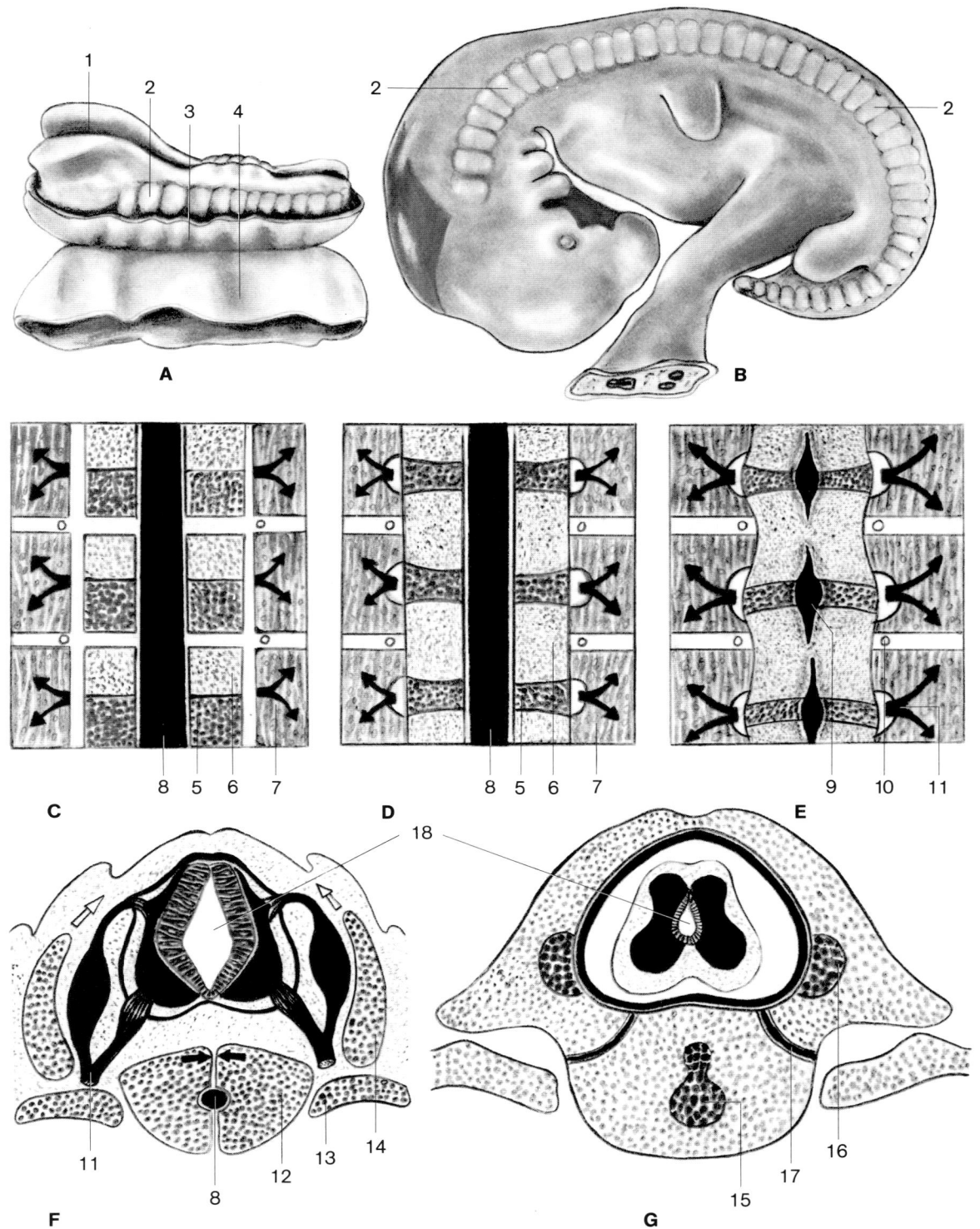

Figure 3A–G

A   Left lateral view of a 22-day-old embryo
B   Left lateral view of a 34-day-old embryo
C–E   The three stages of formation of the sclerotome
F   The three parts of the sclerotome
G   The cartilaginous vertebra with its three primary ossification
    centers

1 neural groove *2* somites *3* amnion (cut edge) *4* cut wall of the
yolk sac *5* densely packed region of the sclerotome *6* loosely packed
region of the sclerotome *7* myotome *8* notochord *9* nucleus
pulposus *10* metameric artery *11* spinal nerve *12* hemicentrum
13 bud of costal process *14* bud of posterior arch *15* median
primary ossification center of centrum *16* lateral primary ossification
center of posterior arch *17* Schmorl's intermediate cartilage
18 central canal

III. Postnatal Development

The formation of the spine continues after birth. Spinal growth and adaptation to the erect position are achieved in the postnatal period.

A. Maturation and Growth of the Vertebrae

Schmorl's intermediate cartilage evolves toward the fusion of the median and lateral primary ossification centers and thus disappears between the ages of 4 and 8 years, depending on the subject. Fusion of the lateral primary ossification centers occurs during the first year of postnatal life. Consequently, full dehiscence of the vertebral arches of the spine exists at birth. Fusion begins in the lower thoracic spine and extends cranially and caudally to involve the entire spine at about the age of 7 years. Thus the apparent radiological absence of fusion of the posterior sacral arches should not be referred to as spina bifida in a given child before the age of 8 years.

After birth, *secondary ossification centers* appear in the superior and inferior surfaces of the vertebral bodies and in the vertebral processes. The secondary centers of the vertebral bodies are also known as the annular epiphyses or as *cartilaginous* and then *osseous margins of Schmorl and Junghans*. Up to the age of 2 years the cranial and caudal surfaces of the centrum or vertebral body are covered by cartilage with an annular ridge seen on roentgenography as a notch on the angles of the centrum, giving a steplike image. Islets of bone appear in the annular ridge of the cartilaginous margin at about the age of 2 years in the thoracolumbar region (T10 to L1) and involve the entire spine at about the age of 10 years. These secondary centers have often been considered as discoid plates homologous to the epiphysis of the long bones of the limbs and from which the spine grows. However, according to Schmorl and Junghans each of these centers is an ossification anulus belonging to the intervertebral discs and forming coupled units, i.e., cartilaginous disc-plates constituting a mobile, elastic, shock-absorbing physiological entity, as opposed to the rigid vertebral bodies. The osseous margins are seen as an opaque line, detached from the superior and inferior surfaces of the vertebral bodies with an anterior thickening near the angles of the vertebral bodies.

Fusion of these bony ridges occurs progressively, beginning at the age of 14 years and terminating in the lumbar region no later than the age of 17–18 years. The other secondary ossification centers are located in the spinous processes (paired centers in the cervical region), transverse processes, superior and inferior articular processes, and lumbar mamillary processes. These centers appear between the ages of 11 and 18 years and their fusion is complete when growth stops between the ages of 21 and 25 years. The atlas presents a secondary ossification center in the anterior arch. The axis possesses a secondary center for the ossification of the odontoid process, a center for the inferior surface of its vertebral body, and a pair of ossification centers for its spinous process. The seventh cervical vertebra displays a well-developed costal ossification center anterior to the transverse processes. Fusion of the different sacral segments occurs in the caudocranial direction but is complete only at the age of 30 years in most adults, with the absence of definitive fusion persisting in some cases.

B. Adaptation to the Erect Position

Study of the spinal column in the evolution of the vertebrate animals shows that adaptation to quadrupedia is achieved by the appearance of *cervical lordosis* and that adaptation to the erect position in the higher anthropoid animals and man is related to the presence of *lumbosacral lordosis*. At birth cervical lordosis is fully established, whereas in our opinion lumbosacral lordosis is incomplete (Louis 1964). Despite the rapid development in the fetus of a lumbosacral angle forming the promontory at the level of the vertebral bodies, this angle seems to be due to the progressive regression of the volume of the sacral vertebral bodies rather than the existence of a true angulation between the lumbar and sacral spine.

In large series of newborn infants and adults, we measured the angles formed by the inferior articular column of L5 with the posterior plane of the L5 vertebral body. The mean angle was 168° at birth and 145° in adult Europeans (France) and 150° in adult black Africans (Senegal). It was deduced from these results that lumbosacral lordosis undergoes completion after birth and that the lumbosacral isthmic region (generally L5, sometimes L4 or L3) displays a further average incurvation of 18°–23° during growth.

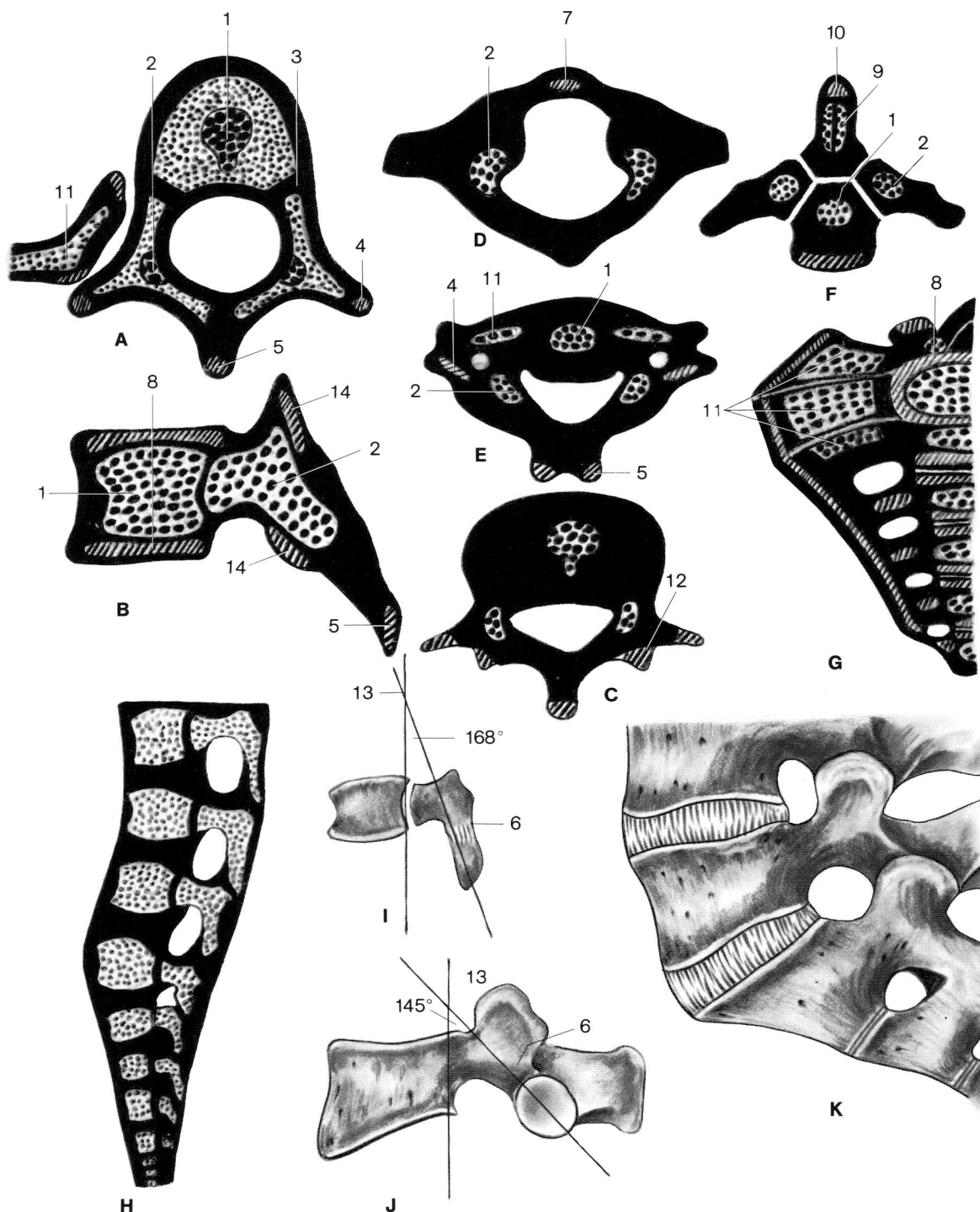

Figure 4 A–K

A, B   Primary and secondary ossification centers of the thoracic vertebrae

C   Ossification of the lumbar vertebrae

D   Ossification of the atlas

E, F   Ossification of the axis

G   Ossification of the sacrum

H, I   The lumbosacral column and fifth lumbar vertebra of the neonate

J, K   The lumbosacral column and fifth lumbar vertebra of the adult

1 median primary ossification center   *2* lateral primary center
3 Schmorl's intermediate cartilage   *4* secondary ossification center of transverse process   *5* secondary center of spinous process   *6* vertebral isthmus   *7* secondary center of the anterior arch   *8* marginal ridge or annular epiphysis   *9* primary ossification centers of the odontoid process   *10* secondary center of the odontoid process   *11* primary costal center   *12* secondary center of mamillary process
13 lumbosacral isthmic angle   *14* secondary ossification center

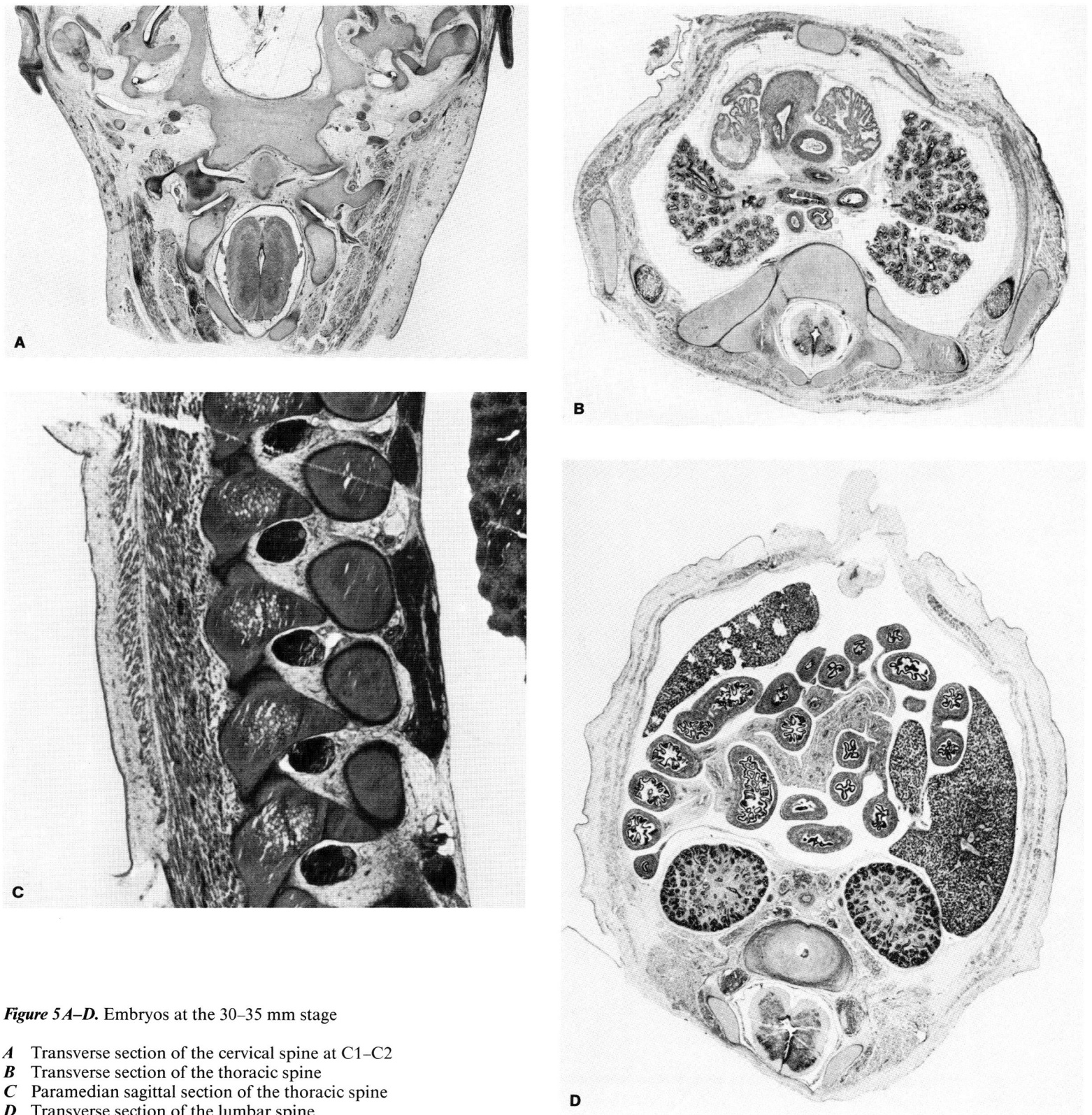

Figure 5 A–D. Embryos at the 30–35 mm stage

A   Transverse section of the cervical spine at C1–C2
B   Transverse section of the thoracic spine
C   Paramedian sagittal section of the thoracic spine
D   Transverse section of the lumbar spine

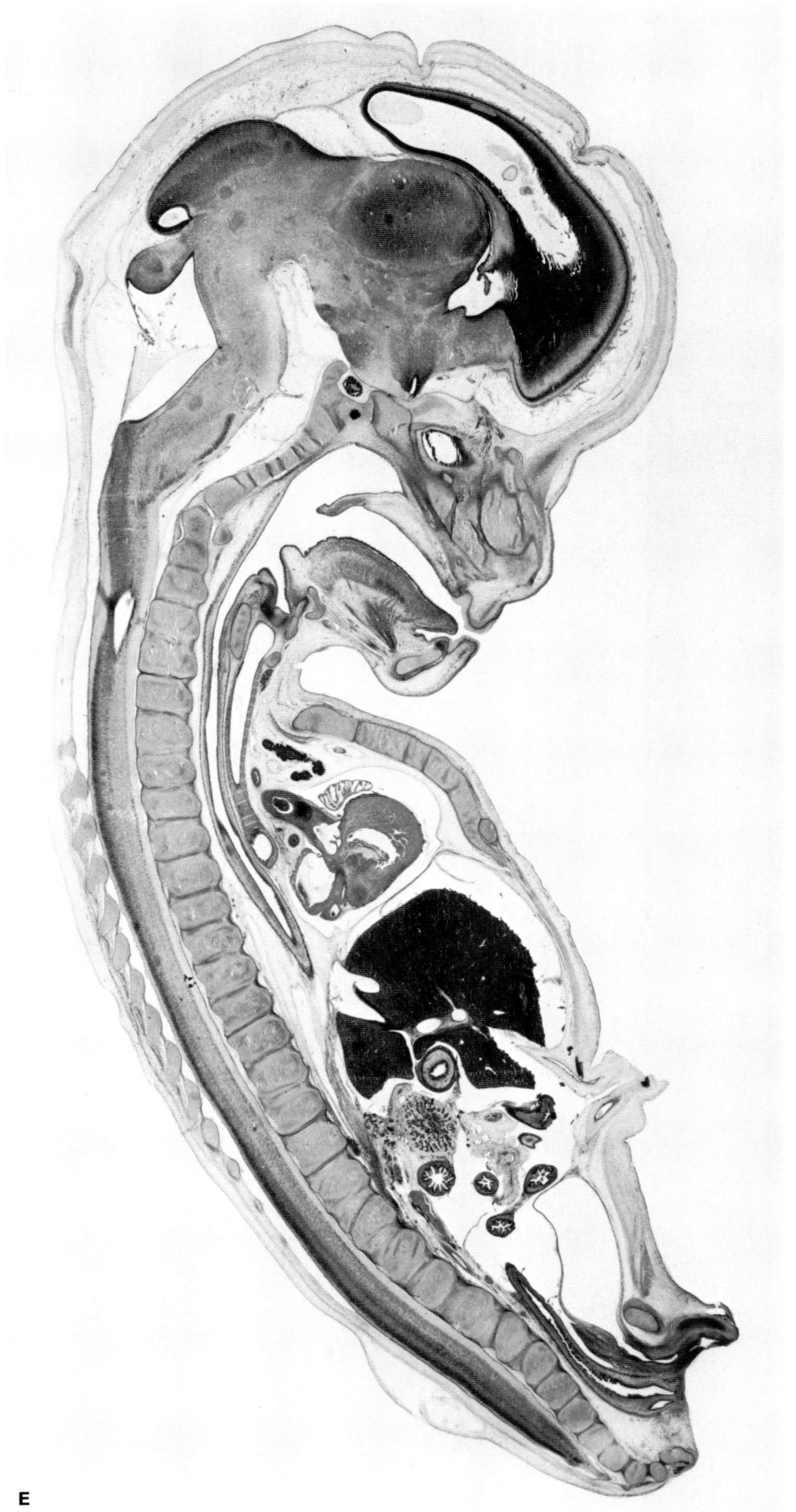

Figure 5 E

Median sagittal section of a 35-mm embryo
($\times 6.5$)

E

IV. Malformations of the Vertebrae

A. Dysraphia of the Notochord

The persistence of the neurenteric canal or simply its replacement by an adhesion of the digestive tube to the notochord leads to the absence of fusion of the two halves of the sclerotome known as *anterior rachischisis*. In this malformation the vertebral body is divided into left and right segments resembling the wings of a butterfly. The reader should recall diastematomyelia, where the spinal cord is divided into two segments by the mesodermal tissue and often by a bony septum arising from the posterior surface of the vertebral bodies.

A very severe form of dysraphia is *iniencephaly,* a monstrosity featuring anterior and posterior fissure of the cervical spine, occipital bone, and upper thoracic vertebrae. The central cavity is occupied by very abnormal posterior brain and spinal cord with a digestive adhesion or fistula. The appearance of iniencephaly is characteristic: the head is in retroflexion with absence of the nuchal region and continuity of the scalp directly on the dorsal skin.

Vertebral dysmorphia or "mosaic spine" is a less severe form of dysraphia of the notochord, although the morphological aspect of a more or less large spinal segment is highly disturbed by the existence of right and left compensated hemivertebrae. These lesions can be accounted for by a defect in the anterior fusion of the vertebral bodies causing a shift in the level of fusion between the right and left hemisclerotomes.

B. Abnormal Segmentation of the Sclerotomes

The perichordal mesenchyme may present anomalies of segmentation due to disturbed induction of the somites, leading to numerical anomalies, transitional anomalies, or congenital vertebral fusion.

Numerical anomalies can be regional and compensated, thus resembling the transitional anomalies. These anomalies are distinct from the true numerical anomalies represented by an extra vertebra (sixth lumbar or eighth cervical vertebra) or a missing segment (sacrum, coccyx, Klippel-Feil syndrome).

The *transitional anomalies* can be interpreted as the result of an error involving the level of induction of the regional morphology. For example, the pelvis phylogenically and ontogenically ascends the spine, successively coming into contact with the vertebrae lying higher up (Regalia 1880). According to the level of arrest of the coxal bone, the sacral vertebrae will develop more or less superiorly. The position of the coxal bone relative to the spine induces the formation of the sacrum. The transitional anomalies vary greatly from the cranium to the coccyx. *Occipitalization of the atlas* features the more or less complete fusion of the atlas to the base of the occipital bone. An exceptional finding is the *occipital vertebra* where the occipital bone presents bony features resembling the posterior arch of the atlas.

A uni- or bilateral *cervical rib* is a cervicothoracic transitional anomaly resulting from the individualization and full development of a costal ossification center in the seventh cervical vertebra. In some cases the cervical rib is reduced to a posterior bony portion with a thick band of fibroconjunctive tissue extending anteriorly to the sternum. A *lumbar rib* is a common anomaly, presenting as a supernumerary ossicle or true rib at the ossification center of the transverse processes of L1. *Lumbosacral transitional vertebrae* correspond to either the lumbalization of S1 or the sacralization of L5. This anomaly is uni- or bilateral and occurs in about 7% of births. These transitional vertebrae present a giant transverse process resembling the ala sacralis and forming a neoarticulation with the sacrum and sometimes the coxal bone. The underlying intervertebral disc and the corresponding posterior articulations are often atrophic. In some cases the transverse process is fused to the ala sacralis. The *sacrococcygeal region* is a frequent site of anomalies resulting from the uni- or bilateral separation of the lowermost sacral segment or the fusion of one or both sides of the sacrum to the coccyx. A *"vertebral tail"* is a very rare anomaly due to lengthening and straightness of the coccygeal segments.

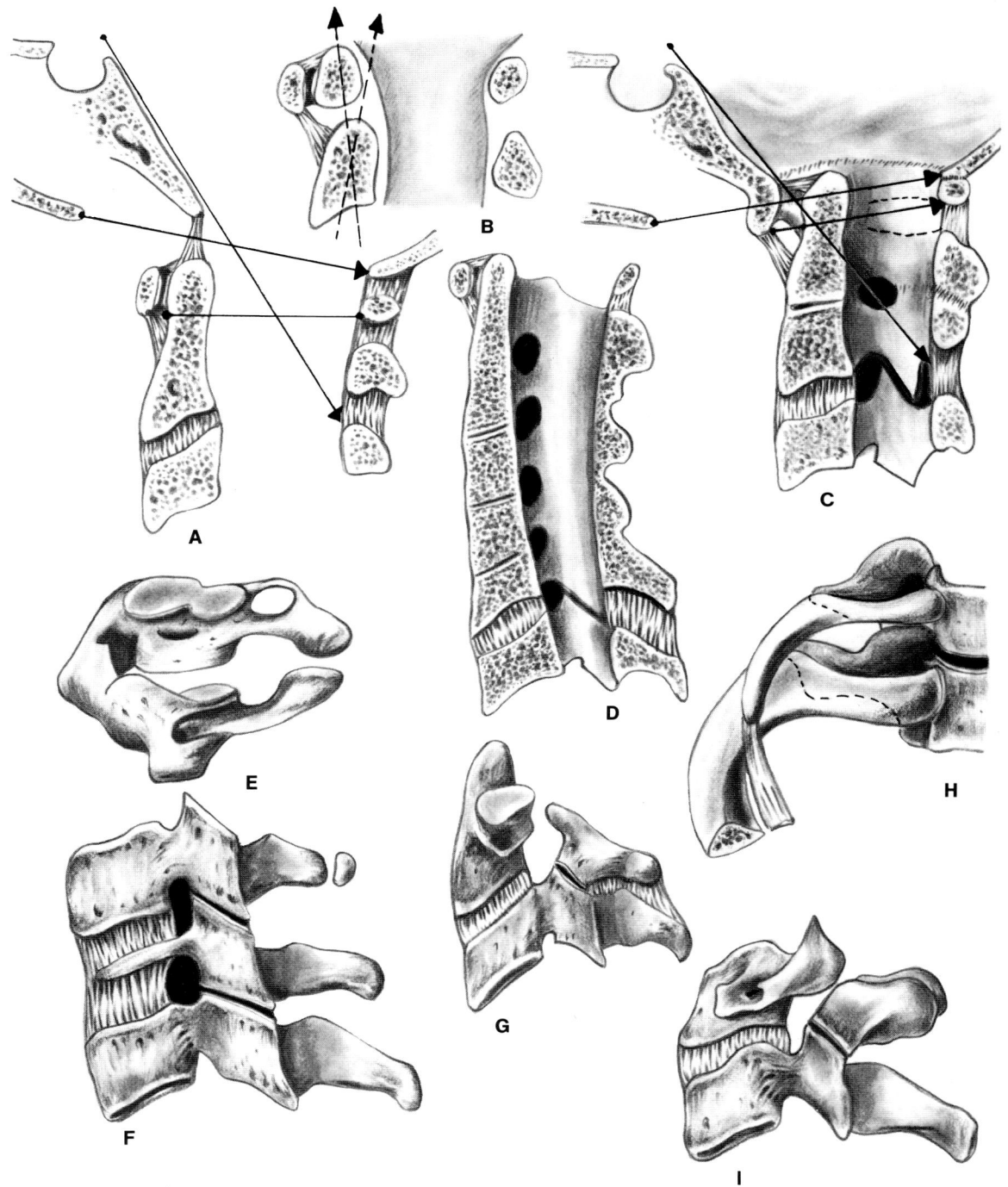

Figure 6 A–I

A   The normal craniovertebral junction
B   Os odontoideum
C   Basilar impression
D   Klippel-Feil syndrome
E   Failure to close of the posterior arch of the atlas and bony anulus for the vertebral artery

F   Platyspondylia and spinous ossicle
G   Spondylolysis of the axis
H   Cervical rib
I   Spondylolysis of C6

Basilar impression, featuring the invagination of the upper cervical spine into the foramen magnum, can be considered a transitional anomaly, and occurs when the odontoid process rises above Chamberlain's line, drawn from the posterior margin of the hard palate to the dorsum of the foramen magnum. This malformation is often accompanied by occipitalization of the atlas, Klippel-Feil syndrome, atlantoaxial instability, and Arnold-Chiari syndrome (protrusion of the cerebellar tonsils and medulla oblongata below the foramen magnum).

Congenital vertebral fusion results from the absence of segmentation of two or more sclerotomes with complete or partial loss of the densely packed cells which normally form the intervertebral disc. This anomaly can be found at all levels of the spine. Congenital vertebral fusion is accompanied by the complete or partial absence of the intervertebral disc. The fusion may involve only the vertebral bodies, in which case kyphosis develops, or the vertebral bodies and posterior arches, with axial shortening of the involved vertebral segment and stenosis of the intervertebral foramina. *Klippel-Feil syndrome* is a special case of vertebral fusion. Patients with this syndrome have a short neck, very low hairline, and rounded back. The syndrome may be associated with pterygium colli (mandibulothoracic web) or Sprengel's deformity (congenital elevation of the scapula). The several cervical vertebrae fused into a single block are interrupted only by the vertebral canal and stenotic intervertebral foramina. The absence of the intervertebral discs and posterior articulations renders the involved segment totally rigid.

C. Vertebral Hypoplasia and Agenesis

Destruction of the cells of part or all of the sclerotome which is to form a given vertebral body can lead to its arrested development, for example, *agenesis of the odontoid process* and platyspondylia. Arrested development of the anterior or posterior part of the loosely packed region of the sclerotome leads respectively to the formation of a dorsal or ventral hemivertebra, causing congenital kyphosis. In both cases the over- and underlying intervertebral discs fuse in the missing region of the vertebral body. A *lateral* noncompensated *isolated hemivertebra* can only be accounted for by agenesis of the left or right half of the sclerotome. This malformation results in congenital scoliosis. Complete or partial *aplasia of a posterior arch* is an exceptional finding. Agenesis of the caudal bud, situated at the caudal part of the primitive streak, leads to a series of malformations involving not only the lumbosacral spine but also the lower limbs, urogenital organs, and rectum. These malformations include agenesis of the sacrum, ectrosomia (congenital lack of the lower body segment), and symmelia or sirenomelia (fusion of the lower limbs).

D. Abnormal Ossification

A malformation known as *os odontoideum* occurs when the odontoid process remains separated from the body of the axis. The ossification centers of the sacral crest may fuse with the spinous process of L5, which undergoes hypertrophy to form spina bifida occulta of S1 and S2. Ossicles result from absence of fusion of the secondary ossification centers in the tip of the spinous processes, the articular processes, and in the anterior annular margin of the vertebral bodies. Certain minor malformations of the *articular processes* are due to aplasia, dysplasia, or malposition disturbing the orientation, symmetry, and dynamic functional capacity of the articular facets.

E. Abnormal Caliber of the Vertebral Canal

Caliber anomalies include *stenosis* of the vertical or lumbosacral canal. The congenital form of stenosis is less frequent than the acquired variety, due to arthrosis in particular. *Widening of the canal* is an exceptional finding; when accompanied by dilatation of the conus medullaris, it sometimes involves a sacral termination of the spinal cord. Diastematomyelia and vertebral dysmorphia are also associated with an enlarged vertebral canal.

F. Congenital Spondylolysis and Spondylolisthesis

Although true congenital spondylolisthesis due to agenesis of the articular facets of the sacrum does exist, spondylolysis is no longer considered to be a congenital lesion. On the contrary, spondylolysis results from fatigue fracture related to static conditions that are frequently transmitted hereditarily.

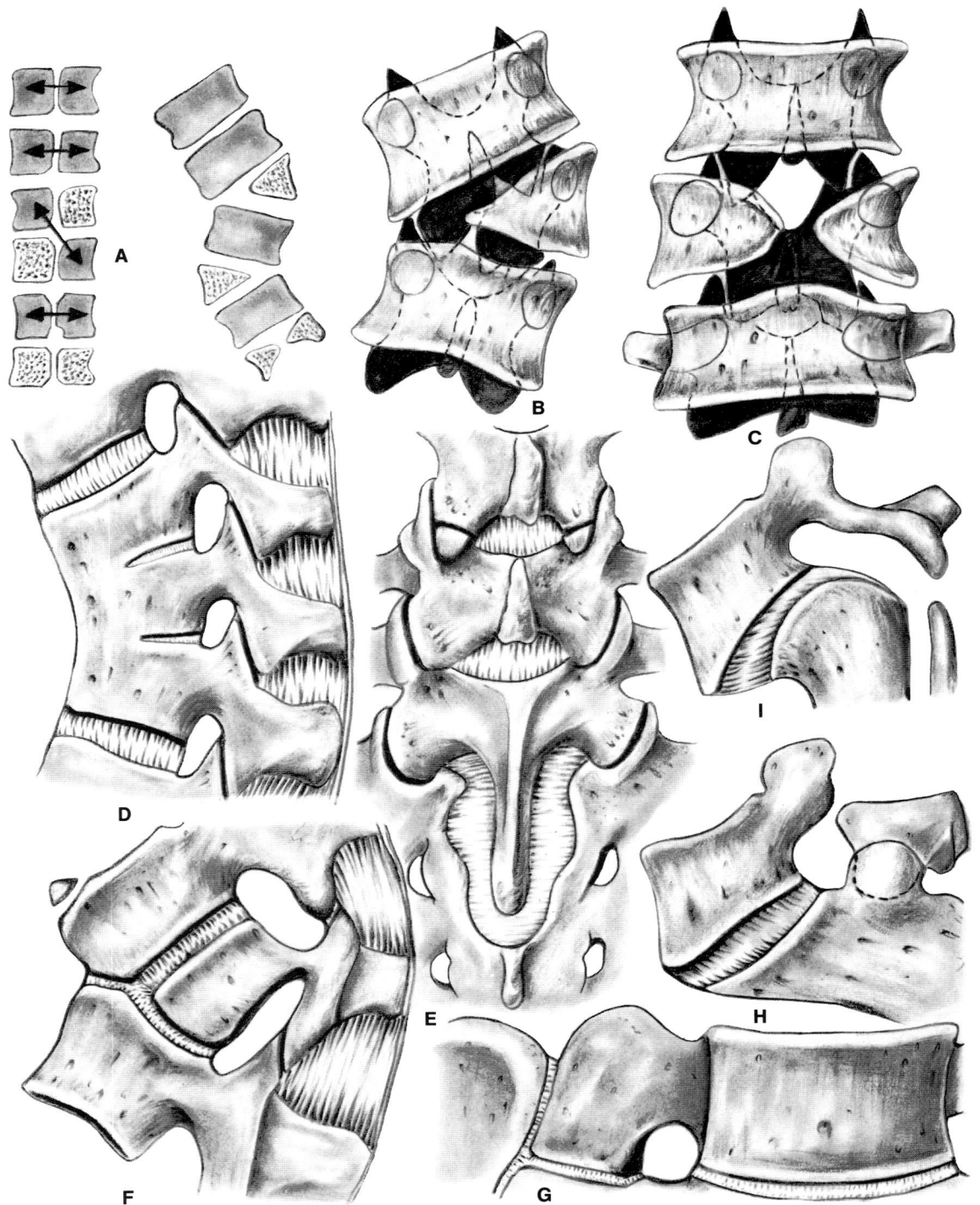

Figure 7A–I

A The mechanism producing vertebral dysmorphia
B Lateral hemivertebra
C Anterior rachischisis
D Vertebral fusion
E Articular ossicles and hypertrophy of the L5 spinous process with spina bifida of S1 and S2

F Dorsal hemivertebra and defective fusion of the annular epiphysis
G Lumbosacral transitional anomaly
H Spondylolysis of L5
I Spondylolisthesis of L5 due to agenesis of the sacral facets

2 Morphology of the Spine

I. Cervical Spine

The cervical spine or cervical column extends from the cranium to the thorax. The seven cervical vertebrae are denoted C1 to C7 in descending order. The first and second cervical vertebrae present special features regarding form, function, and name: C1 is called the atlas and C2 the axis. In the erect anatomical position the cervical spine presents a posterior concavity (lordosis) that disappears on flexion and in certain subjects with a flat or hollow back. The cervical spine is described in terms of the different aspects shown in the plates.

A. Posterior Aspect

The cervical spine presents a deep concave posterior surface between the occipital region and the thorax. The spinous processes lying along the midline are its only palpable structures. The atlas, which is the only cervical vertebra lacking a spinous process, has a posterior tubercle that cannot be palpated since it lies in the depressed region subjacent to the occipital bone. The vertebrae C2 to C6 have bifid spinous processes, whereas C7 displays a simple spinous process. The spinous process of C2 is large and well developed. The spinous process of C3 is practically hidden under that of C2. The spinous processes increase in volume from C3 to C7, the latter being referred to as the vertebra prominens. In fact the spinous processes of C6, C7, and T1 are difficult to distinguish by palpation, since their dimensions are very similar. The line of spinous processes is flanked on each side by two smooth planes of bone, each presenting two surfaces. The first, lying in the paramedian plane and composed of the successive vertebral laminae with a slight lateral oblique slant, is transversely interrupted by the narrow depression of the interlaminar spaces. Only the membranous spaces between the occipital bone and atlas and between the atlas and axis are larger (from 3 mm in extension to 10 mm in flexion). The second plane lies lateral to the first, and is constituted by the articular pillars of the zygapophyses lying in the coronal plane with a width of 15 mm. The articular interfaces are identified transversely by their position flush with the interlaminar spaces. The lateral margin of this bony plane is easily identified by its steplike edge. The plane of the articular pillars is modified by the posterior arch of the atlas passing horizontally through it, creating a bony spicule lying between two depressions, i.e., the suprajacent depression or groove for the vertebral artery and the subjacent groove over which passes the greater occipital nerve (Arnold's nerve).

B. Anterior Aspect

The cervical spine presents a convex anterior surface between the base of the cranium and the thoracic inlet, the origin of which at C3 is hidden by the mass of facial bone. The anterior cervical spine can be divided into a central corporeal region and two lateral transverse regions. The corporeal segment begins under the basilar part of the occipital bone with the transverse prominence of the anterior arch of the atlas covering the odontoid process or dens of the axis. The subsequent vertebral bodies are aligned over each other, separated by the intervertebral spaces with the intervertebral discs slightly protruding anteriorly with respect to the central part of the vertebral bodies. This medial region, narrow at its summit (15 mm wide) and progressively wider toward the lower cervical vertebrae (25–30 mm wide at C7), presents an anterior convexity in the vertical and horizontal planes. The lateral transverse regions are flat and lie in the frontal plane, resembling the rungs of a ladder at the level of the upper halves of the vertebral bodies: these are the transverse processes, limited laterally by their anterior tubercles. One of these, the carotid tubercle of C6 (Chassaignac's tubercle), is an excellent surgical landmark since it protrudes anteriorly with respect to that of C7. Between the transverse processes are located the intertransverse sulci for the vertebral artery, its accompanying veins and vegetative nerve, and the spinal nerve. At C1 and C2 this lateral region widens laterally allowing the articular pillars to extend the plane of the underlying transverse processes. Thus these lateral regions are narrowest at C5 (15 mm wide) and wider at the two ends (35 mm at C1 and 25 mm at C7).

C. Craniovertebral Articulations

The head rests on the cervical spine by articulating with the occipital bone, the atlas, and the axis.

The *atlantoccipital articulation* joins the elliptic and convex occipital condyles with the superior articular cavities of the atlas (glenoid cavities). The articulation has a capsule and three ligaments, i.e., the lateral ligament and the anterior and posterior atlantoccipital membranes. The articular interfaces describe a transverse oval-shaped area.

The *atlantoaxial articulation* comprises three joints, one median and two lateral. The median joint is between the dens of the axis and anterior arch of the atlas anteriorly and the transverse ligament of the atlas posteriorly. This transverse or cruciform ligament has two vertical bands which attach to the anterior edge of the foramen magnum and the posterior surface of the body of the axis. The articular interfaces form a vertical cylinder. The lateral joints are between the inferior articular facets of the atlas and the superior articular facets of the axis. These articular surfaces are sligthly convex with an interface describing a portion of a sphere. The joint is strengthened by an articular capsule reinforced medially by an inferior lateral ligament (Arnold's ligament) and two anterior and posterior atlantoaxial ligaments homologous to the suprajacent atlantoccipital membranes.

The *occipital bone* is joined to the axis by powerful ligaments: the membrana tectoria, extending from the anterior edge of the foramen magnum to the posterior surface of the body of the axis behind the cruciform ligament; the alar ligaments, which join the occipital condyles to the tip of the dens of the axis; and the apical ligament of the dens, which extends from the tip of the process to the anterior margin of the foramen magnum.

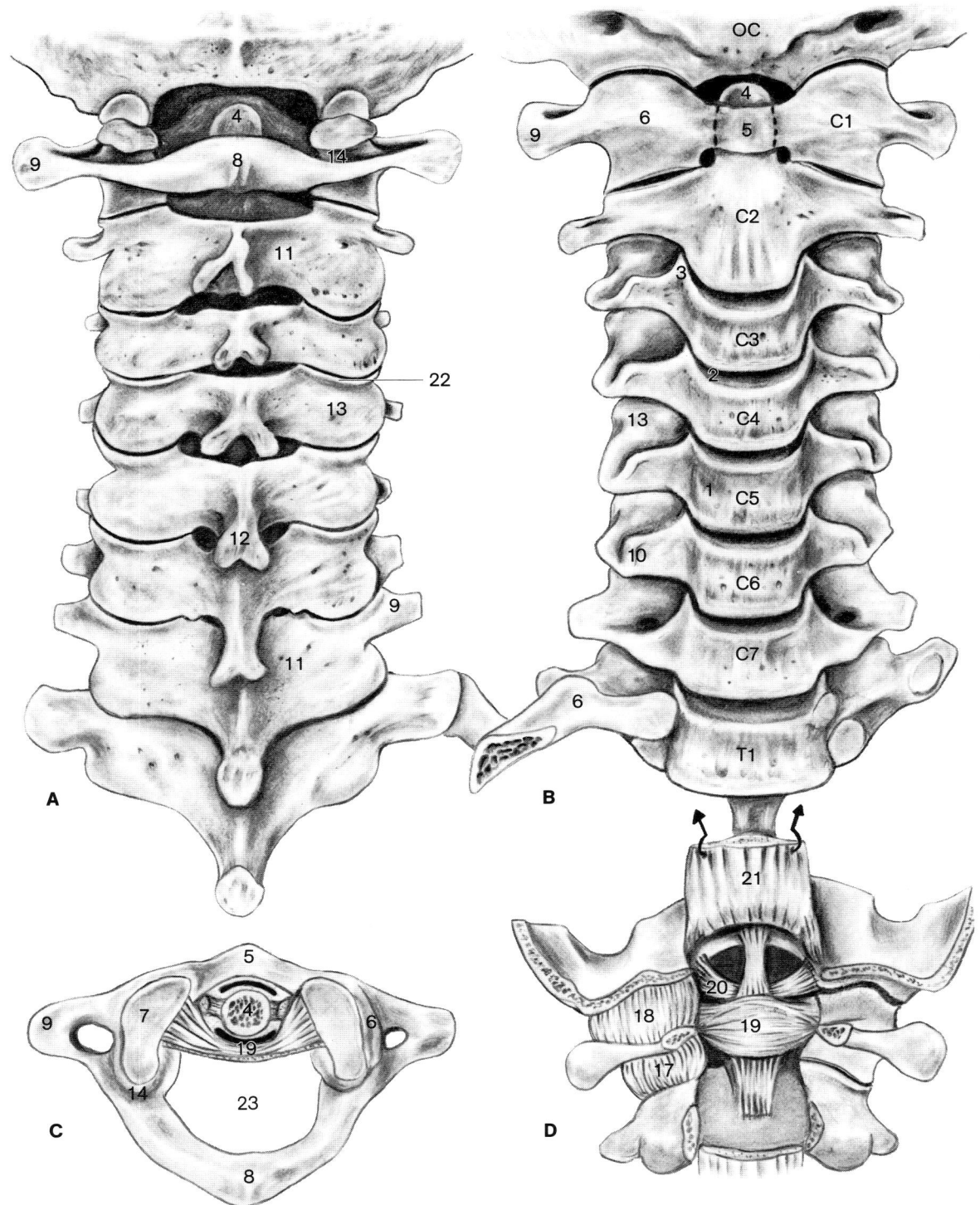

Figure 8 A–D

A   Posterior aspect of the cervical spine (columna cervicalis)
B   Anterior aspect of the cervical spine
C   Superior aspect of the atlas
D   Posterior aspect of the craniovertebral articulations

1 corpus vertebrae   *2* spatium intervertebrale   *3* uncus   *4* dens axis
5 arcus ant., tuberculum anterius   *6* massa lateralis   *7* fovea
articularis sup.   *8* arcus post., tuberculum post.   *9* processus
transversus   *10* tuberculum caroticum   *11* lamina arcus vertebrae
12 processus spinosus   *13* zygapophysis   *14* sulcus arteriae vertebralis
15 foramen transversarium   *16* foramen magnum   *17* capsula
articularis articulationis atlanto-axialis lateralis   *18* capsula
articularis articulationis atlanto-occipitalis   *19* lig. cruciforme atlantis
20 lig. alaria   *21* membrana tectoria   *22* junctura zygapophysealis
23 foramen vertebrale

D. Lateral Aspect

Seen in profile, the cervical spine presents two protruding columns corresponding to the articular and transverse processes aligned along the longitudinal axis of the spine and well separated from C2 to T1 but superimposed from C2 to the occipital bone. From the inferior surface of the axis to the superior surface of the first thoracic vertebra the articular processes, resembling beveled cylinders, lie over one another to form the posterior or zyapophyseal articulations. The resulting articular interfaces slant obliquely downward and posteriorly to form a $30°-50°$ angle with the horizontal plane. The articular pillar of C6 is distinguished from that of the other cervical vertebrae by its bayonet-shaped region separating the superior and inferior articular facets. Similarly, the articular pillar of the axis differs by its wide region of fusion with the vertebral body and a markedly constricted bayonetlike region between the superior and inferior articular facets. Thus these two vertebrae display a sort of isthmic region which is a possible site of spondylolysis. The transverse processes of C1 and C2 lie flush with the articular pillars and present a single tubercle, whereas the lower-lying transverse processes arise anterior to the articular pillars. The transverse processes from C3 to C7 display anterior and posterior roots connecting the process to the flank of the vertebral body and anterior part of the articular pillar respectively. The foramen transversarium lies between these roots and receives the vertebral artery, its accompanying veins, and the vertebral nerve. These transverse processes display two grooves, one anterior and one lateral to the intervertebral foramen, and present an anterior and posterior tubercle. The direction of the transverse processes follows that of the spinal nerves and thus varies, i.e., the upper processes have an oblique downward and lateral slant, while the lower ones have a progressively more anterior direction.

E. Sagittal Section

The sagittal section reveals the presence of canals passing through the cervical spine.

The vertebral canal, called the cervical canal in this region, begins at the level of the foramen magnum and continues downward by the juxtaposition of the vertebral foramina. In the upper cervical spine the vertebral canal is oval-shaped and large (35 mm × 30 mm), but it becomes triangular and smaller with an anterior base and rounded angles in the lower thoracic spine (25 mm × 16 mm). The anterior wall or base corresponds to the posterior surface of the vertebral bodies and intervertebral discs. The posterolateral walls are formed by the laminae and ligamenta flava. The vertebral canal contains the spinal cord, spinal nerves, their vessels, and meningeal structures. At each intervertebral space the cervical canal communicates on the right and left with the intervertebral foramina. The latter, from C2 to T1, are bounded by the vertebral pedicles, posterior articulations, and intervertebral discs. The intervertebral foramina lie in the anterolateral angles of the vertebral canal. The first two foramina lie laterally and are bounded by the atlantooccipital and atlantoaxial membranes, the osseous ridge of the foramen magnum, the posterior arch of the atlas, and the vertebral arch of the axis. The spinal nerves and vessels pass through these foramina.

F. Articulations of the Inferior Cervical Vertebrae

The cervical vertebrae from C2 to T1 articulate with each other by three joints at each level, i.e., the intervertebral disc anteriorly and the two posterior or zygapophyseal joints.

The *intervertebral disc* is inserted on the cartilaginous plates of two adjacent cervical vertebrae, the upper and lower plates being opposite in shape: the superior surface of the cervical vertebral body is deeply concave transversely, due to the characteristic semilunar ridges or uncus on the lateral margins, and the inferior surface is reciprocally convex, due to the lateral indentations (lacinia lateralis). The inferior surface of the vertebral body is concave anteroposteriorly since it has an anterior lip or rostrum. The disc's peripheral portion, the anulus fibrosus, contains overlapping laminae; the fibers of contiguous laminae lie at an oblique angle to each other. The central zone of the disc is filled with a highly aqueous gel under pressure between the last laminae of the anulus fibrosus, often taking on a nearly spherical shape: this central core is the nucleus pulposus. The disc is surrounded anteriorly by an anterior longitudinal ligament and posteriorly by a posterior longitudinal ligament; these ligaments are intimately bound to the disc. After the age of 30 years the disc frequently fissures between the uncus and lacinia lateralis, thus simulating the articular cavity of an uncovertebral joint (Trolard).

The *posterior articulations* between the articular processes have an interface at $30°-50°$ to the horizontal plane; the interface is ovoid in shape, with a transverse greater axis. Numerous ligaments extend a greater or lesser distance from the capsule. The intertransverse ligaments, between the transverse processes, are rather loose scattered fibers in the cervical region. The strong ligamenta flava connect the middle of the anterior surface of a lamina to the superior margin of the subjacent lamina and extend transversely from the anterior surface of one articular capsule to another, presenting a small dehiscence on the midline. The interspinous and supraspinous ligaments are reinforced in the cervical region by the powerful ligamentum nuchae, a veritable median sagittal septum of the neck.

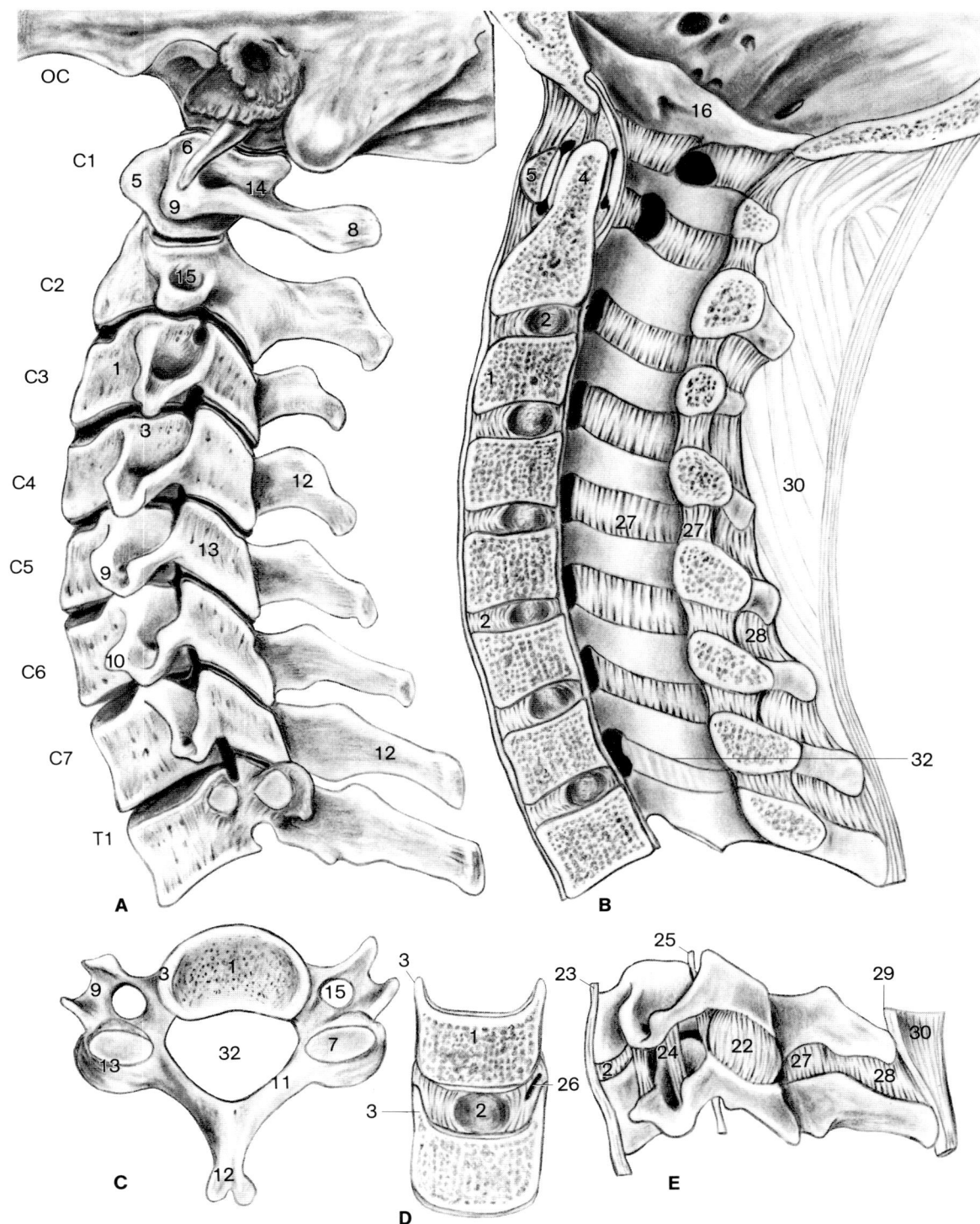

Figure 9 A–E

A   Lateral aspect of the cervical spine (columna cervicalis)
B   Median sagittal section of the cervical spine
C   Superior aspect of a cervical vertebra (vertebra cervicalis)
D   Coronal section of the cervical intervertebral disc (discus interverte-
bralis cervicalis)
E   Lateral aspect of the intervertebral joints

1 corpus vertebrae *2* discus intervertebralis: anulus fibrosus, nucleus
pulposus *3* uncus *4* dens axis *5* arcus ant., tuberculum ant.

6 massa lateralis *7* fovea articularis sup. *8* arcus post.,
tuberculum post. *9* processus transversus *10* tuberculum caroticum
11 lamina arcus vertebrae *12* processus spinosus *13* zygapophysis
14 sulcus arteriae vertebralis *15* foramen transversarium
16 foramen magnum *22* capsula articulationis zygapophysialis
23 lig. longitudinale ant. *24* lig. intertransversarium
25 lig. longitudinale post. *26* articulatio uncovertebralis *27* lig.
flavum *28* lig. interspinale *29* lig. supraspinale *30* lig. nuchae
31 foramen intervertebrale *32* foramen vertebrale, canalis cervicalis

G. Radiology

The *anterior aspect* of the cervical spine is explored by antero-posterior roentgenography with the mouth open for C1 and C2 and by standard anteroposterior films to visualize C3 to T1. Opening the mouth allows examination of the symmetry of the craniovertebral articulations and the morphology of the axis and dens and of the lateral masses of the atlas. The anteroposterior view of the lower cervical spine shows the anterior column of the vertebral bodies and intervertebral discs on the midline with clear visualization of the uncovertebral articulations. On either side, the columns of the posterior articulations appear as two uniform bands without an articular interface and limited laterally by a regular undulated line.

The *lateral aspect* as seen on profile roentgenography allows visualization of the curvature of the entire cervical spine, the anterior discocorporeal column, the posterior articular columns, and the successive spinous processes. The anterior column shows the rectangular shape of the vertebral bodies from C3 to T1, the conic form of C2, and the flattened oval-shaped anterior arch of the atlas. The intervertebral discs are seen as biconvex structures slanting downward and anteriorly; their height is equal to half that of a vertebral body. The posterior columns appear superimposed to form a single image like a stack of diamond shapes. The laminae are seen interposed between the articular pillars and the section of the spinous processes. Finally, profile films allow evaluation of the form and caliber of the cervical canal between the posterior surface of the vertebral bodies and the anterior margin of the laminae.

The *oblique or three-quarter view* is particularly instructive for the study of the intervertebral foramina which normally present a regular oval shape and are of constant size over the entire cervical spine. These foramina are limited posteriorly by the posterior articulations, anteriorly by the uncovertebral articulations, and above and below by the vertebral pedicles.

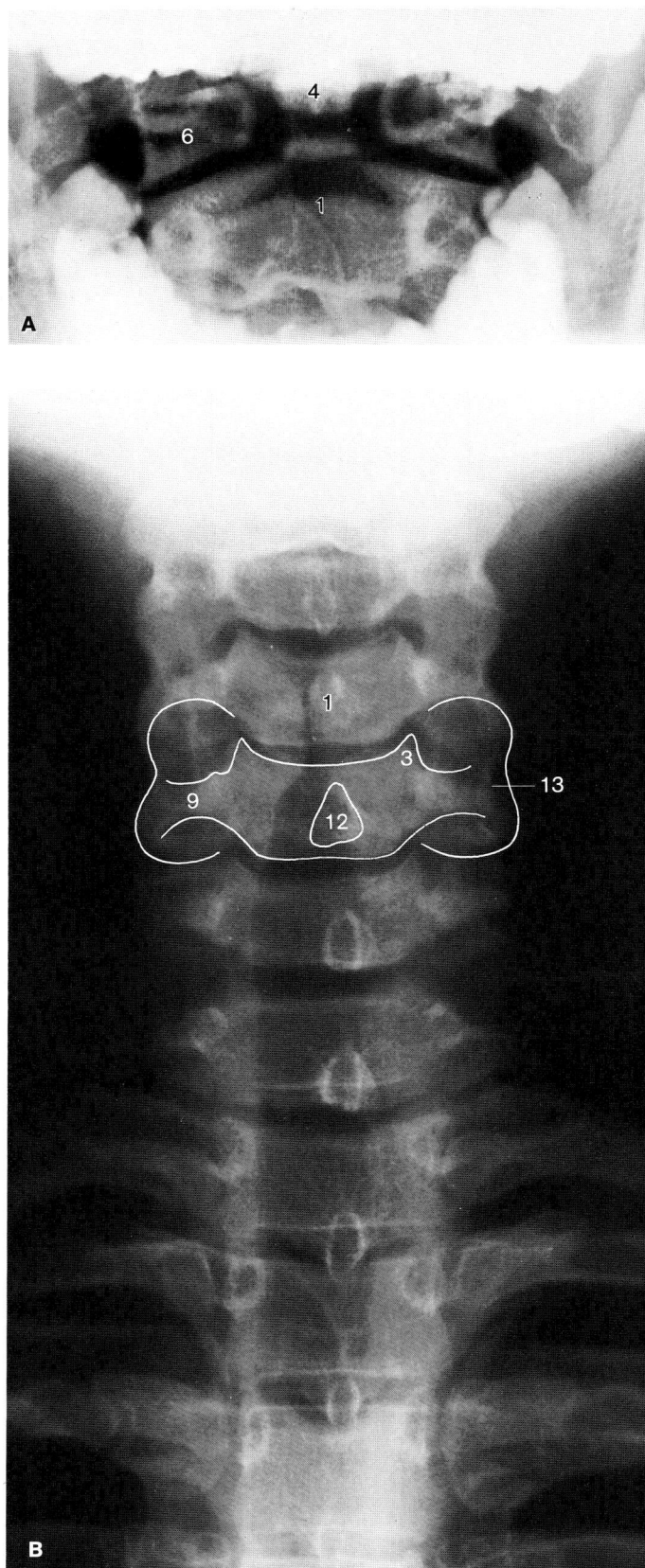

Figure 10 A, B

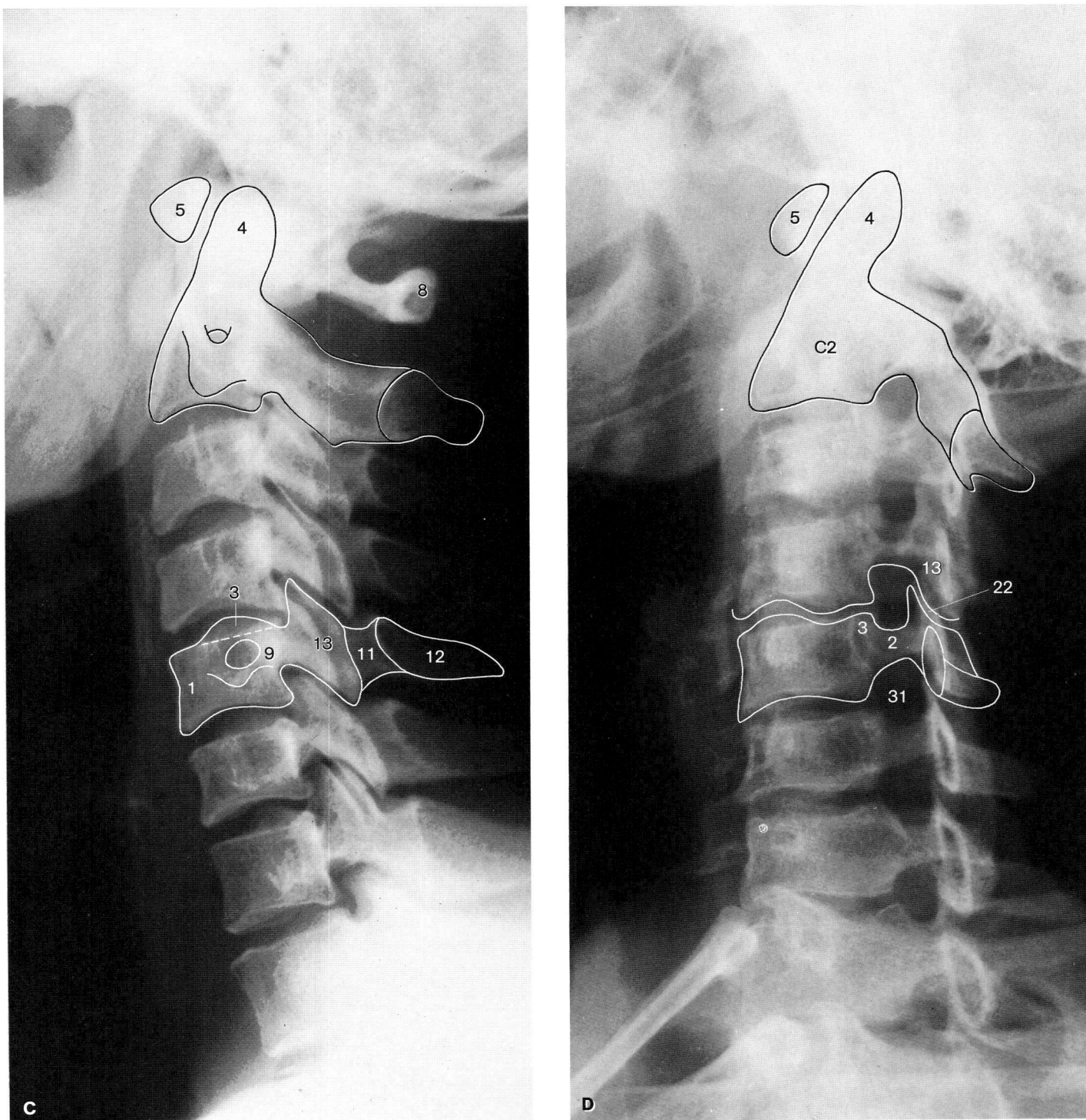

Figure 10 C, D

A   Anteroposterior X-ray of the axis and atlas with the mouth open
B   Anteroposterior X-ray of the cervical spine
C   Profile X-ray of the cervical spine
D   Oblique (three-quarter) X-ray of the cervical spine

1 corpus vertebrae 2 spatium intervertebrale 3 uncus corporis
4 dens axis 5 arcus ant., tuberculum ant. 6 massa lateralis 8 arcus
post., tuberculum post. 9 processus transversalis 11 lamina arcus
vertebrae 12 processus spinosus 13 zygapophysis 16 foramen
magnum 22 articulationes zygapophyseales 31 foramen intervertebrale

II. Thoracic Spine

The thoracic spine is that part of the vertebral column supporting the rib cage, and with the sternum forms the skeleton of the thorax. It consists of twelve vertebrae denoted T1 to T12. The whole of the thoracic spine has a posterior convexity (kyphosis) which is more or less pronounced in different individuals and practically absent in subjects with a flat or hollow back. It is described in terms of the different aspects shown in the plates.

A. Posterior Aspect

The transition from the cervical to the thoracic spine occurs through a change in curvature which causes the posterior surface from T1 to T6 to slant obliquely toward the surface, presenting a median crest and lateral grooves. The midline crest of the spinous processes is palpable under the skin of the back and thus can be used to identify the vertical axis of the spine and the level of each vertebra. Congenital anomalies of alignment of the spinous processes should not be mistaken for vertebral rotation.

The spinous crest is thickened by the unituberous processes in its superficial portion but is narrow in its middle region with a "saw-tooth" appearance due to the triangular interspinous spaces. The spinous crest widens at its base to continue with the laminae or posterior arches. The mean height of the spinous crest is 18–25 mm.

The frontal plane of the lateral grooves comprises three parts, i.e., the laminar, articular, and transverse regions. The paramedian laminar region is constituted by the vertebral laminae overlapping each other like tiles on a roof, the superior lamina being posterior to the inferior one. Accordingly, the interlaminar spaces are virtual and cannot be used as a route of approach except to perform a spinal tap on or near the midline with the needle slanted markedly upward. The laminar region of the lateral grooves is barely 5 mm wide, rendering hemilaminectomy difficult unless the procedure includes suppression of the contiguous articular region lying laterally.

The position of the posterior or zygapophyseal articulations can be identified by drawing a circle 1 cm in diameter with its center at the inferolateral angle of the lamina. The third portion of the lateral grooves is discontinuous since it is composed of the transverse processes inserted between the zygapophyseal articulations and slanting posteriorly and laterally at a 40° angle. The length of the transverse processes and thus the width of the lateral grooves are greater at T1, diminishing progressively to T12. Hence the overall width of the thoracic spine in the adult decreases from a mean of 75 mm at T1 to 55 mm at T12.

B. Anterior Aspect

When viewed in its anterior aspect, the thoracic spine is characterized by the protrusion of the vertebral bodies in front of the plane of the transverse processes. The juxtaposition of the vertebral bodies separated by the intervertebral spaces forms a sagittal column with an anterior concavity. The dimensions of the thoracic spine vary from top to bottom. The anteroposterior depth of the vertebral bodies increases regularly from T1 to T12 (from 15 mm to 32 mm on average), whereas the transverse width decreases from T1 to T4 (from 30 mm to 25 mm) and then increases to T12 (45 mm). Accordingly, the transverse section from T1 to T3 is reniform with a greater transverse axis, whereas the lower thoracic vertebrae display a heart-shaped horizontal section just slightly larger transversely than anteroposteriorly. The costal facets arise from the posteroinferior and superior regions of the lateral surfaces of the vertebral bodies. On each side the vertebral bodies bear two costal demifacets, except T11 and T12 which have only one pair.

Finally, except for T11 and T12, the tips of the transverse processes have an anterolateral costal facet.

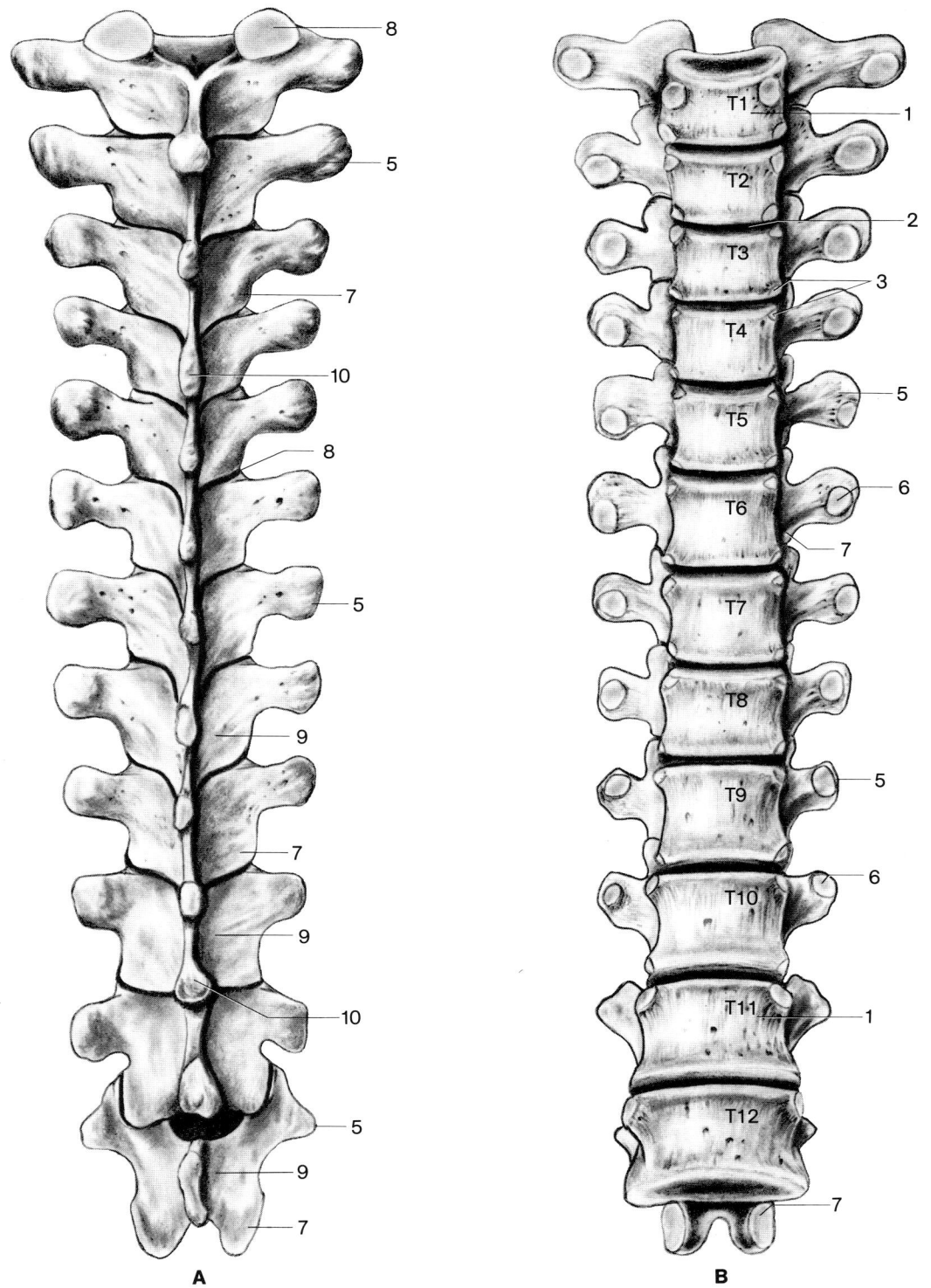

Figure 11 A, B

A Posterior aspect of the thoracic spine
B Anterior aspect of the thoracic spine
(columna thoracica)

1 corpus vertebrae 2 spatium intervertebrale 3 fovea costalis sup., inf.
5 processus transversus 6 fovea costalis transversalis 7 processus

articularis inf. 8 processus articularis sup. 9 lamina arcus vertebrae
10 processus spinosus

C. Lateral Aspect

The anterior concavity of the thoracic spine is clearly visible when viewed in profile. The juxtaposition of the corresponding parts of the thoracic vertebrae forms vertical columns of homologous structures. The anterior column comprising the vertebral bodies and intervertebral spaces progressively widens toward the lower part of the thoracic spine. The costal facets arise from the posterior part of the vertebral bodies on each side of the intervertebral space. This anterior column is transversely depressed in the middle region of the vertebral bodies and widest at the intervertebral spaces, which are about one quarter the height of the vertebral bodies. The vertebral pedicles and intervertebral foramina are aligned posterior to the anterior column. The vertebral pedicles arise from the upper half of the vertebral bodies. The intervertebral foramina are bounded by the pedicles, the posterior surface of the intervertebral spaces, and the anterior surface of the zygapophyseal articulations. The inferior part of the intervertebral foramina is occluded by the heads of the ribs. The left and right posterior columns formed by the articular processes lie posterior to the intervertebral foramina. The articular interfaces display a pronounced obliquity, lying at about 65° to the plane of the intervertebral spaces. The transverse processes project from the articular pillars between the superior and inferior articular facets. The tip of each transverse process from T1 to T10 bears an oval costal facet. The short transverse processes of T11 and T12 do not articulate with the ribs. Viewed in profile the region of the laminae is so narrow that only the succession of the spinous processes merits description. The inferoposterior slant of the spinous processes increases from T1 to T6 and then decreases down to T12. The projection of the spinous processes on the vertebral bodies is sufficiently constant to allow the following topographical correlations:

- From T1 to T3 the tip of each spinous process projects over the upper half of the underlying vertebra.
- From T4 to T6 the tip of each spinous process lies over the lower half of the underlying vertebra.
- From T7 to T9 the tip of each spinous process projects over the upper half of the subjacent vertebra.
- From T10 to T12 the tip of each spinous process is level with the subjacent intervertebral space.

D. Sagittal Section

A sagittal paramedian section of the thoracic spine demonstrates the intervertebral discs and ligaments uniting the vertebral segments. The entire anterior column is clearly visible showing the alternate rectangular sections of the vertebral bodies and intervertebral discs between the anterior and posterior longitudinal ligaments. The anterior column with its posterior convexity has a greater anteroposterior width in the lower thoracic region. In each disc the nucleus pulposus lies immediately behind the center of the anulus fibrosus. In the illustration, the posterior arch has been sectioned flush with the laminae and ligamenta flava. The laminae are shaped like drops of water, pointed at the top and rounded at the bottom. The ligamenta flava can be seen inserted on the anterior surface and superior edge of the laminae. The interspinous and supraspinous ligaments connect adjacent spinous processes. The vertebral canal, called the thoracic canal in this region, lies between the anterior column and posterior arches of the vertebrae and presents a regular cylindrical shape with a mean diameter of 16 mm. Between the vertebral pedicles the vertebral canal communicates with the intervertebral foramina, which are bounded anteriorly by the posterior surface of the discs and posteriorly by the portion of the ligamentum flavum lining the anterior surface of the posterior (zygapophyseal) articulation.

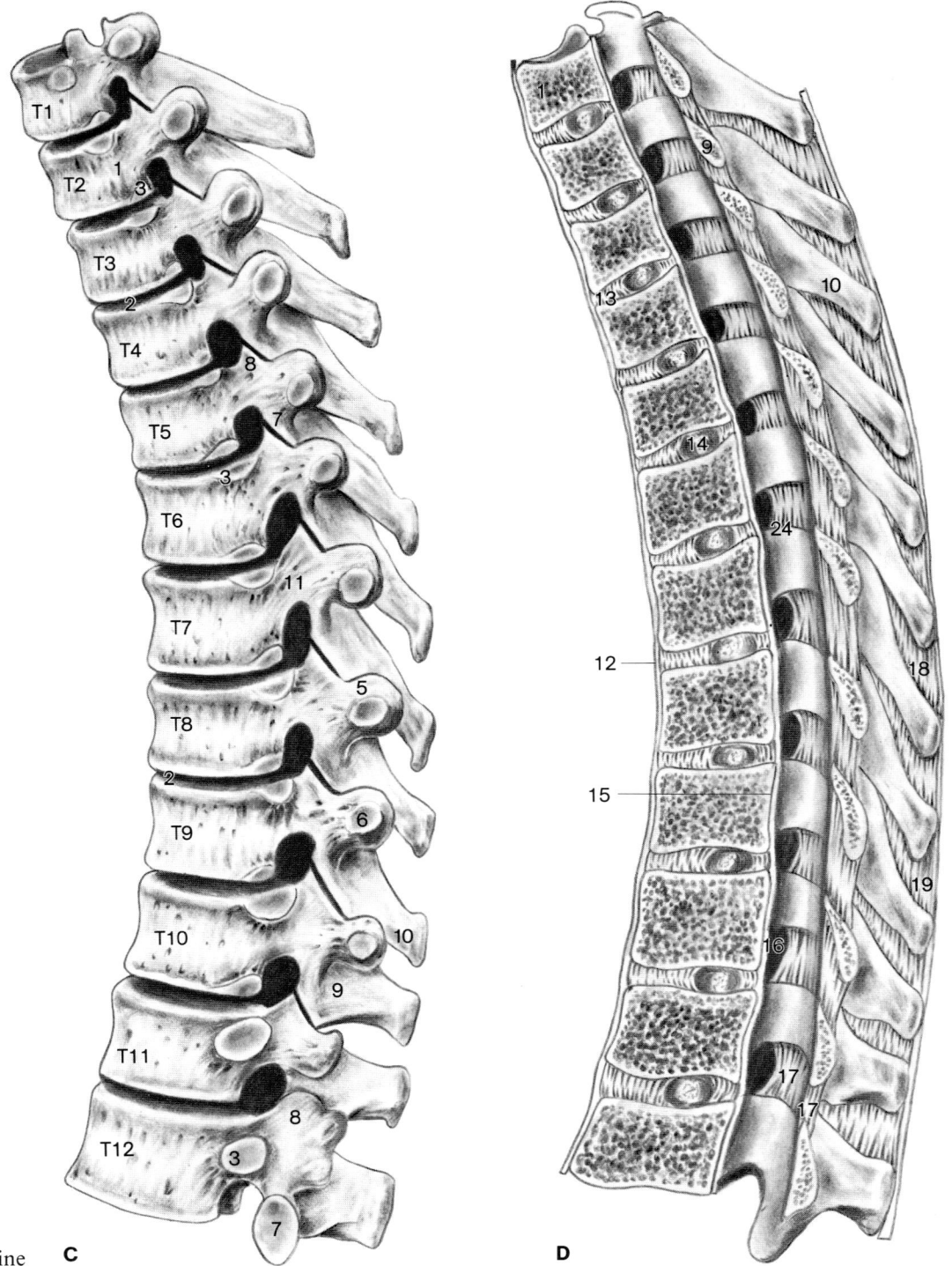

Figure 11 C, D

C Lateral aspect of the thoracic spine (columna thoracica)

D Median sagittal section of the thoracic spine

1 corpus vertebrae 2 discus intervertebralis 3 fovea costalis sup., inf.
5 processus transversus 6 fovea costalis transversalis 7 processus articularis inf. 8 processus articularis sup. 9 lamina arcus vertebrae
10 processus spinosus 11 pediculus arcus vertebrae

12 lig. longitudinale ant. 13 anulus fibrosus 14 nucleus pulposus
15 lig. longitudinale post. 16 foramen intervertebrale 17 lig. flavum
18 lig. interspinale 19 lig. supraspinale 24 canalis thoracicus

E. Intervertebral Articulations

The *vertebral bodies* are joined together by the intervertebral discs and longitudinal ligaments. The discs are biconvex interosseous ligaments inserted on the cartilaginous plates covering the superior and inferior surfaces of the vertebral bodies. The outer part of each disc, called the anulus fibrosus, is composed of laminae with oblique fibers; the fibers of two contiguous laminae lie at an oblique angle to each other. The deepest layers delineate an almost spherical central space containing a gelatinous substance known as the nucleus pulposus, situated nearer to the posterior part of the disc. The anterior longitudinal ligament extends over the anterior and lateral surfaces of the vertebral bodies and intervertebral discs as a continuous longitudinal band. Surgical rasping of this ligament is difficult since it adheres strongly to the intervertebral discs and neighboring part of the vertebral bodies. The posterior longitudinal ligament lies on the posterior surface of the vertebral bodies and intervertebral discs. The ligament is crenate, being narrow and nonadherent at the center of the vertebral bodies and widened and adherent in the region of the intervertebral discs.

Between the *articular (zygapophyseal) processes* are arthrodiae whose planar articular facets covered by cartilage are markedly oblique (on average at 65° to the plane of the intervertebral discs). The articular facets are joined together by a fibrous capsule reinforced anteriorly by the ligamentum flavum and posteriorly by a posterior ligament. A synovial membrane lining the inner surface of the capsule presents folds which have often been mistaken for a small intra-articular meniscus on anatomical slices.

Ligaments connect the *other parts of the posterior arches,* i.e., the ligamenta flava between the laminae, the interspinous ligaments joining the spinous processes, the supraspinous ligament lying along and adherent to the spinous processes, and the intertransverse ligaments connecting the tip of the spinous processes.

F. Costovertebral Articulations

The vertebrae and ribs articulate with one another through two joints: the articulation with the head of the rib and the costotransverse articulation.

The *articulation of the head of the rib* joins the head of the rib, with its superior and inferior planar facets separated by the anteroposterior crest, to the vertebral depression comprising the two vertebral demifacets above and below the intervertebral disc which forms the base of the depressed vertebral region. The joint is reinforced by the articular capsule limited anteriorly and posteriorly by the anterior and posterior radiate ligaments. These fan-shaped ligaments extend from the head of the rib to the two vertebral bodies and intervertebral disc. The posterior radiate ligament extends to the anterior surface of the suprajacent intervertebral foramen and to the pedicle of the subjacent vertebra. An interosseous ligament, also known as the intra-articular ligament of the head of the rib, extends from the crest of the costal head to the intervertebral disc, thus dividing the joint into two secondary articulations with two synovial compartments. In some cases the two compartments communicate posteriorly. The head of the rib represents a surgical landmark for identification of the intervertebral disc.

The *costotransverse articulation* joins the articular part of the tubercle of a rib to the tips of the transverse process. The articular facets involved in this joint are roughly circular, representing the segment of a cylinder with a greater horizontal axis. The costal facet of the transverse process is concave, that of the tubercle of the rib being reciprocally convex. The joint is reinforced by a synovial lined capsule and by the superior and lateral costotransverse ligaments. The superior ligament is composed of three bands connecting the posterior surface of the neck of the rib to the inferior margin of the transverse process, the anterior surface of the transverse process, and the inferior margin of the suprajacent transverse process. The lateral ligament extends from the tip of the transverse process to the superolateral ridge of the tubercle of the rib.
The eleventh and twelfth ribs differ from the others by the absence of the costotransverse articulations. The heads of the first, eleventh, and twelfth ribs articulate with single vertebral facets without insertion on the intervertebral disc.

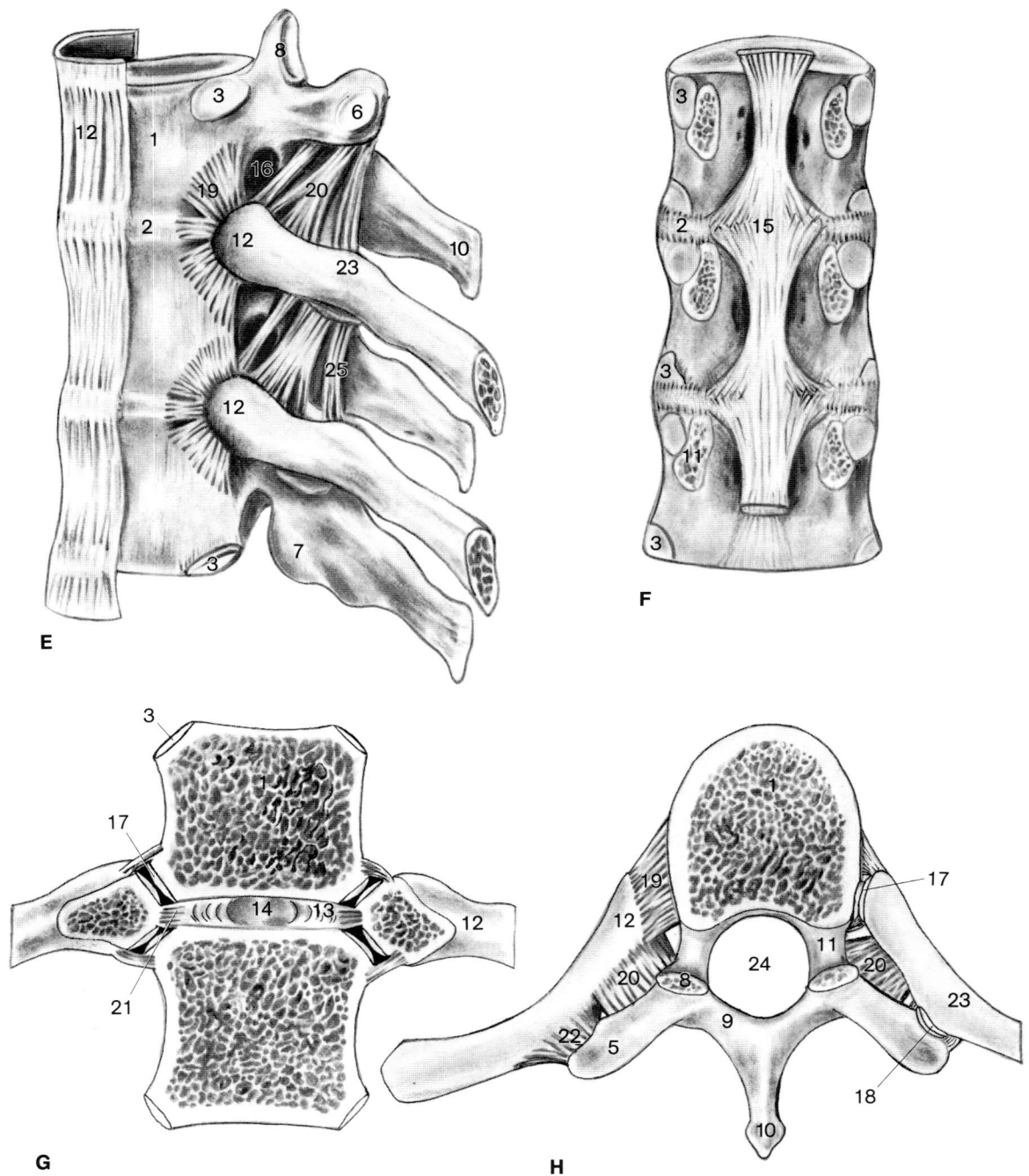

Figure 11 E–H

E   Lateral aspect of the costovertebral articulations (articulationes costovertebrales)
F   Posterior aspect of the vertebral bodies
G   Coronal section of the costovertebral articulations
H   Superior aspect of the costovertebral articulations

1 corpus vertebrae   2 discus intervertebralis   3 fovea costalis sup., inf.   5 processus transversus   6 fovea costalis transversalis

7 processus articularis inf.   8 processus articularis sup.   9 lamina arcus vertebrae   10 processus spinosus   11 pediculus   12 caput costae   13 anulus fibrosus   14 nucleus pulposus   15 lig. longitudinale post.   16 foramen intervertebrale   17 articulatio capitis costae   18 articulatio costotransversaria   19 lig. capitis costae radiatum   20 lig. costotransversaria sup.   21 lig. capitis costae interarticulare   22 lig. costotransversaria lateralis   23 tuberculum costae   24 foramen vertebrale canalis thoracicus   25 lig. intertransversarium

G. Radiology

The anteroposterior and profile views are the two essential radiological positions for the examination of the thoracic spine.

1. Anteroposterior View

Although all the elements of the thoracic vertebrae can be seen on anteroposterior films, the vertebral bodies are easier to identify than the posterior arches.

The *vertebral bodies* appear as rectangular structures decreasing in size from T1 to T3 and increasing in size from T4 to T12. The superior and inferior surfaces of the vertebral bodies are linear and horizontal. When the X-rays are directed obliquely, the surfaces no longer form a single line but two lines corresponding to the anterior and posterior hemicircumferences of the vertebral body. The concave lateral margins of the vertebral bodies near the upper and lower surface give insertion to the heads of the ribs straddling the intervertebral spaces. The column formed by the vertebral bodies is normally symmetrical and rectilinear without protrusion of any of its component.

The multiple contours of the *posterior arches* can be identified through the image of the vertebral bodies. The pedicles and spinous processes are the least difficult to identify. The X-rays project the section of the pedicles onto the superior angles of the vertebral bodies, and the pedicles thus appear as oval structures with a lateral depression in the region of the costovertebral articulation. The tubercle of the spinous process is seen on the midline near the inferior surface of the vertebral body, and the transverse process is also easy to identify, since it extends lateral to the upper half of the vertebral body. The costotransverse joint is clearly visible as two oblique lines corresponding to the articular facets. The articular processes and laminae are more difficult to identify. The superior articular processes extend above the shadow of the pedicles, and the inferior processes project below the pedicles in the lower angle of the vertebral bodies. The laminae are found between the spinous and articular processes.

2. Lateral View

The lateral view gives the most information about the thoracic spine, except that the left and right halves of the vertebrae cannot be distinguished. Lateral roentgenograms should be examined from the vertebral bodies toward the spinous processes.

The *vertebral bodies* appear as rectangular structures with concave superior, inferior, and anterior margins.

The *posterior arches,* although slightly camouflaged by the ribs, can be identified in the region of the posterior surface of the vertebral bodies. The pedicles extend out from the superior half of the posterior margin of the vertebral bodies. The articular processes are located above and below the posterior end of the pedicles and form a small posterior column. The sections of the laminae continue inferiorly and posteriorly with the spinous processes.

The *mobile segments* of the thoracic spine are clearly visible on lateral X-rays. The oval intervertebral foramen and the posterior articulation lie posterior to the narrow intervertebral space.

The *vertebral canal* is also clearly seen on lateral films. The anterior wall of the canal is represented by the posterior margin of the vertebral bodies, slightly camouflaged by the root of the pedicles. The posterior wall is delineated by the anterior margin of the section of the laminae extended by the spinous processes.

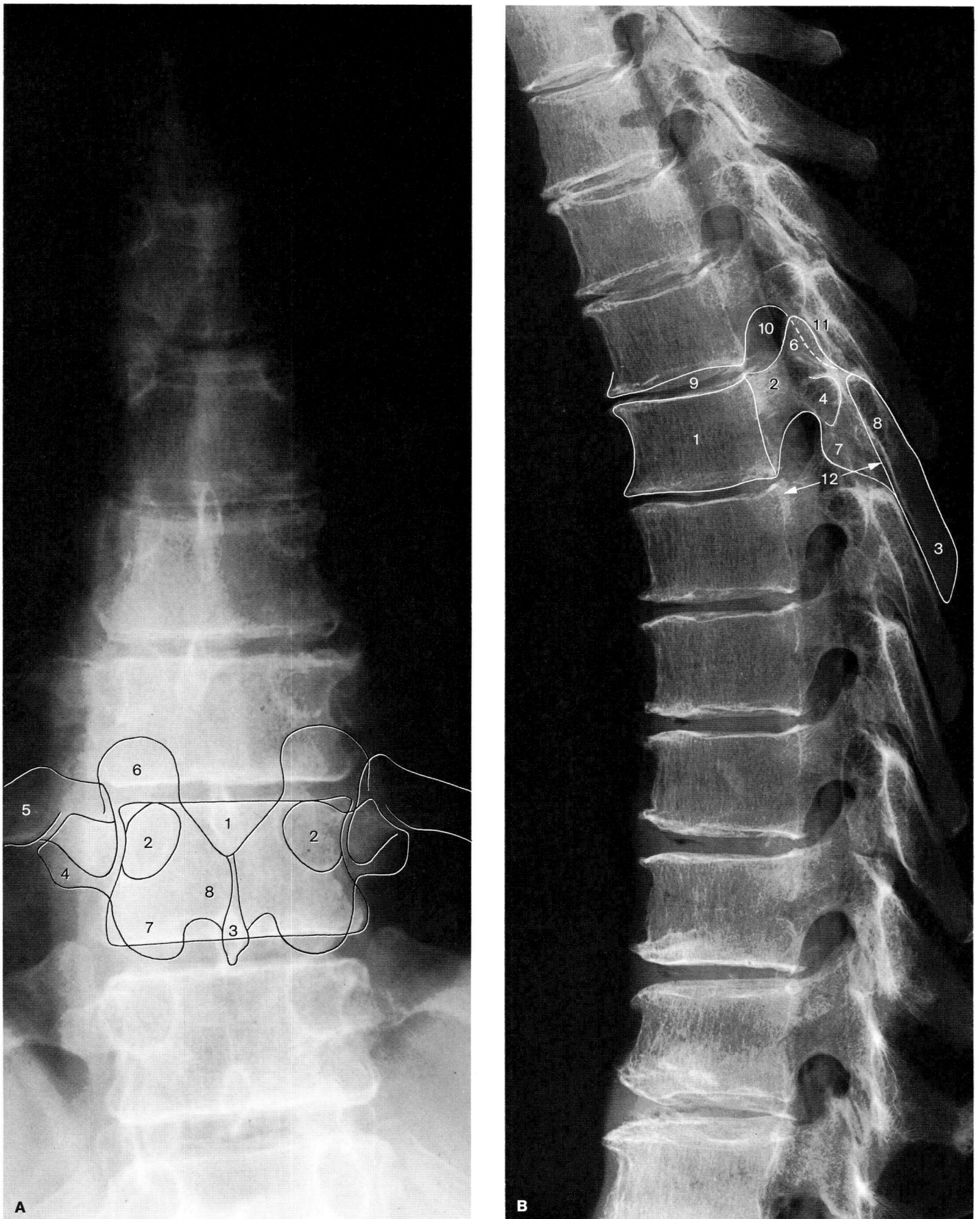

A

B

Figure 12 A, B

A Anteroposterior X-ray of the thoracic spine

B Lateral X-ray of the thoracic spine from an autopsy specimen with dearticulation of the ribs

1 corpus vertebrae 2 pediculus arcus vertebrae 3 processus spinalis 4 processus transversus 5 os costale 6 processus articularis sup. 7 processus articularis inf. 8 lamina arcus vertebrae 9 discus intervertebralis 10 foramen intervertebrale 11 articulationes zygapophyseales 12 canalis vertebralis

III. Lumbosacral Spine

The segment of the vertebral column subjacent to the thoracic cage and inserting into the pelvic girdle to support the abdominopelvic cavity is called the lumbosacral spine. This spinal segment comprises the five lumbar vertebrae denoted L1 to L5, followed by the five sacral vertebrae fused to form a single unit, the sacrum, and finally the coccyx. The lumbosacral spine is described in terms of the different aspects shown in the plates.

A. Posterior Aspect

Three parts of the lumbosacral spine can be described from top to bottom: the polyarticulated lumbar column with a posterior concavity (lordosis), the fused sacrum displaying a posterior convexity (kyphosis), and the appendicular coccyx extending down from the sacrum.

The *lumbar column* has larger dimensions than the spinal segments lying above. A median region and three lateral regions on each side can be described. On the midline, the crest of spinous processes lies in the median sagittal plane and displays a narrow (3–4 mm) middle region with a base on the vertebral arch and a thick free tip (8–10 mm). The spinous processes have slightly greater dimensions in the horizontal plane than in the vertical plane (about 25 mm and 20 mm respectively). In some subjects the lumbar spinous processes are unusually long, thus decreasing the dimensions of the interspinous spaces, which are shieldlike in shape with two rectilinear margins and a V-shaped base. The spaces open on lumbar flexion and become virtual on extension or hyperlordosis. The grooves formed by laminae, lying on each side of the spinous crest, are bounded laterally by the posterior (zygapophyseal) articulations. The interlaminar spaces, which are normally occupied by the thick ligamenta flava, are of greater height than in the other regions of the spine. These spaces are largest (8–15 mm) on flexion or kyphosis and smallest on extension. The transverse width of the laminae is about 8 mm, thus allowing hemilaminectomy. The L5-S1 interlaminar space displays the largest transverse and craniocaudal dimensions, which decrease progressively between the subjacent vertebrae. The laminar groove is connected laterally to the posterior columns comprising the articular processes and the interarticular zones, also known as the isthmic regions. This lateral part of the vertebral arches is composed of a series of oval structures, the posterior or zygapophyseal articulations, between which are the depressions corresponding to the isthmic regions. The pronounced mamillary processes lie just lateral to the posterior articular interfaces. Finally, the posterior surface of the lumbar spine is extended laterally by the deeper plane of the transverse processes. The successive transverse processes form a steplike bony plane extending about 10 mm lateral to the posterior pillars. The transverse processes arise between the isthmus and the superior articular facet. At the limit separating the isthmus and transverse process is a small bony outgrowth called the accessory process. The articular facets ware 10–12 mm high in the craniocaudal direction and 10–15 mm wide transversely. The transverse processes of L4 are the smallest, thus allowing identification of a transitional vertebra.

The *sacrum* is distinguished from the lumbar column by the absence of interlaminar spaces and zygapophyseal articulations, by its oblique slant posteriorly, and by its domed shape. The median sacral crest lying on the midline prolongs the lumbar spinous crest. The sacral crest bifurcates at the sacral hiatus at the level of S4. The sacral grooves, transversely flat and convex in the craniocaudal direction, are widest (20 mm) at the upper sacrum, narrowing to 10 mm in the region of the sacral cornua. The four sacral foramina constitute the lateral boundary of the sacral grooves. The sacral foramina are flanked laterally on each side by the alae sacrales.

The *coccyx,* a flat bone in the shape of a triangle with a superior base, is the most caudal part of the spine.

B. Anterior Aspect

Viewed from in front, the *lumbosacral spine* resembles a cone whose base rests on that of an inverted quadrangular pyramid. The region of the bases at the L5-S1 intervertebral space forms the sacral promontory. Above the promontory the lumbar spine displays an anterior convexity, whereas below, the anterior surface of the sacrum presents an anterior concavity.

The *lumbar spine* is formed by the successive vertebral bodies, appearing reniform on transverse section. When viewed head on, the vertebral bodies resemble posteriorly flattened cylinders increasing in size from L1 to L5. The mean dimensions of L1 are height 25 mm and width 40 mm, whereas L5 is 28 mm by 50 mm. The intervertebral spaces are about one third the height of the vertebral bodies.

The *anterior surface* of the sacrum is concave. The middle region, flanked by the sacral foramina, is flat. Transverse crests arise between the four vertically aligned foramina on each side. The lateral surfaces of the sacrum correspond to the alae sacrales.

The flat triangular *coccyx* extends down from the tip of the sacral concavity.

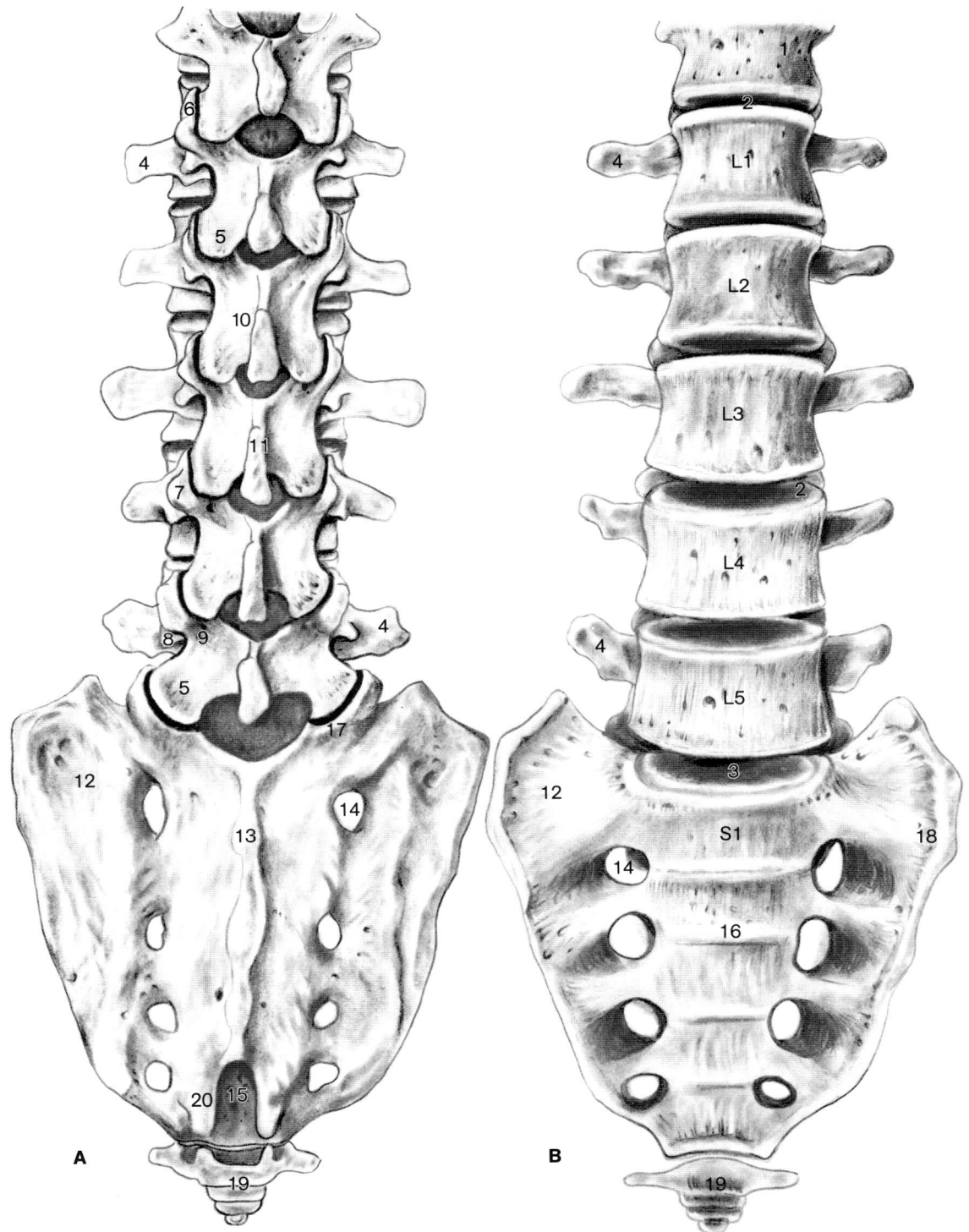

Figure 13 A, B

A Posterior aspect of the lumbar spine (columna lumbalis)
B Anterior aspect of the lumbar spine

1 corpus vertebrae *2* spatium intervertebrale *3* basis ossis sacri (promontorium) *4* processus costarius *5* processus articularis inf. *6* processus articularis sup. *7* processus mamillaris *8* processus accessorius *9* isthmus *10* lamina arcus vertebrae *11* processus spinosus *12* pars lateralis ossis sacri *13* crista sacralis mediana *14* foramina sacralia dorsalia, pelvinia *15* hiatus sacralis *16* linea transversa *17* processus articularis sup. *18* facies auricularis ossis sacri *19* os coccygis *20* cornu sacrale

C. Lateral Aspect

Viewed in profile the lumbosacral spine is clearly S-shaped with an anterior lumbar convexity and anterior sacral concavity. The transition occurs in the region of the promontory.

In the *lumbar region* the vertebral bodies are circularly and horizontally depressed in their center, and their diameter increases at the superior and inferior surfaces. Thus the intervertebral spaces containing the intervertebral discs are easy to identify by sight and especially on palpation. The intervertebral spaces are narrower posteriorly due to the lumbar lordosis, and this must be taken into account when exploring the discs or manipulating the lumbar vertebral bodies. The intervertebral foramina separated by the pedicles are aligned posterior to the anterior column. Thus the intervertebral foramina are limited above and below by the pedicles, anteriorly by the posterior surface of the discs, and posteriorly by the zygapophyseal articulation. These foramina are larger (18 mm × 8 mm) than those in the upper segments of the spine. However, the two final foramina at L4-L5 and L5-S1 are slightly smaller, although their corresponding spinal nerve roots are larger. The posterior columns formed by the successive articular processes and isthmic regions lie posterior to the intervertebral foramina. The overall direction of the posterior columns is one of posterior concavity, according to the degree of regional lordosis, but on close inspection these columns are in fact sinusoidal. They give rise laterally to the transverse processes, displaying a slight posterior tilt with respect to the coronal plane, and posteriorly to the mamillary and accessory processes. The lumbosacral profile is limited posteriorly by the spinous processes. The interspinous spaces can be identified by palpation and thus give the horizontal level of the corresponding disc and zygapophyseal articulations.

In the *sacral region,* the lateral view of the spine demonstrates the anterior protrusion of the sacral plate slanting downward and forward. The lateral part of the sacrum, known as the ala sacralis, lies below the sacral plate and presents an articular facet participating in the sacroiliac articulation. In continuity with the anterior lumbar column the body of the sacrum progressively tapers and is terminated by the coccyx. The zygapophyseal articulation of L5-S1 continues the posterior columns of the lumbar spine. This articulation presents an angulation equivalent to that of the promontory on the pelvic side of the sacrum. The successive posterolateral sacral tubercles are homologous to fused posterior articulations. The posterior profile of the sacrum is terminated by the sacral crest.

D. Sagittal Section

A sagittal section of the lumbosacral spine to the left of the spinous processes shows the osteofibrous continuity of the different segments.

The anterior column is formed by the successive rectangular vertebral bodies of L1 to L4, the trapezoidal body of L5, and the inverted and curved cone of the sacral body. The intervertebral discs, present only above the sacrum, are biconvex in their middle region near the nucleus pulposus. The anulus fibrosus is tapered on the concave side of the sacrum and thickest on the convex side. The angular lumbosacral junction forms the promontory, a veritable keystone of the lumbosacral curvature. The degree to which the components of this angle are wedge-shaped varies from subject to subject, but generally involves the body of L5, the L5-S1 disc, and the inclination of the sacral plate. The promontory forms a mean angle of 118° in women and 126° in men (Bleicher and Beau).

The vertebral canal, referred to as the lumbosacral canal in this region, is triangular on section with an anterior base. The canal widens from L1 to the L5-S1 intervertebral disc and then narrows again down to the sacral hiatus. The intervertebral and sacral foramina form porthole-shaped communications with the anterolateral angles of the vertebral canal. The posterior plane of the canal is constituted by the alternate laminae and ligamenta flava, backed by the spinous processes and interspinous spaces containing the interspinous ligaments. The interspinous and interlaminar spaces can be used as the route of access to the vertebral canal during spinal puncture by directing the needle horizontally parallel to the greater axis of the spinous processes.

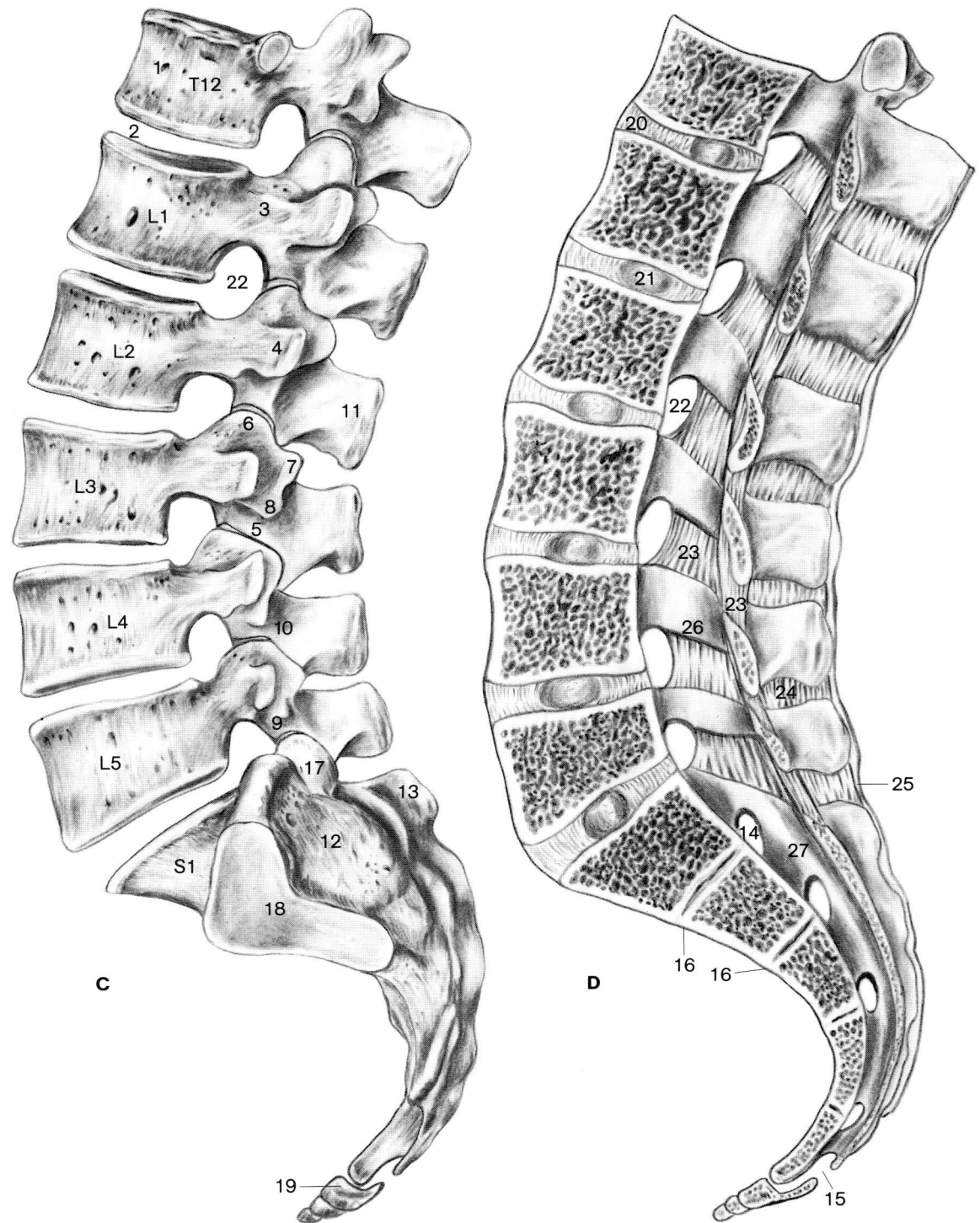

Figure 13 C, D

C Lateral aspect of the lumbar spine (columna lumbalis)
D Median sagittal section of the lumbar spine

1 corpus vertebrae *2* spatium intervertebrale *3* pediculus *4* processus costarius *5* processus articularis inf. *6* processus articularis sup. *7* processus mamillaris *8* processus accessorius *9* isthmus *10* lamina arcus vertebrae *11* processus spinosis *12* pars lateralis ossis sacri *13* crista sacralis mediana *14* foramina sacralia dorsalia, pelvinia *15* hiatus sacralis *16* linea transversa *17* processus articularis sup. *18* facies auricularis ossis sacri *19* os coccygis *20* discus intervertebralis: anulus fibrosus *21* discus intervertebralis: nucleus pulposus *22* foramen intervertebrale *23* lig. flavum *24* lig. interspinale *25* lig. supraspinale *26* canalis lumbalis *27* canalis sacralis

E. Lumbosacral Articulations

The lumbar vertebrae articulate with each other and the sacrum by means of the intervertebral discs and zygapophyseal joints. The sacrum articulates with the coxal bones at the sacroiliac joints and with the coccyx at the sacrococcygeal joint.

The *intervertebral discs* of the lumbosacral region are the largest of the entire spine. In the adult these discs attain 10–15 mm in height and their base measures 50 mm × 30 mm. The discs are inserted by their anulus fibrosus on the reniform cartilaginous plates of two adjacent vertebrae. Anteriorly and posteriorly lie the anterior and posterior longitudinal ligaments. The anulus fibrosus containing overlapping laminae like the layers of an onion is particularly strong, since the fibers of contiguous laminae lie obliquely to each other. The innermost laminae delineate a spherical central cavity containing the highly hydrophilic nucleus pulposus, composed of mucopolysaccharides and collagen fibrils. Between the nucleus pulposus and anulus fibrosus there is no smooth surface, but a histological transition zone, so that in this region the nucleus pulposus cannot be described as a sort of ball bearing sealed within the anulus fibrosus. The nucleus is located posterior to the geometric center of the intervertebral disc.

The *zygapophyseal articulations* are of the trochoid type, as the upper facets are hollow segments of a vertical cylinder whereas the lower facets are slightly convex. The facets are covered by cartilage, and the superior and inferior facets occupy the anterolateral and posteromedial parts of the articulation respectively. The articular interface is vertical in the craniocaudal direction, but curved with its center near the base of the spinous processes in the horizontal plane. The facets of the posterior articulation at L5-S1 are less curved than the suprajacent articulations. The interface of the L5-S1 posterior joint displays a posterior concavity lying at a 45 ° angle to the coronal and sagittal planes. The zygapophyseal articulations are reinforced by a synovial lined capsule, the ligamentum flavum anterior to the articulation, a posterior ligament strengthening the capsule from behind, and other ligaments inserting on these articulations. The latter include the interspinous and supraspinous ligaments and the intertransverse ligaments between the accessory processes.

The *sacroiliac joints* articulate the auricular facets of the sacrum with the coxal bone. These articulations are curved around a geometric center located near the posterolateral tubercles of the sacrum. The articular surface of the sacrum is a concave groove and that of the coxal bone is reciprocally convex to fit perfectly with the former.
In addition to a capsule and synovial membrane the sacroiliac articulations present plurifascicular ligaments, i. e., the ventral sacroiliac ligaments anteriorly and the interosseous and dorsal sacroiliac ligaments posterior to the joint. These ligaments are bilaminar, having deep and superficial layers. Ligaments at some distance from the articulation consolidate the union between the lumbosacral spine and coxal bones.

These ligaments include the iliolumbar ligaments, extending from the transverse processes of L4 and L5 to the iliac crest, and the sacrosciatic ligaments. The dorsal sacrosciatic ligament connects the posterior iliac spines and the lateral margins of the sacrum and coccyx to the tuberosity of the ischium and the ischial ramus. The ventral sacrosciatic ligament, anterior to the dorsal ligament, extends from the lateral margins of the sacrum and coccyx to the sciatic spine.

The *sacrococcygeal joint* comprises a pseudodisc reinforced by anterior, posterior, and lateral ligaments.

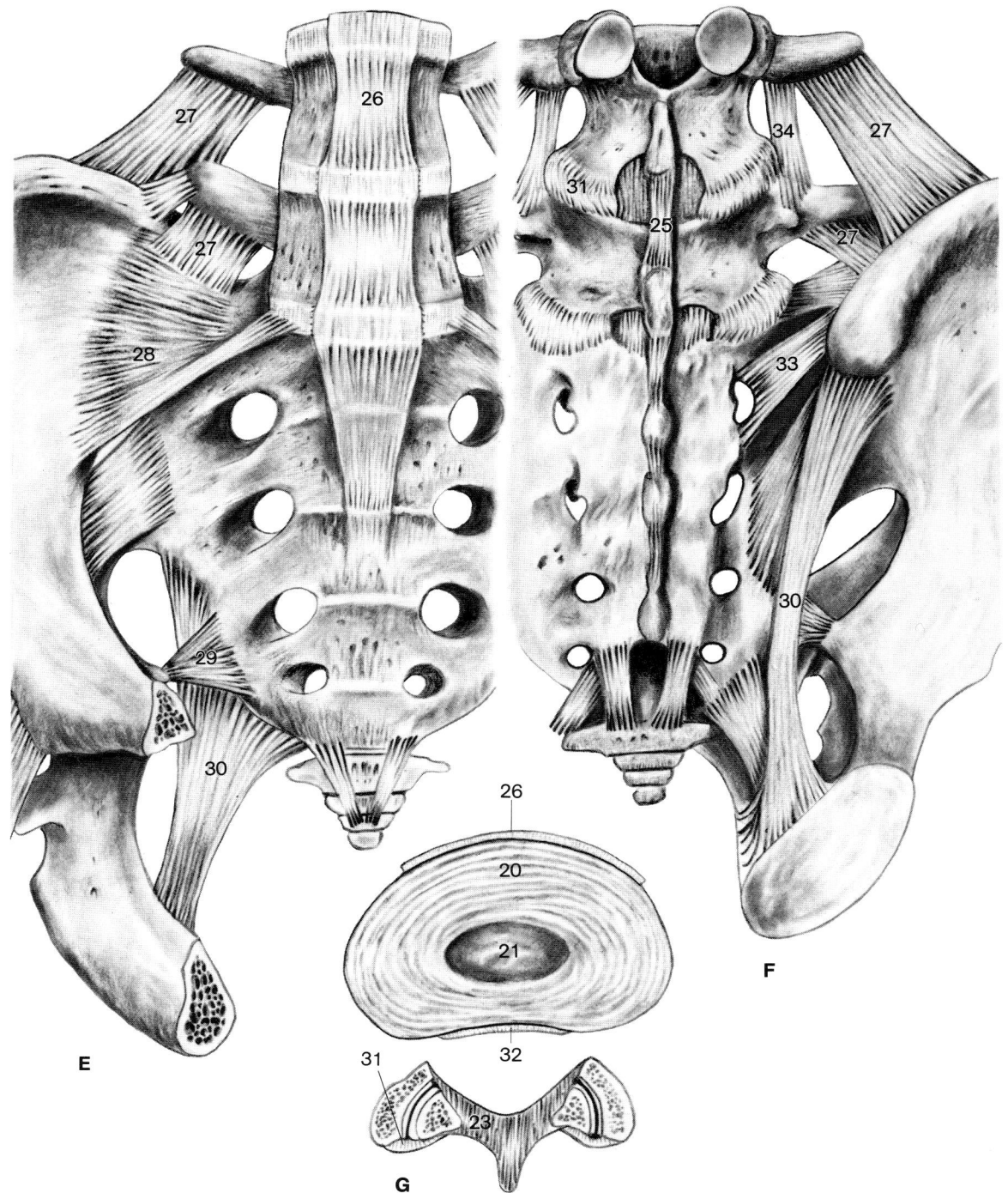

Figure 13 E–G

E Anterior aspect of the lumbosacral and sacroiliac articulations (ligamenta pelvis)
F Posterior aspect of the lumbosacral and sacroiliac articulation
G Horizontal section of an intervertebral space (spatium intervertebrale)

20 discus intervertebralis: anulus fibrosus *21* discus intervertebralis: nucleus pulposus *23* lig. flavum *25* lig. supraspinale *26* lig. longitudinale ant. *27* lig. iliolumbale *28* lig. sacroiliacum ventrale *29* lig. sacrospinale *30* lig. sacrotuberale *31* capsula articulationis zygapophysealis *32* lig. longitudinale post. *33* lig. sacroiliacum dorsale *34* lig. intertransversarium

F. Radiology

The main planes of examination of the lumbosacral spine are anteroposterior, lateral, and oblique (three-quarter) roentgenographic views, discography, and axial sections (computerized axial tomography and standard axial tomography).

1. Anteroposterior View

On anteroposterior films the numerical correspondence of each vertebra should first be sought in order to identify a transitional anomaly. In the region of the *sacrum* the superior plate, anterior sacral foramina, and sacroiliac joints can be seen.

The *bodies* of the lumbar vertebrae appear as rectangular structures with concave lateral margins. The superior and inferior surfaces of the vertebral bodies are seen as a single horizontal line when the X-rays are parallel to them, but as two liplike lines when the X-rays are oblique.

The component structures of the *vertebral arch* are visible through the transparent shadow of the vertebral bodies. The pedicles are projected at the level of the superior angles of the vertebral bodies, and are oval vertical structures above L4 but triangular at L4 and L5. On each side of the vertebral bodies the transverse processes are projected onto the lateral surface of the pedicles. The posterior tubercle of the spinous process is visible in the region of the inferior surface of the vertebral body. The articular processes and laminae form a characteristic X-shaped image. The superior angles or superior articular processes are projected above the pedicles and the inferior angles or inferior articular processes can be identified below the inferior margin of the vertebral bodies. The center of the X is located over the spinous process with the laminae lying on each side.

The *mobile vertebral segment* can be identified by the intervertebral spaces corresponding to the intervertebral discs and by the posterior zygapophyseal articulations. The interlaminar space is clearly visible between the spinous processes.

2. Lateral View

The *lumbosacral curvature* should first be examined on profile films. The direction of the sacrum with respect to a vertical line gives a good estimation of the degree of lumbosacral lordosis, e.g., a nearly horizontal sacrum reflects hyperlordosis.

The *sacrum,* in addition to its tilt and curvature, presents traces of the intersacral spaces and sacral plate on lateral X-rays. It is continued downward by the coccyx, with a variable sacrococcygeal angle.

The *vertebral bodies* appear as quadrangular structures with concave sides. The vertebral body of L5 is often trapezoidal, corresponding to the keystone of the lumbosacral lordosis.

The superior and inferior surfaces of the vertebral bodies appear as two lemniscuslike lines.

The *posterior arches* begin at the pedicles arising from the upper half of the posterior margin of the vertebral bodies. The superior and inferior articular processes occupy the superior and inferior angles of the posterior edge of the pedicles, constituting a vertical pillar whose middle region corresponds to the isthmus. The laminae appear superimposed over the images of the isthmus. The spinous processes extend horizontally behind the articular pillar at the level of the inferior surface of the vertebral body.

The *mobile segments* of the lumbosacral spine are easily identifiable by the intervertebral spaces corresponding to the intervertebral discs and by the posterior articulations lying in the same horizontal plane.

The semilunar *intervertebral foramina* project between the pedicles, the posterior margin of the intervertebral spaces, and the posterior articulations.

The *vertebral canal* is relatively easy to identify between the posterior margin of the vertebral bodies and the anterior edge of the laminae, whose section is projected above the isthmus. The distance between these two structures yields the caliber of the canal.

3. Lumbar Discography

Opacification of the nucleus pulposus gives highly useful information. In normal young subjects, the aspect of the nucleus is variable: a regular solid sphere, a sphere with amputation in its anterior half near the equator (shirt-button image), or a quadrangular structure. In older individuals without an apparent vertebral anomaly, certain nuclei are replaced by an irregularly laminated cavity (Rabischong).

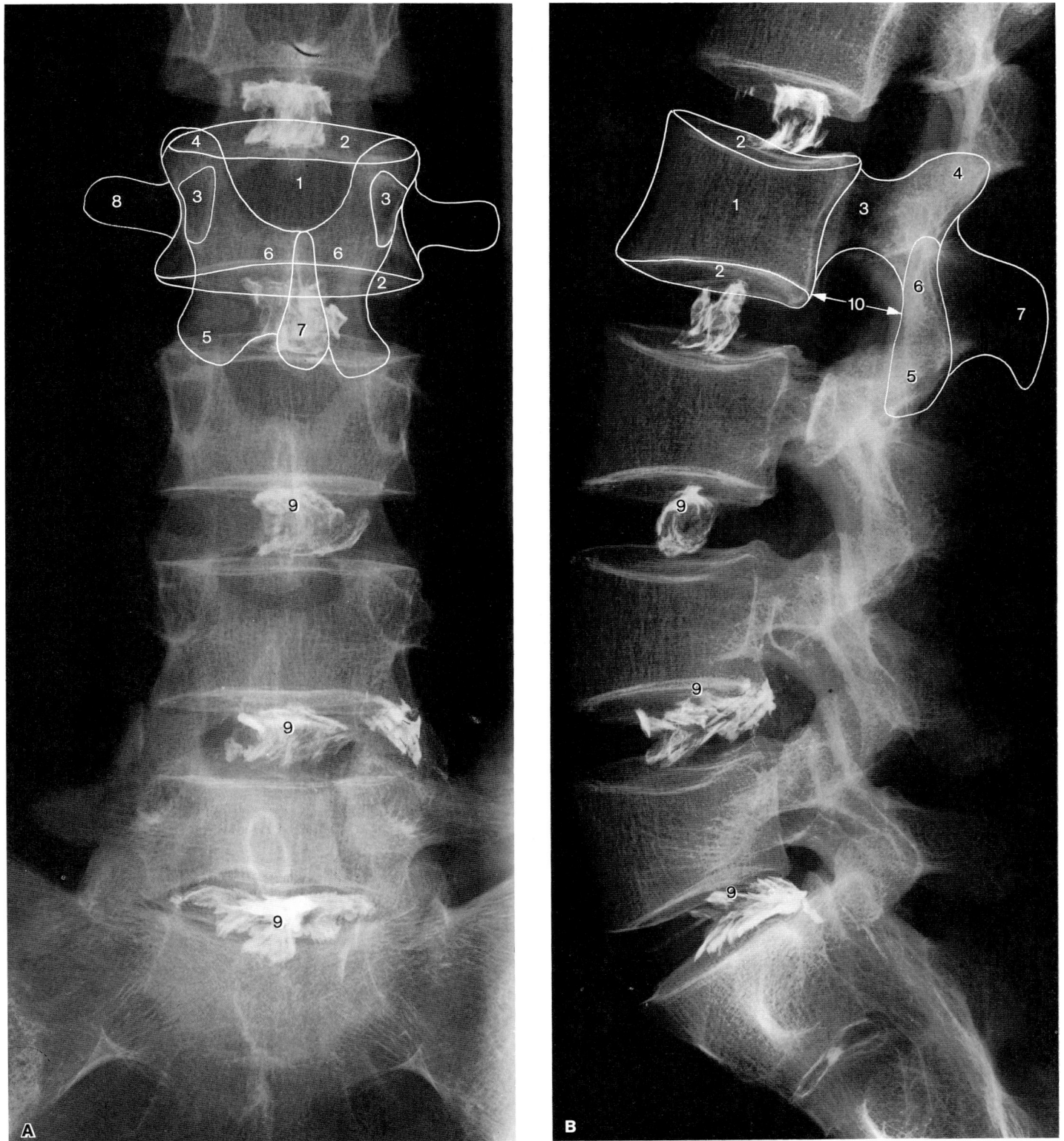

Figure 14 A, B

A   Anteroposterior X-ray (anatomical specimen with discography)
B   Lateral X-ray (anatomical specimen with discography)

1 corpus vertebrae   *2* extremitas cranealis and extremitas caudalis
3 pediculus arcus vertebrae   *4* processus articularis sup.   *5* processus articularis inf.   *6* lamina arcus vertebrae   *7* processus spinalis
8 processus transversalis   *9* nucleus pulposus   *10* canalis vertebralis

4. Oblique View

Right or left oblique films are particularly indicated for the study of the isthmus (pars interarticularis) and the posterior articulations.

The *isthmus,* the narrow part of the vertebral arch between the articular processes and lamina, appears at the inferior and medial margin of the pedicle. The image of the posterior arch in fact resembles that of a little dog on oblique films. The snout corresponds to the transverse process, the ear to the superior articular process, the eye to the pedicle, the collar to the isthmus and the forelimb to the inferior articular process. In the absence of spondylolysis of the isthmus the supra- and subjacent articular interfaces are parallel, but do not lie along the same line.

The *posterior articulations* clearly show their interface due to the posterolateral obliquity of the joints. Degenerative or traumatic alterations of these articulations can thus be identified, since the articular interface is normally 2–3 mm wide and the articular facets, bordered by a thin cortical line, lie perfectly opposite each other without translation or overlapping.

5. Axial View

Viewed transversely, the lumbar vertebrae clearly display the vertebral bodies and posterior arches comprising the pedicles, the laminae, and the articular, spinous, and transverse processes. The presence of a vertebral tumor can be confirmed and perfectly localized by axial roentgenography. The cross section of the vertebral canal can be measured in the anteroposterior, transverse, and oblique directions. Finally, the posterior articulations are well visualized, allowing identification of eventual osteophytes impinging on the vertebral canal or intervertebral foramina.

6. Structure of the Vertebrae

Like all skeletal structures, the vertebrae are adapted to the constraints imposed by their function. The vertebrae are compact bones, consisting of cancellous tissue surrounded by thin cortical bone.
Study of the trabecular structure of the cancellous bone shows the presence of laminar systems with fixed orientation. One vertical trabecular system traversing the vertebral body from the superior to the inferior surface displays a slight convexity toward the periphery, and is intersected by a second, horizontal system. The horizontal trabeculae extend from the vertebral arch (laminae and spinous and transverse processes), funnel through the pedicles, and spread out fanlike to the walls of the vertebral body. The third system is composed of two bundles of oblique trabeculae. The superior bundle, spread out on the superior plate of the body, passes through the pedicle to fan out toward the walls of the inferior articular process. The inferior trabecular bundle extends from the low-er plate of the vertebral body to the superior articular process. The fourth, horizontal arciform system is contained within the vertebral arch, passing through the laminae to connect the two transverse processes. Finally, the fifth system comprises vertical arciform trabeculae localized within the pillars of the articular processes. The structure of the vertebrae thus confirms the existence of three vertical columns (vertebral body and articular processes) with a system of intersecting trabeculae passing through the pedicles. There is thus a functional synergy among the three vertical columns, as the constraints on each merge to produce a force acting on all three. The anterior part of the vertebral bodies presents a weak area between the two oblique trabecular bundles, thus facilitating wedge compression of the bodies during trauma.

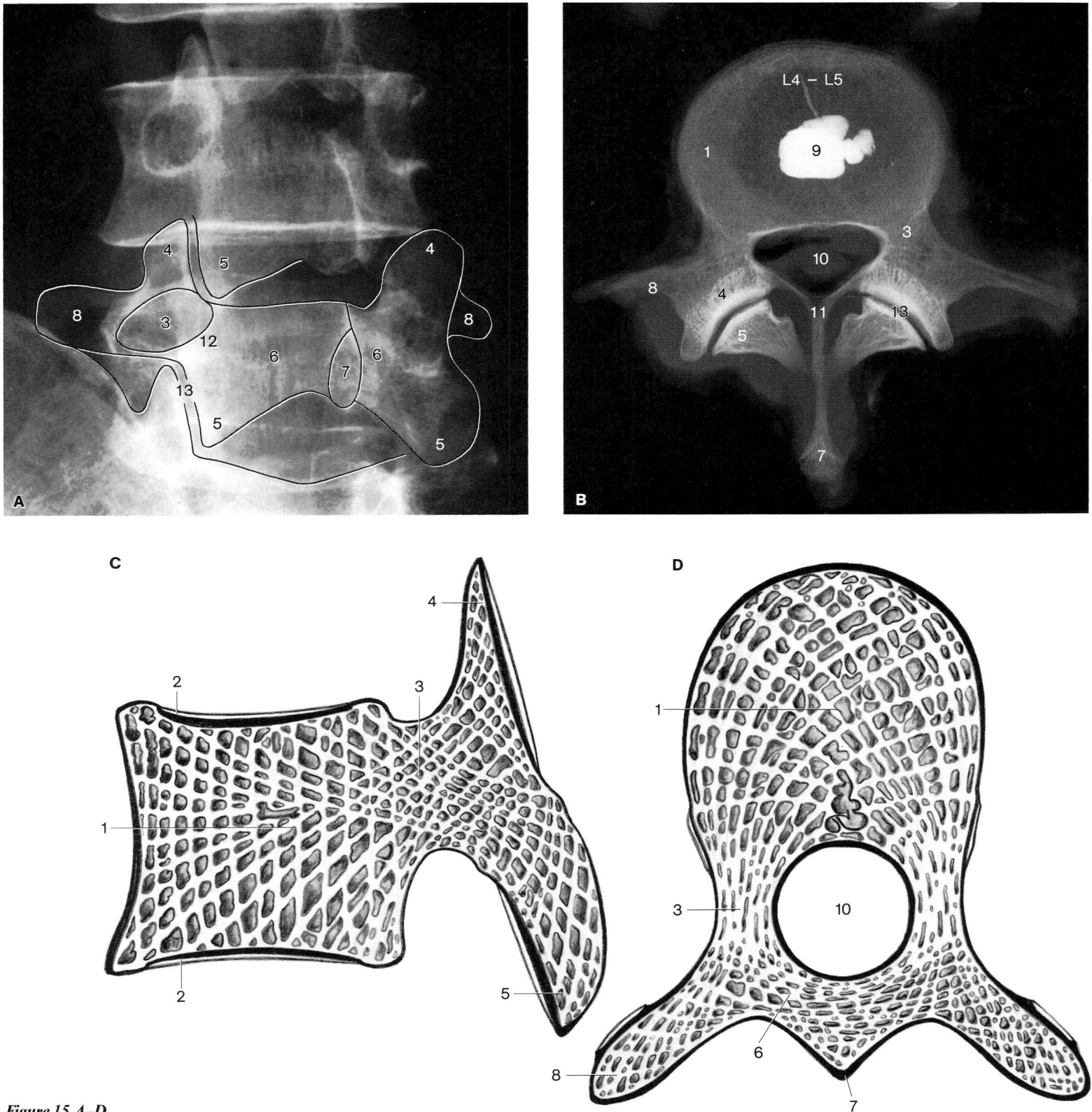

Figure 15 A–D

A   Oblique X-ray of the lumbosacral spine showing the little dog image

B   Horizontal section through the L4-L5 intervertebral disc after opacification of the nucleus pulposus

C, D   Schematic illustration of vertebral structure

1 corpus vertebrae   2 extremitas cranialis and extremitas caudalis
3 pediculus arcus vertebrae   4 processus articularis sup.   5 processus articularis inf.   6 lamina arcus vertebrae   7 processus spinalis
8 processus transversalis   9 nucleus pulposus   10 canalis vertebralis
11 lig. flavum   12 isthmus (pars interarticularis)   13 structura zygapophysealis

IV. Spinal Myology

Full understanding of the vertebral muscles is necessary not only for the comprehension of spinal statics and dynamics but also for the elaboration of a coherent plan of functional rehabilitation. Furthermore, during operation the surgeon must not alter the quality of these muscles, in order to avoid postoperative syndromes which may be invalidating. The vertebral muscles are arranged in two layers, i.e., the posterior layer of extensor muscles and the anterolateral layer of essentially flexor muscles.

A. Posterior Muscles

The posterior muscles are found in three spinal segments, the nuchal region, the trunk, and the pelvic region.

1. Nuchal Muscles

The nuchal muscles lie in four layers from the superficial to the deep regions.

Trapezius. The trapezius extends from the external occipital protuberance to the spinous process of T12, the lateral third of the clavicle, and the acromion and spine of the scapula. This muscle is involved in the movements of extension and rotation.

Splenius and Levator Scapulae. The splenius extends from the ligamentum nuchae and the spinous processes of C7 to T5 to the mastoid (splenius capitis) and the transverse processes of C1 to C3 (splenius colli). The levator scapulae joins the superomedial angle of the scapula to the transverse processes of C1 to C5. These muscles are involved in extension and lateral flexion.

Complexus Muscles. The greater complexus (semispinalis capitis) has its origin on the transverse processes of T6 to C4 and the spinous process of C7 and inserts on the occipital bone. The lesser complexus (longissimus capitis) connects the transverse processes of T1 through C3 to the mastoid. The longissimus cervicis extends from the transverse processes of T5 to T1 to those of C7 to C3. The cervical part of the sacrolumbar muscle (iliocostalis cervicis) originates on the posterior arches of C7 to C3. All these muscles participate in the movements of lateral extension and flexion.

Deep Muscles. The rectus capitis posterior minor extends from the posterior tubercle of C1 to the occipital bone, and the rectus capitis posterior major joins the spinous process of C2 to the occipital bone. The obliquus capitis inferior originates on the spinous process of C2 and inserts on the transverse process of C1. The tubercle of the atlas is connected to the occipital bone by the obliquus capitis superior. The transversus spinalis extends from the sacrum to C2 between the transverse processes and the four suprajacent spinous processes. Finally, the interspinalis cervicis inserts on the spinous

processes extending upward from the sacrum to the atlas. All the deep muscles are involved in extension. The rectus capitis posterior major and the obliquus capitis inferior and superior also participate in the movements of rotation.

2. Muscles of the Trunk

These muscles of the trunk are also arranged in four layers.

Latissimus Dorsi. The origin of the latissimus dorsi is on the posterior third of the iliac crest, the sacral crest, and the spinous processes of L5 to T6. The muscle joins the lumbar aponeurosis (fascia thoracolumbalis) and inserts on the bicipital groove of the humerus. It is the elevator of the trunk.

Rhomboideus. The rhomboideus muscle originates on the spinous processes of C7 to T4 and inserts on the spinal margin of the scapula.

Serratus Posterior. The serratus posterior superior originates on the spinous processes of C7 to T3 and inserts on the first three ribs. The serratus posterior inferior extends from the spinous processes of C3 to T11 and inserts on the last four ribs. An intermediate fascia lies between these two muscles, which are involved in respiration.

Erector Spinae. Five muscle bodies form the erector spinae extending from the spinous processes to the ribs:

1. The interspinalis thoracis and lumborum.
2. The spinalis thoracis and lumborum, originating on the spinous processes of L2 to T11 and inserting on those of T10 to T1.
3. The transversospinalis.
4. The longissimus lumborum and thoracis, which originates as part of the common mass of the transversospinalis and iliocostalis extending from the lumbar spinous processes, sacral crest, sacral groove, and coxal bone to insert on the posterior arches of the ribs and the transverse processes of the thoracic and lumbar vertebrae.
5. The iliocostalis lumborum and thoracis, extending from the common mass of muscle to insert on the lumbar transverse processes and the last ten ribs.

The components of the erector spinae are extensor muscles.

3. Extensor Muscles of the Pelvic Region

Acting on the sacrum by the intermediary of the pelvis, the gluteal muscles (gluteus maximus, medius, and minimus) and posterior femoral muscles (semitendinus, semimembranosus, and biceps femoris) are extensors.

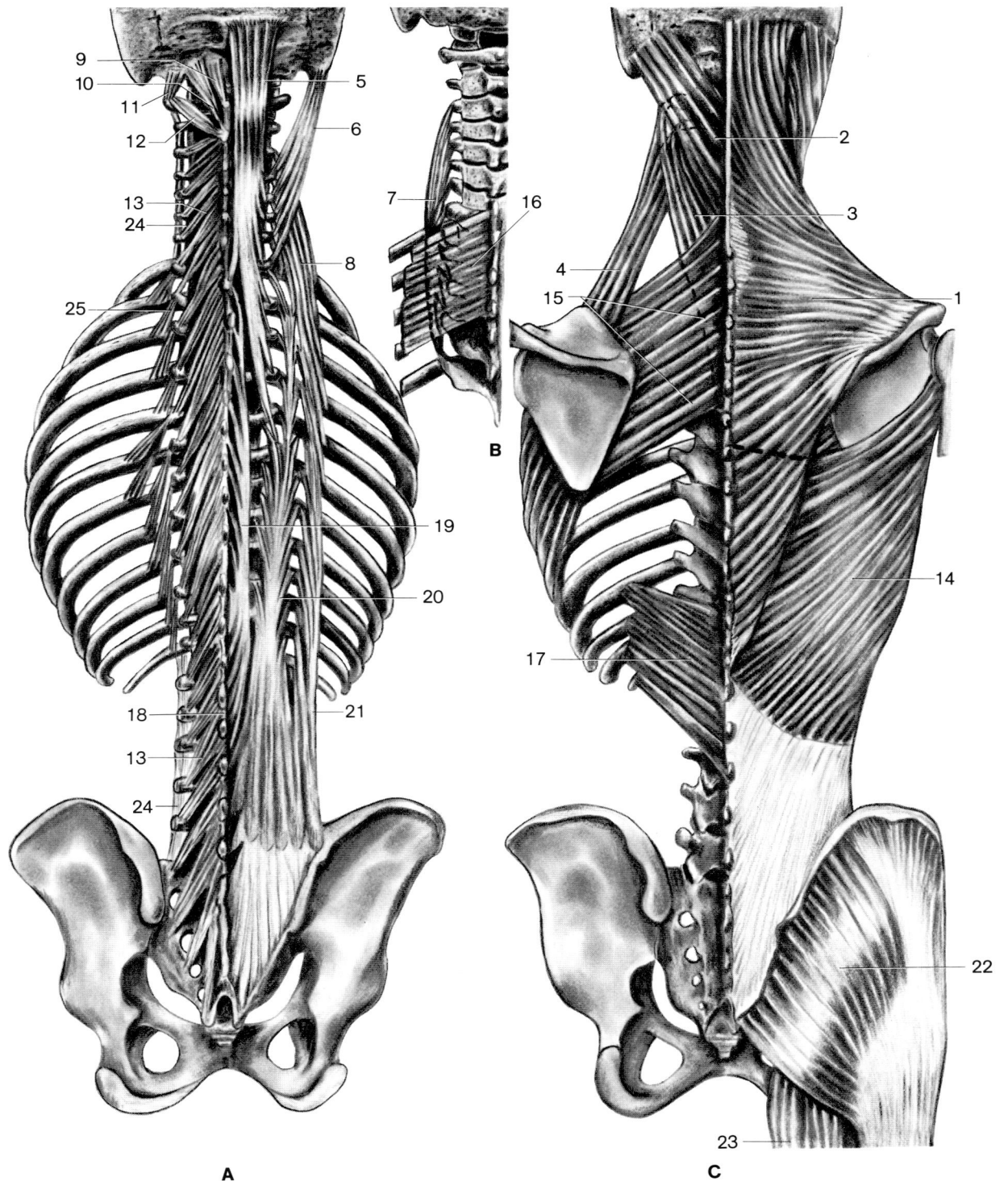

Figure 16 A–C

A, B   The deep posterior extensor muscles of the spine
C   The superficial posterior extensor muscles of the spine

1 m. trapezius   *2* m. splenius capitis   *3* m. splenius cervicis
4 m. levator scapulae   *5* m. semispinalis capitis   *6* m. longissimus
capitis   *7* m. longissimus cervicis   *8* m. iliocostalis cervicis *9* m. rectus
capitis post. minor   *10* m. rectus capitis post. major   *11* m. obliquus
capitis sup.   *12* m. obliquus capitis inf.   *13* m. transversospinalis

14 m. latissimus dorsi   *15* m. rhomboideus major and minor
16 m. serratus post. sup.   *17* m. serratus post. inf.   *18* m. interspinales
19 m. spinalis thoracis   *20* m. longissimus lumborum and thoracis
21 m. iliocostalis lumborum and thoracis   *22* m. glutaeus maximus
23 post. femoral muscles (semitendinus, semimbranosus, and biceps
femoris)   *24* mm. intertransversarii laterales lumborum and posteriores
cervicis   *25* mm. levatores costarum breves

B. Anterolateral Muscles

The anterolateral muscles of the spine lie in the neck, the thorax, and abdominal region.

1. Muscles of the Neck

The neck muscles form a superficial and a deep layer.

Superficial Layer. The sternocleidomastoideus originates on the sternum and medial end of the clavicle and inserts on the mastoid. This muscle participates in the flexion, lateroflexion, and rotation of the head.

Deep Layer. The scaleni muscles extend from the cervical tranverse processes to the first two ribs. The scalenus anterior originates on the transverse processes of C3 to C6 and inserts on Lisfranc's tubercle of the first rib. The scalenus medius joins the transverse processes of C2 through C7 to the superior surface of the first rib. The scalenus posterior, originating on the transverse processes of C4 to C6, is attached to the lateral surface of the second rib. The scaleni muscles participate in lateroflexion and rotation. The rectus capitis anterior and lateralis extend from the atlas to the base of the cranium. The longus colli originating from C1 to T3 extends to the lateral parts of the vertebrae, the vertebral bodies and transverse processes. The longus capitis originates on the transverse processes and extends from C6 to the base of the occipital bone. These muscles make possible the movements of flexion and lateroflexion. The deep neck muscles also include the intertransversarius.

2. Muscles of the Thorax

The three layers of *intercostal muscles* occlude the intercostal spaces. These muscles include the intercostalis externus, which is continued posteriorly by the levator costarum; the intercostalis internus; and the intercostalis intimus, which blends posteriorly with the subcostalis.

The *diaphragm* comprises three bundles according to their site of insertion. The pars sternalis inserts on the xiphoid appendix, the pars costalis is inserted on the last six ribs and their costal cartilage, and the pars lumbalis, arising from the lumbocostal arches and the diaphragmatic pillars, inserts on the spine and twelfth rib. The right and left medial pillars (crus mediale, dextrum and sinistrum) form the boundaries of the aortic hiatus (hiatus aorticus). The lateral pillars (crus laterale) form the arches of the psoas muscle (arcus lumbocostalis medialis) and quadratus lumborum (arcus lumbocostalis lateralis). Diaphragmatic muscle fibers are also inserted on the centrum tendineum. In addition to its respiratory function, the diaphragm lends support to the spine by intra-abdominal pressure.

3. Muscles of the Abdomen

The abdominal muscles lie in two layers.

Anterolateral Muscles. The rectus abdominis extends along the midline from the pubis to the anteroinferior part of the thorax. In its lower portion the rectus abdominis is doubled by the pyramidalis. The lateral muscles of the abdomen lie on each side of the midline; from the superficial to the deep regions they include the obliquus externus abdominis, the obliquus internus abdominis, and the transversus abdominis. The terminal aponeuroses of these muscles form a sheath around the rectus abdominis (vagina musculi recti abdominis). These long muscles extend from the anterior arch of the last eight ribs toward the iliac crest, the pubis, and ligamentum inguinale. The anterolateral muscles contribute to increase the intra-abdominal pressure and to flex the thoracolumbar spine by applying a movement of rotation, i.e., unilateral contraction pulls the anterior surface of the trunk toward the side of the contracted muscle.

Posterior Iliolumbar Muscles. This muscle group comprises the intertransversarii laterales, mediales lumborum, the quadratus lumborum, and the iliopsoas. The quadratus lumborum originates on the iliac crest and transverse processes of the lower lumbar vertebrae and inserts on the twelfth rib and transverse processes of the upper lumbar vertebrae. The iliopsoas descends from the dihedral angle formed by the transverse processes and bodies of the lumbar vertebrae and from the internal iliac fossa, passes through the crural arch (ligamentum inguinale), and inserts on the lesser trochanter. The quadratus lumborum inclines the spine on the side of muscle contraction, whereas the iliopsoas flexes the lumbar spine by inducing rotation toward the side opposite the muscle contraction.

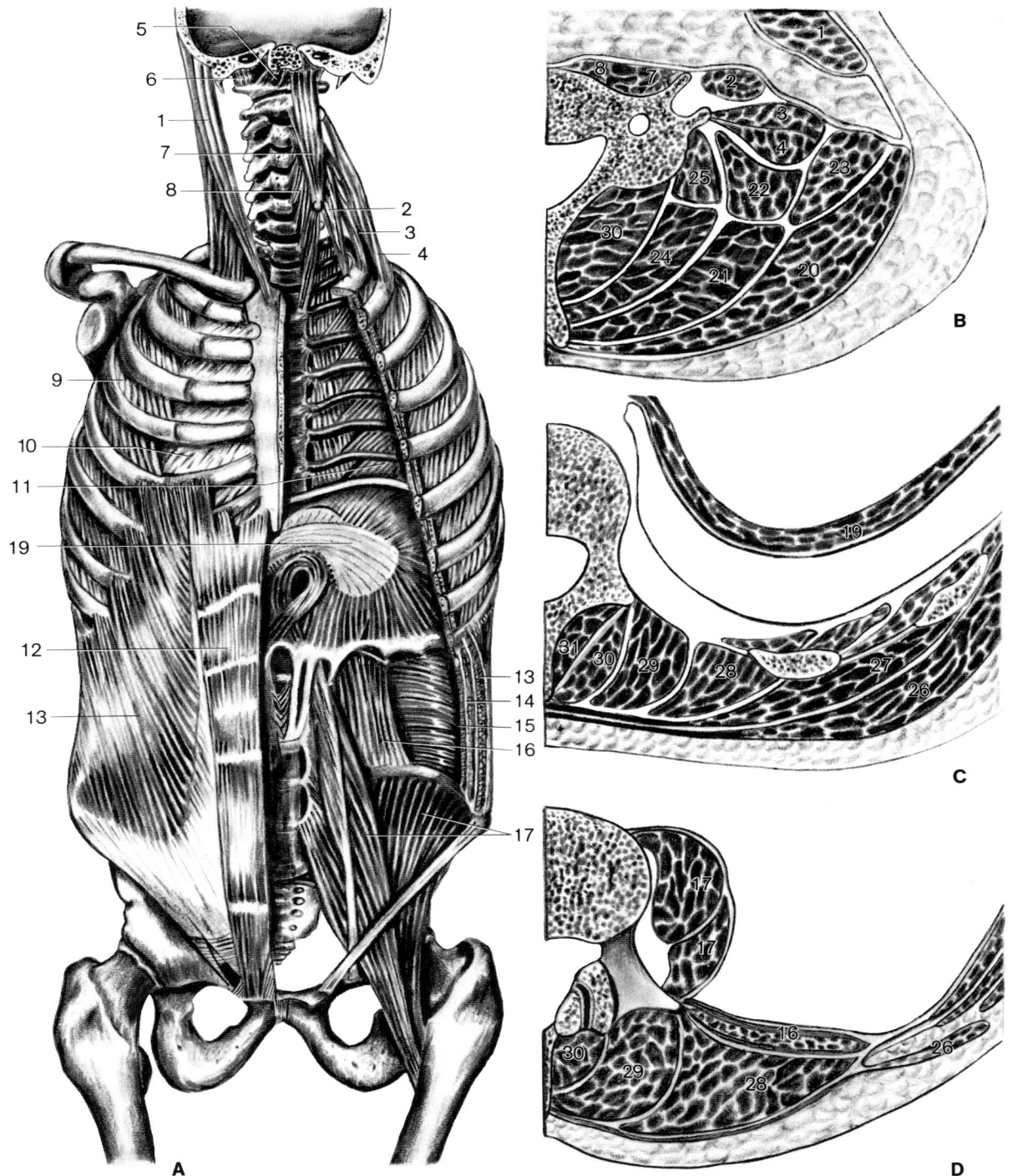

Figure 17 A–D

A

B

C

D

A Anterior aspect of the spinal muscles
B Horizontal section through the muscles of the neck
C Horizontal section through the thoracolumbar muscles
D Horizontal section through the lumbar muscles

1 m. sternocleidomastoideus *2–4* m. scalenus ant., medius, post.
5 m. rectus capitis ant. *6* m. rectus capitis lateralis *7* m. longus capitis
8 m. longus colli *9* m. intercostales externi *10* m. intercostales interni

11 m. intercostales intimi *12* m. rectus abdominis *13* m. obliquus externus abdominis *14* m. obliquus internus abdominis *15* m. transversus abdominis *17* m. iliopsoas *19* m. diaphragma *20* m. trapezius *21* m. splenius capitis *22* m. splenius cervicis *23* m. levator scapulae *24* m. semispinalis capitis *25* m. longissimus capitis *26* m. latissimus dorsi *27* m. serratus post. inf. *28* m. iliocostalis *29* m. longissimus *30* m. transversospinalis *32* m. spinalis thoracis

3 Spinal Static Function

I. Normal Spinal Curvatures

The static function of the spine is that by which the spine participates in the equilibrium of the trunk and head by means of the spinal curvatures.

A. Theories on the Formation of Spinal Curvatures

Phylogenic Theory. The comparative anatomy of the vertebrates allows us to reconstruct the various stages in the evolution of the spine. In this respect, three major periods can be distinguished, corresponding to three different groups of vertebrates, i.e., the fish, the tetrapods, and the anthropoids including man. The spine of fish is simple and uniform, with a ventral concavity. As the tetrapods began to walk on dry land the various segments of their spine underwent progressive modifications. The disappearance of the ribs from the first vertebra posterior to the head formed the cervical region and thus allowed greater mobility of the head, which had to extend on the neck to face horizontally. In this way the cervical curvature appeared with its posterior concavity. The disappearance of the ribs caudal to the thoracic region created the lumbar segment. The vertical erection of the body in the anthropoids and man to allow the standing position and bipedal locomotion required modification of the lumbar curvature, which became concave posteriorly.

Ontogenic Theory. Study of vertebral development in the human from the embryo to childhood allows us to retrace the major phylogenic stages. The aquatic conditions of intrauterine development are associated with a single ventral concavity of the spine. In the first year of postnatal life the cervical spine is bent back upward when the child is seated or crawling on all four limbs. When the child begins to take its first steps the lumbar curvature changes to lordosis.

Mechanical Theory. The different spinal curvatures seen in profile can be accounted for by the mobility or fixity of the vertebral segments in question. The two more or less fixed regions of the spine, i.e., the thoracic and pelvic regions, retain their primitive curvature with anterior concavity. Conversely, holding the head and trunk upright modifies the two mobile regions, i.e., the cervical and the lumbar spine, so that the spine lies posterior to the center of gravity of the body. The spinal curvature with its posterior concavity in the cervical and lumbar regions allows the powerful spinal muscles to counterbalance the anterior forces of gravity.

B. Features of the Curvatures

The fully developed spine does not display a curvature in the coronal plane except in some cases where there is a small left concavity at the level of the aortic arch. Four curvatures alternate in the sagittal plane, i.e., lordosis of the cervical spine (posterior concavity), kyphosis of the thoracic spine (posterior convexity), lumbar lordosis, and sacrococcygeal kyphosis. The transitions between the first three curvatures are regular and smooth whereas the lumbosacral junction displays a prominent anterior angle known as the lumbosacral angle of the promontory (120°–130°). In the upright position the vertical line drawn up from the center of the polygonal base of equipoise passes through the bodies of the cervical vertebrae, the body of T12, the posterior surface of the body of L3, and the sacral plate. Hyperflexion causes the cervical and lumbar lordoses to disappear. The spinal curvatures become more accentuated with age and lumbar lordosis is more pronounced in women.

Finally, by physical calculation it can be shown that a column with four alternate curvatures is 17 times more resistant to stress than a rectilinear column ($R = C^2 + 1$).

C. Influence of the Pelvis

Given the state of equilibrium of the pelvis and thus of the spine on the two femoral heads, there exists a relation between the lumbar curvature and the position of the hips. In collaboration with Henry we studied (1978) this relation by examination of the femorolumbosacral angle in 500 subjects. This angle, formed by the posterior edge of the sacral plate and the vertical line passing through the tip of the acetabulum, varies from $-7°$ to $+55°$ with a mean of 21°. A negative angle corresponds to hyperlordosis. In the supine position, elevation of the outstretched lower limbs initially induces lumbar hyperlordosis and then kyphosis.

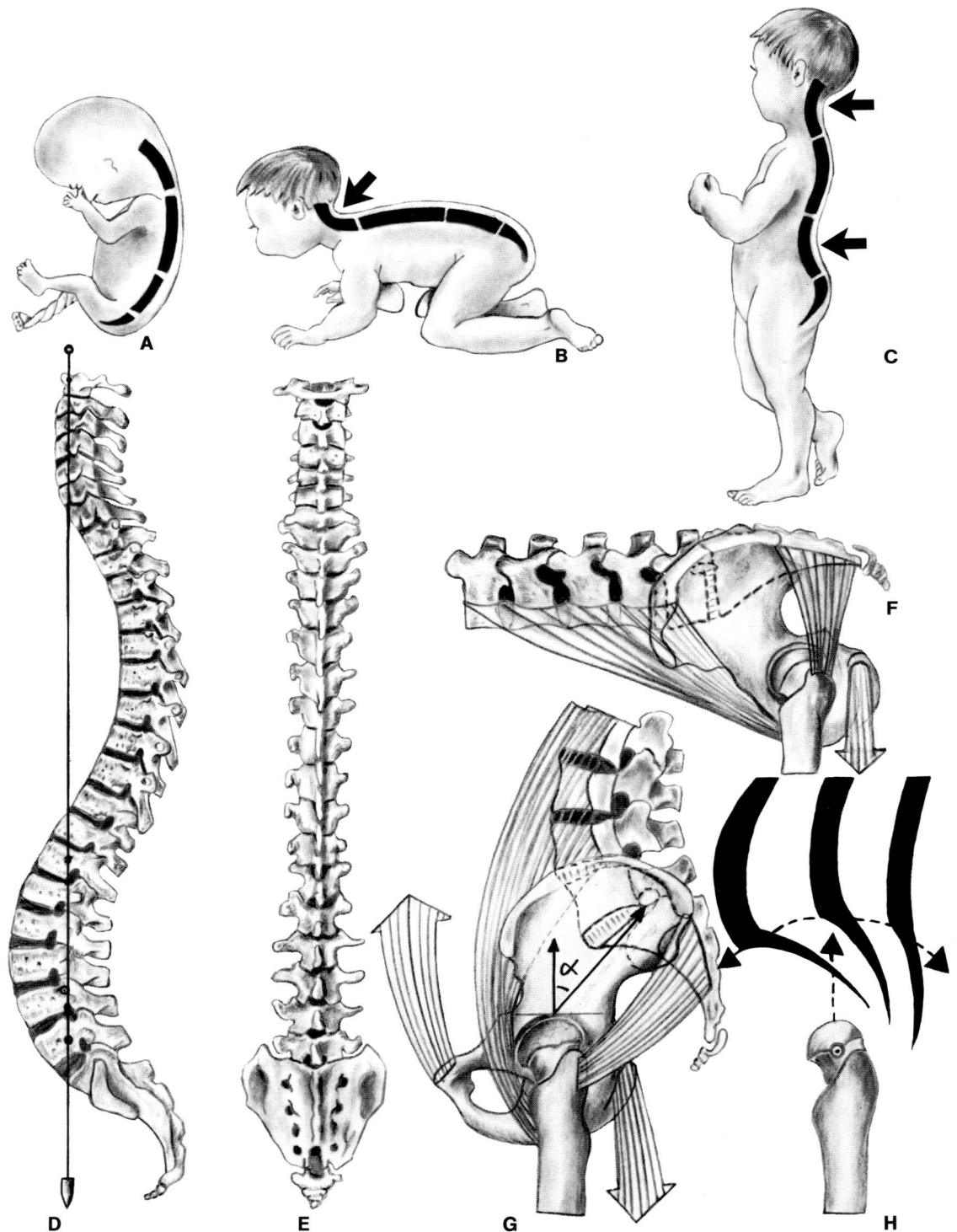

Figure 18 A–H

A   The fetal spine showing a single curvature with anterior concavity
B   The neonatal spine showing the appearance of the first lordosis involving the cervical spine induced by erection of the head
C   The spine with its four definitive curvatures after induction of lumbar lordosis by the erect position
D   The normal sagittal curvatures of the spine
E   Absence of a coronal curvature in the normal spine

F   The lumbar spine in the quadrupedal position with the femurs at 90° to the spinal axis and disappearance of lumbar lordosis
G   The femorolumbosacral angle (α) showing the position of the hips relative to the lumbosacral junction
H   Different lumbar curvatures according to the position of the lumbosacral junction relative to the hips

II. Variations of the Spinal Curvatures

In addition to the normal pattern of the spinal curvatures, a certain number of congenital or acquired variations with or without accompanying pathological phenomena can be described. Delmas and Raou described a spinal index by which one aspect of these modifications of curvature can be quantified. The index *(I)* is computed by measuring the lenght *(L)* of the anterior surface of the spine from the atlas to the sacral plate and the height *(H)* of the spine in a straight line from the atlas to the sacral plate. The index is then $I = H \times 100/L$. Normally the index is close to 95 ($\pm$ 1). An increased index signifies that the spine is practically linear whereas a decreased index reflects the accentuation of the spinal curvatures. Rectilinear spines are less mobile than those with pronounced curvatures, which are more dynamic. However, clinical and radiological features of the spine also allow the characterization of a certain number of variations in the sagittal and coronal planes.

A. Sagittal Variations

Thoracic hyperkyphosis or round back features the exaggeration of the posterior convexity of the thoracic region near T7. This postural attitude corresponds to hyperflexion of the thoracic spine.

Lumbar hyperlordosis creates an overly hollow lumbar region with anterior projection of the abdomen. This postural attitude reflects the existence of lumbar hyperextension.

Kypholordosis corresponds to the simultaneous exaggeration of thoracic kyphosis and lumbar lordosis, thus decreasing the height of the spine. In such cases the index of Delmas is less than 93. This type of spine is highly dynamic, but deteriorations, due to extreme positions of all the spinal joints, arise sooner than would otherwise be the case.

Anterior projection of the neck, often accompanying thoracic hyperkyphosis, can also be an isolated finding. In the latter case it is probably caused by a poor postural attitude, maintaining the face toward the ground rather than toward the horizon. This produces fatigue of the cervicothoracic junction.

Hollow back corresponds to an attitude of very slight lordosis of the thoracic segment contrasting with the normal kyphosis in this region. From the dynamic standpoint forced flexion of the cervical spine is difficult in subjects with hollow back. This postural attitude rapidly leads to cervical sprain syndrome.

Flat back is similar to the preceding variation in that the thoracic spine has lost its normal kyphosis and the other spinal curvatures are diminished. Patients with flat back display an index of Delmas greater than 97. This postural attitude often evolves toward the cervicothoracic sprain syndrome.

Total kyphosis of the spine is reminiscent of the fetal curvatures lacking cervical and lumbar lordosis, but where the spine is almost entirely convex posteriorly. This deformity is compensated by retroversion of the pelvis.

Total lordosis, as opposed to total kyphosis, features lordosis extending from the lumbar region to the cervicothoracic junction with the site of maximum curvature in the region of the inferior thoracic spine.

Vertebral inversion is a rare deformity where the normal sites of lordosis are replaced by kyphosis. The curvatures are in opposition to the dynamic characteristics of the different regions of the spine and thus rapidly lead to pathological overexertion with deterioration of the osteoarticular structures.

B. Coronal Variations

Poor postural attitudes during growth in normal subjects can lead to lateral deviation of the spine in the coronal plane. This deformity is postural scoliosis, which can however evolve toward fixation and thus true structural scoliosis. The main types of scoliosis are the following:
Thoracic scoliosis generally presents with a single right-sided convexity from T4 to T12. A small compensatory lumbar curve in the opposite direction, called the minor curve, is found below. The deformity is often accompanied by a pronounced costal gibbosity on the side of the thoracic convexity due to vertebral rotation.

Figure 19 A–N

A	Physiological sagittal curvature
B	Thoracic hyperkyphosis
C	Lumbar hyperlordosis
D	Kypholordosis
E	Anterior projection of the neck
F	Hollow back
G	Flat back
H	Total kyphosis
I	Total lordosis
J	Vertebral inversion
K	Thoracic scoliosis
L	Lumbar scoliosis
M	Thoracolumbar scoliosis
N	Combined thoracic and lumbar scoliosis

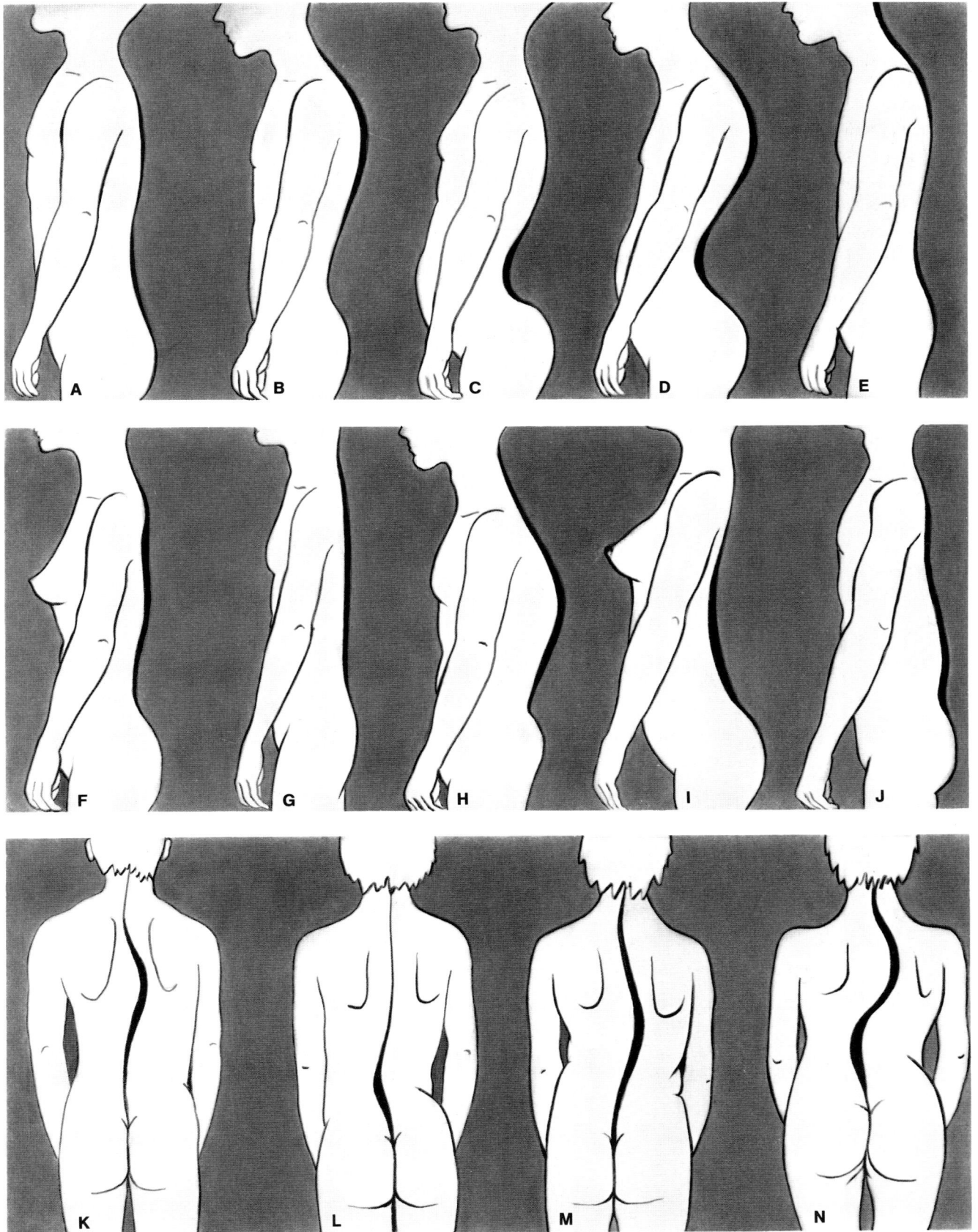

Figure 19 A–N

Lumbar scoliosis presents as a main primary convexity on one side of the lumbar spine with a suprajacent minor compensatory curve. This type of scoliosis is only a small deformity but after the age of 40 years evolves toward painful syndromes.

Thoracolumbar scoliosis presents with a main convexity centered at T10. Two minor compensatory curves exist above and below the major convexity. This deformity often leads to vertebral disequilibrium, i.e., a vertical line passing through the center of gravity of the head no longer intersects the sacral plate, thus leading to overexertion of the muscle groups opposing the disequilibrium. The final result is damage due to excessive pressure on the articular surfaces on the inside of the curvature.

Combined thoracic and lumbar scoliosis with two major curves presents as two reciprocal convexities in the thoracic and lumbar regions. Since the two curves are generally of the same magnitude, the resulting disequilibrium is of minor importance and the deformity is less apparent. Conversely, the shortening of the trunk is pronounced.

Cervicothoracic scoliosis is relatively rare. The deformity is unaesthetic, since the head no longer lies in the axial prolongation of the trunk.

Good static function thus corresponds to a well equilibrated spine with physiological curvatures, i.e., within normal limits. Orthopedic therapy should be aimed at the best and earliest possible reduction of the spinal deviations in order to avoid the often unaesthetic and painful or disruptive consequences involving the major cardiovascular and dynamic vertebral functions.

4 Spinal Stability

I. Vertical Stability

Stability of the spine is that quality by which the vertebral structures maintain their cohesion in all physiological positions of the body.

Instability, or loss of stability, is a pathological process which can lead to displacement of vertebrae beyond their normal physiological limits. The factors influencing stability differ according to whether the spine is studied vertically along its major axis or horizontally, perpendicular to the major axis.

A. Elementary Structure of the Vertebrae

From the atlas to the sacrum it is possible to identify those structures in the complex morphology of the vertebrae that support the forces of gravity. The atlas (C1) can be likened to two lateral masses joined by two arches. The axis (C2) can be reduced to three pillars, a vertical conical pillar lying medially and anteriorly (dens and body) and two lateral oblique pillars in the form of parallelepipeds. These three pillars are fused above in the body of C2 and diverge below. With respect to stability the axis does not have true pedicles and the structures referred to as such are actually isthmuses since they are interarticular structures. The structural features of C3 to L4 are analogous to those of the axis, i.e., these vertebrae are composed of three pillars: the anterior pillar formed by the vertebral body and the two pillars formed by the articular processes lying posteriorly. The three pillars are reinforced by horizontal bars, namely the pedicles and laminae. A similar configuration is found at L5 except that the vertebral body is cuneiform and the posterior pillars are angled at the isthmic zones. The sacrum provides three points of support for the three pillars, i.e., the sacral plate and two sacral facets. The gravitational forces are then transferred from the sacrum to the pelvic girdle by the two auricular facets.

B. Overall Stability of the Spine

The juxtaposition of the various vertebral structures makes it possible to follow the lines of gravitational force from the cranium to the pelvis. The cranium transfers its weight to the spine through two pillars lying in the same coronal plane. The two pillars become three columns in the body of the axis, which is thus a veritable carrefour for the transmission of the forces. The forces are then transferred down the three columns, which are arranged in a triangle with an anterior apex. The more voluminous anterior column takes on the aspect of a quadrangular pyramid formed by the alternating vertebral bodies and intervertebral discs down to the sacral plate. The two posterior columns lying in a coronal plane are composed of the successive articular processes. At C2 and L5 these columns present an isthmic angulation facilitating spondylolysis. The sacrum also constitutes a carrefour of the descending forces, since it receives them at three points but transmits them to the pelvis and lower limbs through two lateral points. This vertical system of columns is reinforced by horizontal struts which, at the level of each vertebra, solidly join the columns to each other. The struts are the two arches of C1, the posterior arch of C2, and the pedicles and laminae of the vertebrae lying below C2. The spinous and transverse processes do not participate in the system of spinal stability.

Under static and dynamic conditions the spinal curvatures modify the axis of the vertical columns but in no way change the principles of axial stability. Understanding of this system finds application in vertebral trauma and surgical stabilization of the spine. The instability due to spinal trauma is proportional to the number of ruptured columns. Surgical stabilization subsequent to vertebral excision or fracture-dislocation requires the reconstruction of one to three columns, depending on the lesion.

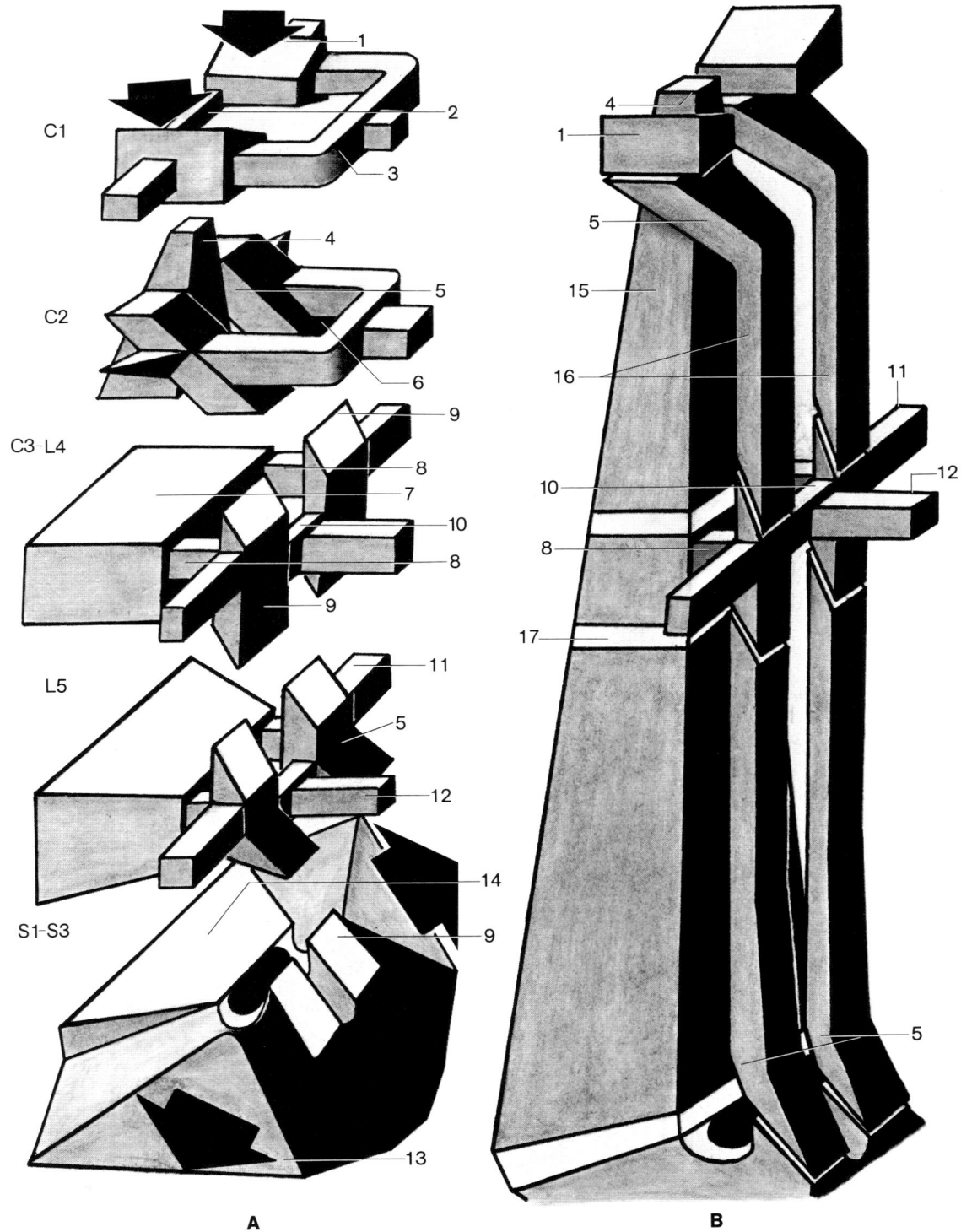

Figure 20 A, B

A   Elementary structure of the vertebrae

B   Overall structure of the spine

1 massa lateralis *2* arcus ant. *3* arcus post. *4* dens *5* isthmus
6 foramen vertebrale *7* corpus vertebrae *8* pediculus arcus vertebrae
9 processus articularis *10* lamina arcus vertebrae *11* processus
transversus *12* processus spinosus *13* facies auricularis *14* basis
ossis sacri *15* columna ant. *16* columna post. *17* discus intervertebralis

II. Horizontal Stability

When the spine is submitted to forces perpendicular to its greater axis, the points of weakness are located in the mobile, articular zones. It is of interest to consider the elements which stabilize the vertebrae during the movements of flexion-extension and rotation-inclination. Differences in the constitution of the intervertebral articulations call for the craniovertebral joints to be considered separately from the other vertebral joints.

A. Craniovertebral Articulations

During forced flexion of the head, the anterior surface of the odontoid process butts against the anterior arch of the atlas. The excess anterior displacement of the atlas is resisted by the ligamentum cruciforme atlantis, the membrana tectoria, and the ligamenta alaria. During extension the odontoid process acts as a buttress preventing posterior sliding of the atlas. Similary, contact between the posterior margin of the foramen magnum, the posterior arch of the atlas, and the spinous process of the axis limits extension of the head. The membrana atlanto-occipitalis anterior and the ligamentum transversum stretch during extension. During rotation of the atlas on the axis the ligamenta alaria, the lateral parts of the membrana tectoria, the articular capsules, and the ligamenta flava act as brakes. Lateral inclination is limited by the contact between the articular facets on the side of inclination and by the tension of the capsules, intertransverse ligaments, and the lateral part of the membrana tectoria on the opposite side. In summary, the means of vertebral stability in the horizontal articular plane are the bony buttresses and ligamentous brakes.

B. Other Vertebral Articulations

From C2-C3 to L5-S1 the same mechanisms of horizontal stability exist. These are envisaged below by study of the extreme elementary movements of the vertebrae.

Flexion. During flexion, stability is ensured by the coupled action of the osteoligamentous articular buttresses and the ligamentous brakes. The ligaments acting as a brake to extreme vertebral flexion are those located posterior to the nucleus pulposus, i.e., the posterior part of the anulus fibrosus, the ligamentum longitudinale posterior, the articular capsule, the ligamentum flavum, the ligamentum interspinale, and the ligamentum supraspinale. The buttresses of flexion are the articular processes whose facets oppose the horizontal sliding. Thus, vertebral instability on flexion can occur only after fracture of the articular process or rupture of the ligamentous brakes, which may lead to luxation.

From our laboratory experiments on fresh cadavers we conclude that all the ligaments posterior to the nucleus pulposus must be ruptured to produce abnormal vertebral displacement. Partial rupture of these ligaments is not sufficient to create instability.

The coexistence of two structures, the articular buttresses and ligamentous brakes, constitutes an efficacious system of mobility with stability. The oblique planes of the articular facets allow sliding, which leads to angulation between two vertebrae, but the limit of elasticity of the ligaments prohibits luxation of the articular facets.

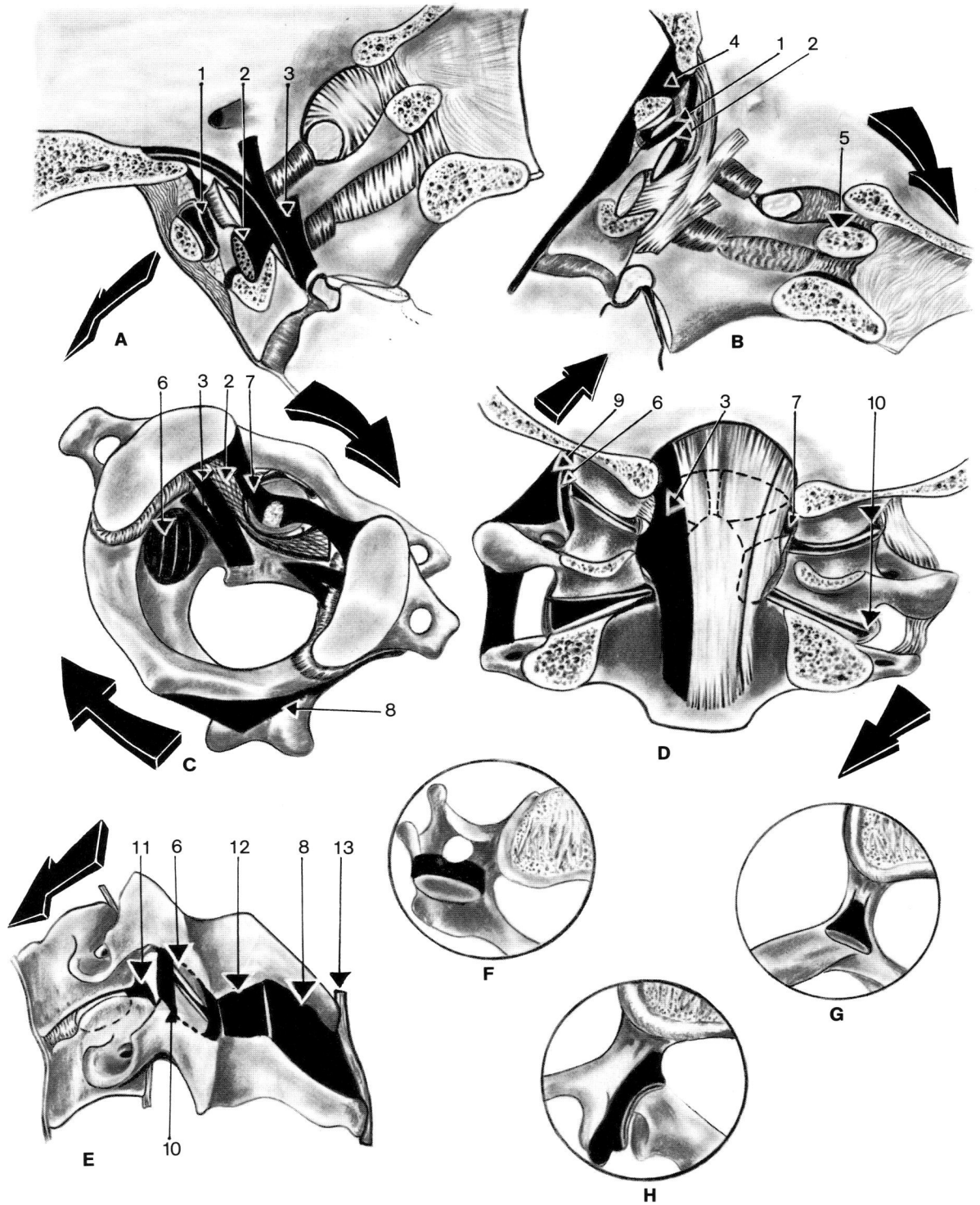

Figure 21 A–H

A Flexion of C1 and C2
B Extension of C1 and C2
C Rotation of C1 and C2
D Lateral inclination of
    C1 and C2
E Inferior cervical flexion
F Cervical articular buttress
G Thoracic articular buttress
H Lumbar articular buttress

1 dens *2* lig. transversum and cruciforme atlantis *3* membrana tectoria *4* membrana atlanto-occipitalis ant. *5* arcus post.
6 capsula articularis *7* lig. alaria *8* lig. interspinale *9* lig. laterale

10 processus articularis *11* pars post. anuli fibrosi *12* lig. flavum
13 lig. supraspinale

Extension. During forced extension the bony buttresses and ligamentous brakes are again brought into play. In contrast to flexion, the ligamentous brakes involved in extension are those situated anterior to the nucleus pulposus, i.e., the anterior longitudinal ligament and the anterior part of the anulus fibrosus. The bony buttresses limiting extension lie at the three angles of a triangle with an anterior base, i.e., the most posterior parts of the articular and spinous processes come into contact with each other in full extension of the cervical, thoracic, or lumbar spine. The zones of posterior contact can be evidenced on both X-rays and autopsy specimens. A neofacet lacking articular cartilage often appears on the postero-inferior part of the upper articular processes (in the isthmic region), reflecting excess extension or lordosis, especially of the lumbar spine. Similarly, the margins of adjacent spinous processes reciprocally fit together, the upper process resembling an inverted V over the lower process.

Rotation and Inclination. The movements of rotation and lateral inclination almost always occur in coupled fashion. Inclination of the articular facets at 45°–80° with respect to the plane of the intervertebral space imposes simultaneous sliding and rotation. When the lower right articular facet advances upward and forward, the left articular facet slides downward and backward. Practically all the structures participating in vertebral union are involved in checking the movements of rotation and inclination. The oblique fibers of the laminae of the anulus fibrosus stretch to limit rotation and inclination. Once again, the bony buttresses limiting these movements are the articular processes, especially those in the lumbar region. In the thoracic and cervical regions other bony structures have this function. In the thoracic spine lateral inclination and rotation are considerably limited by the costovertebral joints, despite the facility of such movement afforded by the circular orientation of the articular facets in this region. In the cervical spine the vertebral unci and transverse processes limit these movements. Bony contact of the uncovertebral pseudoarticulations is the first phenomenon which occurs to limit rotation and lateral inclination. Other reciprocal pseudoarticulations between the lower surface of the cervical transverse processes and upper articular processes limit the amplitude of inclination and rotation. To our knowledge only one other report in the literature (Veleanu 1971) has referred to this particular anatomical phenomenon. These transversoarticular pseudojoints are characterized by the inverted V shape of the posteroinferior surface of the transverse processes which fits over the anterosuperior margin of the upper articular processes from C2 to T1.

In conclusion, vertebral stability brings into play practically all the bony and ligamentous components of the spine. Accordingly, theories of spinal stability giving emphasis to only one component in preference to the others appear to us to be oversimplifications, which may limit both the understanding of the pathophysiological mechanisms of spinal instability and their management. Such theories include the theory of the posterior wall comprising the vertebral bodies and intervertebral discs (Rieuneau and Decoulx), the posterior ligamentous complex of Holsworth, and the role of the articular processes (Ramadier) and of the middle segment, i.e., the posterior discocorporeal wall, vertebral pedicles, and articular processes (Roy-Camille).

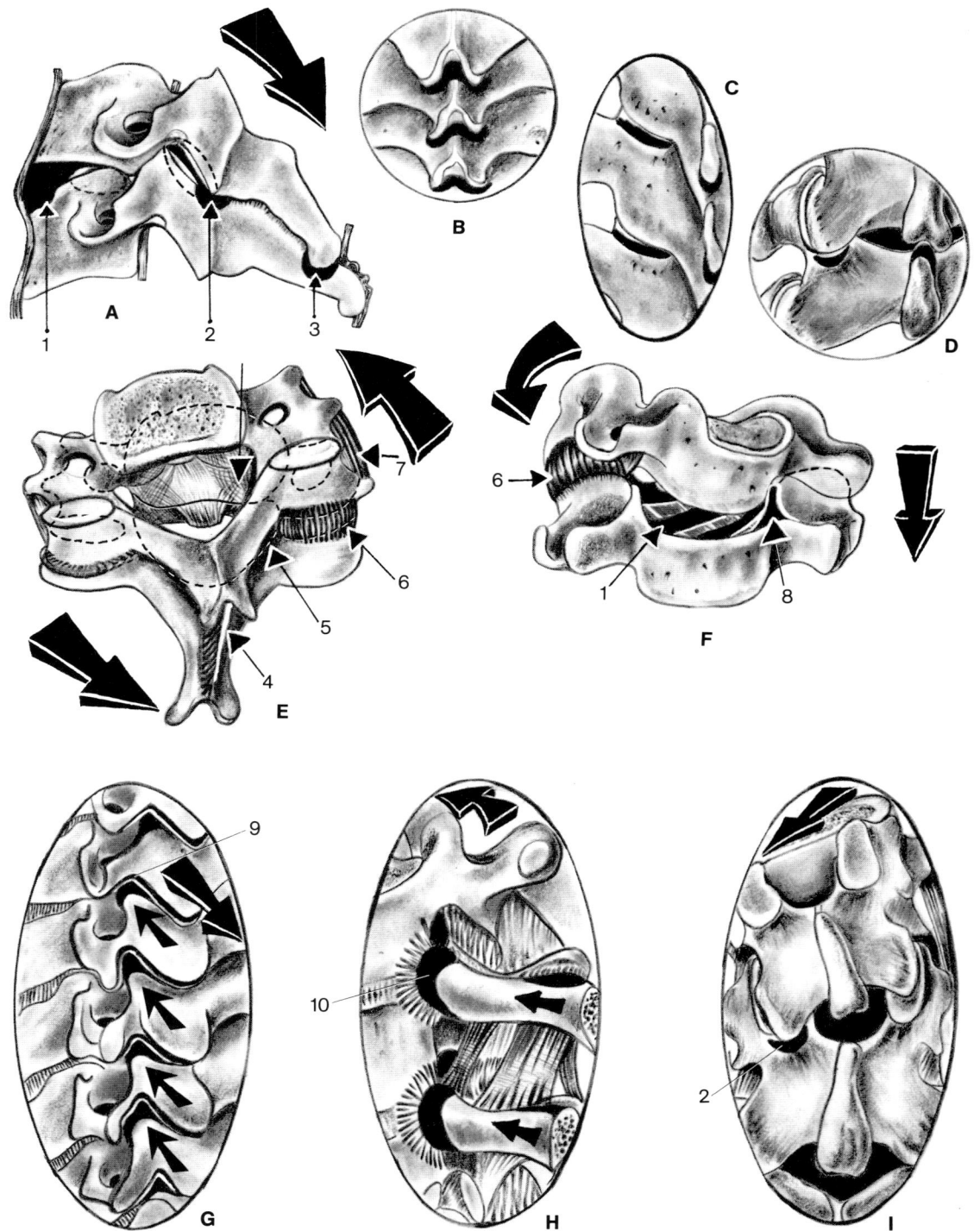

Figure 22 A–I

A   Cervical vertical extension
B   Cervical buttresses
C   Thoracic buttresses
D   Lumbar buttresses
E, F Cervical rotation-inclination
G   Cervical buttresses
H   Thoracic buttresses
I   Lumbar buttresses

1 annulus fibrosus *2* articular buttress *3* spinous buttress *4* lig. interspinale *5* lig. flavum *6* capsula articularis *7* lig. intertransversum   *8* uncus *9* articulatio transversoarticularis *10* articulatio capitis costae

5 Spinal Dynamic Function

I. Articular Mechanics

The spine, owing to its polyarticulated structure, possesses a great dynamic potential. Its structure, comprising different articular stages or mobile segments of Schmorl and Junghans, can be divided into two distinct vertebral regions, namely the craniovertebral junction, without a disc, and the subjacent spine, with intervertebral discs.

A. Craniovertebral Junction

The head rests on the cervical spine in an unstable manner, since its center of gravity lies in front of the spine. Balance is reestablished by the predominance of the extensor over the flexor muscles in the nuchal region.

The *first mobile segment* comprises the two atlanto-occipital joints which are transversely aligned and whose facets are shaped like shoe soles, with the greater axis slanting anteriorly and medially. The geometric volume that can be perfectly inscribed between the articular interfaces is an ovoid with a greater horizontal axis and a lesser sagittal axis. The articular facets represent sections through this volume. Thus, the mobility of these joints occurs essentially by flexion-extension about the transverse axis. Minor movements of lateral inclination and rotation are also possible. The geometric center of these movements is located at the level of the anterior quarter of the foramen magnum.

The *second mobile segment,* between C1 and C2, consists of two groups of articulations, the median and lateral atlantoaxial joints. The cylindrical median articulations between the odontoid process on the one hand and the osteofibrous anulus of the anterior arch and the transverse ligament on the other hand form a trochoid articulation allowing rotation around a vertical axis passing through the tip of the dens. Very small movements of elongation and shortening along the vertical axis and minute adaptive displacement to flexion-extension are also possible. The lateral articulations are inscribed on a portion of a sphere whose geometric center, located below the superior surface of C3, lies on the prolongation of the axis of the odontoid process. The articulations function synchronously with the median joints to allow what is essentially rotation. During this movement helicoidal displacement occurs, since the atlas moves from its zenith at the top of the segment of the sphere at zero rotation to its lowest position when fully rotated.

The base of the odontoid process is the embryological equivalent of the C1–C2 intervertebral disc. Accordingly, trauma of the upper cervical spine in flexion or extension facilitates rupture of the odontoid process in the horizontal plane of flexion-extension between the two lateral atlantoaxial joints.

B. Intervertebral Discs

The mechanical qualities of the 23 intervertebral discs are derived from their structure. Sealed between the upper and lower surfaces of two adjacent vertebrae, the discs consist of three parts: the anulus fibrosus, the nucleus pulposus, and cartilaginous plates. The anulus fibrosus is composed of a laminar mass whose circular layers lie in the horizontal plane. The fibers in a given layer lie in the same direction whereas those of two contiguous layers lie obliquely to each other. The nucleus pulposus occupies the central core of the anulus fibrosus and although spherical, does not resemble a solid structure like a ball bearing sealed within the disc, as has been too often described. The contents of the nucleus are highly hydrophilic (about 85% water) and the internal resting pressure, ranging from $1.5\,kg/cm^2$ when recumbent to $10\,kg/cm^2$ when standing (Nachemson), forces the walls of the deepest laminae of the anulus fibrosus into their spherical shape. In fact, the nucleus pulposus also displays a loosely packed fibrillar structure continuous with that of the anulus fibrosus, without a clear boundary between the two. The cartilaginous plates represent a zone of transition between the disc and body of the vertebra, allowing the insertion of the fibrils of the anulus fibrosus and the diffusion of fluids from the vertebral vascular bed to nourish or fill the nucleus pulposus. The discs have no vascular supply after birth. When submitted to prolonged compression the pressure within the nucleus pulposus increases, thus inducing an identical counterpressure in the anulus fibrosus and a slight decrease in the height of the disc due to fluid leakage. Conversely, at rest the height of the discs increases owing to maximum filling of the nucleus pulposus. Accordingly, a given individual is taller after a long rest than after a long period of effort. The mechanical properties of the disc allow movements of compression when loaded, stretching when distended, rotation about the nucleus, lateral inclination, and translation. However, although an isolated disc allows a wide range of movements between two vertebrae, the presence of the posterior zygapophyseal articulations limits these movements to a spatial sector proper to each region of the spine.

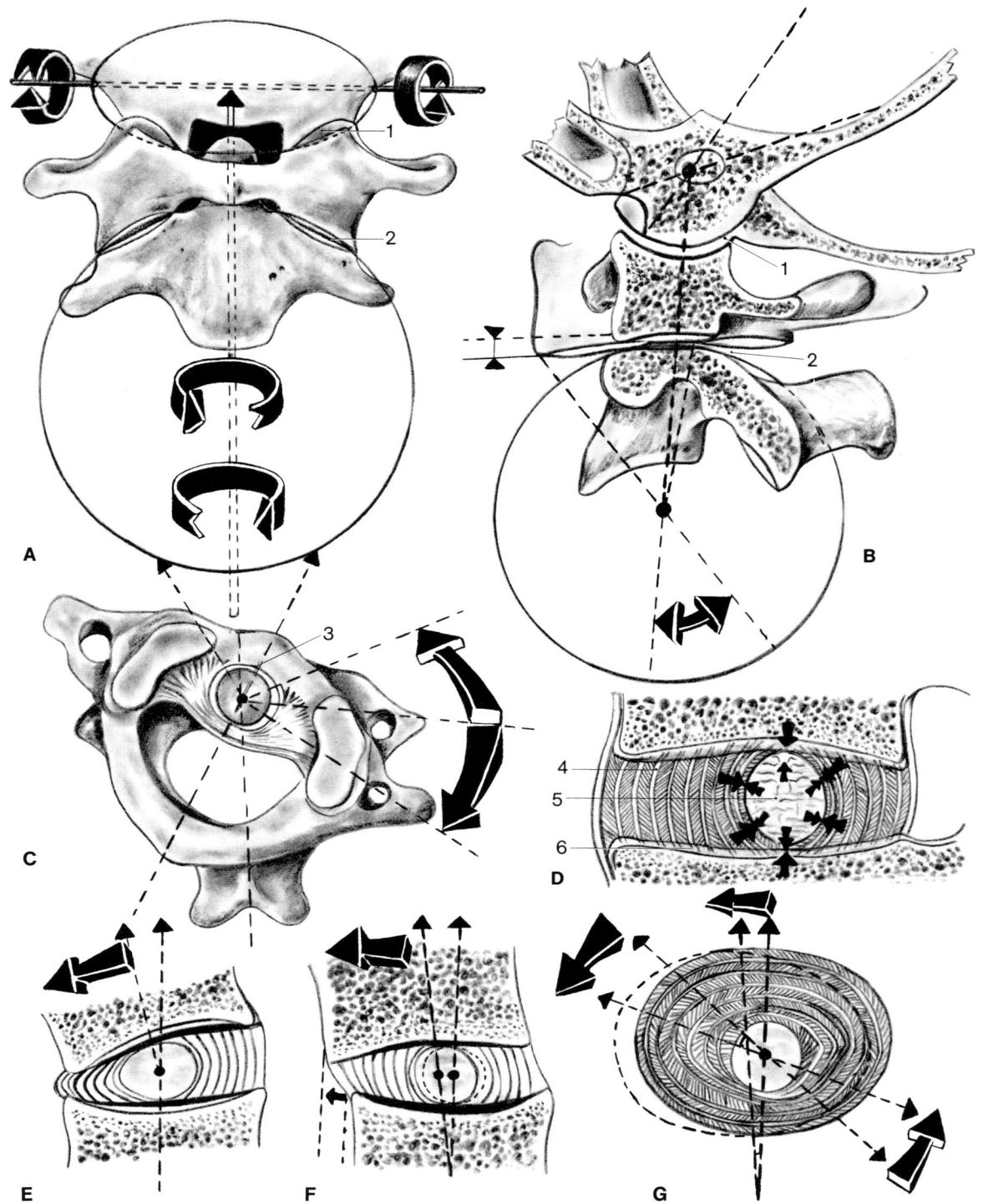

Figure 23 A–G

A Anterior aspect of the craniovertebral junction
B Sagittal section of the craniovertebral junction
C Superior aspect of the median atlantoaxial articulation
D Sagittal section of the intervertebral disc
E Inclination of the disc

F Translation of the disc
G Rotation of the disc

1 articulatio atlantooccipitalis *2* articulatio atlantoaxialis lateralis
3 articulatio atlantoaxialis mediana *4* anulus fibrosus *5* nucleus
pulposus *6* lamina cartilaginosa

The articular mechanics of the vertebrae with discs from C3 to S1 are dependent upon the coexistence of three joints in each mobile segment, i.e., the intervertebral disc and the two zygapophyseal articulations. The two types of associated movements, flexion-extension and inclination-rotation, display special regional features in the cervical, thoracic, and lumbar segments of the spine.

C. Flexion-Extension

The movements of flexion and extension are the resultant of the elementary movements between pairs of adjacent vertebrae, and occur in the sagittal plane. The most common concept that is proposed to explain the mechanism of these movements is the assimilation of flexion-extension to rotation around a transverse axis passing through the center of the nucleus pulposus. Overlay tracings of dynamic roentgenograms are sufficient to illustrate the erroneous nature of this concept. Using two cervical vertebrae as an example, three explanatory mechanisms can be envisaged. Sagittal movements of these vertebrae could occur by translation (sliding) along the slope of the articular facets. However, it is obvious that this type of movement would lead to variation in the height of the intervertebral space that would not be allowed by the intervertebral disc. A second hypothesis would be to imagine a rolling (seesaw) movement of the upper vertebra on the superior surface of the nucleus pulposus. However, in this situation the coaptation of the articular facets would be perturbed beyond physiological limits. Thus a third hypothesis must be advanced to account for the mechanical conditions of the disc and the zygapophyseal articulations. The displacement of flexion-extension is indeed a circular movement about a transverse axis, but the axis is not situated at the level of the nucleus pulposus but lies below, in the body of the lower vertebra. The cartilage-lined articular facets produce an articular interface inscribed on the arc of a circle with the same center. The superior surface of the disc is also inscribed on an arc with the same center. The movement of the upper vertebra thus describes an arc with arcuate sliding of the articular facets and pendulous displacement of the disc about the same geometric center. Our studies based on tracings of roentgenograms from 15 postmortem spines in flexion and the then extension confirmed this mechanical theory. Our conclusions are thus in agreement with earlier studies by Fick (1911), Strasser (1913), Penning (1968) and Lysell (1969), who also described an axis of rotation in the body of the vertebra subjacent to the intervertebral disc. This contradicts the more classical and widely held opinion of Exner (1954) and Hjortsjo (1959) according to which the center of movement is in the nucleus pulposus. Many authors have proposed that the center varies during a given movement and describe an area comprising the different instantaneous centers of rotation (Gonon 1978).

In our studies we observed this same articular mechanism throughout the spine, but the location of the centers of movement varied according to the region of the spine. In the case of the C2–C3 articulation the center of movement is the lowest, i.e., in the body of C4. Below the C2–C3 intervertebral joint, the center of each cervical intervertebral articulation lies in the inferior part of the lower vertebra. In the thoracic and lumbar regions the center of movement is located in the central part of the superior surface of the lower vertebra. One consequence of this low position of the centers of flexion-extension is the anterior sliding or antelisthesis during hyperflexion of one vertebra on the subjacent vertebra. At the C2–C3 joint, physiological displacement is 2.5–3.5 mm; from C4 to C7 it is 1.5–2 mm; and from T1 to L5 it is 0.5–1.5 mm. Thus reference can be made to pathological displacement (instability) only when the displacement exceeds these physiological limits.

D. Inclination-Rotation

Lateral inclination is simultaneously accompanied by rotation (and vice versa) owing to the pronounced obliquity of the posterior articular facets. When a vertebra inclines to one side, the inferior articular facet on that side moves backward and slides downward to the bottom of the articular interface, whereas the inferior articular facet on the opposite side glides upward and forward, thus producing the accompanying rotation. The center of inclination is located midway between the right and left articular facets. The features of rotation vary according to the regions of the spine. Rotation of the cervical spine does not describe an arc of a circle but rather a segment of an ellipse.

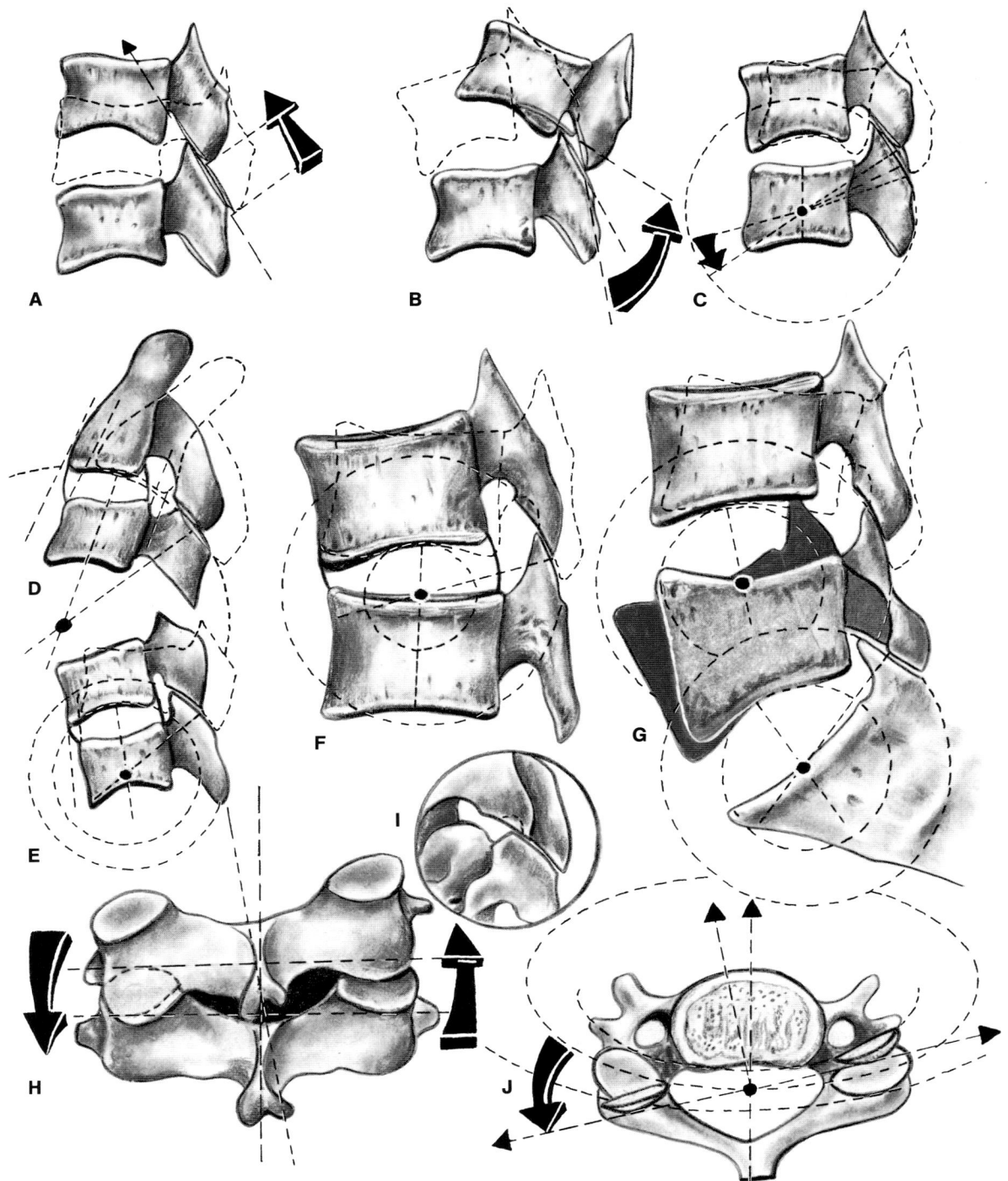

Figure 24 A–J

A   Spinal movement by sliding along the articular facets (erroneous theory)

B   Spinal movement around a spherical nucleus pulposus (erroneous theory)

C   Arcuate spinal movement around a transverse axis whose center lies well below the intervertebral disc (correct theory)

D   Flexion-extension at C2–C3: angulation and translation (sliding)

E   Flexion-extension at C5–C6: angulation and translation (sliding)

F   Flexion-extension at D8–D9

G   Flexion-extension at L4–L5–S1

H–J   Cervical inclination and rotation

In the *thoracic region* inclination of the vertebrae is accompanied by rotation and vice versa. This dynamic synergy is the result of two combined mechanisms. On the one hand, as in the case of the cervical spine, the inclination of the articular facets (at 75°–85° to the horizontal) triggers rotation during the angulation, since the articular facet that glides upward moves forward while the facet that slides downward moves backward. On the other hand, the powerful vertical and oblique costotransverse and intertransverse ligaments create a phenomenon of simultaneous inclination and rotation due to the interplay of asymmetrical tensions. Lateral inclination also produces a component of extension. This mechanism, accompanied by the progressive cuneiformity of the vertebrae as their size increases craniocaudally, produces the association of lateral inclination, rotation, and extension in scoliosis. In the thoracic spine, the axis of rotation in the horizontal plane is inscribed on the arc of a circle whose center is located in the middle of the superior surface of the vertebra.

In the *lumbar region* the orientation of the articular facets differs greatly from that of the upper segments of the spine. Lateral inclination is made possible by a rolling movement between the vertical rail-like superior articular facets. Rotation is greatly restricted since in the horizontal plane the articular facets are inscribed on a posteriorly open parabolic curve. The axis of rotation runs through the spinous processes, thus imposing on the intervertebral disc a movement of oscillation with shearing.

E. Orientation of the Articular Facets

Consideration of the different types of articular facet relative to just the horizontal plane reveals a striking continuous series of geometric figures on which the facets are inscribed, reflecting their capacities to allow rotation.

The *odontoaxial articular facets* are inscribed on a perfect circle passing through the vertical axis of the odontoid process. This configuration is the most adapted to rotation.

The *thoracic facets* are also inscribed on the arc of a circle whose center is located below the nucleus pulposus. This configuration also facilitates rotation.

The *upper cervical facets* are inscribed on the arc of a circle but its center lies well in front of the vertebrae, allowing fairly ample rotation.

The *lower cervical facets* lie in the coronal plane and thus afford greater extension-flexion than inclination-rotation.

The *facets of the lumbar vertebrae* are inscribed on parabolic curves with a posterior opening and thus resemble a segment of the groove of a pulley. This configuration is the least adapted to rotational movements.

The *lumbosacral facets,* however, are inscribed on a more open curve and thus are less inhibitory to rotation than those of the upper lumbar vertebrae.

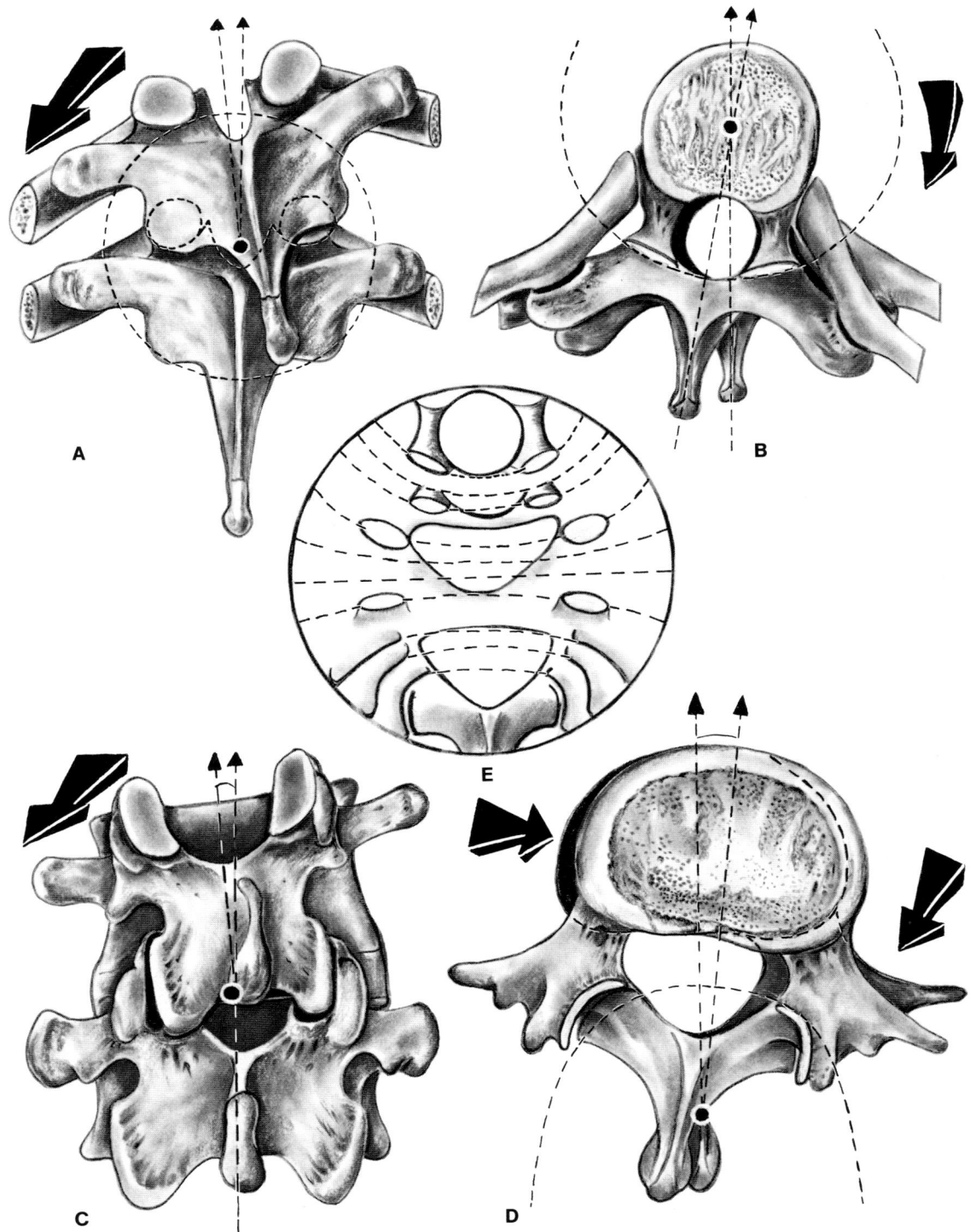

Figure 25 A–E

A   Lateral inclination of the thoracic vertebrae
B   Rotation of the thoracic vertebrae
C   Lateral inclination of the lumbar vertebrae
D   Rotation of the lumbar vertebrae
E   The series of geometric orientations of the vertebral articular facets

II. Regional Amplitude

Each mobile segment composed of two adjacent vertebrae is capable of only low-amplitude movements. The summation of these movements yields the amplitude of displacement of the cervical, thoracic, and lumbar regions. The combined range of movements of the three spinal regions corresponds to the overall amplitude of spinal mobility in flexion-extension, axial rotation, and lateral inclination.

A. Flexion-Extension

1. Cervical Spine

Occipital bone-C1:	20°	C4–C5:	20°
C1–C2:	0°	C5–C6:	22°
C2–C3:	15°	C6–C7:	18°
C3–C4:	15°	C7–T1:	10°

Total flexion: 45°; total extension: 75°; total flexion-extension: 120°

2. Thoracic Spine
Total flexion: 30°; total extension: 20°; total flexion-extension: 50°

3. Lumbar Spine

L1–L2: 11°		L4–L5: 24°	
L2–L3: 12°		L5–S1: 18°	
L3–L4: 18°			

Total flexion: 53°; total extension: 30°; total flexion-extension: 83°

4. Amplitude of the Entire Spine
Total flexion: 128°; total extension: 130°; total flexion-extension: 258°

B. Axial Rotation

1. Cervical Spine
Right and left rotations:

Occipital bone-Cl:	$2 \times 12° = 24°$
C1–C2:	$2 \times 23° = 46°$
C2–C3:	$2 \times 6° = 12°$
C3–C4:	$2 \times 6° = 12°$
C4–C5:	$2 \times 7° = 14°$
C5–C6:	$2 \times 6° = 12°$
C6–C7:	$2 \times 6° = 12°$
C7–T1:	$2 \times 6° = 12°$
Total rotation:	$2 \times 72° = 144°$

2. Thoracic Spine

T1–T2: 6°	T5–T6: 6°	T9–T10 : 4°
T2–T3: 6°	T6–T7: 8°	T10–T11: 6°
T3–T4: 6°	T7–T8: 4°	T11–T12: 4°
T4–T5: 6°	T8–T9: 4°	T12–L1 : 10°

Total rotation: $2 \times 35° = 70°$

3. Lumbar Spine

L1–L2: 2°	L3–L4: 3°	L5–S1: 4°
L2–L3: 3°	L4–L5: 4°	

Total rotation: $2 \times 8° = 16°$

4. Amplitude of the Entire Spine
Total rotation: $2 \times 115° = 230°$

C. Lateral Flexion

Right and left lateral flexions:

1. Cervical Spine

Occipital bone-C1: $2 \times 3° = 6°$		C4–C5: $2 \times 6° = 12°$	
C1–C2:	0°	C5–C6: $2 \times 4° = 8°$	
C2–C3:	$2 \times 5° = 10°$	C6–C7: $2 \times 4.5° = 9°$	
C3–C4:	$2 \times 6° = 12°$	C7–T1: $2 \times 5° = 10°$	

Total lateral flexion: $2 \times 33.5° = 67°$

2. Thoracic Spine
Total lateral flexion: $2 \times 20° = 40°$

3. Lumbar Spine
Total lateral flexion: $2 \times 20° = 40°$

4. Amplitude of the Entire Spine
Total lateral flexion: $2 \times 73.5° = 147°$

These data are mean values. Certain subjects possess a more flexible spine than others owing to constitutional factors, physical training, or age. The data were derived in part from the studies of Lysell, David and Allbrook, Tanz, Gregersen and Lucas, and Kapandji.

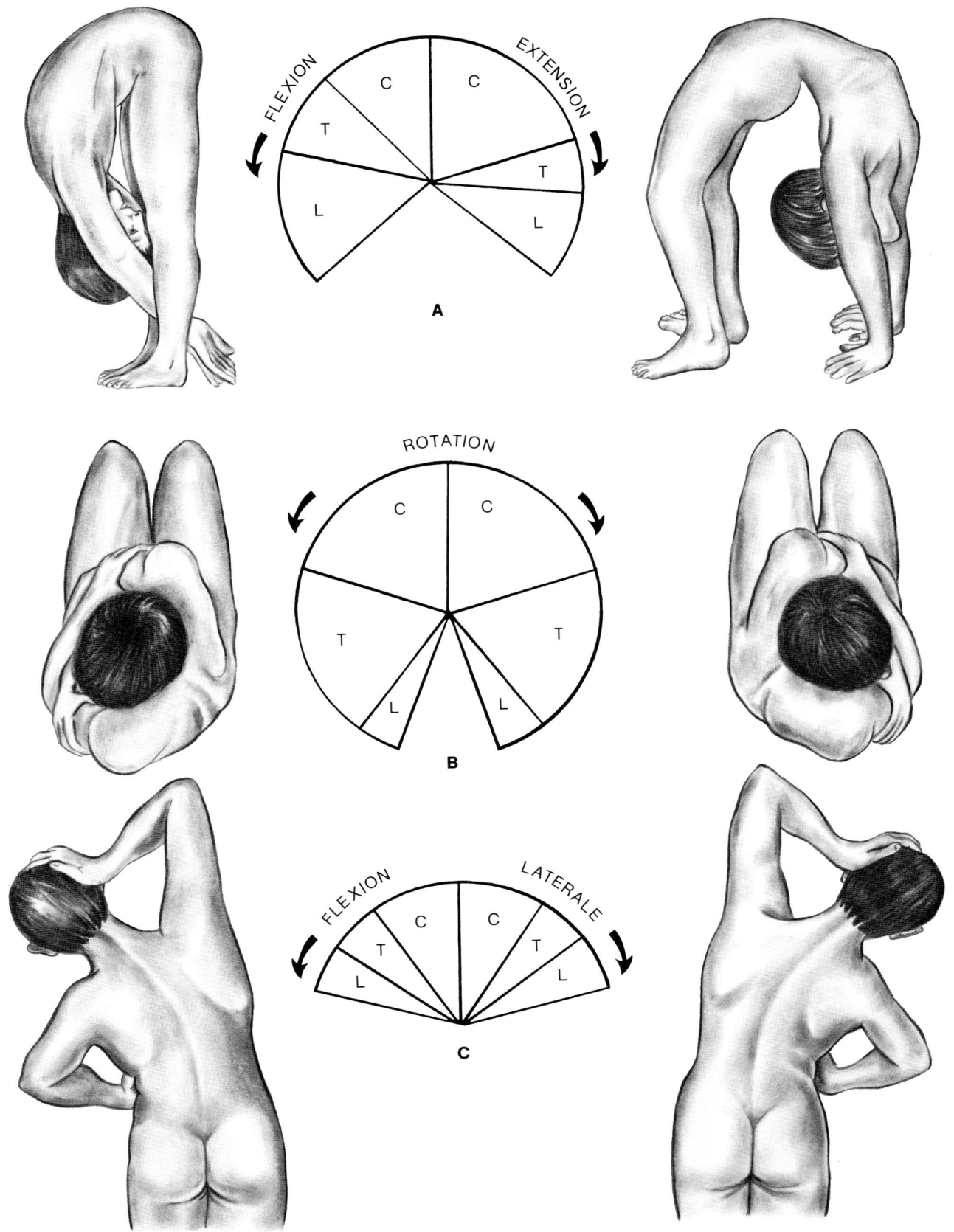

Figure 26 A–C

A   Amplitudes of flexion-extension
B   Amplitudes of axial rotation
C   Amplitudes of lateral flexion

III. Adaptation of the Spine to Effort

With the human body in different positions the spine is submitted to gravitational and muscular forces, and also exterior forces when the body acts on the outside world. The complexity of the mechanical phenomena brought into play leaves many unanswered questions at present. Our approach will therefore be to consider the theoretical aspects, then laboratory data, and finally anatomoclinical observations.

A. Theoretical Aspects

1. The "Spinal Lever"

The theories of levers are classically applied to estimate the physical constraints to which the spinal structures are submitted. According to Brueger and Kapandji the spine can be likened to two pillars, i.e., the anterior pillar formed by the vertebral bodies, which is passive, and the pillar formed by the posterior arches, which is active owing to the insertions of the spinal muscles. The fulcrum of the lever would be the posterior articulations. This system of leverage would act as a damping device sparing the intervertebral disc when submitted to the axial forces of gravity. Another type of lever is more often proposed to estimate the physical constraints of the spine. In this case, the fulcrum would be at the nucleus pulposus with a short posterior arm on which the forces of the spinal muscles (M) would act and a longer anterior arm receiving the gravitational forces (P). By computation, with the body in the erect position at rest, the force P acting on the L5–S1 joint would be 45 kg, M would be 90 kg and the total pressure on the intervertebral disc would be $P + M = 135$ kg. With the body bent forward and the knees extended, a 10-kg weight applied to the arms yields a total pressure of 250 kg acting on the disc; with the trunk erect and the knees flexed this total pressure would be 145 kg. However, this model rapidly becomes unrealistic if computation is made when an 80-kg weight is to be lifted, i.e., the disc would be submitted to a force of 1 ton, which exceeds the resistance of this structure. Despite these considerations, lifting a weight with the knees flexed and the trunk erect affords the greatest sparing of the anatomical structures of the spine and that is therefore the recommended position. To arrive at more plausible estimated forces the role of intra-abdominal pressure has had to be invoked. During an intense effort the abdomen does indeed act like an inflated structure absorbing a large part of the forces transmitted by the trunk, thus reducing the forces acting on the spine by 30%–50% (Kapandji).

2. Theory of Articular Triangulation

Our conception of the spine as being composed of three vertical columns leads us to consider the synergy of three joints in each mobile segment during effort. These three joints are the intervertebral disc and the two zygapophyseal articulations. With the exception of the biarticular atlantoaxial segment, all the mobile spinal segments are triarticular. At each level the posterior articulations lie in a plane nearly perpendicular to that of the disc. This notion also applies to C1–C2 where the odontoatlantoid articulations are perpendicular to the atlantoaxial joints. This configuration creates an orthogonal articular system whose mode of participation during effort differs according to the orientation of the axis of the spine relative to the forces acting upon it. In the vertical position the forces of gravity and weight-bearing coupled with opposing muscular forces produce a compressive effect on the discs and a shearing effect on the posterior articulations. Conversely, when lifting a weight with the trunk in the horizontal position the different forces produce essentially compression of the posterior articulations and a shearing effect on the discs, although the required rigidity of the spine is nevertheless accompanied by an accessory effect of axial compression of muscular origin. Consequently, during the movements and efforts exerted by the spine the posterior articulations share with the discs in bearing the constraints applied to the vertebrae. Thus there exists a modulated system of leverage involving these different structures. Accordingly, the total area of the discal and zygapophyseal articular surfaces in each mobile segment increases in the craniocaudal direction to meet the increasing physical constraints. We calculated the mean total articular surface area at different spinal levels as follows: C1, 3.8 cm^2; C7, 4.1 cm^2; T6, 7 cm^2; L1, 12 cm^2; S1, 18 cm^2. Furthermore, the caliber of the flexor and extensor muscles of the trunk similarly increases caudally down to the gluteal muscles. This concept of triangulation allows better understanding of the role of the articular processes and their pathological alterations. They should not be considered merely as being involved in the orientation of spinal movements, but also as weight-bearing structures subject to the pathological alterations of effort (sprain, arthrosis).

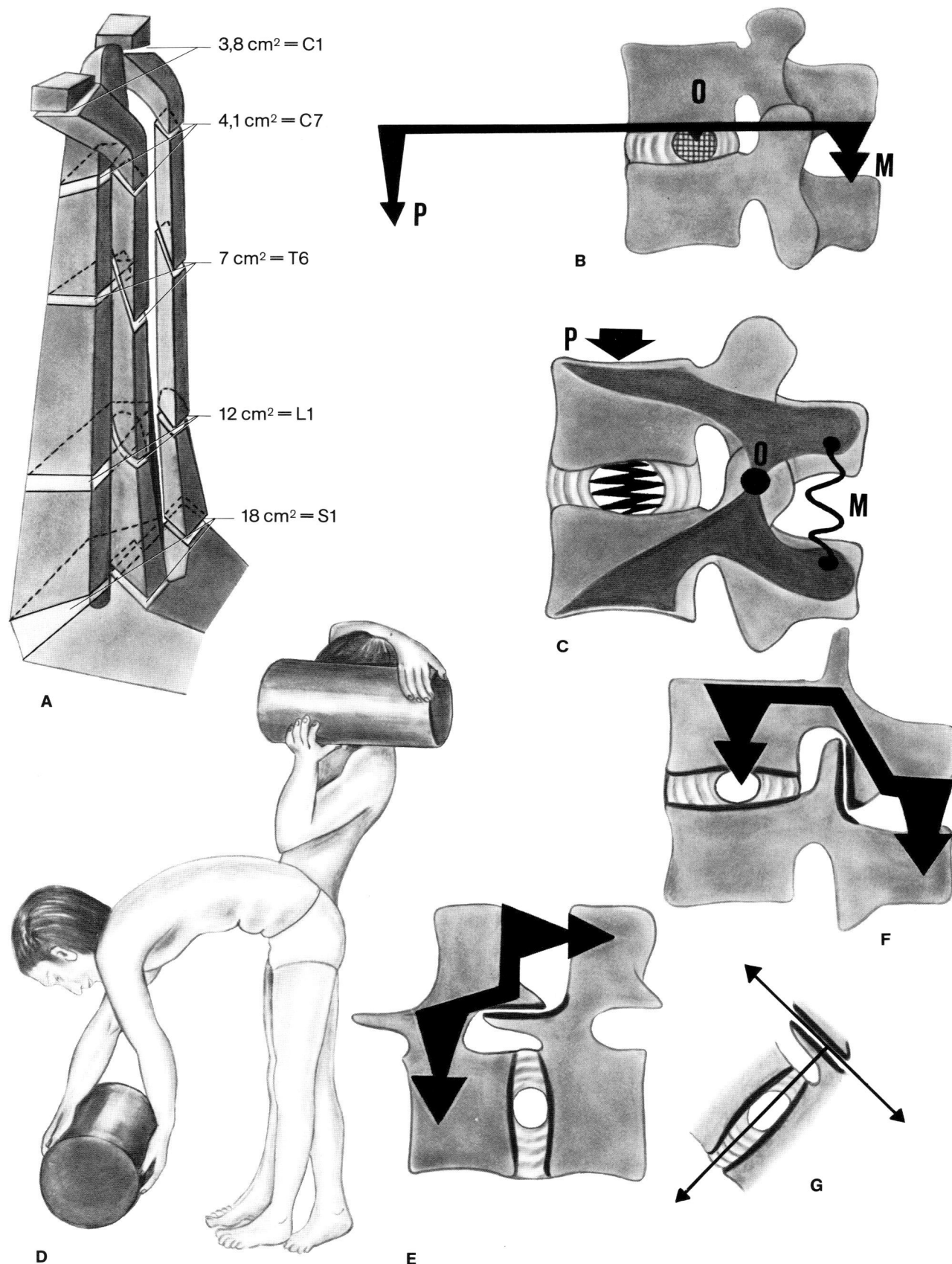

Figure 27 A–G

A   Spinal architecture comprising three columns with articular triangulation at each level. The numbers indicate the articular surface area at each level

B   The spinal lever. *O*, balance; *P*, resultant gravitational force; *M*, resultant spinal muscular forces

C   Damping lever (according to Kapandji)

D   Efforts of lifting and maintaining a load

E–G   Forces acting at the articulations between vertebrae in flexion, upright stance, and the intermediate position, according to the triangulation concept

B. Experimental Data

Many studies have been devoted to determining the resistance of the spinal structures and the pressures to which they are submitted.

1. Resistance of the Spinal Structures

The data given below are those of Evans (1969), based on laboratory studies of anatomical specimens. In the erect position the lumbosacral spine ruptures under a mean axial load of 300 kg in preserved anatomical specimens and 180 kg in fresh postmortem specimens. Rupture of the lumbosacral spine also occurs when a transverse force causing flexion attains 135 kg. The lumbar intervertebral discs will rupture under a compressive force ranging from 265 to 540 kg/cm². We personally tested the resistance of intervertebral union in 15 fresh anatomical specimens. When the disc is sectioned the posterior-union between two vertebrae ruptures under a horizontal force in flexion or extension of 35–45 kg. The resistance of the intervertebral discs varies as a function of age and the presence or absence of degenerative lesions. In young subjects, the tearing force required to rupture the intervertebral disc in flexion or extension exceeds 120 kg, whereas in older subjects with degenerative lesions of the disc rupture occurs at a force of 25 kg (cervical spine) to 50 kg (lumbosacral spine).

2. Intradiscal Pressures

Studies by Nachemson performed in vivo have given much valuable data in this domain. In the cadaver, as in the recumbent relaxed subject, the pressure within the intervertebral disc is 1.5 kg/cm². In the seated position, the intradiscal pressure at L3–L4 is 10–15 kg/cm² with a tangential component of 60–80 kg/cm² acting on the posterior part of the disc. In the standing position these pressures are 30% lower than in the seated position. Bearing a load obviously increases the intradiscal pressure, e.g., a 20-kg load increases the intradiscal pressure from the resting value of 15 kg/cm² to 20 kg/cm². Multiplication of these pressures by the surface area of the discs yields a true weight of 135 kg for the L3–L4 disc when seated, which attains 200 kg under a 20-kg load. Tension of the abdominal cavity by Valsalva's maneuver (forced expiration against the closed glottis) increases the intradiscal pressure by 5%–35%. Wearing a corset brace reduces this pressure by 25% and solid posterior fusion causes a 30% decrease. According to our theory of articular triangulation, one can conceive of the importance of the constraints to which the posterior articulations are submitted when a share of the load of the discs is transferred to them with the trunk in flexion or extension.

C. Anatomoclinical Observations

Aging of the vertebral structures is reflected on roentgenography by the well-known signs of discarthrosis and degenerative lesions of the posterior articulations. Since there often exists a direct relation with the efforts allowed by the spine, the study of the site of the lesions of arthrosis gives a precise idea of the vertebral constraints.

1. Hyperflexion and Hyperkyphosis

Vertebral hyperflexion increases the load on the anterior part of the intervertebral discs, the horizontal surfaces of the vertebral bodies, and the superior part of the articular facets. The same mechanical conditions induce the static disturbances of hyperkyphosis with production of anterior osteophytes of the discs and anterosuperior osteophytes of the posterior articulations.

2. Hyperextension and Hyperlordosis

Hyperextension transfers forces toward the posterior arch and accessorily to the posterior part of the intervertebral disc. Thus, in cases of hyperlordosis, it is not surprising to observe signs of age-related arthrosis localized essentially on the posterior articulations with zones of neocontact between normally distant structures, i.e., between the spinous processes, between the inferior part of the articular facets and the subjacent laminae, and between the superior part of the articular facets and the pedicular or isthmic regions.

3. Rotation, Lateral Flexion, and Scoliosis

Lateral flexion with rotation increases the load on the lateral part of the discs, the uncovertebral pseudoarticulation and the homolateral posterior articulation, with neocontact between the cervical transverse process and the tip of the superior articular facet. At an advanced age, the deformity of scoliosis shows signs of arthrosis at the level of the abnormal spinal concavity with dislocation due to shearing of the most horizontally inclined disc and arthrosis of the posterior articulation. Cervical uncarthrosis reflects overworking of the cervical vertebrae in lateral flexion and rotation.

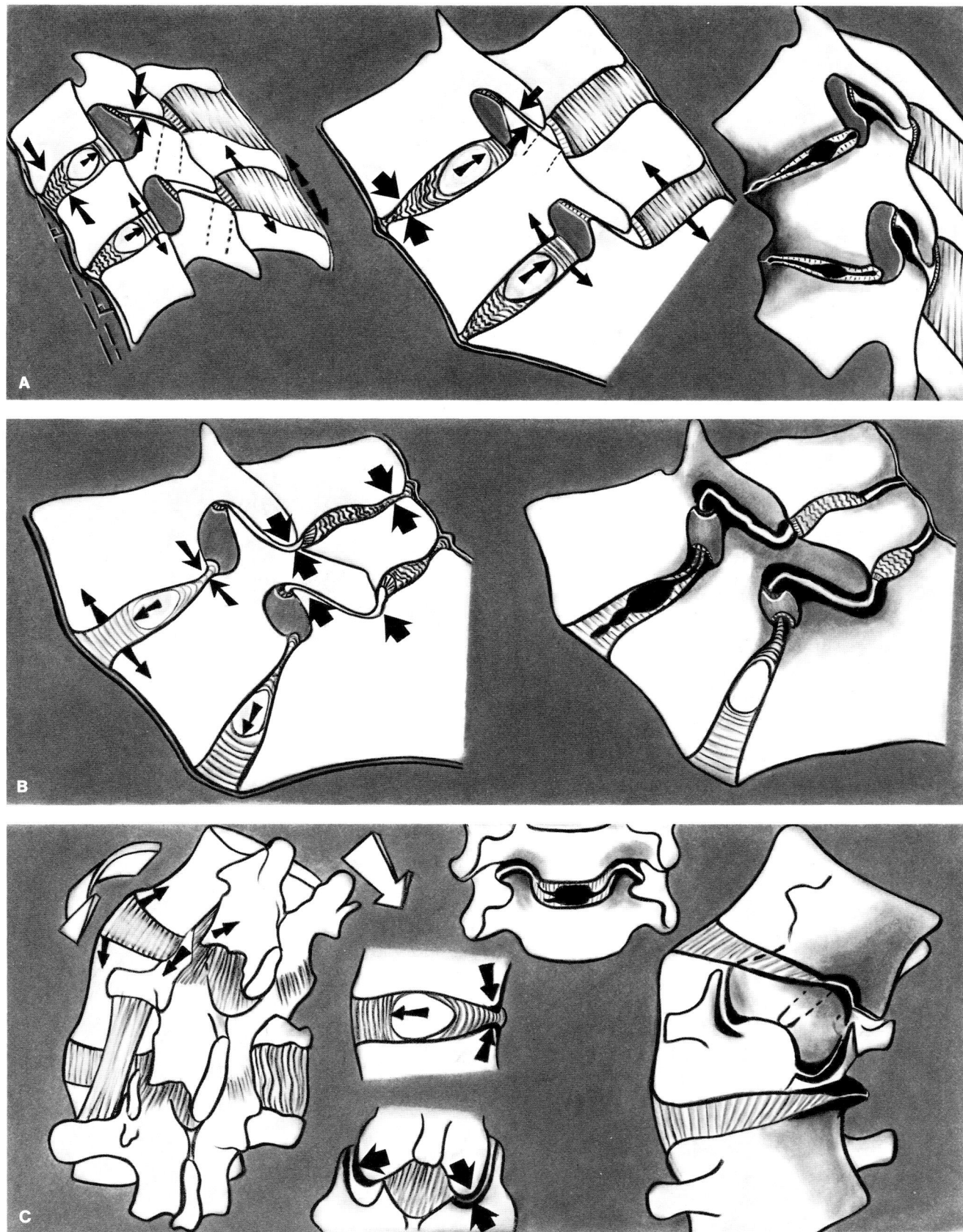

Figure 28 A–C

A Spinal constraints in hyperflexion and signs of arthrosis in hyper-kyphosis

B Spinal constraints in hyperextension and signs of arthrosis in hyper-lordosis

C Spinal constraints in lateral flexion and rotation with signs of arthrosis in scoliosis and uncarthrosis

6 Spinal Function: Neural Protection

I. Vertebral Canal

In addition to its locomotor functions (statics, stability, and dynamics) the spine ensures the passage and protection of the neural elements and their annexes by the vertebral canal and intervertebral foramina. The vertebral canal is a veritable tunnel lying along the greater axis of the spine, formed by the successive vertebral foramina alternating with the fibrous structures of intervertebral union from the foramen magnum to the sacral hiatus.

A. Walls

The anterior and posterior walls of the vertebral canal are separated from each other by the lateral angles. The *anterior wall* of the canal is a plane surface comprising the posterior surface of the vertebral bodies and intervertebral discs and the posterior longitudinal ligament. The height of the posterior surface of the vertebral bodies increases regularly from C3 to L5 to form a continuous wall at the sacral level. Similarly, the posterior surface of the discs increases from 2 mm at C2 to 8 mm at S1 (23 discs). The flat posterior edge of the disc in young subjects forms a more or less protruding ridge with advancing age. The internal and ventral venous plexuses of the vertebrae run longitudinally on each side of the posterior longitudinal ligament, forming transverse anastomoses between the middle of the vertebral bodies and the posterior longitudinal ligament. The anterior wall of the vertebral canal constitutes a risk of compression of the neural structures (spinal cord and nerve roots) in cases of trauma, tumor, or Pott's disease due to angular kyphosis, bony splinters, tumor invasion, or abscess. The *posterior wall* of the canal, forming a dihedral angle or anteriorly open groove, is composed of the alternating laminae and ligamenta flava. Access to the spinal canal is easiest via the posterior wall by laminectomy, the interlaminar approach, or spinal puncture. The interlaminar spaces, narrow in the cervical region (median or lateral occipital puncture) and practically blind in the thoracic region owing to the overlapping of the laminae, can easily be used as a route of surgical approach only in the lower lumbar spine (L3 to S1). The right and left *lateral angles* of the vertebral canal are formed by the pedicles and intervertebral foramina. The angle on each side is dihedral, referred to as an "interdiscoligamentous defile" by Latarjet and Magnin, since it is sufficiently narrow for the spinal nerve root contained within to be compressed by a prolapsed disc or arthrosis (uncarthrosis and arthrosis of the zygapophyseal joints). Such compression occurs between the posterior wall of the disc and the anterior surface of the posterior articulations lined by the ligamentum flavum. These angles are also occupied by the internal longitudinal venous plexuses, which must be avoided or cauterized in surgery of the vertebral canal.

B. Lumen

The vertebral canal and its lumen obviously fit perfectly with the spinal curvatures in the sagittal plane (cervical and lumbar lordosis and thoracic and sacral kyphosis). The mean sacrovertebral angle at the lumbosacral junction is 120° in men and 128° in women (Bleicher and Beau). The inner form of the vertebral canal varies according to the spinal region and the plane of section. In the horizontal plane the vertebral canal has an oval cross section (35 mm × 30 mm) in the region of the foramen magnum; a triangular section with rounded angles (23 mm × 14 mm) in the cervical region; a circular section (16 mm) in the thoracic segment; and a triangular section flattened in the anteroposterior direction (26 mm × 17 mm at L5–S1) in the lumbosacral region. The lumen of the vertebral canal has three enlarged zones, the occipitocervical junction, the lower cervical segment, and the lumbosacral region, and three narrow zones, the upper cervical, middle thoracic, and sacral regions. The zones of enlargement correspond to the spinal regions with the greatest mobility, where the contents of the vertebral canal must consequently display a certain degree of dynamic flexibility. In the narrowest segments of the vertebral canal the neural components are more frequently exposed to traumatic, infectious, or tumoral compression (i.e., in the thoracic and sacral regions). In the course of flexion-extension of the spine the length of the vertebral canal (mean length: 70 cm) changes. Forced extension shortens the canal by decreasing the interlaminar spaces and compressing the posterior part of the intervertebral spaces. Conversely, hyperflexion increases the length of the vertebral canal by the same mechanism operating in the opposite direction. Our measurements have shown that between these two extreme positions the length of the vertebral canal can vary by 5–9 cm, depending on the flexibility of the individual's spine.

The normal range of individual variation in the caliber of the vertebral canal, especially in the cervical and lumbar regions, must be known in order to interpret pathological vertebral stenosis correctly. The following table is reproduced from the studies of Delmas and Pineau:

Spinal level	Transverse diameter		Anteroposterior diameter	
	Mean (mm)	Range (mm)	Mean (mm)	Range (mm)
C1	28.9	24–36	30.7	25–29
C2	23.3	19–26	16.3	13–22
C3	23.3	19–28	14.5	10–19
C4	23.9	20–29	13.9	11–18
C5	24.7	21–29	13.9	9–19
C6	25	21–29	13.8	10–18
C7	24.2	21–29	13.9	11–18
T1	20.8	18–25	14.8	12–18
L1	22.9	19–27	17.3	13–22
L2	22.9	20–28	16.3	12–21
L3	22.8	19–28	15.9	11–20
L4	23.1	18–29	15.9	9–21
L5	25.9	20–35	17.1	10–24

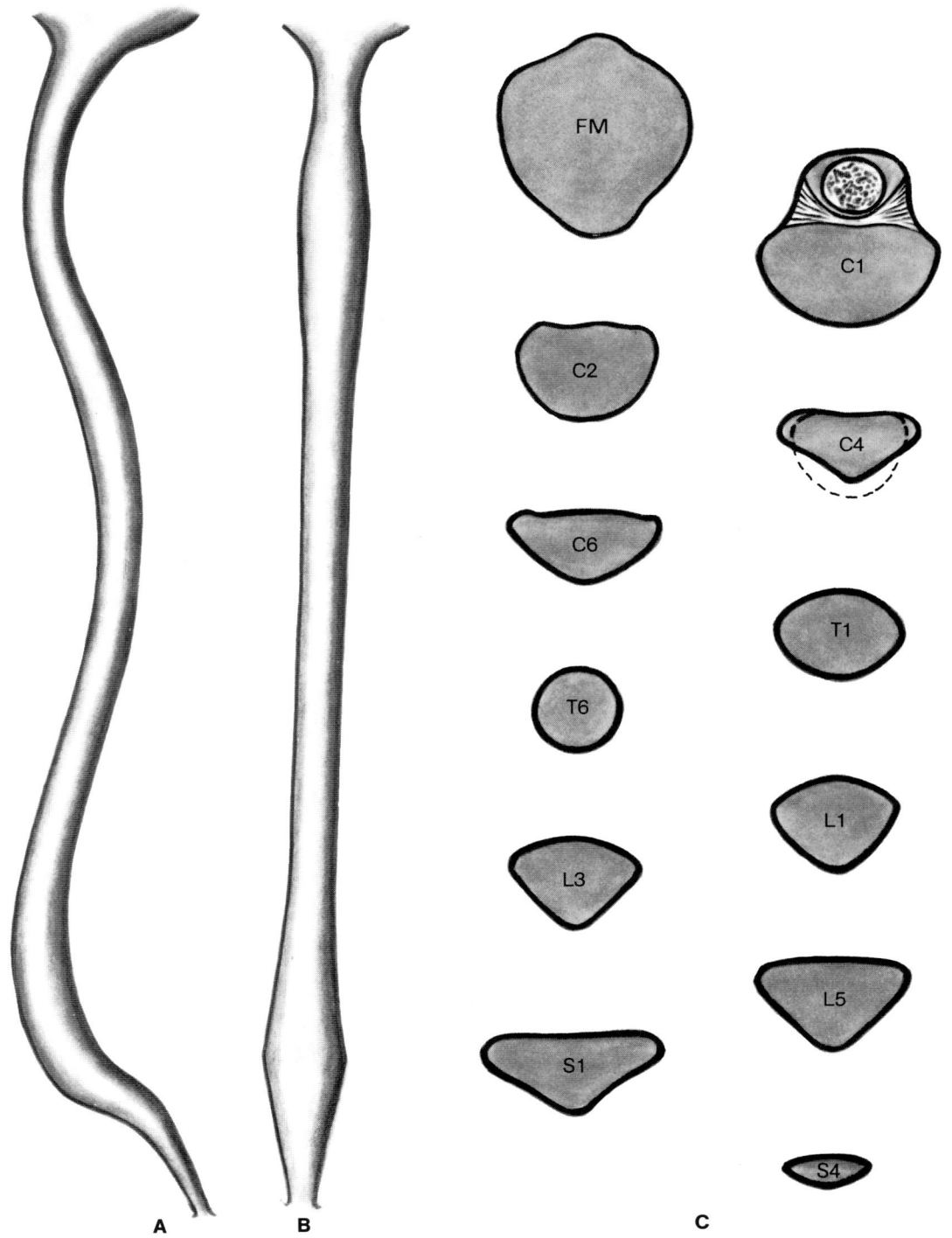

Figure 29 A–C

A Sagittal section of the vertebral canal
B Coronal section of the vertebral canal
C Horizontal sections of the vertebral canal

II.The Intervertebral Foramina

Along with the vertebral canal the intervertebral foramina provide passage and protection for the spinal nerves and their accompanying vertebral blood vessels. Although the term intervertebral foramen refers to any spinal orifice or canal through which a spinal nerve passes, it should be underlined that there exists a common type of foramen from C2 to S1, i.e., 23 paired foramina at the 23 intervertebral discs, and two variant types, one at each extremity of the spine. The intervertebral foramina are arranged in symmetrical pairs at each metameric level. Five sectors can be distinguished when studying the orifices giving passage to the spinal nerves.

A.Upper Cervical Region (Occipital Bone to C2)

The first two pairs of cervical nerves, contrary to the other spinal nerves, do not run through completely osteoarticular foramina, but rather through partly osteoarticular and partly fibrous orifices. The first cervical nerve (C1), along with the vertebral artery, passes through an orifice in the atlantooccipital membrane on the posterior surface of the atlantooccipital joint. The passage of the second cervical nerve (C2) is by an orifice on the posterior surface of the atlantoaxial joint through the atlantoaxial membrane. These orifices are influenced by the articular movements in this region and thus elongation of the nerves can occur during extreme movements.

B. Lower Cervical Region (C2 to C7)

The intervertebral foramina from the axis to the seventh cervical vertebra are of a common type. They are limited superiorly and inferiorly by the pedicles, anteriorly by the postero-inferior half of the vertebral body and the posterolateral surface of the intervertebral disc with its uncovertebral pseudo-articulation, and posteriorly by the zygapophyseal joints accompanied by the ligamentum flavum on their anterior aspect. In fact, the bony margins of each foramen are sufficiently dense for it to be considered as a canal. Each intervertebral foramen opens internally at the level of the lateral angles of the vertebral canal and externally in the zone flush with the transverse foramen, and is thus extended by the spoutlike transverse process. Each foramen resembles the sole of a shoe, the inferior part representing the heel. The mean dimensions of the foramina are 12 mm in height and 6 mm in width. The length of the foramina ranges from 6 mm to 8 mm with a slightly oblique downward, forward, and lateral slant. The cervical intervertebral foramina are modified by spinal movements, i.e., opening on anterior flexion, and lateral flexion and rotation towards the side opposite the foramina; narrowing on extension, and lateral flexion and rotation towards the homolateral side. The foramina may be pathologically narrowed by discal lesions (prolapse), osteoarticular lesions (arthrosis, fracture-luxation) of the zygapophyseal or uncovertebral articulations, and by tumors of the bone or neural tissue. Lesions involving the cervical intervertebral foramina, veritable topographical crossroads, thus give rise symptoms which can be osteoarticular, radicular, and vascular (the vertebral artery and its radiculomedullary branches).

C. Thoracic Region (C7 to T12)

The thoracic intervertebral foramina display common features due to the presence of the ribs from C7–T1 to T11–T12. The vertebral pedicles form the upper and lower boundaries of each foramen. The anterior margin is constituted by the lower half of the vertebral body and the posterior surface of the intervertebral disc. The posterior limits correspond to the zygapophyseal joints and the ligamentum flavum. The foramina present an oblique oval form with mean dimensions of 12 mm by 7 mm. However, the presence of the rib head at the inferior part of each foramen narrows the size by one third. The length of the foramina corresponds to the thickness of the pedicles, i.e. 6 mm on average. The foramina lie horizontally and thus a transverse straight line can be drawn from the right to the left foramen at each level. The spinal nerve occupies only one fifth of the volume of its foramen.

D. Lumbar Region (T12 to S1)

The lumbar intervertebral foramina have the same limits as those in the thoracic region but are larger and lack a rib at the outlet. In the lumbar region the foramina resemble the auricle of the ear, with mean dimensions of 18 mm by 13 mm. The L5–S1 intervertebral foramen is slightly smaller despite the fact that the fifth lumbar nerve contained therein is larger than the other spinal nerves. The length of the lumbar foramina (more closely resembling canals) corresponds to the thickness of the pedicles (8–15 mm). The foramina slant obliquely downward and outward in the coronal plane. Extreme flexion and hyperextension cause the foramina to enlarge and narrow respectively. Their internal opening on the lateral angles of the vertebral canal corresponds to the interdiscoligamentous defile of Latarjet and Magnin. Pathological stenosis is most apt to produce radicular lesions in this region. Anterior radicular lesions result from prolapse of the intervertebral disc or tumors of the vertebral body, whereas posterior lesions are produced by arthrosis of the posterior articulations or spondylolysis of the isthmic regions with or without spondylolisthesis.

E. Sacral Region

The fusion of the sacral segments results in transformation of the intervertebral foramina into four pairs of sacral foramina, each foramen resembling a T-shaped tunnel with an internal orifice at the lateral angles of the sacral canal and two external orifices, one on the ventral and one on the dorsal aspect of the sacrum. The foramina decrease in size from S1 to S4 (from 13 mm to 4 mm on average). The sacral hiatus fulfils the function of the last foramen, giving passage to the fifth sacral and the coccygeal nerve roots.

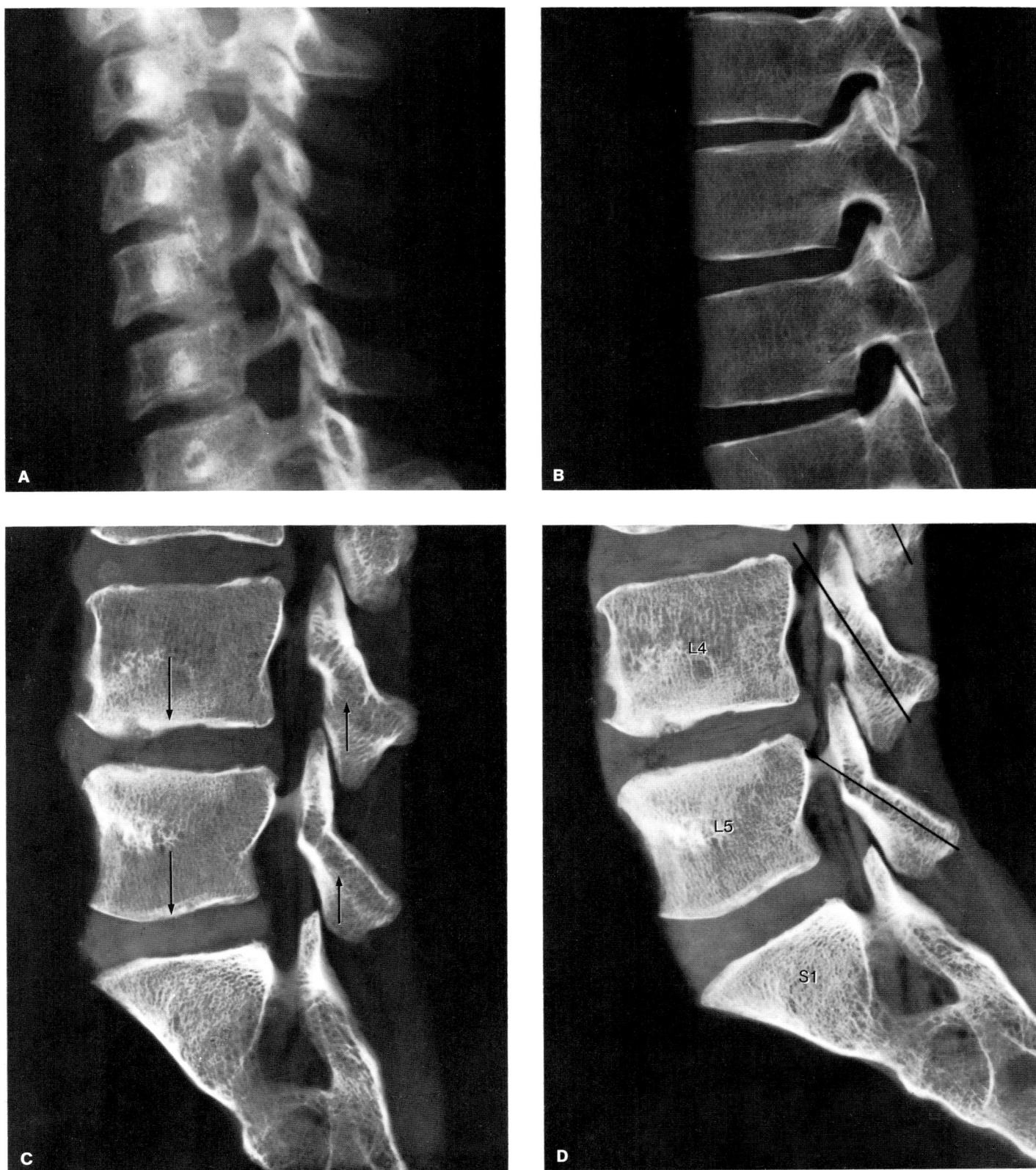

Figure 30 A–D

A   Cervical intervertebral foramina
B   Thoracic intervertebral foramina
C   Lumbar intervertebral foramina on hyperflexion
D   Lumbar intervertebral foramina on hyperextension

III. Vertebral Pedicles

From the anatomical standpoint the vertebral pedicles do not represent special structures for the protection of the intraspinal neural formations. However, since the pedicles are used in surgery to receive posterior screws it is necessary to understand their morphology and topography fully. The different regional types of pedicle are described below in craniocaudal order.

A. Pedicles of the Axis (C2)

The pedicles of the axis correspond in reality to interarticular isthmic regions, forming two small anteroposterior columns slanting slightly upward and forward. If they are extended posteriorly they project above the inferior facet of the axis, forming a horizontal oval area measuring 12 mm × 6 mm. The best direction for driving a bone screw into the pedicle, from a point of entry 10 mm above the center of the inferior articular facet, is 20° upward and 20° medially. The depth of penetration into the bone should be 25–30 mm.

B. Lower Cervical Pedicles (C3 to C7)

The cervical pedicles slant obliquely forward and medially at a 30° angle. Their posterior projection forms a 10 mm by 7 mm oval area. Screw penetration should be initiated at a point 3–4 mm above the center of the superior articular facet. When penetration is to extend to the body of the vertebra, the screw should be directed inward at a 20° angle in the horizontal plane perpendicular to the axis of the articular pillar. In fact, the risk of injury to the spinal nerve or vertebral artery is so great that pedicular screwing should not extend beyond the anterior plane of the articular bone mass, i.e., mean penetration of 14 mm in a strictly sagittal plane.

C. Upper Thoracic Pedicles (T1 to T3)

The pedicles of the the upper thoracic vertebrae display a vertical oval section. Like the cervical pedicles, they are located in the space between the superior and inferior articular facets and extend upward to the level of the inferior quarter of the superior facet. They slant obliquely inward at 20°–30° and downwards at 15°. Their thickness, greater at T1 than T3, ranges from 10 mm to 6 mm. Penetration by a pedicular screw should be from a point 3 mm below the center of the superior articular facet with an oblique direction 20° inward and 10° downward, and should be to a depth of 25–30 mm.

D. Middle Thoracic Pedicles (T4 to T10)

The pedicles in the middle thoracic region lie in a practically sagittal plane, slanting 10° inward and 10° downward. When extended posteriorly, their projection forms a vertical oval area on the articular pillar between the superior and inferior facets and overlaps part of the superior facet. An easy way to identify the articular facets is to inscribe a 10-mm diameter circle on the posterior arch of the thoracic vertebra in the angle formed by the inferior margins of the transverse process and the lamina. The thoracic pedicles are only 4–6 mm thick. The point for screw penetration is 3 mm below the center of the superior articular facet, i.e., on the horizontal ridge of the lamina which extends the posterosuperior margin of the transverse process (often presenting a small fossa due to hyperextension). The screw should be directed in a strictly sagittal plane perpendicular to the plane of the lamina, with penetration of 30–40 mm.

E. Thoracolumbar Pedicles (T11 to L2)

These pedicles are larger (8 mm on average) and lie in the sagittal plane without slanting laterally. They present a slight tilt of 5° with respect to the horizontal plane. Their projection forms a vertical oval area on the vertebral arch midway between the upper and lower articular facets. The site for screw penetration is the same as that of the middle thoracic pedicles. The thoracolumbar pedicles present a landmark of the lumbar type, i.e., an isthmic zone limited laterally by a semicircular notch which corresponds to the posteroinferior margin of the pedicle. Bone screws should always enter the pedicle 3–4 mm above and medial to this point. It is appropriate to use 35–45-mm screws.

F. Lower Lumbar Pedicles (L3 to L5)

The lower lumbar pedicles lie in a strictly sagittal plane perpendicular to the axis of the vertebral canal, and thus fan out like the spokes of a wheel due to the presence of lumbosacral lordosis. Their coronal section is triangular with an outer sagittal edge and an inner hypotenuse slanting downward and outward. The spinal nerves run along the inner and outer edges. The thickness of the pedicles ranges from 10 mm to 20 mm, being greatest in the lower vertebrae. The point of penetration of a pedicular screw is located at the intersection of two lines; the vertical line passing through the sagittal part of the articular interface above the pedicle and the horizontal line passing through the inferior end of the articular interface. Another landmark is the outer isthmic notch. Screw penetration should begin 3–4 mm above this point in a sagittal plane without inclination relative to the horizontal plane at L3 and L4 and at 5°–10° downward at L5. The depth of penetration should be 38–48 mm.

G. Sacral Pedicles

The pedicle of S1 is by itself sufficiently thick to take a bone screw, as it is extended on its outer surface by the ala sacralis. The inferior limit of the S1 pedicle corresponds to the first sacral foramen. To avoid injury to the S1 nerve root, which runs from the medial half of the L5–S1 posterior articulation to the outer margin of the first sacral foramen, the following procedure should be used: The screws should be driven into the ala sacralis from a point in the region lateral to the L5–S1 articulation and first sacral foramen and above the second sacral foramen; their direction should be 45° laterally and 45° inferiorly. In order not to penetrate beyond the sacroiliac articulation the screws must be 45–55 mm long.

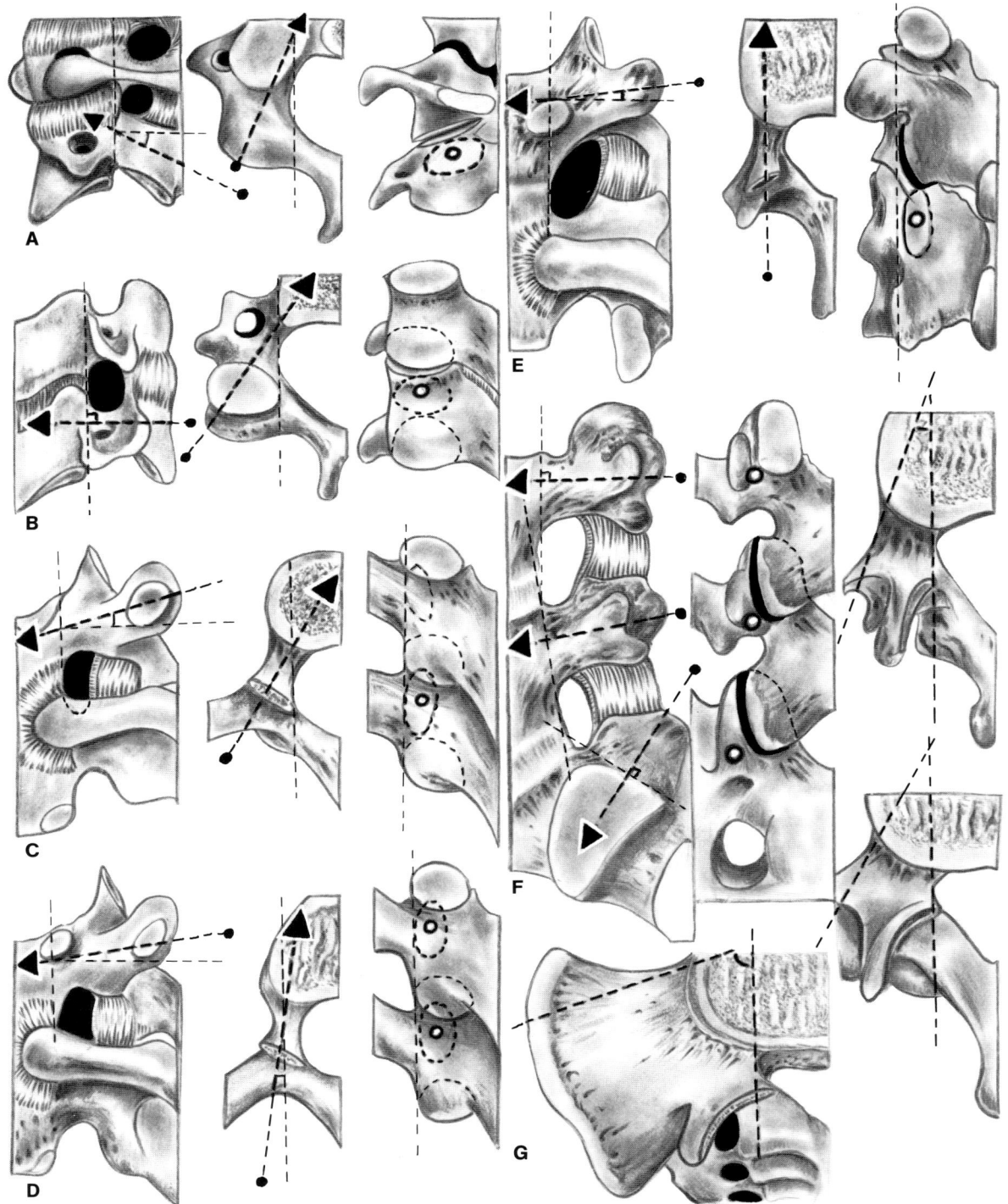

Figure 31 A–G

A The pedicles of C2
B The pedicles of the lower
    cervical vertebrae
C The upper thoracic pedicles
D The middle thoracic pedicles
E The thoracolumbar pedicles
F The lumbosacral pedicles
G The ala sacralis

7 Radiculomedullary Axis

I. Radiculomedullary Morphology

The spinal cord (medulla spinalis) and spinal nerve roots (radices nervorum spinalium) are those parts of the nervous system protected by the vertebral canal.

The *spinal cord* forms a long cylindrical cord whose caliber varies due to the presence of two enlarged zones in the cervical and lumbar regions (intumescentia cervicalis and lumbalis) corresponding to the nerves of the upper and lower limbs. The mean length of the spinal cord is 45 cm, to which must be added the 25 cm of the filum terminale, and its mean weight is 30 g. It is of friable consistency, hence its fragility to trauma including surgery. It follows the spinal curvatures exactly and terminates in most cases at the level of the L1–L2 intervertebral disc. Its mean caliber of 10 mm allows considerable room in the enlarged regions of the vertebral canal, but at the level of the thoracic spine narrowing of the canal by one third suffices to compress the cord. The external surface of the cord is marked by six longitudinal sulci, i.e., the anterior median fissure (fissura mediana anterior), deep enough to accommodate the anterior spinal artery; the median posterior sulcus (sulcus medianus posterior), much shallower; and two lateral sulci (sulcus lateralis posterior and anterior) on each side, through which emerge the rootlets of the spinal nerves (fila radicularia).

Each medullary segment, known as a myelomere, gives off nerve rootlets which in turn give rise to the *spinal nerve roots*. The spinal cord consists of 31 myelomeres and thus gives rise to 31 pairs of spinal nerve roots: eight cervical, twelve thoracic, five lumbar, five sacral, and one coccygeal. The spinal nerve roots display an enlargement, the spinal ganglion, after which the dorsal and ventral roots (radix dorsalis and radix ventralis) fuse to form the spinal nerve (nervus spinalis). The spinal ganglion and the origin of the spinal nerve lie in the intervertebral foramina. Due to the apparent ascension of the spinal cord within the vertebral canal (resulting from unequal growth of these two structures), the direction and length of the spinal nerve roots vary according to their level of emergence. In the cervical region the nerve roots are short and practically horizontal with evenly spaced fila radicularia. In the thoracic region the nerve roots run obliquely downward and are longer (equivalent in length to the height of one to two vertebral bodies), the inferior fila radicularia implanting on the superior filum. The lumbosacral region displays vertical nerve roots increasing in length down to the filum terminale with short joined fila radicularia. On emergence from the intervertebral foramina the spinal nerves divide into a large ventral ramus and small dorsal ramus, which are anastomosed to the vegetative ganglions by the communicating rami (rami communicantes). Caudal to the conus medullaris the spinal nerve roots group together to form the cauda equina.

Macroscopically, the spinal cord is divided into two distinct parts, the peripheral white matter (substantia alba) and the central gray matter (substantia grisea). The center of the gray matter is traversed by a canal extending the entire length of the spinal cord, the ependymal or central canal (canalis centralis). The gray matter is arranged in the form of the letter H with an intermediate zone (pars intermedia) and two ventral and dorsal horns (cornu ventrale, cornu dorsale). The pars intermedia gives rise to a lateral horn (cornu laterale) in the region between the T2 and L2 nerve roots. The central canal divides the pars intermedia into two anterior and posterior gray commissures (commissura grisea). The superficial sulci and horns of the gray matter segment the white matter into three pairs of columns, known as the ventral, lateral, and dorsal funiculi (funiculi anteriores, laterales, and posteriores). The left and right halves of the white matter are connected at the base of the anterior median fissure by the white commissure (commissura alba), whereas posterior to the pars intermedia the white matter is separated by the median dorsal septum (septum dorsale medium).

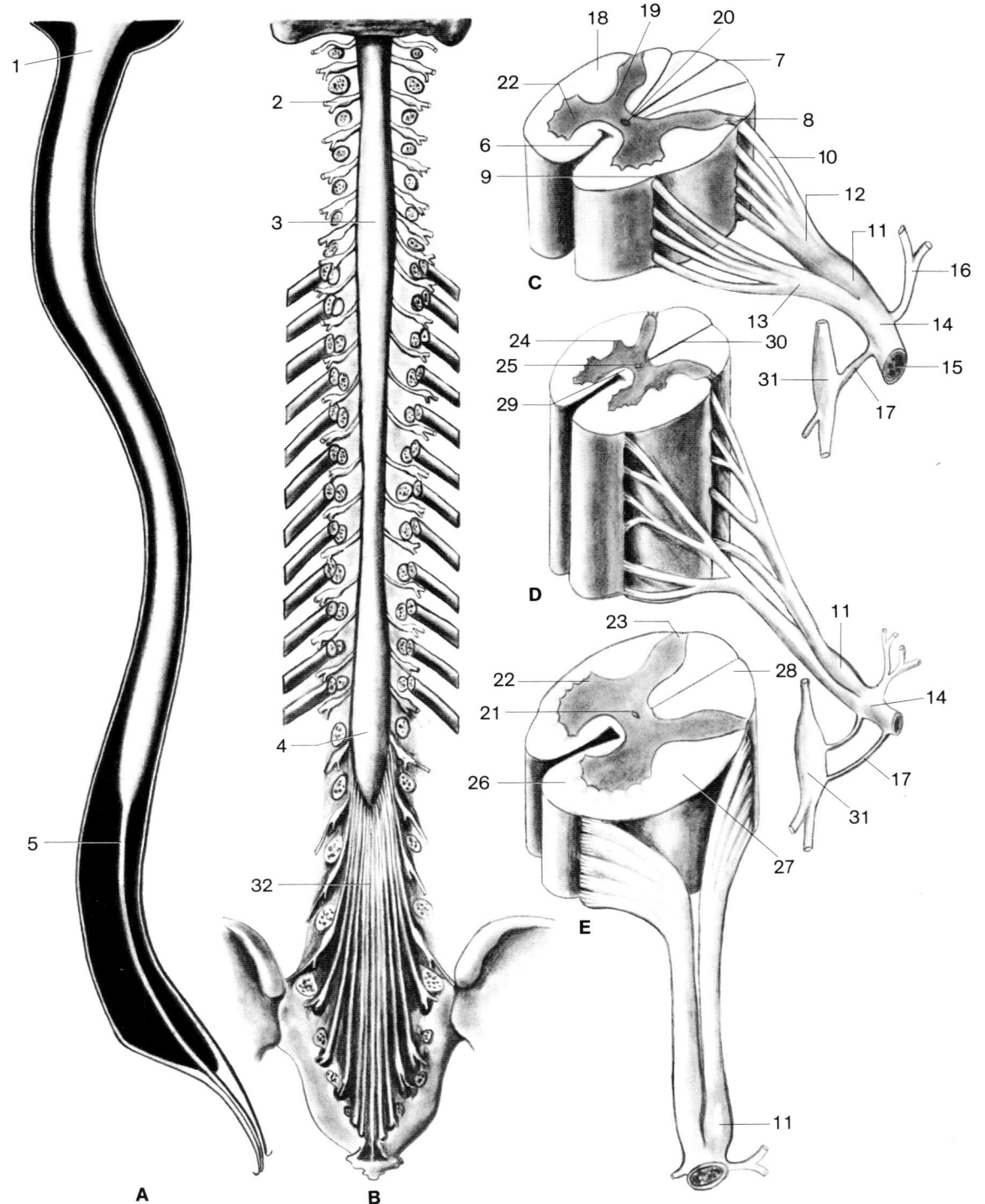

Figure 32 A–E

A Lateral view of the spinal cord in the vertebral canal
B Posterior view of the spinal cord and spinal nerve roots in the vertebral canal and intervertebral foramina
C Cervical myelomere and cervical spinal nerve
D Thoracic myelomere and thoracic spinal nerve
E Lumbar myelomere and lumbar spinal nerve

1 medulla spinalis 2 radices nervorum spinalium 3 intumescentia cervicalis 4 intumescentia lumbalis 5 filum terminale 6 fissura mediana ant. 7 sulcus medianus post. 8 sulcus lateralis post. 9 sulcus lateralis ant. 10 fila radicularia 11 ganglion spinale 12 radix dorsalis 13 radix ventralis 14 n. spinalis 15 ramus ventralis 16 ramus dorsalis 17 rami communicantes 18 substantia alba 19 substantia grisea 20 ependyma, canalis centralis 21 pars intermedia 22 cornu ventrale 23 cornu dorsale 24 cornu laterale 25 commissura grisea 26 funiculus ant. 27 funiculus lateralis 28 funiculus post. 29 commissura alba 30 septum dorsale medium 31 ganglia autonomica 32 cauda equina

II. Morphology and Topography of the Spinal Meninges

The meninges are the envelopes of the central nervous system and afford protection and nourishment. They form a fully closed covering around the brain and spinal cord within the cranium and vertebral canal. Classically, three meninges are described: the pia mater, intimately lining the external surface of the neural strutures; the dura mater, covering the deep surface of the cranial bones and vertebrae; and the arachnoid membrane (arachnoidea), interposed between them in the form of large transparent sheets delimiting spaces filled with cerebrospinal fluid (CSF: liquor cerebrospinalis). In fact modern descriptions refer to two meninges, the soft meninx (leptomeninx) and hard meninx (dura mater), which are derived from different embryological structures. The leptomeninx corresponds to the association of the pia mater and arachnoidea and presents a very loose alveolar structure constituting the subarachnoid spaces (cavum subarachnoidale) containing the CSF. The epidural space (cavum epidurale) lies between the deep surface of the bone and dura mater; it may be the site of fluid collection (hematoma, purulent fluid), and can be used to introduce anesthetics (epidural anesthesia). Normally, there exists between the dura mater and arachnoidea a virtual space, the subdural space (cavum subdurale), which can be used surgically to open the dura mater without causing leakage of the CSF. Meningeal hemorrhage develops in the subarachnoid spaces.

Iodated contrast material can be introduced into these spaces by needle puncture, thus allowing myelography between the foramen magnum and conus medullaris and lower down, radiography of the cauda equina (saccoradiculography). At the level of the lateral columns of the spinal cord the leptomeninx forms the denticulate ligament (ligamentum denticulum), which is a coronal septum with one margin adherent to the spinal cord along its entire length and a crenated margin inserting on the dura mater midway between the orifices of emergence of the spinal nerve roots. This ligament stabilizes the spinal cord within the sleeve of dura mater. The emergence of the spinal roots through the dura mater constitutes another means of stabilization of the spinal cord. The site of emergence is on the lateral part of the dura mater and forms a fixed point of the nerve roots due to their adherence to these structures. The emergence of the nerve roots resembles a double-barrelled funnel for the dorsal and ventral roots with an arcuate fold at the inferior margin. The spinal ganglion and spinal nerve are enveloped in the same sheath of dura mater which is extended out of the spine by the neurolemma.

The dura mater sheath, continuous with the cranial dura mater, originates at the level of the foramen magnum and descends the vertebral canal to terminate below the conus medullaris. The anterior surface of the dural envelope is loosely adherent to the posterior longitudinal ligament and is extended below the conus medullaris by the coccygeal ligament containing the filum terminale, which is attached caudally to the posterior surface of the fourth sacral segment.

The termination of the dural envelope varies according to individuals. Our study of 115 anatomical specimens (1961) allowed identification of four types of termination relative to the sacral intervertebral spaces:

Termination at S1–S2:	43%
Termination at the center of S2:	32%
Termination at S2–S3:	23%
Termination at S3–S4:	2%

This topographical distribution by orthogonal projection onto the walls of the vertebral canal differs from the radiological topography.

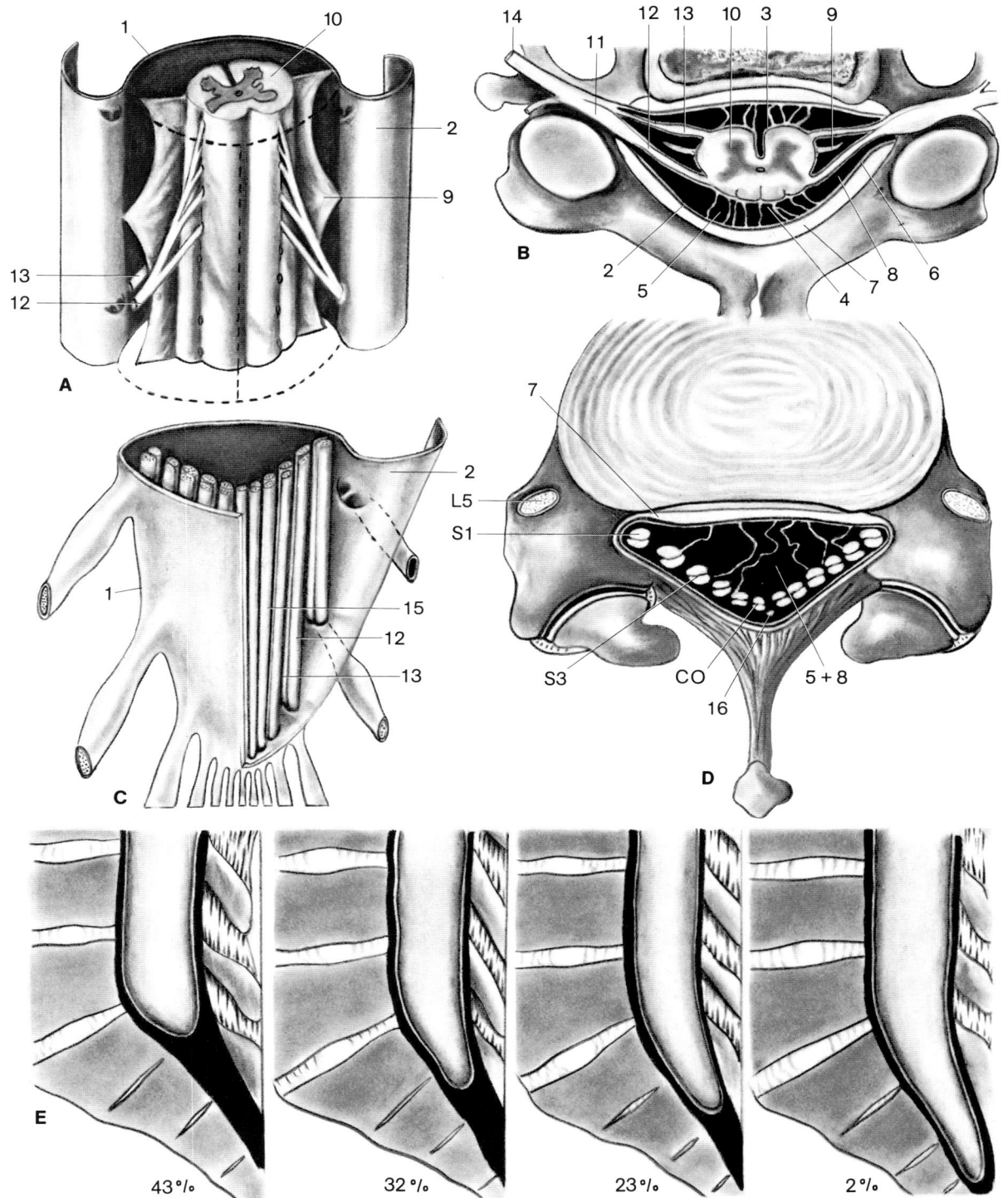

Figure 33 A–E

A   Posterior aspect of the spinal cord after opening of the dura mater
B   Horizontal section of the cervical canal
C   Posterior aspect of the cauda equina after opening of the dura mater
D   Horizontal section of the vertebral canal through the L5–S1 disc
E   The four topographical types of termination of the dural envelope

1 meninges *2* dura mater spinalis *3* pia mater spinalis *4* arachnoidea spinalis *5* cavum subarachnoidale *6* cavum subdurale *7* cavum epidurale *8* liquor cerebrospinalis *9* lig. denticulatum *10* medulla spinalis *11* ganglion spinale *12* radix dorsalis *13* radix ventralis *14* n. spinalis *15* cauda equina *16* filum terminale

III. Vertebromedullary Topography

Knowledge of vertebromedullary topography is based on the works of Chipault (dating back to 1893), who used the spinous processes as points of reference. However, spinal pathology and surgery require more precise description. Accordingly, the descriptions given below are derived from 115 anatomical specimens and based on the geometric projection of the myelomeres on the intervertebral discs, vertebral bodies, and laminae. The topography of the myelomeres is dependent upon the level of termination of the spinal cord.

A. Spinal Cord Termination

The cone-shaped termination of the spinal cord is identified by the origin of the filum terminale and is located between the T12–L1 and L2–L3 intervertebral discs. Schematically, five common types of spinal cord termination can be described: (1) the T12–L1 disc, (2) the center of the body of L1, (3) the L1–L2 disc, (4) the center of the body of L2, and (5) the L2–L3 disc.

We encountered two exceptional sites of spinal cord termination, at L4 and S4. The latter was an operative finding in a 50-year-old woman whose spinal cord had retained its embryonic horizontal metameric position. In Europeans the most frequent site of termination is at the center of the body of L1 (44%), whereas in Africans the most common level of termination is lower by half a vertebral body, i.e., at the L1–L2 intervertebral disc (52%). The mean level of termination in these two populations is at the center of the L1–L2 disc (36%). No relation exists between the level of spinal cord termination and age, sex, or height.

Topography of spinal cord termination

Subjects	T12–L1 disc	Center of L1	L1–L2 disc	Center of L2	L2–L3 disc
Adult Europeans (%)	16	44	20	16	4
Adult Africans (%)	8	8	52	24	8
Total (%)	12	26	36	20	6
Children		4	5	6	

B. Myelomeres

Given the importance of individual variations, the mean topography corresponding to the most frequent site of termination will be described first, i.e., individuals presenting a spinal cord ending at the L1–L2 intervertebral disc. Thereafter, discussion will be devoted to the means of determining the extreme topography of the less frequent types, based on the *mean topography*, which is as follows:

– C1: foramen magnum and atlantooccipital space
– C2: odontoid process and atlas
– C3 to T11 (except C8): these myelomeres are located at the level of the vertebral immediately cranial to their numerical equivalent

– C8 and T12: intervertebral disc above the vertebra above that numerically corresponding to the myelomere; the C6–C7 disc for the C8 myelomere and the T10–T11 disc for the T12 myelomere
– L1, L3, and S1: center of the body of T11, T12, and L1 respectively
– L2: T11–T12 disc
– L4, L5: straddling the T12–L1 disc
– S2 to S5: lower third of the L1 vertebral body
– Spinal cord termination (coccygeal root): L1–L2 disc

Extreme Topography. Certain differences between Europeans and Africans can be noted. In Africans the cervical and upper thoracic myelomeres display a more variable position, often lying higher up than in Europeans; one vertebra higher for the lower four cervical myelomeres and half a vertebra higher for the upper cervical and upper thoracic myelomeres. The lower thoracic and lumbosacral myelomeres present the same variations in Europeans and Africans, although the lowest myelomeric sites are more frequent in the latter. The extreme variations of the myelomeres (corresponding to about 25% of spines) can be deduced from the mean topography (75% of spines) by adding or substracting half a vertebra for the cervical myelomeres ($\pm$ 0.5 cm) and dorsal myelomeres ($\pm$ 1 cm) and one vertebra for the lumbar and sacral myelomeres ($\pm$ 2.5 cm).

C. Topographical Types

Comparative studies of the termination of the spinal cord and dural envelope according to subjects led us to identify different types of spine. In general, it can be stated that the lowest site of termination of the dural envelope is accompanied by the lowest site of spinal cord termination.

Although by no means absolute, this is a useful guide in calculating the type of medullary termination when radiological opacification of the dural termination is available. The two most frequent topographical varieties are the L1–S1 type (termination of the spinal cord above the L1–L2 intervertebral disc and termination of the dural envelope above the S1–S2 disc), more frequent in Europeans, and the L2–S2 type (spinal cord termination below the L1–L2 disc and dural termination below the S1–S2 disc), more common in Africans. The other varieties of termination are the L1–S2, L2–S1, and L3–S3 types.

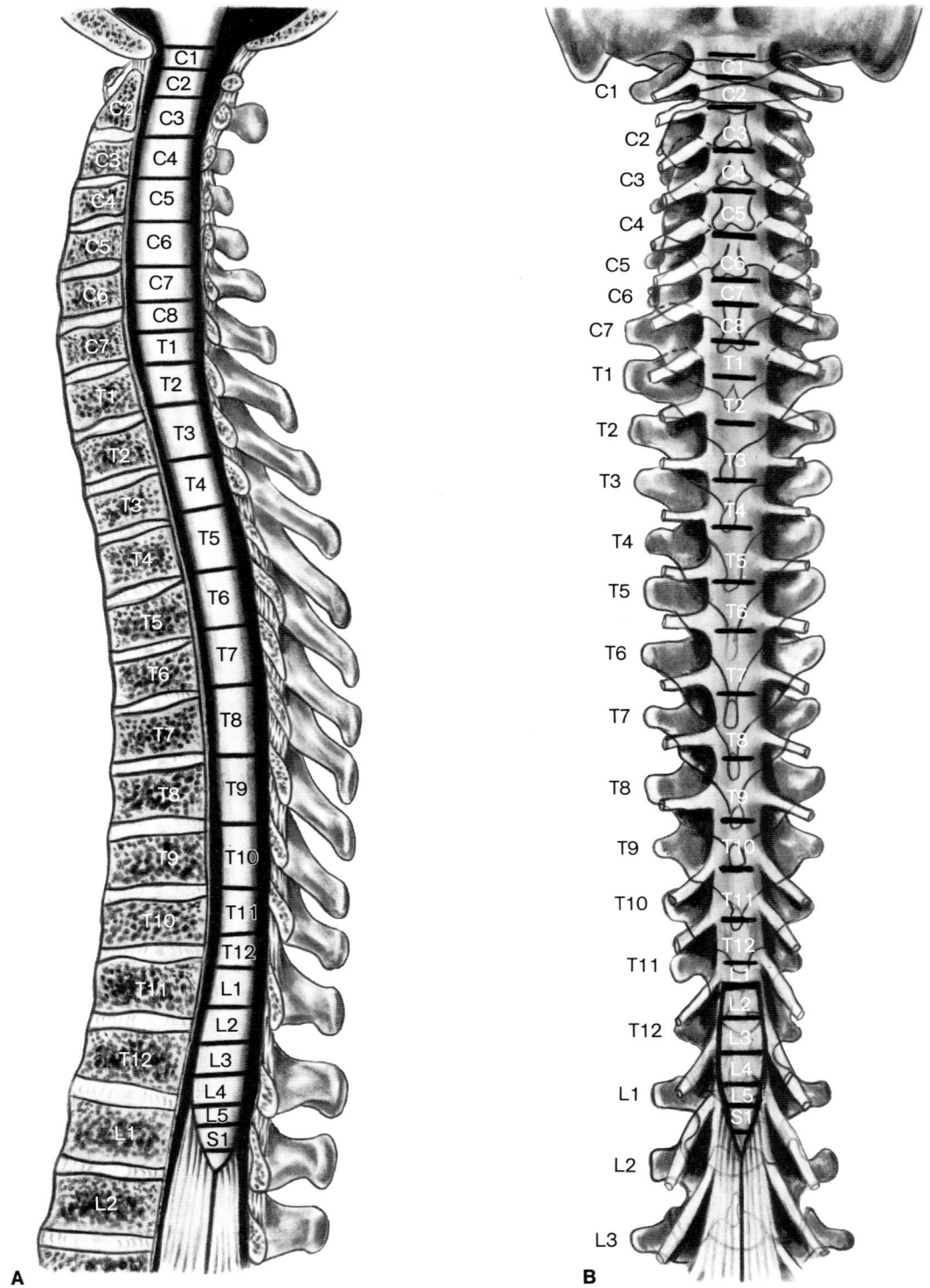

Figure 34 A, B

A Vertebromedullary topography
on a median saggital section
of the spine

B Vertebromedullary topography
as seen by transparency through
the posterior aspect of the spine

IV. Vertebroradicular Topography

Three zones allow determination of the topography of the spinal nerve roots: their medullary origin on the myelomeres, their point of passage through the dura mater, and their position in the corresponding intervertebral foramen.

A. Dural Emergence of the Nerve Roots

The level at which each spinal nerve root traverses the dural envelope is dependent upon the type of dural termination, and thus the level of emergence of each root can be deduced for a given type of dural termination. This topographical point is fairly reliable. Furthermore, at the level of dural emergence of the nerve root the two rami are clearly separate, the anterior corresponding to the motor and the posterior the sensory nerve root. Accordingly, this landmark can be used to achieve a selective sensory radicotomy, especially in the lumbosacral region. If the point of reference of dural emergence is taken as the intervertebral disc corresponding to the intervertebral foramen from which the nerve root escapes, then two main types of dural emergence can be described, according to the level of dural termination at S1–S2 (S1 type) or S2–S3 (S2 type).

The S1 type of dural termination has the following features:
- Roots C1 to C7 emerge below the plane of the corresponding disc, i.e., 1–2 mm below the inferior edge of the disc.
- The emergence of C8 is exactly in the plane of the corresponding C7–T1 disc.
- Roots T1 to T12 emerge above the plane of the corresponding disc: the lower the nerve root the higher its point of emergence, i.e., half a vertebra above the disc at the bottom of the thoracic spine.
- The L1 root emerges at the level of the center of the body of L1, the L2 root above the center of the body of L2, the L3 root at the level of the upper third of L3, the L4 root at the level of the upper quarter of L4, and the L5 root at the level of the upper fifth of the body of L5.
- The dural emergence of the S1 root is immediately above the level of the L5–S1 disc, i.e., more than one vertebra above its intervertebral foramen. The most caudal nerve roots, S2, S3, S4, S5, and the coccygeal (CO), traverse the dural envelope in very close proximity to each other at the level of the dural termination, i.e., at the posterior surface of the body of S1.

The S2 type of dural termination displays these features:
- Roots C1 to C3 traverse the dural envelope below the corresponding disc.
- Roots C4 to C6 emerge at the level of the corresponding discs.
- Roots C7 to T5 emerge above the corresponding discs near the center of the suprajacent vertebral body.
- Roots T6 to L3 traverse the dural envelope at the level of the center of the vertebral body above the corresponding disc.

- The L4 root emerges at the level of the upper third of the L4 body; the L5 root traverses the dural envelope at the level of the upper quarter of L5.
- The S1 root traverses the dural envelope at the level of the lower edge of the L5–S1 disc.
- The S2 root emerges from the dural envelope at the level of the lower part of S1; roots S3 and S4 emerge above and below the level of the middle third of S2.

These topographical relations vary a few millimeters according to the degree of spinal flexion and in certain operative positions.

B. Nerve Roots in the Intervertebral Foramina

Cervical Region. The intervertebral foramina are lacking for the first two pairs of cervical nerves, which emerge from the spine through an osteofibrous orifice lying medial to the posterior articulations. The five remaining cervical pairs (C3 to C8) escape through their corresponding intervertebral foramina (75% occluded by the nerve root) with a very slight oblique slant downward and forward, except C8 which runs horizontally.

Thoracic Region. The small-caliber thoracic nerve roots occupy only one fifth the volume of their intervertebral foramina. They run in contact with the upper pedicle of the foramina, above the level of the intervertebral disc. The upper thoracic nerves display a practically recurrent ascending course. The middle thoracic nerves lie horizontal in the intervertebral foramina, and the lower thoracic nerves display a clearly descending course in the upper part of the foramina.

Lumbar Region. Although large, the lumbar spinal nerves occupy only one third the volume of their intervertebral foramina, which they traverse diagonally from the medial surface of the superior pedicle to the lateral surface of the inferior pedicle.

Sacral Region. The sacral nerve roots form a "chicken-foot" structure in the sacral canal. The ventral rami emerge through the anterior sacral foramina and the dorsal rami through the posterior sacral foramina. The coccygeal roots and fifth pair of sacral nerve roots escape through the sacral hiatus.

A fairly rare type of radicular emergence is the existence of a common trunk for roots L5 and S1 in the region where they traverse the dural envelope, although the spinal nerves separate and run through their respective intervertebral foramina. The modifications of neural topography resulting from precise spinal movements are discussed later in the section devoted to neuromeningeal dynamics. In the lateral recesses of the spinal canal the spinal nerve roots are exposed to compression by a prolapsed intervertebral disc and in the intervertebral foramina may be compressed anteriorly and posteriorly by degenerative uncovertebral and zygapophyseal lesions respectively.

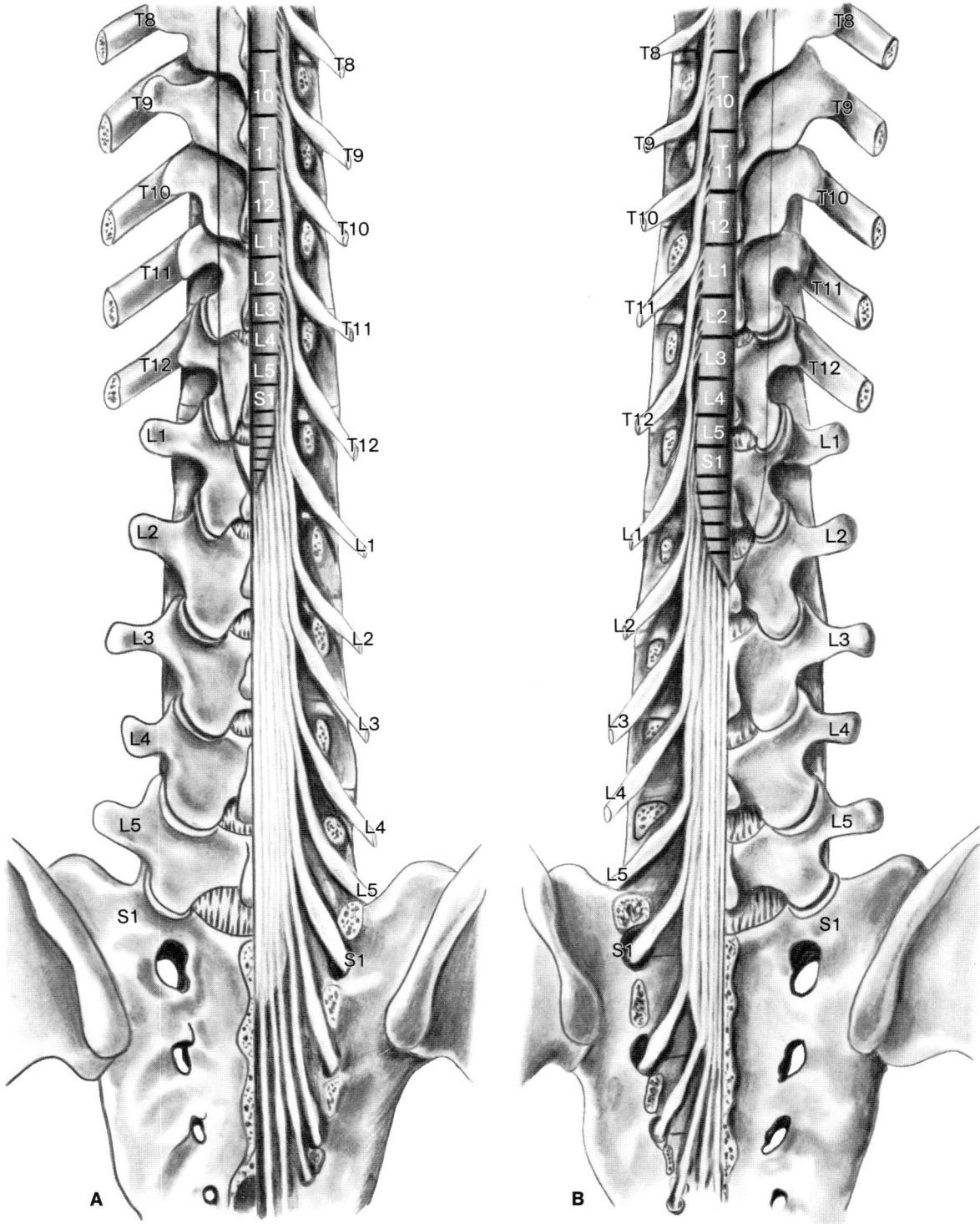

Figure 35 A, B

A Posterior aspect of the radiculomedullary topography in the L1–S1 type

B Posterior aspect of the radiculomedullary topography in the L2–S2 type

V. Neuromeningeal Roentgenography

A. Cervical Myelography

Opacification of the cervical subarachnoid space (cavum subarachnoidale) with modern iodated products of reduced toxicity for the neural tissue yields remarkably clear images of the neuromeningeal structures, incomparably better than those obtained by air myelography. Four radiological views, profile, anteroposterior, and right and left oblique, are necessary to view the full circumference of the vertebral canal and its contents.

Profile. The opaque column of CSF, limited by the dura mater, follows perfectly the form of the vertebral canal with the smooth curved margins of the cervical lordosis. In many normal subjects over 35 years of age this opaque column is marked by slight notches at the level of the posterior margin of the intervertebral discs and anterior margin of the ligamenta flava between the laminae. The spinal cord can be identified within the opaque column as a lighter band separated by 2–3 mm CSF in front and behind.

Anteroposterior and Oblique. These two views give practically the same image except that the oblique films give a better picture of the emergence of the nerve roots on one side. The opaque column of the subarachnoid space displays crenated lateral contours facing each intervertebral foramen due to the emergence of the spinal nerve roots (transfictio radicularia durae matris). The anterior and posterior roots of each spinal nerve traverse the dura mater through two contiguous but distinct orifices, thus displacing the dura mater and subarachnoid space 4–7 mm outward. Distal to the site of dural emergence, a narrow sleeve of subarachnoid space accompanies the nerve roots and spinal ganglion out to the origin of the spinal nerve near the outlet of the intervertebral foramen. This arachnoid sheath common to the nerve roots (vagina arachnoidealis communis radicarum) is very lightly opacified on myelography. Within the opaque column it is easy to identify the lighter band corresponding to the cervical cord and its swelling separated from the lateral walls of the dura mater by a right and left band of CSF 4–6 mm wide. The latticelike clarity of the fila radicularia is clearly identifiable through these lateral columns and can be seen to run towards the arachnoid sleeve common to the nerve roots.

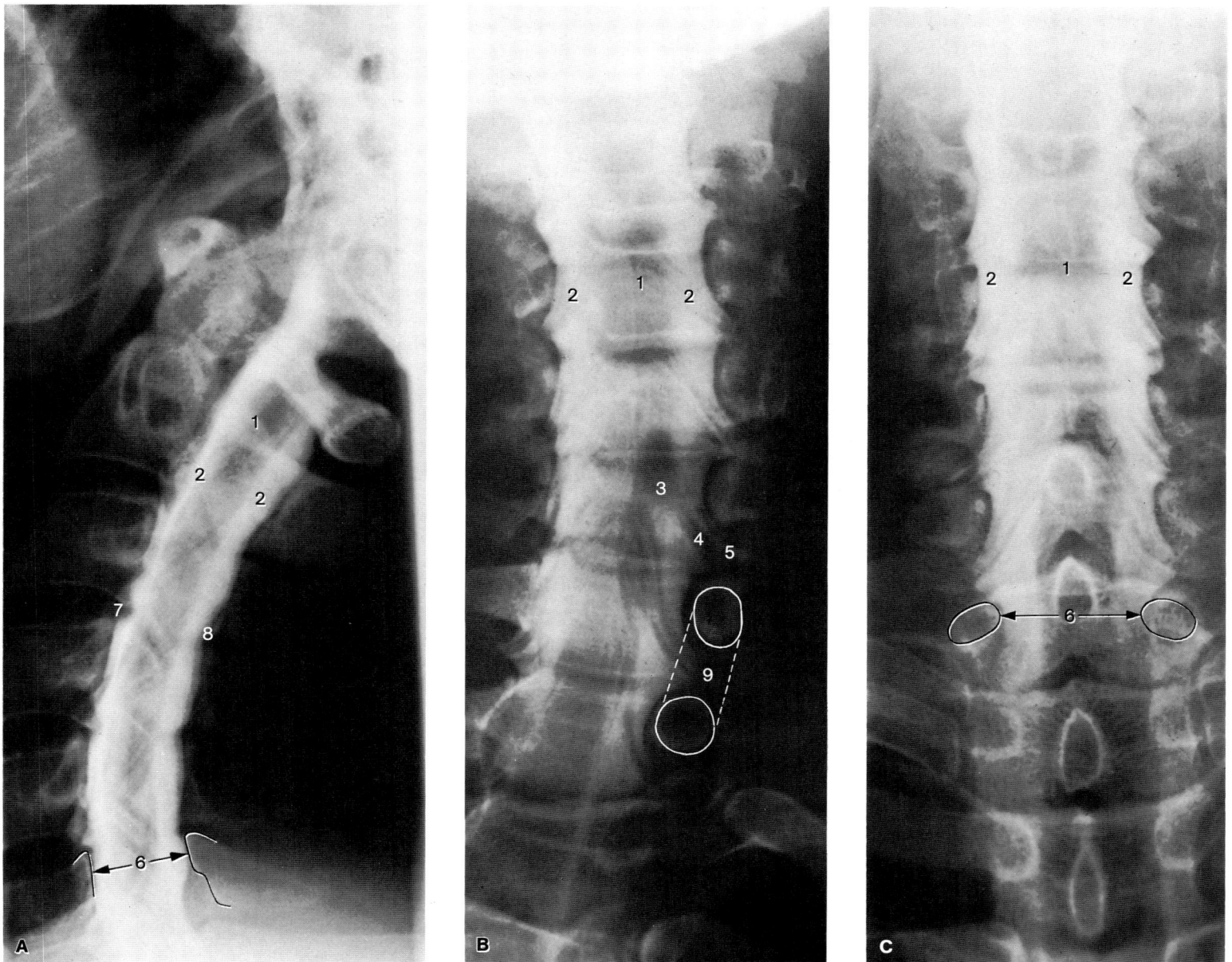

Figure 36 A–C

A   Profile myelography (metrizamide)
B   Left oblique myelography
C   Anteroposterior myelography

1 medulla spinalis   *2* cavum subarachnoideale   *3* fila radicularia
4 transfictio radicularia durae matris   *5* vagina arachnoidealis communis radicorum   *6* canalis vertebralis   *7* discus intervertebralis
8 lig. flavum   *9* foramen intervertebrale

B. Thoracic and Lumbosacral Myelography

Iodate opacification of the subarachnoid space (cavum sub-arachnoideale) in the thoracic and lumbosacral regions gives images very similar to those obtained in the cervical spine.

The *spinal cord* appears as a light band at the anterior part of the opaque column. The spinal cord is separated from the anterior wall of the vertebral canal by only a thin opaque band of CSF, whereas posteriorly the layer of CSF is 6–8 mm thick. The termination of the spinal cord is clearly visible near the L1–L2 intervertebral disc.

The *lumbosacral nerve roots* group together below the spinal cord termination to form the cauda equina, thus yielding a vertically striated image. Seen in profile the opacified column perfectly follows the form of the vertebral canal down to L5, but below this level the dura mater terminates in the form of a cone so the opaque column occupies only the posterior part of the sacral canal. A prolapsed L5–S1 intervertebral disc can thus protude into this dead space without altering the image of the opaque column. When the dural termination is lower (S2 or S3), the dead space is no longer situated at L5–S1 but below. The margins of the opaque column are crenated by the dural emergence of the nerve roots (transfictio radicularia durae matris), prolonged by the arachnoid sheath common to the nerve roots (vagina arachnoidealis communis radicorum). Each point of dural emergence of the nerve root forms two contiguous orifices. At their base the funnel-like dura mater and subarachnoid space are radiologically subdivided by the passage of the anterior and posterior nerve roots to form small supra- and subradicular fossae (Salamon and Louis). The supraradicular fossa is a regular narrow opaque line above the translucent intermingled nerve roots. The subradicular fossa appears as an opaque triangle lying below the nerve roots. The disappearance of these fossae or the common arachnoid sheath is the earliest and most subtle sign of radicular compression due to a prolapsed intervertebral disc.

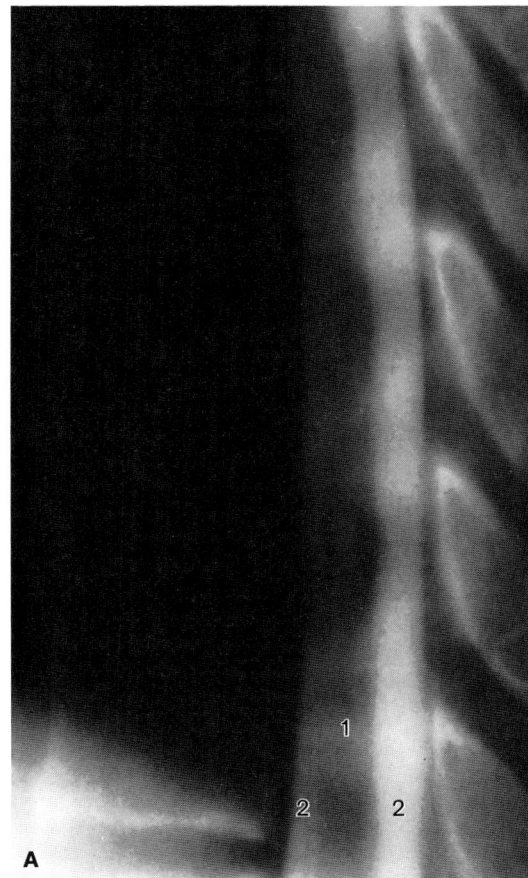

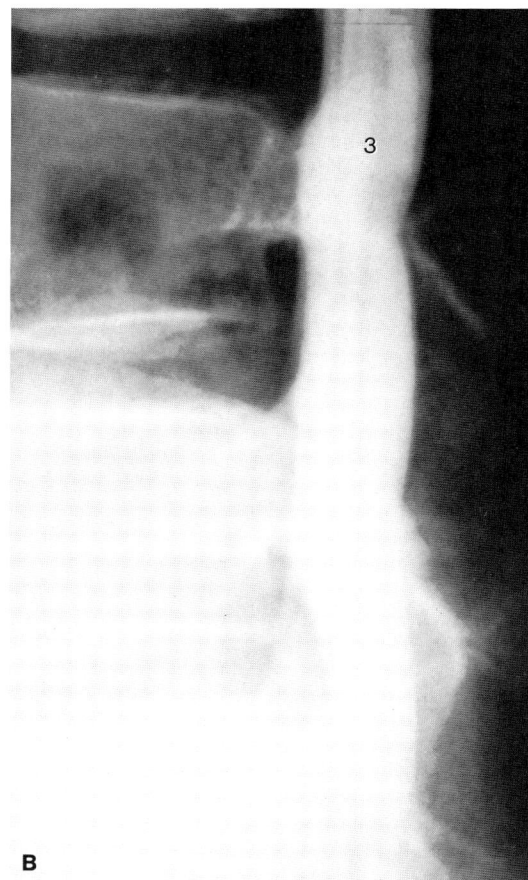

Figure 37 A, B

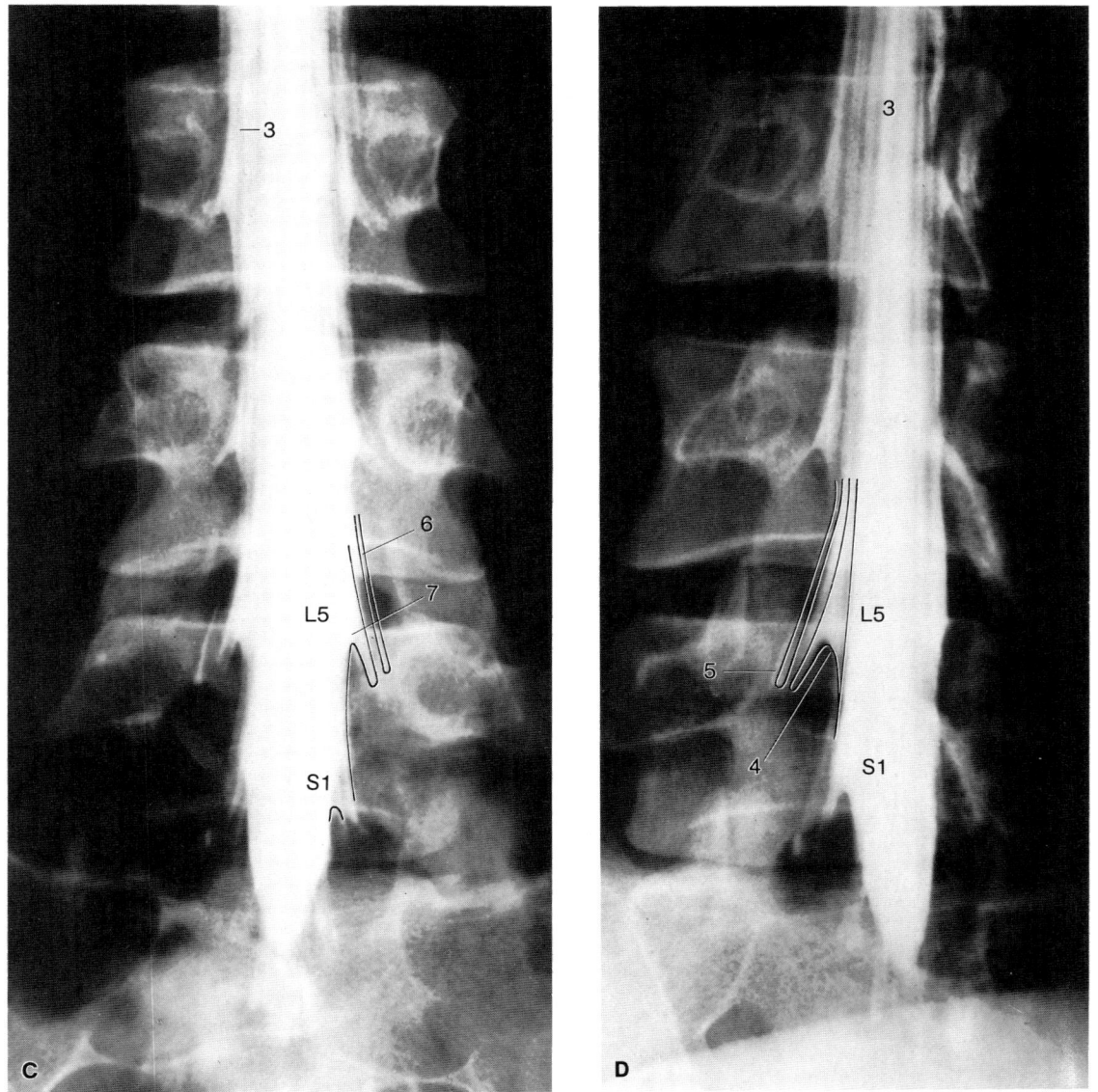

Figure 37 C, D

A   Profile thoracic myelography (metrizamide)
B   Profile lumbosacral radiography of the cauda equina (metrizamide)
C   Anteroposterior radiography of the cauda equina
D   Oblique (three-quarter) radiography of the cauda equina

1 medulla spinalis   *2* cavum subarachnoideale   *3* cauda equina
4 transfictio radicularia durae matris   *5* vagina arachnoidealis communis radicorum   *6* fossa radicularia sup.   *7* fossa radicularia inf.

C. Axial Tomography of Dural Envelope and Spinal Nerve Roots

1. Myelography. Myelography allows identification of a relatively infrequent anomaly of radicular emergence leading to radicalgia due to minor protrusion of the intervertebral disc. This anomaly is the common trunk of the L5 and S1 nerve roots, about 1 cm in length outside the dural envelope and dividing at the entrance to the L5–S1 intervertebral foramen to give rise in to its two branches, the L5 and S1 spinal nerves, which run through their respective intervertebral foramina.

2. Horizontal Sections. Horizontal sections of the opacified envelope in the lumbosacral spine give a normal and reliable picture by computerized axial tomography subsequent to radiography of the cauda equina.

The *section at L2–L3* shows that the nerve roots in the cauda equina are not arranged haphazardly but in a precise order, i.e., a row of roots in the coronal plane with an anterior concavity and the coccygeal nerve root in the center. The nerve roots emerging highest from the canal lie the farthest from the center. This slice clearly shows the narrowness of the lateral recess of the vertebral canal, which is thus a common site of radicular compression due to a discal lesion or degenerative lesion of the posterior articulation.

The *section at L3–L4* also demonstrates the orderly arrangement of the cauda equina within the dural envelope. The L3 nerve root has traversed the dural envelope and can be seen to lie in the intervertebral foramen, whereas the L4 root, still within the dural envelope, is the most external of the intradural nerve roots, i.e., the first to be exposed to lateral prolapse of the intervertebral disc. The L3 root is free in the intervertebral foramen and can escape anterior to the hernia, but the L4 root is blocked in the dural envelope and cannot escape the compression.

The *section at L4–L5,* similar to the preceding one, shows the dural emergence of the suprajacent nerve root (L4), which is free in the intervertebral foramen. The L5 nerve root, emerging below, is still blocked in the outer part of the dural envelope.

The *section at L5–S1* shows the high termination of the dura mater, since the conus medullaris of the subarachnoid space is narrow and lies posteriorly against the ligamentum flavum. A large dead space exists between the posterior surface of the L5–S1 intervertebral disc and the dural termination and thus a prolapsed disc can impinge on this space without modifying the opacified image of the subarachnoid space. This finding explains the lack of reliability of radiography of the cauda equina in the identification of a herniated L5–S1 disc in cases of a superior termination of the dural envelope (Louis 1961, 1966). This section also shows the special anterolateral direction of emergence of the S1 nerve root, whereas the suprajacent roots emerge laterally. This anterior course of the S1 root brings it near the L5–S1 intervertebral disc, whereas initial emergence behind the other roots would have led to considering this root less prone to minor discal prolapse.

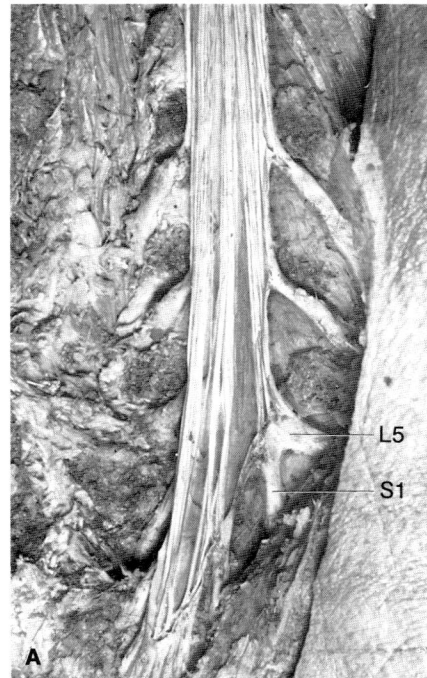

Figure 38 A–E

A   Posterior aspect of an anatomical specimen after laminectomy, showing the common trunk of L5 and S1
B   Horizontal section at L2–L3 with opacification of the subarachnoid space
C   Horizontal section at L3–L4
D   Horizontal section at L4–L5
E   Horizontal section at L5–S1

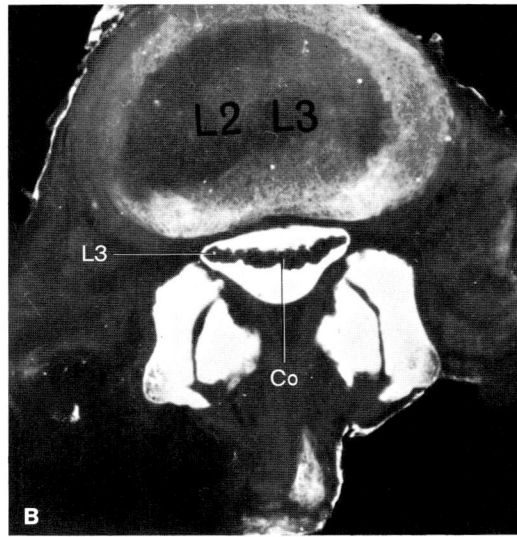

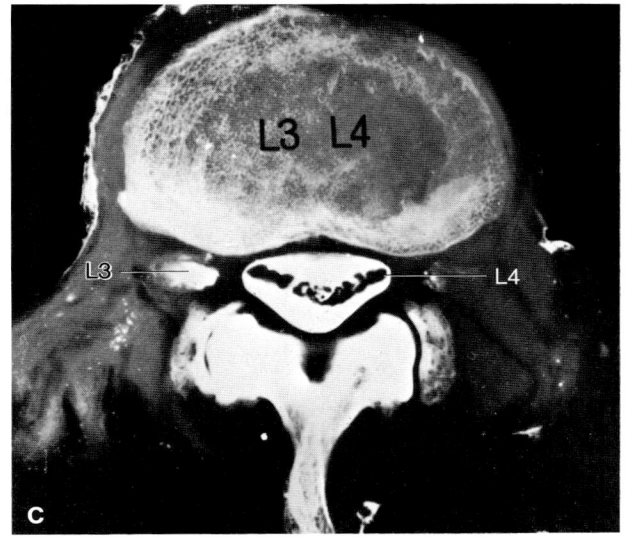

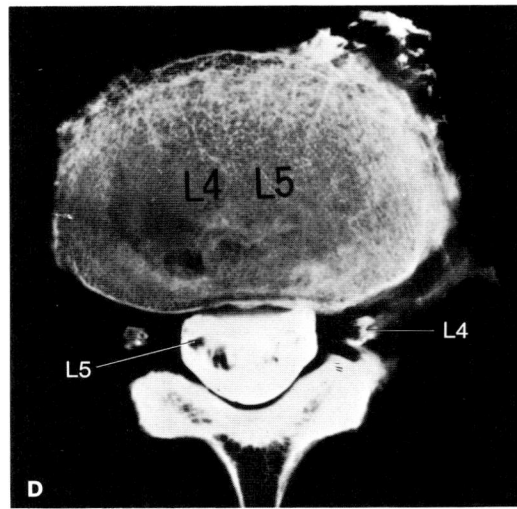

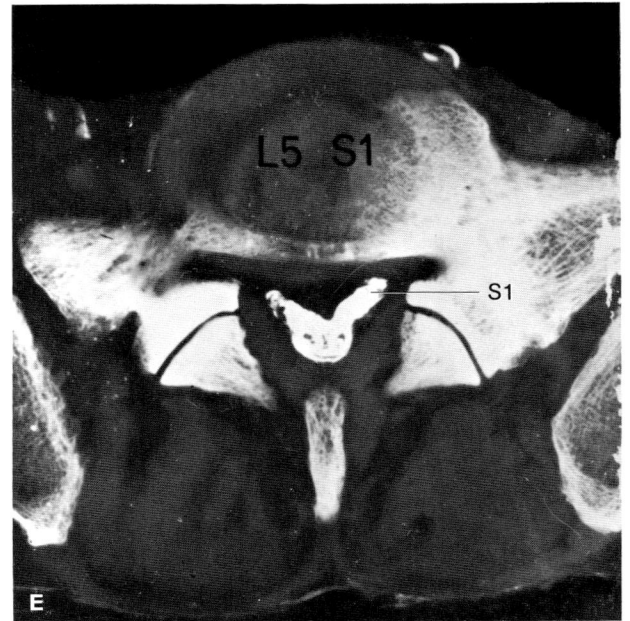

Figure 38 B–E

VI. Systematization of the Spinal Cord

The gray matter corresponds to the neuronal cell bodies grouped together in the center of the spinal cord, while the white matter is formed by the cell processes (dendrites and axons) lying in the peripheral part of the cord. Systematization of the medulla spinalis thus corresponds to the study of the functional sectors of the gray and white matter.

A. Gray Matter

The functional distribution of the gray matter can be explained by the embryological development of the spinal cord. The lamina alaris gives rise to the neurons relaying afferent somatosensory impulses, the lamina basalis to efferent somatomotor impulses, and the sulcus limitans to visceromotor and viscerosensory impulses.

1. Dorsal Horn or Somatosensory Zone

At this level the following structures can be successively described:
– The dorsolateral fasciculus (Lissauer's tract) which is the zone of passage of the sensory fibers of the dorsal spinal root towards the dorsal horn.
– The nucleus of the apical column (Waldeyer).
– The nucleus of the substantia gelatinosa (gelatinous substance of Rolando).
– The nucleus of the central posterior column (Crosby's dorsal funicular nucleus).
– Bekhterev's nucleus and the thoracic nucleus (Clark's column) occupy the isthmic zone (neck of the posterior horn). As opposed to the preceding nuclei, the thoracic nucleus is present in only that part of the spinal cord extending from C8 to L3.

2. Intermediate or Visceral Zone

The sulcus limitans gives rise to the intermediate zone of the gray matter displaying a vegetative visceral function. The dorsal sector of this zone is viscerosensory and the ventral sector visceromotor. Two nuclei can be identified in this zone:

– The intermediomedial nucleus extending the entire length of the spinal cord.
– The more external intermediolateral nucleus, which is discontinuous and cannot be found in the spinal cord swellings (appendiculer zones) corresponding to the nerves of the limbs (appendices).
  Numerous transverse anastomoses connect these two nuclei. Laruelle has described a partially vegetative and partially somatic column in the sacral spinal cord, i.e., the torsade column (nucleus dracuncularis), which is purportedly involved in the functions of child birth.

3. Ventral or Somatomotor Horn

According to Crosby and Kappers, the ventral horn contains several nuclei corresponding to different muscle groups:

The *median nuclei* correspond to the axial muscles; the mediodorsal nucleus for the extensor muscles of the spine and the medioventral nucleus for the flexor muscles of the head and trunk.

The *lateral nuclei* control the muscles of the shoulder and pelvic girdles and their respective limbs: the lateroventral nucleus for the proximal muscles of the girdles; the laterodorsal nucleus for the distal muscles of the forearms, hands, legs, and feet; and the retrodorsolateral nucleus for the small intrinsic muscles of the fingers and toes. It has been proposed that the neurons controlling extension and flexion lie in the anterior and posterior parts of the nuclei respectively.

The *central column* in each appendicular zone corresponds to the nuclei of the thoracoabdominal diaphragm and pelvic muscles (the phrenic nucleus from C3 to C7 and the lumbosacral nucleus from L2 to S2).

In the *cervical spinal cord* the spinal nucleus of the accessory nerve lies in contact with the medioventral nucleus from C1 to C6.
This heterogeneous distribution of the motor nuclei explains the topography of paralysis in acute anterior poliomyelitis due to viral infection of the ventral horns.

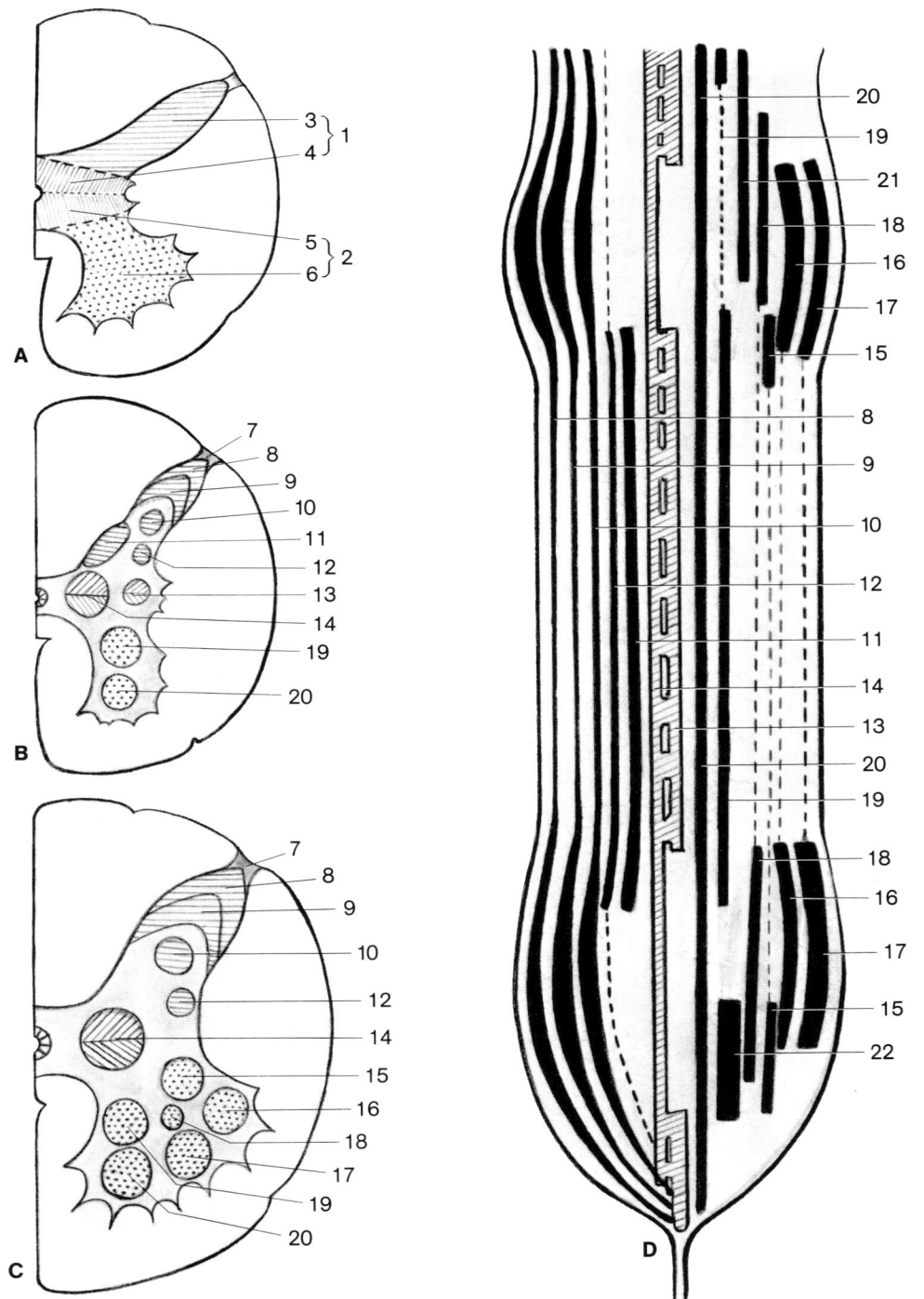

Figure 39 A–D

A   Functional sectors of the gray matter
B   Cellular structure of the thoracic gray matter
C   Cellular structure of the gray matter in the appendicular, cervical, and lumbosacral sectors
D   Parasagittal section of the spinal cord through the columns of the gray matter

1 lamina alaris, sensory   2 lamina basalis, motor   3 somatosensory zone   4 viscerosensory zone   5 somatomotor zone   6 visceromotor zone   7 fasciculus dorsolateralis   8 nucleus apicalis columnae   9 nucleus substantiae gelatinosae   10 nucleus centralis columnae post.   11 nucleus thoracicus   12 nucleus Bekhterevi   13 nucleus intermediolateralis   14 nucleus intermediomedialis   15 nucleus retrolaterodorsalis   16 nucleus laterodorsalis   17 nucleus lateroventralis   18 nucleus phrenicis and nucleus lumbosacralis   19 nucleus mediodorsalis   20 nucleus medioventralis   21 nucleus spinalis n. accessorii   22 nucleus Laruelli dracuncularis

The gray matter also contains reflex somatic and vegetative centers.

4. Reflex Somatic Centers

At each metameric level the spinal cord contains somatic reflex centers comprising reflex arcs between two neurons (one sensory and one motor neuron) and reflex arcs between three or more neurons (one sensory neuron, one or more associative or internuncial neurons, and one motor neuron). These reflexes react to percussion, stretching, or cutaneous stimulation and participate in the regulation of muscle tonus (myotatic or proprioceptive reflex) and defense reflex. An abnormal reflex on clinical examination signifies a lesion of the corresponding myelomere.

5. Vegetative Spinal Centers

Nerve supply to the viscera is ensured by the antagonistic sympathetic and parasympathetic systems. The centers of the parasympathetic system are located in the brain stem and sacral spinal cord. The sympathetic centers are found only in the thoracolumbar spinal cord (C8 to L4). These two systems function in similar fashion. Sensory afferents from the visceral organs and blood vessels display their cell body in the spinal ganglion and a relay in the viscerosensory zone of the neuraxis. The efferent impulses are transmitted by two neurons. The first, the preganglionic neuron, has its cell body in the neuraxis (the visceromotor zone in the spinal cord) and synapses with the second, postganglionic neuron, whose cell body is located in a vegetative ganglion (plexus autonomica) of the laterovertebral or prevertebral plexus. The second neuron terminates on a visceral muscle wall, in the secretory cells, or on the muscle wall of a blood vessel.
A series of sympathetic and parasympathetic centers can be identified in the intermediomedial and lateral columns of the intermediate zone of the gray matter. Knowledge of these centers affords better understanding of the vegetative syndromes due to spinal cord lesions and of the effects of rachianesthesia.

Sympathetic centers include:
- Budge's ciliospinal center (C8 to T3), involved in iridodilation, and the cardioaccelerator center (T1 to T4)
- Pilomotor, sudorific, and vasomotor centers (C8 to L2), involved in thermoregulation
- The bronchopulmonary center (T3 to T5), acting on the caliber and secretion of the bronchi
- The abdominal splanchnic center (T6 to L2), acting on the supramesocolic viscera, colon, and small bowel
- The center of anorectal and bladder continence (L2 to L4)
- The ejaculation center (L1 to L3)

Parasympathetic centers include:
- The center of anorectal expulsion or defecation (S1 to S2)
- The center of bladder expulsion or micturition (S3 to S4)
- The erection center (S2)

B. White Matter

The white matter is made up of three categories of nerve fibers; the radicular fibers, the associative fibers, and the fibers of projection. The different functions of the white matter can be ascribed to these types of fiber.

1. Radicular Fibers and the Reflex Spinal Cord

The sensory and motor neurons running through the spinal nerves and nerve roots and constituting reflex arcs between two or more neurons at each myelomere support the most elementary function of the spinal cord, the reflex. In fact, each radicular fiber articulates with two or three contiguous myelomeres. The human body can thus be divided into motor, sensory, and reflex metameric bands under the control of independent spinal segments.

2. Associative Fibers and the Spinal Cord as an Anatomical Unit

The connection between the reflex units and their horizontal radicular fibers is achieved by longitudinal associative fibers. Those displaying a vegetative function run through the gray matter, while others having a somatic function run through the white matter. There are both short and long fibers. The long descending and ascending fibers between distant myelomeres lie in the fasculi proprii of the posterior funiculi. The descending fibers form the fasciculus semilunaris (comma-shaped tract of Schultze) the fasciculus septomarginalis (oval tract of Flechsig), and the fasciculus triangularis (of Gombault and Philippe). The ascending fibers from the fasciculus proprius posterior (cornucommissural zone of Marie). The short descending and ascending associative fibers lie in the deep parts of the anterior and posterior funiculi to form the fasciculus proprius anterior and lateralis (the juxtagray zones). The associative fibers which link the 31 myelomeres with their reflex functions afford the creation of a spinal entity, a true anatomical and functional unit.

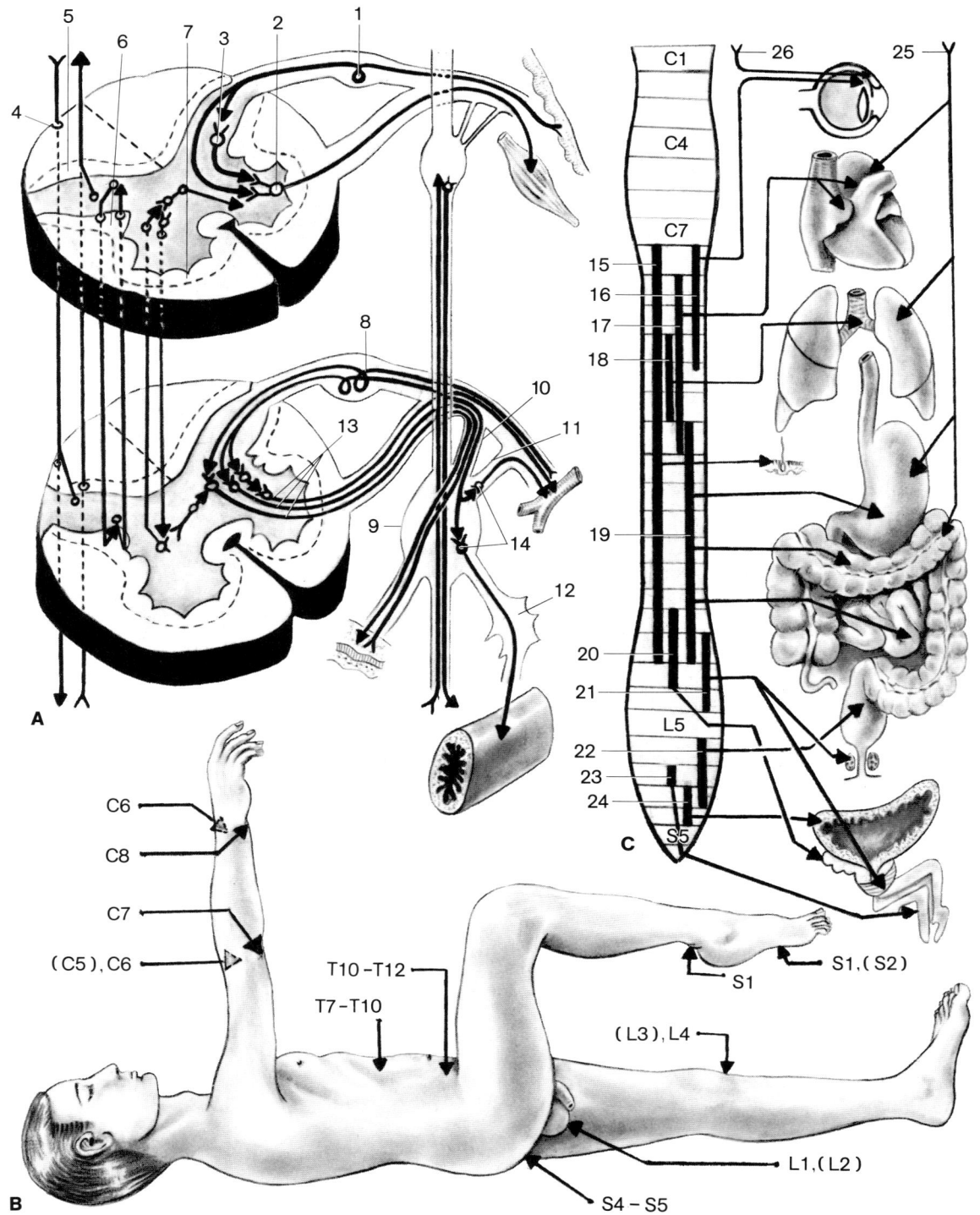

Figure 40 A–C

A Illustration of the medullary reflexes and associative and vegetative tracts
B The main somatic reflexes
C The vegetative centers of the spinal cord

1 sensory neuron *2* motor neuron *3* associative neuron
4 fasciculi proprii (semilunaris, septomarginalis, triangularis)
5 fasciculus proprius post. *6* fasciculus proprius lateralis *7* fasciculus proprius ant. *8* sensory vegetative neuron *9* ganglion trunci sympathici

10 ramus communicans albus *11* ramus communicans griseus
12 plexus autonomica *13* preganglionic neuron *14* postganglionic neuron *15* pilomotor, sudorific, and vasomotor centers
16 Budge's ciliospinal center *17* cardioaccelerator center
18 bronchopulmonary center *19* abdominal splanchnic center
20 ejaculation center *21* center of bladder and anorectal continence
22 defecation center *23* erection center *24* micturition center *25* n. vagus *26* ramus nuclei parasympathetici occulomotorii

Spinal cord function is subordinate to the higher centers in the brain which control each myelomere through ascending and descending fibers of projection.

3. Fibers of Projection: Spinal Cord Subordinate to the Brain

a) Ascending

Sensory messages arriving at the level of each myelomere are transmitted to the brain by the ascending fibers of projection. According to Sherrington and Head the following three types of sensibility can be described.

Exteroceptive sensibility arises from the ectodermal derivatives, essentially the skin. Three tracts are involved in the transmission of this information:
The fasciculus gracilis (Goll's tract) and cuneatus (Burdach's tract) transmit rapid pain. In the spinal cord, this pathway is represented by the peripheral neuron of the spinal ganglion which ascends on the same side as its origin.
The lateral spinothalamic tract transmits thermal sensibility and slow pain.
The ventral spinothalamic tract transmits the coarser protopathic tactile sensibility.
In the last two tracts, the peripheral neuron synapses with a second neuron whose cell body is located in the nucleus of the substantia gelatinosa, the nucleus apicalis columnae, and the central nucleus of the posterior column. The second neuron decussates prior to ascending in the middle part of the ventral funiculus, i.e., ascends on the side opposite its point of origin.

Proprioceptive Sensibility arises in derivatives of the mesoderm, i.e., bones, joints, muscles, and tendons, and is transmitted by two pathways, one conscious and the other unconscious:
The conscious proprioceptive pathway shares the fasciculus gracilis and cuneatus with the pathway for epicritic tactile sensitivity.
The unconscious proprioceptive pathway displays a peripheral neuron which synapses with a second neuron in the posterior horn. This second neuron can be of two types: lying in the thoracic nucleus (Clark's nucleus) and ascending without decussation in the dorsal spinocerebellar tract (Flechsig's tract) of the lateral funiculus, or located in Bekhterev's nucleus and decussating to ascend in the ventral spinocerebellar tract (Gower's tract) on the opposite side.

Interoceptive Sensibility refers to sensory impulses arising in the viscera (endodermal derivates). The peripheral neurons are located in the spinal ganglion and synapse with neurons in the intermediomedial and intermediolateral columns. These neurons then ascend with or without decussation in the spinotectal tract of the anterior funiculus.

b) Descending

The descending fibers, carrying motor impulses from the brain (cerebral cortex and basal ganglions), synapse with neurons in the ventral columns of the gray matter which transmit the impulses to the muscles. Two types of motricity, idiokinetic and holokinetic, can be described.

Idiokinetic motricity arises in the precentral gyrus (ascending frontal circumvolution) and corresponds to motor command of the delicate and precise movements of the small distal muscles of the limbs, facial expression, larynx, and tongue. These nerve impulses descend from the brain in the corticospinal (pyramidal) tract, which follows two routes in the spinal cord: the anterior (direct) pyramidal tract and the lateral (decussating) pyramidal tract. The lateral pyramidal tract arises in the decussation of the pyramids in the medulla oblongata and thus descends in the lateral funiculus on the side opposite its origin. It contains 70%–80% of the pyramidal motor fibers. The innermost fibers carry impulses to the cervical muscles, whereas progressively more lateral fibers transmit impulses to the thoracic, lumbar, and sacral regions. At the level of each myelomere the central neuron of the lateral pyramidal tract synapses with the peripheral neuron in the ventral horn on the same side. The anterior pyramidal tract contains 20%–30% of the pyramidal motor fibers and descends without decussating in the medulla oblongata. The central neuron of the anterior pyramidal tract decussates at the level of each myelomere to reach the ventral horn of the gray matter and muscles on the side opposite the cortical origin of the tract. Thus, almost all the fibers of the pyramidal tract carry impulses to the opposite side of the body with the exception of a small number (5%) of fibers in the ventral pyramidal tract (homolateral fibers).

Holokinetic or extrapyramidal motricity corresponds to the motor command of automatic movements accompanying precise voluntary movements. This type of motricity is transmitted by polyneuronal decussating tracts originating in the cortex and basal ganglia. The rubrospinal tract originates in the mesencephalic red nucleus; the anterior and lateral tectospinal tracts in the quadrigeminal tubercles; the anterior and lateral reticulospinal tracts in the reticular substance; the anterior and lateral vestibulospinal tracts in the vestibular nuclei; and the olivospinal tract in the olivary nucleus of the medulla oblongata.
In short, all the motor tracts decussate and terminate in the ventral horns of the spinal gray matter, referred to as Sherrington's final common pathway.

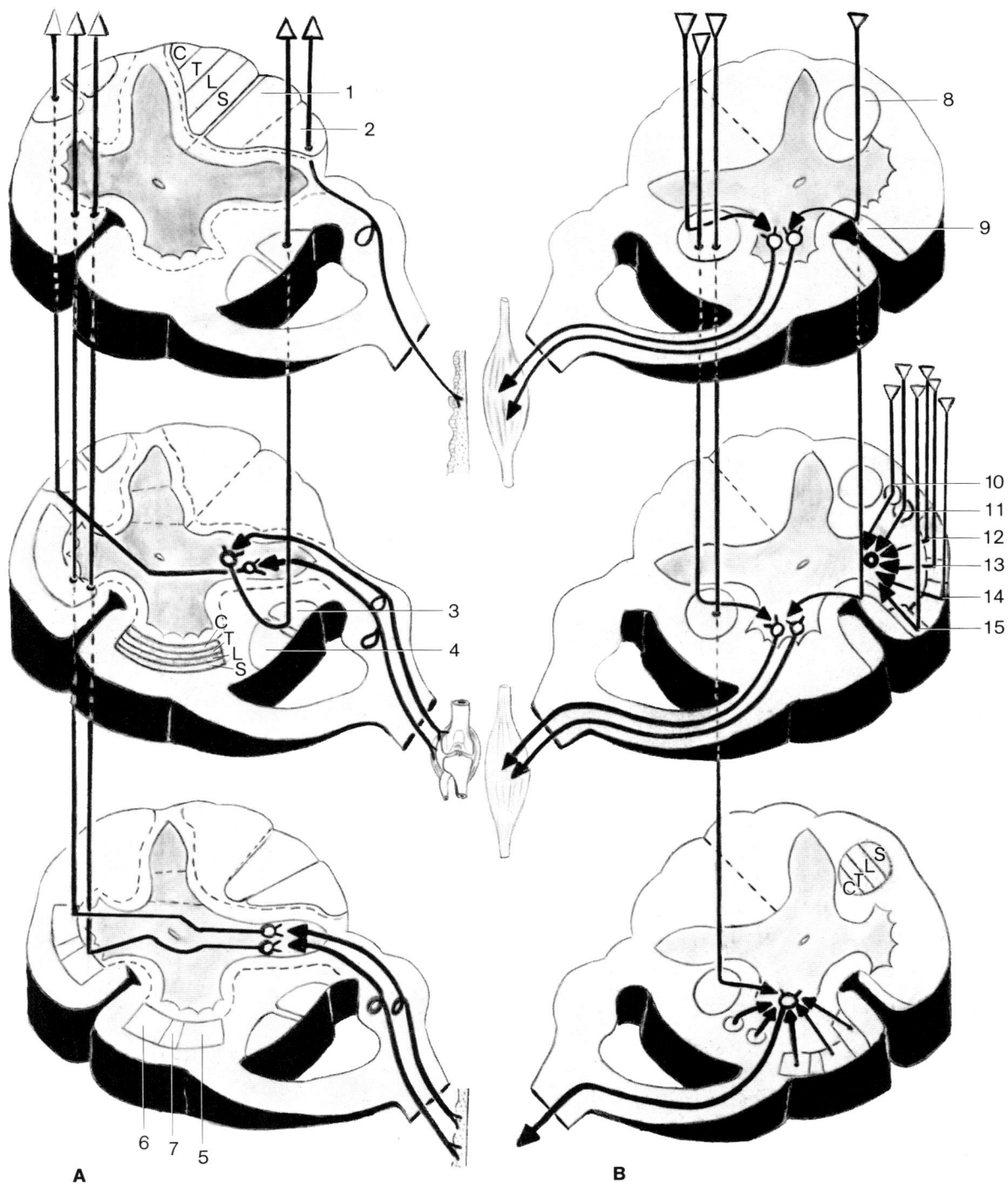

Figure 41 A,B

A   The ascending sensory tracts
B   The descending motor tracts

1 fasciculus gracilis 2 fasciculus cuneatus 3 tractus spinocerebellaris
post. 4 tractus spinocerebellaris ant. 5 tractus spinothalamicus
lateralis 6 tractus spinothalamicus ant. 7 tractus spinotectalis

8 tractus pyramidalis lateralis 9 tractus pyramidalis ant. 10 tractus
rubrospinalis 11 tractus tectospinalis lateralis and reticulospinalis
lateralis 12 tractus vestibulospinalis lateralis 13 tractus olivospinalis
14 tractus vestibulospinalis ant. 15 tractus tectospinalis ant. and
reticulospinalis ant.

C. Applied Pathology

Lesions of the spinal ganglion and the dorsal funiculi, e.g., in the course of tabes dorsalis, cause major disturbances of proprioception with motor incoordination (ataxia). Cavitation in the central region of the spinal cord due to syringomyelia leads to paradoxical sensory dissociation, i.e., only thermoalgesia is abolished owing to the destruction of the spinothalamic decussation in the region of the central canal. In surgery for pain the dorsal spinothalamic tract can be sectioned in the upper cervical region (Frazier's ventrolateral tractotomy). Lesions of the idiokinetic motor pathways (lateral pyramidal tract) above the medulla oblongata cause contralateral hemiplegia, whereas lesions below this level, in the spinal cord, lead to ipsilateral hemiplegia. Unilateral lesions of the spinal cord result in Brown-Séquard's syndrome with paralysis on the side of the lesion and thermoalgesic anesthesia on the opposite side of the body. Infarction in the center of the spinal cord extending to the deep fibers of the lateral pyramidal tract causes motor disturbances of the upper but not the lower limbs (Schneider's syndrome). Lesions involving the full width of the spinal cord in the cervical region cause tetraplegia and in the thoracolumbosacral region paraplegia.

VII. Sensorimotor Areas of the Spinal Cord

The primitive metamerization of the spinal cord allows the identification of areas relating to cutaneous sensitivity (dermatomes) and muscular motricity (myotomes). In fact the metamerization is rather complex, since each cutaneous or muscular area of the spinal cord is related to an average of three spinal segments. Accordingly, an isolated lesion of a spinal nerve only causes partial anesthesia or paralysis in the corresponding part of the body. Total anesthesia and paralysis of a sector of the body straddling two metameres results only from the lesional involvement of at least two contiguous spinal nerves.

A. Dermatomes

The metameric topography of the sensory areas of the spinal cord is shown on the facing page. Knowledge of the following dermatomes is essential to reconstitute the general arrangement of these sensory areas. The upper part of the neck and nuchal region correspond to C2, the scapular girdle to C4, the xiphoid appendix to T6, the umbilicus to T10, the inguinal region to L1, and the perianal region to S3, S4, and S5. In the upper limb the thumb corresponds to C6, the index and middle fingers to C7, and the fourth and fifth fingers to C8. In the lower limb the anterior surface of the thigh and knee corresponds to L3 and L4, the greater toe to L5, and the heel and fifth toe to S1.

B. Myotomes

A given muscle is rarely innervated by a single spinal nerve root (save the intercostal muscles). The muscles generally receive their innervation from two to three nerve roots, of which one is dominant. The following description is limited to the dominant nerve roots of the muscles which are the most useful to know for the interpretation of peripheral neurological syndromes:

- C4 innervates the diaphragm
- C5 innervates the shoulder muscles
- C6 innervates the anterior muscles of the arm
- C7 innervates the posterior muscles of the arm and forearm
- C8 innervates the anterior muscles of the forearm and the thenar eminence
- T1 innervates the muscles of the hypothenar eminence
- T6 to T12 innervate the anterolateral wall of the abdomen
- L1 to L3 innervate the flexor and adductor muscles of the hips
- L3 and L4 innervate the quadriceps muscle
- L5 innervates the extensors of the foot and first toe and the peroneus muscle
- S1 innervates the triceps surae muscles
- L4, L5, and S1 innervate the gluteal muscles
- S1 and S2 innervate the semitendinus, semimembranosus, and biceps femoris
- Only the spinal muscles are innervated by practically all the nerve roots from C1 to S3

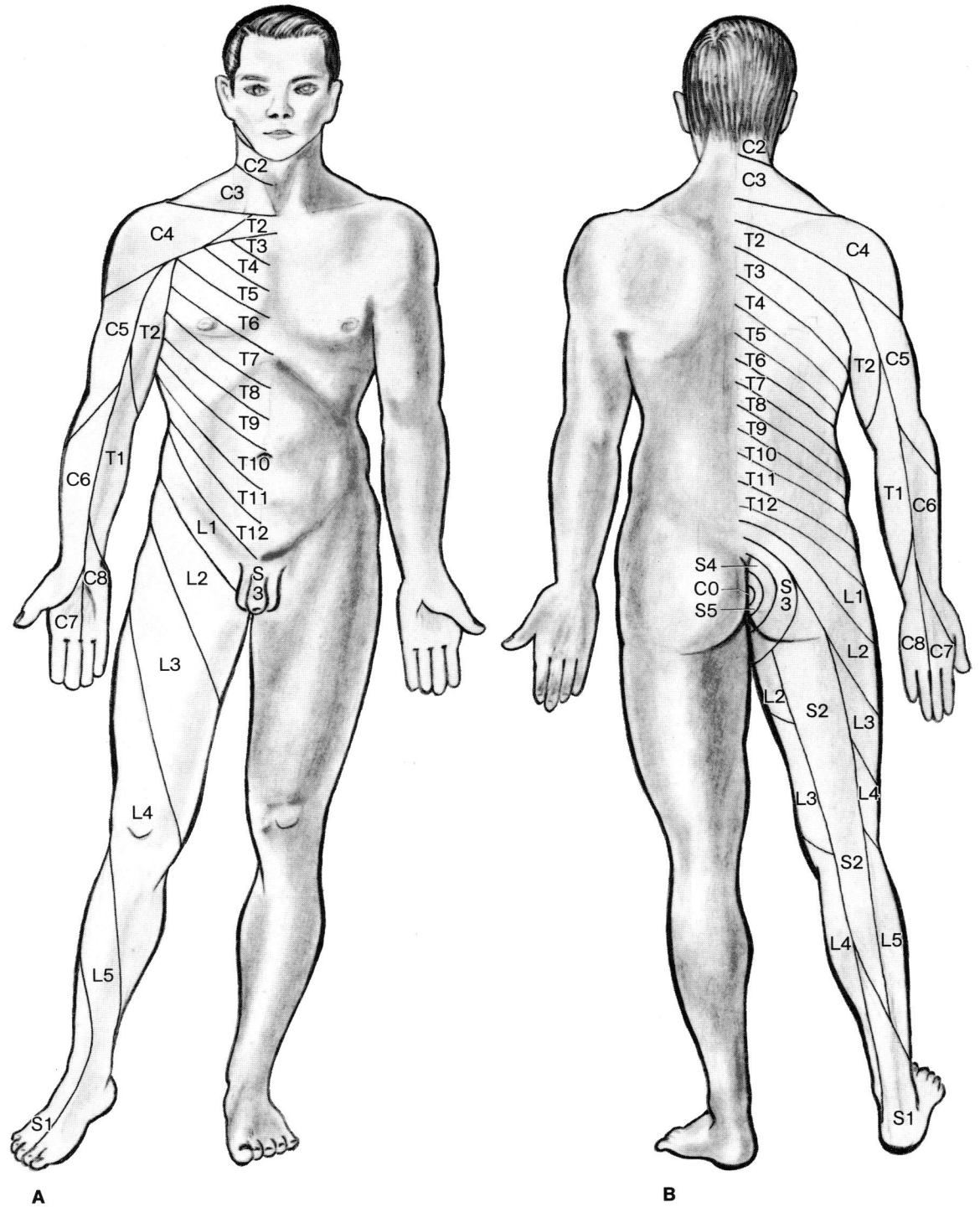

Figure 42 A, B

A   The spinal nerve dermatomes on the anterior aspect of the body

B   The dermatomes on the posterior aspect of the body

VIII. Intrinsic Innervation of the Spine

The osteoarticular ligamentous, meningeal, and vascular constituents of the spine are innervated by the spinal nerves and the laterovertebral sympathetic trunk. These nerve fibers form very fine rami of which full detailed descriptions are lacking. Despite this fact, data from classical and more recent studies allow a sufficiently detailed description for the understanding of different pathological processes. The intrinsic innervation of the spine has a general layout common to all levels of the spine with certain regional variations.

A. General Layout

Three groups of rami innervate the spine: the dorsal rami of the spinal nerves, the meningeal nerve, and rami from the sympathetic trunk.

The *dorsal rami of the spinal nerves* (dorsospinal branch) originate at the outlet of the intervertebral foramina, and are much smaller in caliber than the anterior rami. Each dorsal ramus runs between the transverse processes towards the vertebral arches by skirting the posterior articulations, and after passing over the outer surface of the articulation in contact with the articular capsule divides into medial and lateral rami. The medial ramus innervates the zygapophyseal articulation, the ligamentum flavum, the inter- and supraspinous ligaments, and the medial part of the spinal muscles and the dorsal cutaneous region of the neck, trunk, and buttocks. The lateral ramus supplies the intertransverse ligaments and muscles, iliolumbar ligaments, sacroiliac joints, and the lateral part of the spinal muscles and dorsal skin. These observations are based on studies by Lazorthes (1956), Bradley (1974), Yinchuan (1978), and Bogduk and Long (1979).

The *meningeal nerve* (Luschka's sinuvertebral nerve) arises distal to the intervertebral foramen and in front of the spinal nerve. It is formed by the confluence of two rami, one coming from the sympathetic trunk, the other from the spinal nerve. It traverses the intervertebral foramen and extends to the anterior part of the vertebral canal, giving off branches to the dura mater, the posterior spinal ligament, the superficial and posterior parts of the anulus fibrosus, the intraspinal venous plexuses, and the prearticular part of the ligamentum flavum.

Our work with Serrano Vela (1973) has shown that the anterior spinal ligament and the superficial part of the anulus fibrosus are innervated by *vegetative nerve fibers originating in the sympathetic trunk*. In common with all authors who have studied the innervation of the intervertebral disc, we have found no nerve fibers in the deepest part of the anulus fibrosus or of course in the region of the nucleus pulposus.

B. Regional Variations

1. Cervical

In the cervical region cerebrospinal nerve distribution (dorsal rami) is typically metameric, whereas vegetative nerve distribution is less so. The vegetative fibers emanate from either the sympathetic trunk or the vertebral nerve (Franck's nerve). The latter, originating in the stellate ganglion, innervates and accompanies the vertebral artery through the transverse foramina. This mixed cerebrospinal and vegetative nerve supply clearly grouped around a mobile spinal segment may account for the possible physiopathological subjective interactions between traumatic ligamentous and muscular lesions (cervical sprain or whiplash injury) on one hand, and the symptoms relating to the vertebral artery on the other hand. This type of nerve distribution also sheds light on the phenomenon of referred pain, i.e., pain referred to a cutaneous region at some distance from the exact site of the lesions. A lesion of a ligament or muscle supplied by a dorsal ramus may be cortically sensed in part of the ventral area (radicular dermatome) of the same spinal nerve.

2. Thoracic and Lumbar

Below the upper thoracic spine the horizontal arrangement of the branches of the dorsal rami gives way to a progressively more oblique arrangement. Accordingly, the dorsal rami of T12 terminate in the skin of the superior part of the buttock, thus allowing Maigne to describe the painful syndrome of the thoracolumbar junction with pain referred to the gluteal region. Similarly, the meningeal rami in the lumbar region supply the area of two to three vertebrae. The dorsal rami of the spinal nerves give off a medial branch which runs in the osteofibrous groove, the latter sometimes being replaced by a canal between the mamillary and accessory processes. The medial branch gives off a superior branch to the posterior articulation at the same level as the meningeal ramus, and further down an inferior branch to the subjacent posterior joint. Consequently, the innervation of the posterior articulations is not of the monoradicular type. The deep anterior surface of the posterior joints is also supplied by fibers from the meningeal rami, rendering surgical denervation impossible. Pain from the dorsal rami may be referred to the lumbosacral region, thus mistakenly suggesting the presence of radicular lesions.

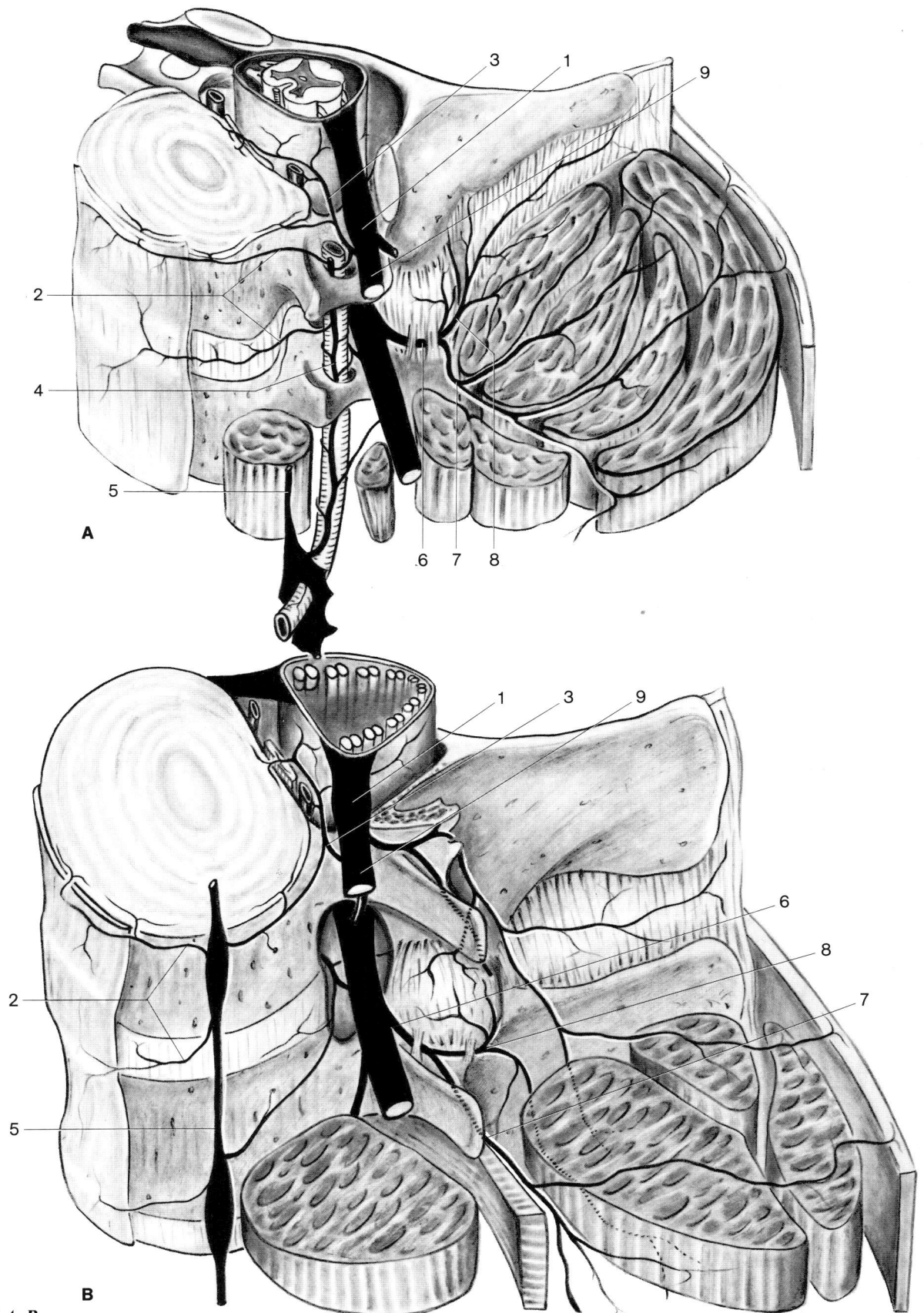

Figure 43 A, B

A   Intrinsic innervation of the cervical spine
B   Intrinsic innervation of the lumbar spine

1 n. spinalis   *2* rami ventralis trunci sympathici   *3* ramus meningeus
4 n. vertebralis   *5* truncus sympathicus   *6* ramus dorsalis n. spinalis
7 ramus lateralis   *8* ramus medialis   *9* ramus ventralis n. spinalis

IX. Osteoneuromeningeal Spinal Dynamics

A. Classical Concepts of Neuromeningeal Dynamics

Much thought has been devoted to the adaptive potential of the neuromeningeal structures within the vertebral canal during movements of the spine. The dynamic possibilities of the spine, especially during extreme movements of flexion-extension or inclination-rotation, are such that it is logical to conclude that the neuromeningeal structures must adapt to these movements. Two types of concept have been advanced in this respect. According to O'Connel, Frykholm, Chamberlain, Young, and Charnley, dynamic adaptation occurs by the physical displacement of the nerves and meninges within the vertebral canal. According to Breig (1960), adaptation is based on the plasticity of the neuromeningeal structures, i.e., the osteoneuromeningeal relations do not vary whatever the direction and amplitude of the spinal movements. This author explained such plasticity as being related to the microscopic undulation of the neuronal processes deep to the pia mater when the vertebral canal is shortened, and to their rectilinear stretching during movements, causing elongation of the vertebral canal.

B. Personal Studies (1964 and 1966)

We examined the problems related to osteoneuromeningeal dynamics by studying over 50 fresh adult cadavers (25- to 45-year-old subjects) 24 h after death and conserved at 4°C without tissue fixation. The initial study technique involved the radiological opacification of the subarachnoid space to identify the spinal nerves and cord with the spine in different positions. Similarly, certain radiological preparations were made by placing metal clips on the meninges after laminectomy, but the errors of parallax inherent to the divergent X-ray beam rendered measurement impossible with displacement of only a few millimeters. We therefore opted for a direct method of measurement, with the vertebral canal opened after removal of the vertebral arches (the pedicles being left intact). Metals pins implanted in the pedicles enabled us to stretch a thread transversely between each pair of pedicles at every spinal level. Knotted threads on the meninges, nerve roots, and spinal cord with the spine erect were placed so that the knots coincided with the interpedicular threads. Movements of the spine including hyperflexion and hyperextension were performed, and observations were made with the naked eye and by photography. A narrow opening over a short spinal segment was used in some cases to verify that the large posterior exposure did not modify the osteoneuromeningeal relations. In this way 24 cadavers yielded valid data.

C. Dynamics of the Vertebral Canal

During movements of flexion the vertebral canal lengthens, as evidenced by the stretching of the posterior surface of the intervertebral discs and the ligamenta flava (Bradford and Sturling 1947). The increased length of the vertebral canal is thus the sum of these intervertebral displacements at each level. Conversely, extension results in a decrease of the length of the vertebral canal (Breig). Although the difference in length of the canal between these two extremes varies according to individuals, it is always in the order of several centimeters (5–9.7 cm). The intraspinal structures must consequently adapt to these changes in length.

When the spine is flexed the posterior surface of each intervertebral disc is flattened. Conversely, during extension the posterior surface protrudes; the magnitude of the protrusion varying according to the age and spinal level of the individual subject (Chamberlain and Young 1939). Furthermore, the ligamenta flava undergo the same modifications as the discs (Taylor 1951), i.e., stretching on flexion and shortening on extension to form a protruding ridge at the posterior surface of the vertebral canal, especially in the lower cervical region. Rotation of the head contracts the vertebral canal at the level of the C1–C2 intervertebral space (Breig).

The following table shows that the amplitude of movement between the erect position and hyperflexion varies considerably according to the level of the intervertebral spaces.

The data given in the table are the mean amplitudes measured in the nine most recently studied spines.

Occ–C1 =	− 1.5 mm	T 2–T 3 =	1.5 mm	T11–T12 =	1 mm
C1–C2 =	0 mm	T 3–T 4 =	1 mm	T12–L 1 =	2 mm
C2–C3 =	1 mm	T 4–T 5 =	1 mm	L 1–L 2 =	2.5 mm
C3–C4 =	2.5 mm	T 5–T 6 =	0 mm	L 2–L 3 =	3.5 mm
C4–C5 =	5 mm	T 6–T 7 =	0 mm	L 3–L 4 =	5 mm
C5–C6 =	6.5 mm	T 7–T 8 =	− 1 mm	L 4–L 5 =	9 mm
C6–C7 =	8 mm	T 8–T 9 =	− 1 mm	L 5–S 1 =	10 mm
C7–T1 =	6 mm	T 9–T10 =	− 1 mm	S 1–S 2 =	0 mm
T1–T2 =	5 mm	T10–T11 =	0 mm		

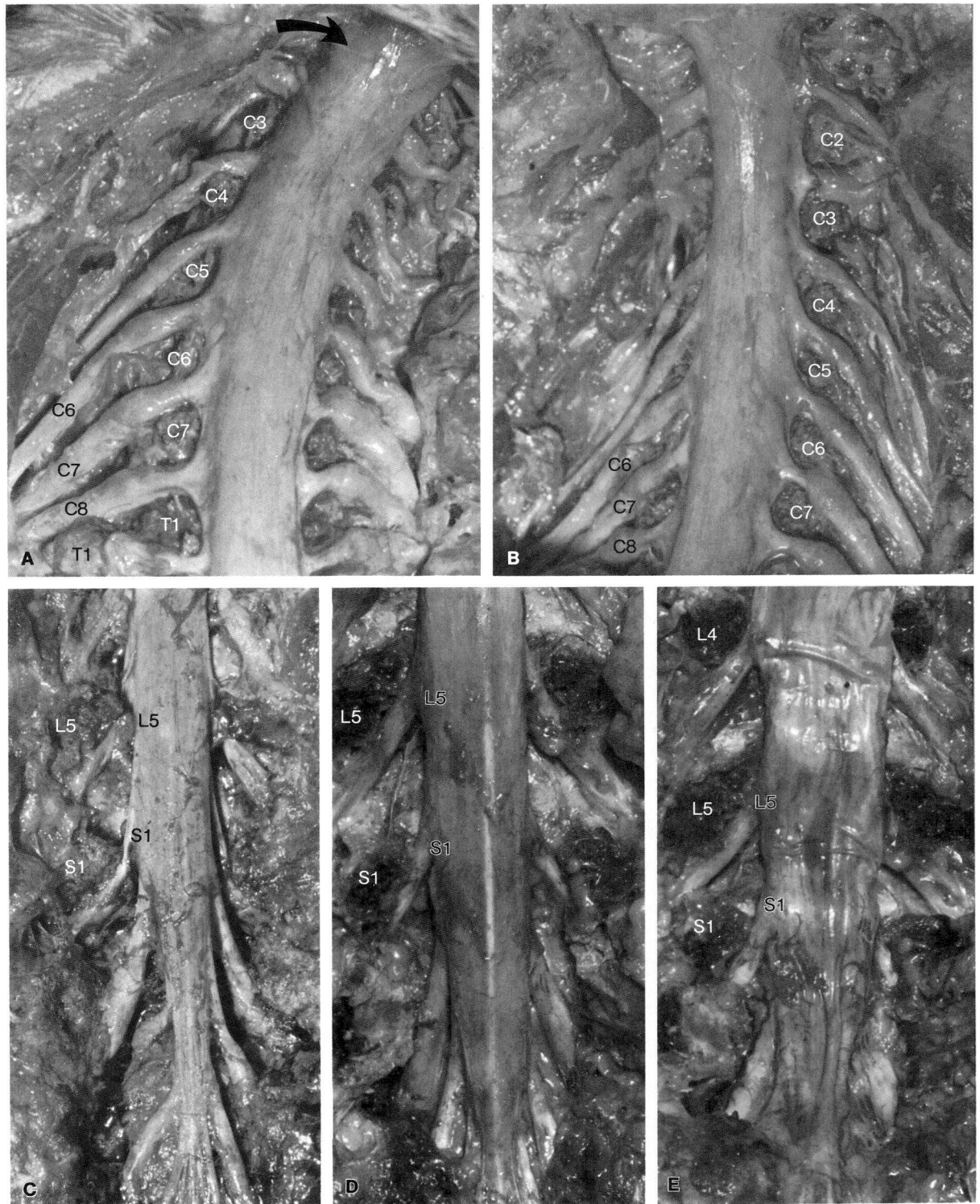

Figure 44 A–E

A Posterior aspect of the cervical dural envelope and cervical nerves in right lateroflexion after removal of the posterior arches

B The same preparation as in *A* with the cervical spine in the erect position. The cut edge of the pedicles is visible between the spinal nerves

C–E Posterior aspect of the dural envelope and spinal nerves in the lumbosacral region in hyperflexion, erect position, and hyperextension. Anatomical specimen after removal of the posterior arches but preservation of the pedicles

The nerves are labeled in *black* and the pedicles in *white*.

In some individuals the mobility of the lumbosacral junction is greater at the level of the L4–L5 intervertebral space than at the L5–S1 level (Delmas and Raou 1952). The lengthening of the vertebral canal between the erect position and flexion varies according to the regions of the spine: mean lengthening in the cervical region is 28 mm, in the thoracic region only 3 mm, and in the lumbar region 28 mm. At the level of certain thoracic intervertebral spaces shortening of the canal occurs on flexion, due to the compression of the corresponding discs. The discs which undergo the greatest stretching on flexion are those in the most mobile spinal regions, i.e., the cervicothoracic and lumbosacral junctions.

In the course of hyperextension the vertebral canal shortens by up to 15 mm in the cervical region and 20 mm in the lumbosacral region in the most flexible spines. The thoracic spine undergoes very little shortening (3 mm).

In the spines we studied, the addition of lengthening in hyperflexion and shortening in hyperextension yields a mean total variability of 97 mm. However, the experimental conditions with suppression of the posterior articulations and posterior ligaments allowed a maximum range of mobility, which is attained in vivo only in cases of acrobatic flexibility or during accidents of hyperflexion or hyperextension.

D. Meningeal Dynamics

During *movements of hyperextension* the dural envelope is marked by transverse plications, mainly in the region of the interlaminar spaces, and its caliber clearly increases transversely and anteroposteriorly. During *movements of hyperflexion* the dural envelope lengthens and its surface becomes smooth and stretched, while its caliber decreases transversely and anteroposteriorly.

Between the positions of extreme hyperextension and hyperflexion the dura mater displays stretching and sliding along the walls of the vertebral canal. These phenomena are similar and most pronounced in the two regions of greatest mobility and lordosis, i.e., the cervical and lumbosacral regions. Conversely, they are practically nonexistent in the poorly mobile thoracic spine displaying kyphosis. For the sake of brevity, only data concerning the lumbosacral dura mater are given below.

A total variation in length of 50.4 mm of the lumbosacral canal (T12 to S1) results in a 39.3 mm change in the length of the lumbosacral dural envelope subjacent to the T12–L1 intervertebral disc (22.5 mm in extension and 16.8 mm in flexion). Thus there is an 11-mm difference between the variations in length of the vertebral canal and dural envelope. This difference is compensated by two phenomena, the cranial ascension of the dural termination and the caudal stretching of the thoracic dura mater. During extension the termination of the dural envelope moves as much as 2 mm caudally, whereas hyperflexion causes a mean displacement in the cranial direction of 5 mm.

The different points of reference (knotted sutures) on the lumbosacral dura mater were displaced on hyperflexion to converge at a given vertebral level, which varied between individuals. Convergence was most of often noted at the level of the L5–S1 intervertebral space and in some cases at the L4–L5 or L3–L4 intervertebral space. In the course of hyperextension in our experiments, the dural points of reference either remained at the same level as in the erect position or displayed caudal displacement of 1–2 mm.

Study of the variations in length of each metameric segment of the spinal dura mater shows significant differences according to the level of the spine. Lengthening and thus stretching of the lumbosacral dural segments increases in the segments closest to the most mobile region, i.e., the L5–S1 region. Accordingly the dural segment at L1–L2 undergoes a 15% variation in length, whereas at L5–S1 this value is 30%. These phenomena can be explained by likening the spinal dura mater to a sort of rope of lumbosacral lordosis so that hyperflexion, which effaces the lordosis, stretches the dura mater, especially at the level of greatest mobility (L5–S1), thus leading to degressive stretching from this point towards the upper and lower ends of the lordotic region.

In the cervical region the site of convergence of the dura mater points of reference is most often near the C5–C6 intervertebral space and in some cases near C4–C5.

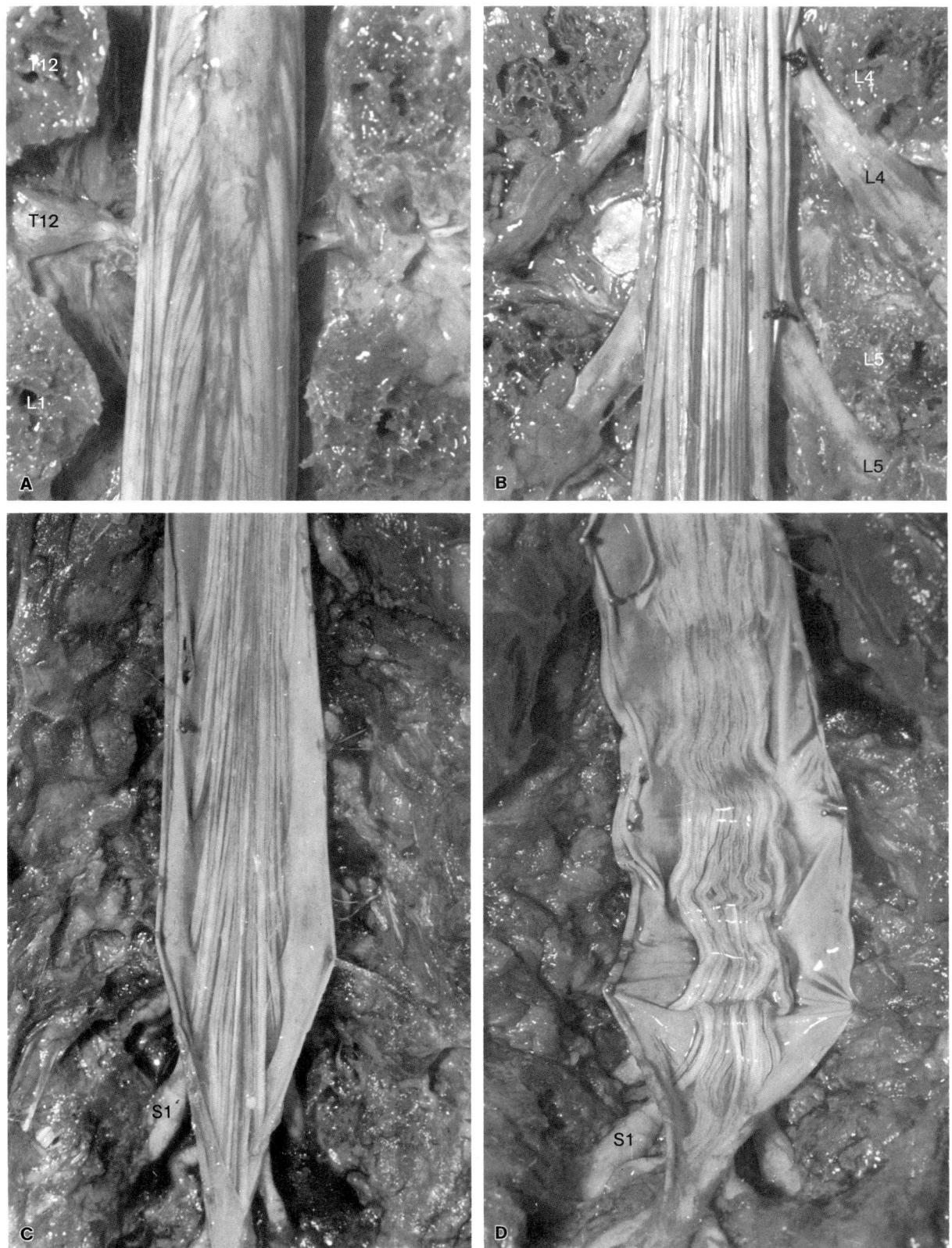

Figure 45 A–D

A   Posterior aspect of the conus medullaris on hyperflexion. Note the horizontalization of the T12 nerve roots deviating with respect to the pedicles

B   Posterior aspect of the cauda equina on hyperflexion. Note the stretching of the nerve roots below L4 and their position against the pedicles

C   Stretched aspect of the roots of the cauda equina on hyperflexion after posterior opening of the dura mater

D   Same specimen as in C, but in extension. Note the distended and undulated appearance of the nerve roots

The nerves are labeled in *black* and the pedicles in *white*.

E. Radicular Dynamics

The following discussion of radicular dynamics begins with the mobility of the lumbosacral nerve roots, followed by the cervical and thoracic roots.

1. Lumbosacral Nerve Roots

During the *movements of extension* the lumbosacral nerve roots display regular undulations and distension in the subarachnoid space. In the epidural region up to the outlet of the intervertebral foramen the tension on each spinal root and nerve relaxes and the nerves diverge with respect to the pedicles.

In the course of *hyperflexion* the spinal roots in the cauda equina undergo more complex phenomena, including changes in length and direction and axial displacement.

Changes in Length. We measured separately the changes in length in the subarachnoid and subdural segments of the spinal nerve roots. The subarachnoid segment (pars subarachnoideale) extends from the medullary emergence of the nerve roots to the point where they traverse the dura mater. The subdural segment corresponds to the region between their dural site of emergence and their point of fusion distal to the spinal ganglion. Although the changes in length are comparable from one subject to another, mean values cannot be given due to individual differences in height and spinal mobility. The following table shows the changes in radicular length measured in one postmortem specimen.

Nerve root	Subarachnoid segment (mm)	Subdural segment (mm)	Total (mm)
L1	− 7	− 10	+ 17
L2	− 2	− 6	− 8
L3	+ 5	− 5	0
L4	+ 8	0	+ 8
L5	+ 11	+ 3	+ 14
S1	+ 18	+ 2	+ 20
S2	+ 28	+ 1	+ 29

In short the L3 nerve root, which retains the same length as in the erect position, constitutes a borderline between the suprajacent roots, which shorten and undulate, and the subjacent roots undergoing progressive stretching in the caudal direction. Accordingly, the roots displaying the greatest stretching, such as S2, present a 16% increase in length when the spine is hyperextended from the resting position.

Axial Displacement. As previously described in the cases of the meningeal structures, the differences between the lengthening of the vertebral canal and nerve roots leads to axial sliding in the cranial or caudal direction, the magnitude of which varies according to individual mobility and the radicular level under consideration. When the most mobile intervertebral disc is one of the three most caudal lumbar discs then the most frequent site of convergence of the nerve roots is at the L4–L5 disc. Accordingly the nerve roots above this level, i.e., above the L4 root, are pulled and slide caudally during hyperflexion, whereas the subjacent nerve roots, i.e., L5, S1, S2, S3, S4, S5, and the coccygeal root, are stretched and slide cranially. The magnitude of sliding varies according to the level of the spine, but can attain 10–12 mm in the intervertebral foramina in the case of roots L5 and S1, as confirmed by the studies of Charnley.

Changes in Direction. We measured the caudal angle formed by the subdural segment of each spinal nerve root in order to compare the changes in direction induced by hyperflexion and hyperextension. The following table illustrates these changes in one case.

Nerve root	Flexion	Extension
T12	100°	50°
L1	90°	52°
L2	60°	44°
L3	40°	44°
L4	30°	40°
L5	16°	32°
S1	13°	34°
S2	17°	28°

These results show that the nerve roots above L3 tend to take on a more horizontal position when the spine passes from extension to flexion, whereas the subjacent nerve roots tend to lie more vertically. This phenomenon is related to the fact that the site of dural emergence of each nerve root constitutes a point of fixation prohibiting sliding of the nerve root where it traverses the dura mater. Consequently, the displacements of the dura mater converge generally near L4–L5, thus pulling caudally the point of dural emergence of the nerve roots above the L4 root, i.e., these roots come to lie more horizontally and diverge with respect to the upper pedicle of their corresponding intervertebral foramen. The inverse phenomenon involves the nerve roots below the L4 root, which are pressed against the inner surface of the upper pedicle of the corresponding intervertebral foramen.

When Lasègue's sign is sought unilaterally, the homolateral lumbosacral nerve roots are stretched and pull the cauda equina and dural envelope toward the side of the maneuver. The nerve roots on the opposite side undergo distension. The tension applied to the sciatic nerve and its branches is transmitted by the intervertebral foramina. The maneuver increases the tension and pressure of the nerve roots against the walls of the vertebral canal, thus causing exacerbation of the pain in cases of radicular compression due to a herniated intervertebral disc. This maneuver performed bilaterally and simultaneously is the equivalent of hyperflexion of the lumbosacral spine.

Subsequent to surgery of the lumbosacral canal, axial mobility of the nerve roots of the cauda equina must be maintained to avoid the painful sequelae of epiduritis. This can be achieved by exercises comprising elevation of the lower limbs alternately while standing.

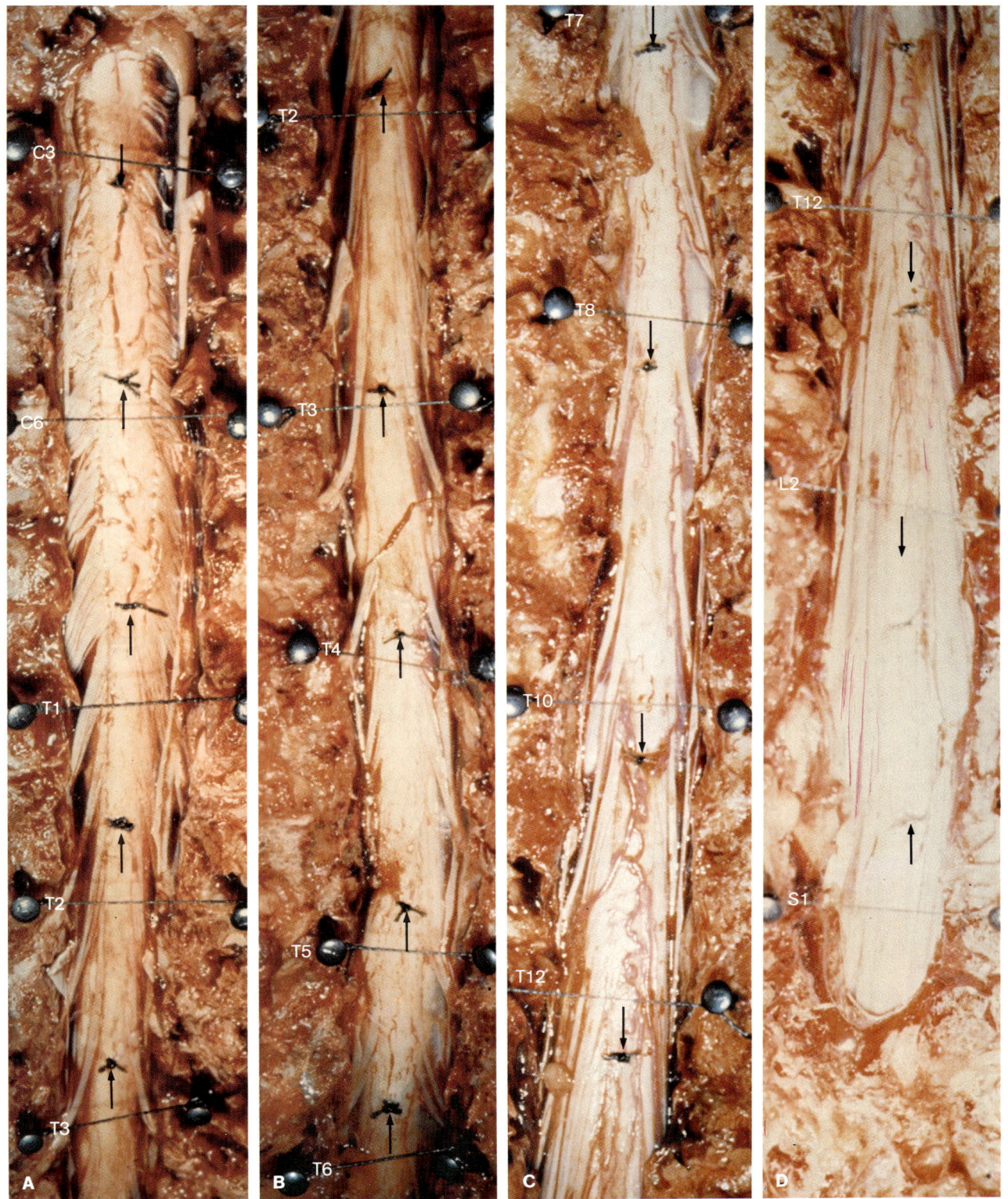

Figure 46 A–D. Experimental total hyperflexion of the spine after removal of the posterior structures. The vertebral canal originates on the *upper left* of the photograph (foramen magnum) and terminates at the sacral canal on the *lower right*. Prior to hyperflexion the points of reference on the spinal cord *(knotted threads)* coincided with the *threads* stretched between the pedicles. Displacement of the myelomeres is towards the C5–C6 and L4–L5 regions

2. Cervical Nerve Roots

The previously described phenomena also occur in the cervical spine: the nerve roots distend with extension, on the same side as lateral flexion, whereas with hyperflexion they stretch, on the side opposite lateral flexion. These phenomena account for the rupture of the nerve roots of the brachial plexus due to trauma with hyperlateroflexion of the head. The point of convergence of axial displacement is at C4–C5 or C5–C6 according to the individual.

3. Thoracic Nerve Roots

The thoracic nerve roots are also affected by spinal movements and display centrifugal axial displacement relative to the zenith of thoracic kyphosis at T6. Hyperflexion stretches the nerve roots and tends to decrease the horizontalization of the subdural segment of roots T1 to T6, whereas roots T7 to T12 display a more horizontal direction of the subdural segment.

F. Medullary Dynamics

The spinal cord, like the nerve roots, must adapt to the variations in length of the vertebral canal (5–9.7 mm). The changes in spinal length and curvature are transmitted to the spinal cord by its continuity with the nonmobile brain at the level of the foramen magnum, by the filum terminale and roots of the cauda equina at the level of the conus medullaris, and by the cervical and thoracic roots, dura mater, and denticulate ligament along the walls of the vertebral canal. The CSF also participates in the mobility of the spinal cord by enveloping it and by acting as a sort of "hydraulic cushion" (Aboulker).

During *forced extension* of the spine the spinal cord displays fine plications near the pia mater and its caliber increases in relation to its length, which decreases without axial sliding.

During *forced flexion* of the spine the different segments of the spinal cord, like those of the dura mater, undergo axial displacement towards the most mobile vertebrae of the cervical (C6) and lumbar (L4) regions. It should be noted that the osteomeningomedullary relations remain unchanged at these levels. The zones of greatest medullary displacement with respect to the walls of the vertebral canal are located at C1 (7 mm caudal displacement), T1 (7 mm cranial displacement), and L1 (10 mm caudal displacement). The zones of least sliding (practically nil) are situated at the zeniths of cervical lordosis (C6) and thoracic kyphosis (T6). The axial sliding due to stretching forces on the spinal cord is accompanied by zones of tension varying according to the myelomeres.

Two regions of the spinal cord, the inferior parts of the cervical (C6 to T2) and lumbar (L4 to the coccyx) swellings, are submitted to the greatest forces of stretching. The former can be accounted for by its correspondence to the zone of greatest cervical mobility (C5 to T1) and the latter by transmission to the conus medullaris of the stretching forces to which the lower lumbosacral roots (below L4) are submitted. When the vertebral canal lengthens 59 mm between the erect position and hyperflexion, the spinal cord is stretched by one tenth its total length, e.g., 43 mm for a 43 cm spinal cord. However, since the stretching of the cord is not equally distributed, the zones of maximum elongation are stretched by one fifth their resting length. Finally, the middle thoracic region of the spinal cord corresponds to a zone of practically zero stretching.

These notions of vertebromedullary dynamics shed light on certain pathological phenomena. Due to a simple exaggeration of these dynamic phenomena involving the cervical and lumbar swellings, vertebral fracture in hyperflexion may cause neurological lesions (quadriplegia or paraplegia, according to the lesional level) without requiring a specific type of bone displacement. Certain neurological lesions subsequent to spinal trauma without radiological evidence of fracture could be accounted for by elongation analogous to that encountered in the course of lesions of the brachial plexus. Finally, certain types of myelopathy inducing structural alterations and consequently abnormal medullary plasticity, and also certain types of arachnoiditis causing pathological adhesions between the meningeal layers, may lead to dynamic disturbances of the spinal cord and nerve roots, ultimately causing pain syndromes and even histological anomalies.

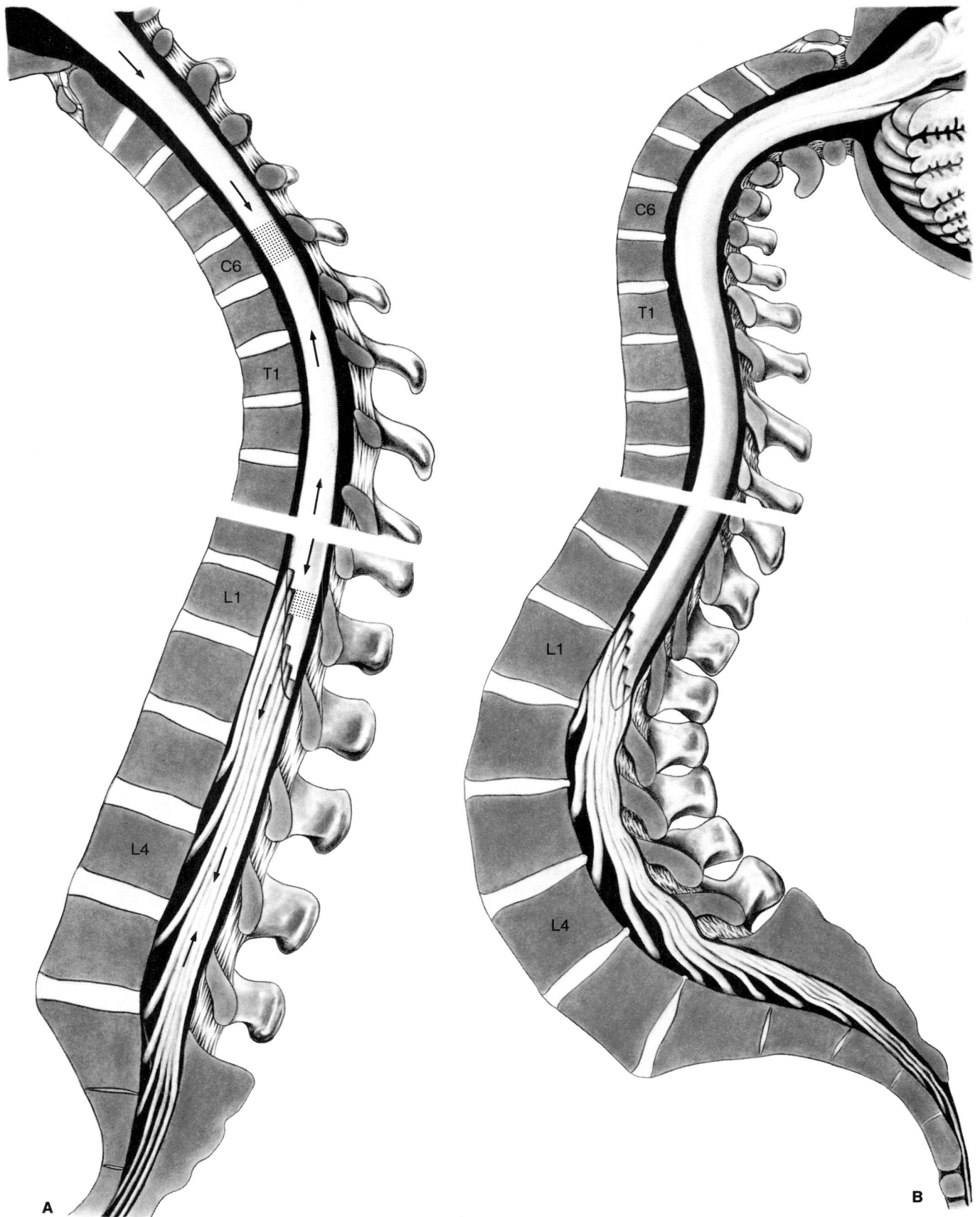

Figure 47 A, B

A Summary of the effects of forced flexion on the vertebral canal, spinal cord, and nerve roots of the cauda equina. *Arrows* indicate the direction of axial sliding and *dotted zones* the medullary regions where maximum stretching occurs

B Summary of the effects of forced extension

8 Spinal Vasculature

I. Major Prevertebral Vessels

The spine functions as a support for the vascular system; the major vascular structures, including the heart, are suspended on its anterior surface.

The data in this chapter are based on numerous classical studies and our work in collaboration with D. Obounou-Akong and R. Ouiminga (Dakar 1969) on the arterial and venous topography of the spine from 110 African postmortem specimens. The great vessels are divided into three sectors, superior, middle, and inferior.

A. Superior Vascular Sector (C1 to T3)

At this level the great vessels are bilateral, thus exposing the anterior surface of the spine. The major *arteries* in this region are:

On the right side, the brachiocephalic trunk, the common carotid artery with its two branches, the internal and external carotid arteries, and the vertebral artery branching off the subclavian artery.

On the left the brachiocephalic trunk is lacking, but the common carotid and subclavian arteries arise separately from the aortic arch.

Regarding the *venous structures,* the great veins lie anterolateral to the arteries, i. e., the right and left brachiocephalic veins and the internal and external jugular veins on each side. The vascular topography in this region imposes anterior and median surgical approaches to the vertebral bodies.

B. Middle Vascular Sector (T4 to L4)

At this level the great vessels are median and thus cover the anterior surface of the spine but expose the lateral surfaces.

Regarding the *arterial vasculature,* the descending aorta lies over the left half of the anterior surface of the spine from T4 to L4.

The *great veins* in this region are the venae cavae, lying over the right half of the anterior surface of the spine. The right pulmonary hilus separates the superior vena cava from the spine (T4 to T7). The inferior vena cava is in uninterrupted contact with the spine from L4–L5 to T8–T9.

The heart lies anterior to the great vessels in the region from T6 to T9. In this region the median position of the great vessels requires that the vertebral bodies be approached surgically via their right and left lateral surfaces.

C. Inferior Vascular Sector (L5 to Coccyx)

At this level the vessels are once again bilateral and symmetrical, leaving the anterior surface of the spine free in the region of the sacral promontory and sacrococcygeal concavity. Accordingly, the best anterior approach to these structures is on the midline. The inferior vasculature comprises the right and left common iliac arteries and veins and the right and left internal iliac arteries and veins.

II. Extraspinal Collateral Vessels

Disposition of the collateral vessels varies in the three vascular sectors.

A. Superior Vascular Sector (C1 to T3)

The main collateral vessels in this sector run longitudinally.

From the *arterial* viewpoint, we should note the following:

The left and right vertebral arteries arise from the subclavian arteries and exceptionally from the aortic arch (1% on the right, 39% on the left) at the level of T1 (in fact between the C6–C7 and T1–T2 intervertebral discs). These arteries penetrate the transverse foramina from C6 to C1 and then pass into the foramen magnum above the posterior arch of the atlas. According to Argenson and Franck (1979), the vertebral arteries may pass through the transverse foramina of C7 (3.5% of cases) or first enter the spine through the transverse foramina of C5 (6% of cases), C4 (1.3% of cases) or C3 (0.1% of cases).

The left and right costocervical trunks arise from the subclavian arteries lateral to the origin of the vertebral arteries at the level of T1. Shortly (5–9 mm) after their origin, these arteries divide to give rise to an ascending branch, the deep cervical artery, and a descending branch, the intercostalis suprema. The deep cervical artery runs between the transverse process of C7 and the head of the rib and then ascends between the deep muscles of the neck, which it supplies. It anastomoses near the atlas with a branch of the vertebral artery. The intercostalis suprema supplies the first two or three intercostal spaces.

The ascending cervical artery, arising from the thyrocervical trunk (itself a branch of the subclavian artery), ascends along the scalenus anterior and prevertebral muscles. Spinal branches of the inferior thyroid artery anastomose with it.

The venous vasculature comprises the following:

- The vertebral veins (most often plexiform) surrounding the vertebral arteries leave the spine through the transverse foramen of C7.
- The descending cervical veins are satellites of the ascending cervical arteries.
- The deep cervical and posterior jugular veins (Walther's veins) run along the deep cervical arteries and end at Pirogoff's venous angle (the junction of the subclavian and internal jugular veins).

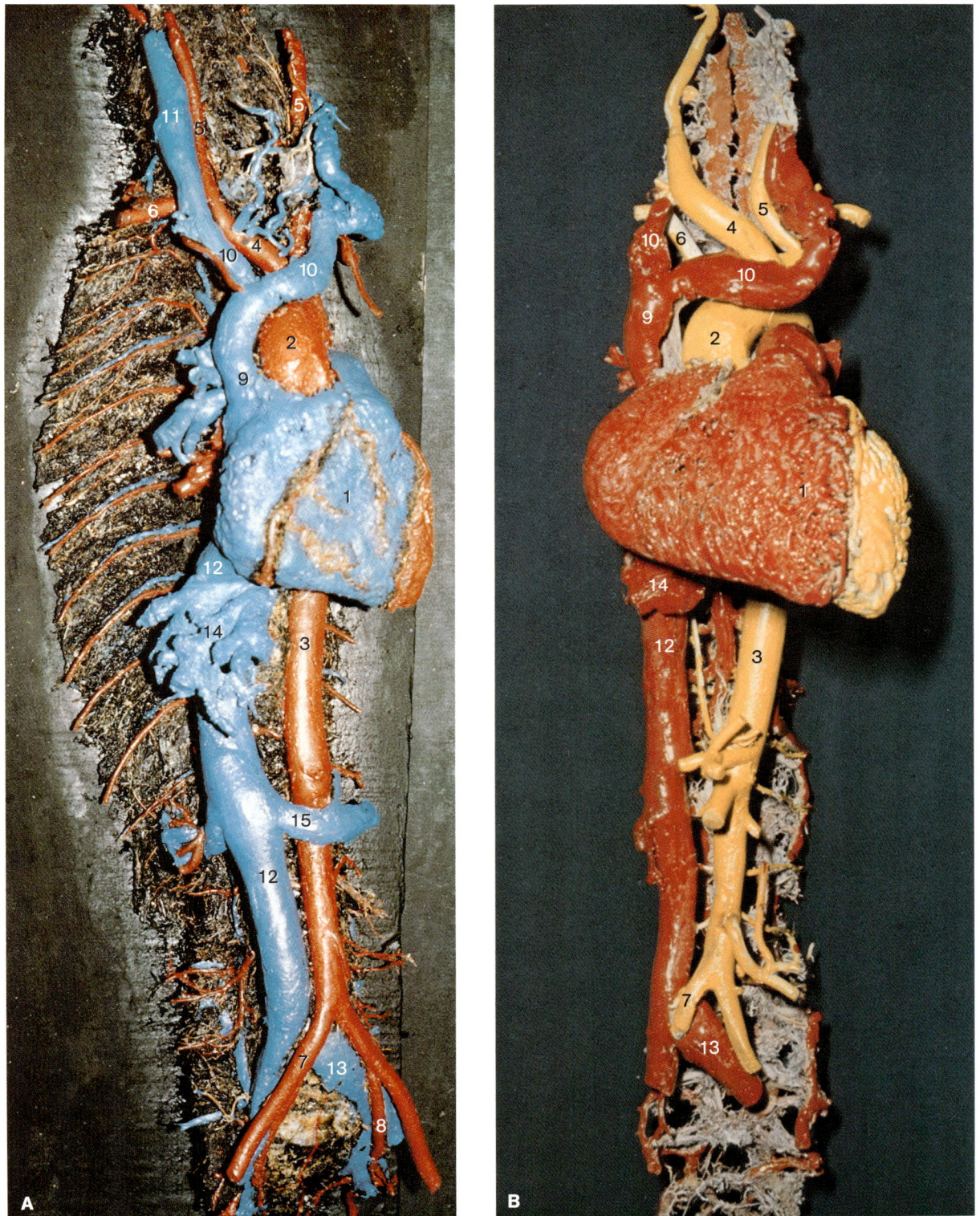

Figure 48 A, B

A   A cast of the prevertebral vessels in an adult African
B   A cast of the prevertebral vessels in a 4-year-old African child

1 cor 2 arcus aortae 3 aorta descendens 4 truncus brachiocephalicus 5 a. carotis communis 6 a. subclavia 7 a. iliaca communis
8 a. iliaca interna 9 v. cava sup. 10 v. brachiocephalicae dextra and
sinistra 11 v. jugularis interna 12 v. cava inf. 13 v. iliaca communis
14 vv. hepaticae

B. Middle Vascular Sector (T4 to L4)

In this region the main topographical distribution of the collateral vessels is metameric and horizontal.

Arterially, the aorta gives off anterior visceral arteries without relation to the spine and posterolateral parietal arteries which run in contact with the vertebral bodies. The latter are the *intercostal and lumbar arteries* in the thoracic and lumbar regions respectively. These parietal arteries arise in pairs, one for each side of a given metamere, in close proximity to the posterior midline of the aorta. From their origin they run towards the lateral surfaces of the vertebral bodies, the intervertebral foramina, and finally the posterior wall of the trunk (intercostal spaces and lumbar regions). The origin of the parietal arteries presents certain variations, i.e., a common trunk giving rise to the right and left arteries, a common trunk giving rise to two arteries on one side, arteries arising above their normal level of origin between a pair of higher arteries, and arteries arising from the flanks of the aorta. Variations in the course of the arteries are of three types: Horizontal arteries arise from the aorta directly at the level of their corresponding intervertebral foramina; this type is most frequent in the region from T6 to L1. Recurrent arteries arise from the aorta well below the level of their corresponding intervertebral foramina; the superior intercostal arteries (T3 to T5) are of this type. Descending arteries arise above the level of their corresponding intervertebral foramina; this type is often found in the lumbar region. In some cases, a single parietal artery bifurcates on the lateral surface of the vertebral bodies to subsequently enter two intervertebral foramina.

At the level of the intervertebral foramina the parietal arteries give off intraspinal branches, *the spinal rami,* and at the level of the posterior foramina (between transverse processes) give off extraspinal branches, the *dorsal rami,* which supply the spinal muscles (running between the longitudinal bundles) and the thoracolumbar skin.

The venous return follows the arterial supply from the periphery to the *parietal intercostal and lumbar veins.* Venous return differs from the arterial supply in its mode of confluence with the great veins; longitudinal veins are interposed between the parietal veins and the venae cavae. The longitudinal veins are the azygos veins in the thoracic region and the ascending lumbar veins in the lumbar region.

There are three azygos vessels in the region of the thoracic spine; the azygos vein (major azygos), the hemiazygos (inferior hemiazygos) and accessory hemiazygos (superior hemiazygos) vein.

Most frequently (55.2% of subjects), the azygos vein arises at the level of the right anterior aspect of T12 from two tributaries, one internal from the inferior vena cava and one lateral formed by the confluence of the twelfth right intercostal and ascending right lumbar veins. The azygos vein runs along the right half of the thoracic vertebral bodies from T12 to T4, where it arches over the right pulmonary hilus to join the posterior surface of the superior vena cava. The azygos vein receives the right intercostal veins on its right flank and the two hemiazygos veins on its left flank at the level of T6 and T7. On the left side, the hemiazygos resembles the lower part of the azygos vein, whereas the accessory hemiazygos vein receives the left intercostal veins from T3 to T6 and descends to join the azygos vein.

This typical distribution can be replaced by one of several variations: left intercostal veins joining the azygos vein directly, without the hemiazygos (9.2% of subjects); a single median major azygos vein (1.3%); the hemiazygos vein replacing the azygos below the level of T7 (1.3%); the azygos originating at the level of L3 and receiving the upper lumbar veins (1.3%); and especially, a major anomaly consisting of the absence of the junction of the inferior vena cava with the right atrium compensated by an oversized azygos vein (1.3%). Surgical ligation of this vein must be avoided.

The ascending lumbar veins are vertical anastomoses between the common iliac veins, the lumbar veins, and the origin of the azygos and hemiazygos veins. The site of anastomosis is deep to the psoas muscle at the level of the lumbar intervertebral foramina.

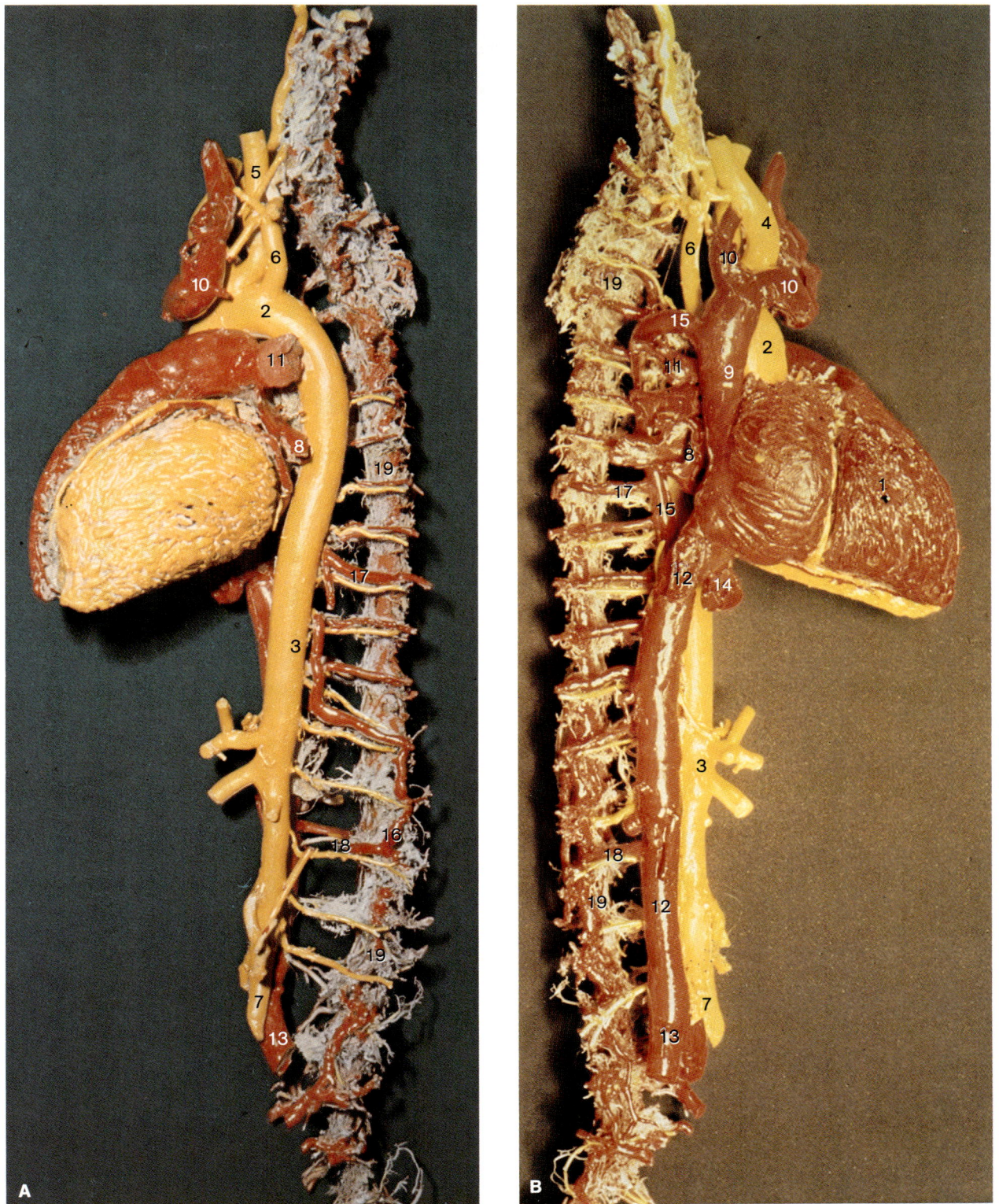

Figure 49 A, B. Plastic cast of the vertebral vessels in a 4-year-old child (aortic system in *yellow* and caval system in *red*). Left lateral aspect (*A*) and right lateral aspect (*B*)

1 cor *2* arcus aortae *3* aorta abdominalis *4* truncus brachio-cephalicus *5* a. carotis communis *6* a. subclavia *7* a. iliaca communis

8 vv. pulmonales *9* v. cava sup. *10* vv. brachiocephalicae *11* aa. pulmonales *12* v. cava inf. *13* v. iliaca communis *14* vv. hepaticae *15* v. azygos *16* v. lumbalis ascendens *17* aa. and vv. intercostales dorsales *18* aa. and vv. lumbales *19* plexus venosi vertebrales interni

C. Inferior Vascular Sector (L5 to Coccyx)

In the lower region of the spine the collateral vessels are distributed vertically.

Three arteries run vertically through the lumbosacral interiliac region:

The *median sacral artery* arises from the posterior surface of the aortic bifurcation between L2 and L5, alone or in conjunction with the third, fourth, or fifth lumbar artery, and exceptionally from the left common iliac artery (1.1% of subjects). It then travels near the midline in front of the sacral promontory, sacrum, and coccyx. In some cases, the median sacral artery gives rise to the fifth lumbar artery and to branches which anastomose anterior to the sacral foramina with the arteries listed below.

The *lateral sacral arteries* arise from the internal iliac artery or its gluteal and ischiatic branches at the level of S1 or S2. There are one to three lateral sacral arteries on each side anterior to the sacral plexus, forming anastomoses with the branches of the median sacral artery.

Veins homologous to the arteries constitute the venous system in this sector.

III. Intraspinal Vessels

The extraspinal collateral vessels give rise to or receive the vascularization of the osteoarticular and neuromeningeal structures of the spine.

This section is based on data from classical studies, our personal observations, and studies by Mineiro (1965) and Crock and Yoshizawa (1977), who have given a particularly good description of the microvascularization of the spine and spinal cord.

Regardless of the spinal region under consideration, there exists a network of arterial and venous collaterals arranged in quadrangular fashion around the vertebrae. Indeed, at all levels of the spine horizontal metameric vessels travel preferentially over the middle of the vertebral bodies at the level of the intervertebral foramina and longitudinal vessels run perpendicular to and anastomose with them.

A. Osteoarticular Vasculature

1. Arterial

Distinction must be made between the arterial vascularization of the vertebral bodies and posterior arches.

The vertebral bodies are supplied by two groups of arterioles: rami arising directly from the parietal arteries and running over the convex surface of the bodies, and rami from the anterior arteries of the vertebral canal which run over the posterior surface of the vertebral bodies. The rami of the parietal arteries (intercostal and lumbar arteries, metameric branches of the vertebral arteries, ascending cervical arteries, and sacral arteries) arise perpendicular to their trunk of origin and run

above and below it over the circumferential surface of the vertebral bodies, penetrating the vertebral bodies through small orifices on their suface. The anterior arteries of the vertebral canal arise at the level of the intervertebral foramina from a branch of the parietal arteries passing anterior to the spinal nerves. The anterior artery rapidly divides to form ascending and descending branches which anastomose with their supra- and subjacent homologues on the same side. Accordingly two anastomotic arterial axes, one on the right and one on the left, are formed on the outer third of the posterior surface of the vertebral bodies, extending the entire length of the spine. Transverse anastomoses between the two axes run over the middle of the vertebral bodies. Rami from this arterial network enter the vertebral bodies through their posterior surfaces. Within the vertebral body, the arterioles are arranged in radiate fashion with axial branches running towards the superior and inferior surfaces. In the cartilaginous plates limiting the intervertebral discs, Crock and Yoshizawa identified arteriolar terminals in the shape of a golf club.

Indeed, in adults the intervertebral disc is devoid of vascularization, receiving nutrients by osmosis. Conversely, in the fetus and young child Mineiro (1965) demonstrated arteriolar terminals in the peripheral and fibrous parts of the disc, but not in the deep parts.

The vertebral arches are supplied by arterioles on each surface, arising from the posterior artery of the vertebral canal and the dorsal rami of the parietal arteries.

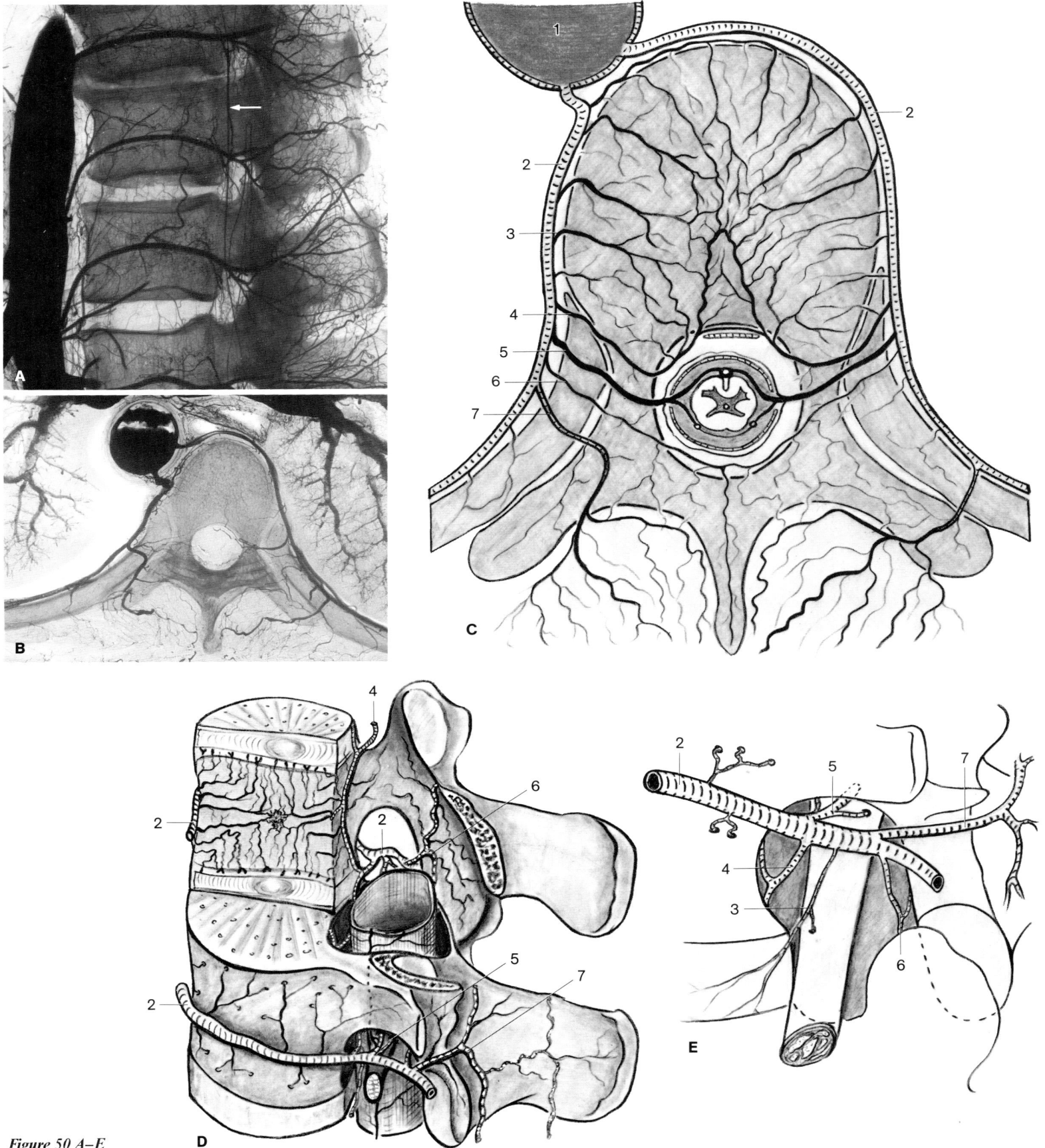

Figure 50 A–E

A   Lateral aspect of the lumbar vertebrae with injection of their arterial vasculature. The *arrow* indicates the anterior spinal artery

B   Horizontal section of the arteries of the thoracic vertebrae after injection

C   The extra- and intraspinal arteries seen on horizontal section

D   Drawing of the extra- and intraspinal arteries

E   The arteries in the intervertebral foramina

1 aorta *2* a. intercostalis post. *3* ramus corporis vertebralis *4* ramus spinalis ventralis *5* ramus spinalis *6* ramus spinalis dorsalis *7* ramus dorsalis

2. Venous

According to Crock and Yoshizawa there exists a capillary bed in the cartilaginous plates which drains into a subchondral venous network. The draining of blood would be through axial rami in a horizontal subarticular venous system comprising large anteroposterior veins near the upper and lower surfaces of the vertebral bodies. This system would then drain through vertical axial rami into the large horizontal centrocorporeal veins which merge with the anterointernal vertebral venous plexuses at the posterior surface of the vertebral bodies. These central veins of the vertebral bodies are largely anastomosed by radiate rami to the veins of the external venous plexuses of the vertebrae.

The *intervertebral discs* display veins only in their most superficial parts.

The *vertebral arches* are drained by a central vein of the spinous process, and by the veins of the laminae which subsequently drain towards the pedicles and the veins of the intervertebral foramina. These veins also form anastomoses with the internal and external vertebral venous plexuses.

B. Neuromeningeal Vasculature

1. Arterial

The spinal cord and nerve roots are supplied by the spinal branches of the vertebral arteries (in some cases the thyrocervical trunk) and the parietal intercostal, lumbar, and lateral sacral arteries. The distribution of the spinal arteries on the surface of the spinal cord follows a horizontal metameric mode, creating a vertical anastomotic system. At the level of a given metamere, the spinal artery arises from a parietal artery at its point of entry to the intervertebral foramen. The spinal artery then runs along the epidural surface of the spinal nerve and finally traverses into the subarachnoid space. The artery divides into two branches; a relatively large ventral radicular branch, which travels along the ventral root to reach the spinal cord, and a more slender posterior radicular branch running along the dorsal nerve root. The ventral branch passes around the anterior column and comes to lie in the median fissure, where it divides to form ascending and descending branches, which anastomose with their supra- and subjacent homologues to form the anterior spinal artery. The dorsal radicular branch divides in contact with the spinal cord to form two short horizontal branches, each of which subdivides to give off ascending and descending branches. These branches anastomose with the ascending and descending branches of the contiguous metameres to constitute two pairs of posterior spinal arteries. The anterior spinal artery constitutes a vertical axis extending the entire length of the spinal cord in the median fissure, and can be considered to originate in front of the medulla oblongata from the confluence of two branches, each arising from the end of the vertebral arteries, or rarely from the inferior cerebellar arteries. The posterior spinal arteries lying on each side of the right and left dorsal nerve rootlets arise from the vertebral arteries at the level of the foramen magnum. These vertical arteries are transversely or obliquely anastomosed at the surface of the spinal cord to form a large-meshed arterial network. Similarly, the five more or less sinuous spinal arteries anastomose with each other at the level of the conus medullaris to form a right and left arterial loop, anastomosing with the radicular arteries of the sacral and coccygeal nerve roots.

Deep arterial distribution to the spinal cord is achieved in two zones. The peripheral zone is supplied by the posterior spinal arteries and the perimedullary arterial circle comprising the anastomoses between the spinal arteries. The central zone receives the sulcocommissural branches of the anterior spinal artery. The sulcocommissural arteries penetrate through the median fissure like the teeth of a comb, alternately on each side of the midline, to reach the intermediate part of the gray matter and the bases of the ventral and dorsal horns. Deep anastomoses exist between these two systems in the region of the posterior gray commissure (Soutoul 1967). The deep part of the lateral column and the margins of the median fissure are supplied with the central zone. Infarction of the central zone of the spinal cord (Schneider's syndrome) accounts for suspended paraplegia, involving the upper but not the lower limbs due to ischemic necrosis of the cervical fibers of the decussating pyramidal tract.

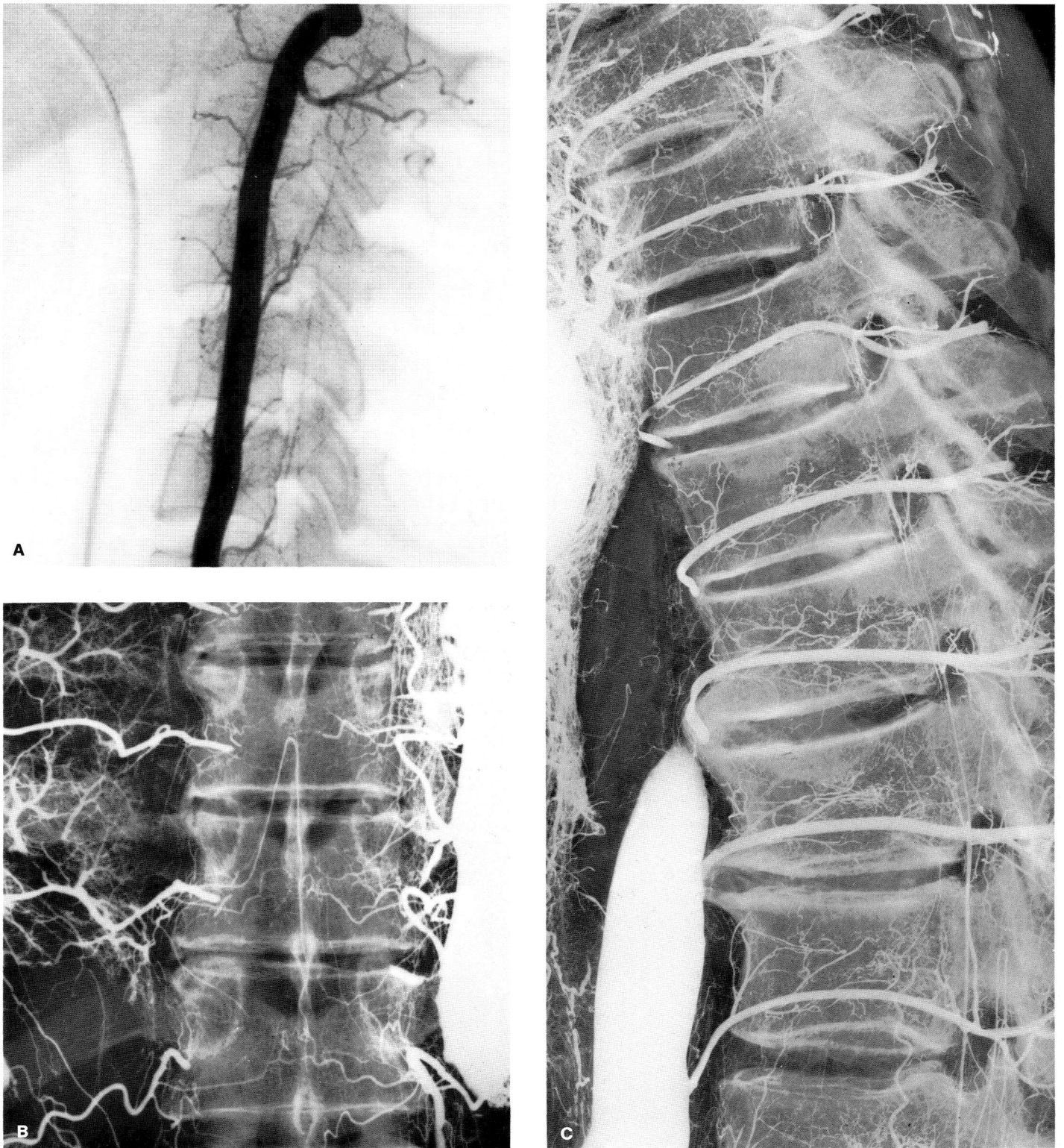

Figure 51 A–C

A Branches of the vertebral artery supplying the spine and cervical spinal cord

B The posterior intercostal arteries and their spinal branches supplying the thoracic spinal cord

C The posterior intercostal arteries and their rami supplying the vertebral bodies and the thoracic and lumbar spinal cord

Classical anatomical studies underline that there are less radiculomedullary or spinal arteries than there are spinal nerves, i.e., only eight to ten arteries supplying the spinal cord. Descriptions of the blood supply to the lumbosacral cord refer to the existence of a single main artery known as Adamkiewicz's artery (1882), which was also identified by Kady (1889) and sometimes referred to as Lazorthe's artery of the lumbar swelling (1957). It arises from an intercostal or lumbar artery (slightly more often on the left side) generally at the level of T8 to L2, and exceptionally from the fourth lumbar or first sacral artery on the left (Obounou and Louis 1969). In the thoracic spinal cord the arterial supply has been described as relatively sparse with only two to three main arteries, most frequently at the level of T9 on the right and T4, T6, and T8 on the left according to our studies. Three or four main arteries enter the cervical spinal cord along with nerve roots C3 to C8, more often on the right than on the left side in our experience. These widely held notions led many authors to consider that major difficulties would be encountered during spinal surgery. Ligation of a main artery, e.g., Adamkiewicz's artery, would lead to acute postoperative ischemia and paraplegia. Similarly, the thoracic spinal cord would be highly prone to the effects of vascular lesions since the scarce main arteries were considered too few in number to supply a relatively long portion of the spinal cord. However, studies on the anastomotic network of the spinal arteries (Lazorthes and Gouaze 1966; Louis 1978) allowed a more realistic assessment of the risks of medullary ischemia, which are lower than initially believed. The arteries of the cauda equina, with anastomoses between their branches in the region of the intervertebral foramina, constitute a system of blood supply supplementary to the anterior and posterior spinal arteries.

Crock and Yoshizawa (1977) pointed out their disagreement with the classical opinion regarding the paucity of arterial supply to the spinal cord. These authors suggested that in the anatomical studies prior to their own work the smallest caliber arteries were not consistently injected and thus only the larger vessels were identified.

Our studies, in agreement with Crock and Yoshizawa, showed the presence of metameric radiculomedullary spinal arteries with variable caliber accompanying each spinal nerve to the spinal cord. The notion of vascular fragility of the spinal cord in general, and of the thoracic cord in particular, should not be perpetuated ad infinitum.

The arteries supplying the dura mater and arising from the spinal arteries form a ladderlike system of longitudinal anastomoses on the outer surface of the dural envelope in front of and behind the points of dural emergence of the nerve roots.

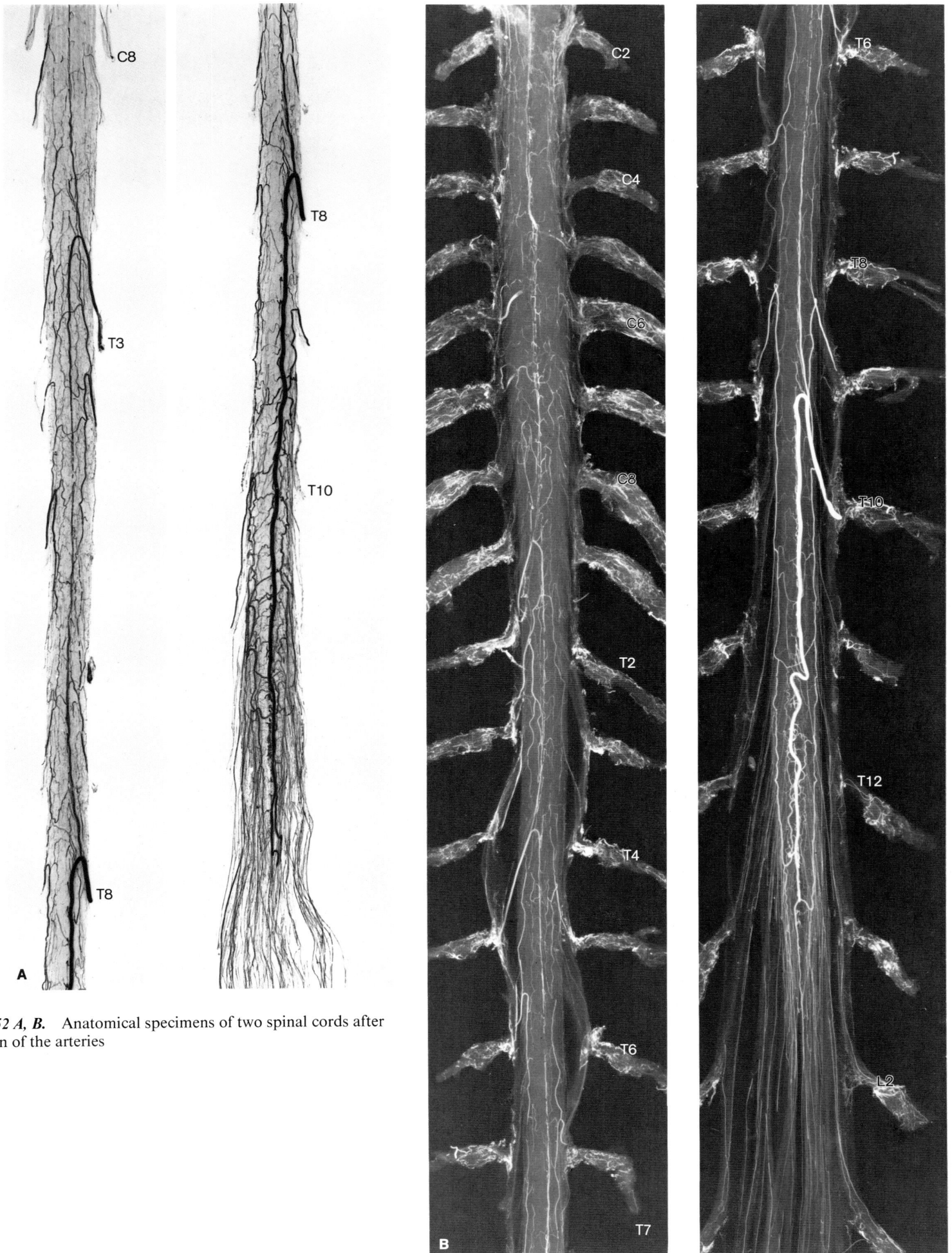

Figure 52 A, B. Anatomical specimens of two spinal cords after injection of the arteries

2. Venous

The veins of the spinal cord radiate from the central region with two main median veins draining blood in opposite directions toward the anterior and posterior spinal veins, lying in the anterior median fissure and posterior median sulcus respectively. At certain regularly spaced levels these sagittal veins anastomose around the central canal (Kadgi 1889; Herren and Alexander 1939; Crock and Yoshizawa 1977). The surface of the spinal cord thus displays a venous network with longitudinal axes and oblique perimedullary anastomoses. The superficial venous system gives rise to dorsal and ventral radicular veins which exit through the dura mater and fuse to form the spinal vein accompanying the spinal nerves up to the intervertebral foramina.
Meningeal veins are located on the outer surface of the dura mater.

IV. Venous Circulation of the Spine

The role of the spinal venous circulation is not just one of simple drainage of the spine. Major studies of this venous system have been made by Walther (1885), Baston (1940), Herlihy (1947), and Cooper (1960). In 1971, in collaboration with Ouiminga and Obounou, we performed an experimental study in monkeys, using the injection of radioactive tracers. The results of this work led to the following conclusions:
The spinal venous circulation drains essentially into the azygos system and accessorily directly into the venae cavae. The level of the arch of the azygos vein represents the junction between the venous circulations flowing in opposite directions, i.e., descending above and ascending below this level. The azygos should be considered the main emissary vein not only of the spinal venous system, but also of the parietal circulation of the trunk articulating with the spinal circulation.
The spinal venous system acts as an intercaval shunt draining blood in the direction of the inferior vena cava in physiological conditions, but reversing the direction of flow (owing to the absence of valves) in cases of obstruction of the superior vena cava. The spinal and parietal venous circulations thus constitute an efficient and vital shunt to overcome any obstacle in the drainage bed of the inferior or superior vena cava.
The spinal venous circulation is capable of draining blood from the pelvic cavity to the cranial sinuses, but in experimental conditions (ligation of the inferior vena cava and azygos vein) only remotely comparable to the physiological condition invoked by Batson (coughing, sneezing, abdominal pressure). Even if it is accepted that pelvic blood can reach the cranial circulation in the occipital plexuses, it is rather improbable that drainage can ascend into the cranial sinuses and cerebral veins, carrying metastatic cells in its flow.

The spinal venous circulation is not limited to the drainage of the hard and soft structures of the spine, but normally participates in draining a significant part of the blood from the tributary organs of the venae cavae and portal system. Our experiments gave the following mean values of the contribution of the spinal system to the venous drainage of the following regions:

Lower limbs	5.7% of drainage towards the azygos vein
Pelvic viscera	6.5% of drainage towards the azygos vein
Supramesocolic viscera	10.8% of drainage towards the azygos vein
Intracranial structures	11.7% of drainage towards the azygos vein

It is highly probable that other organs not investigated in the abovementioned study are drained in similar fashion. The mammary glands belong to the parietal circulation, richly anastomosed to the spinal venous circulation, and venous blood from the thyroid gland may be drained towards the spinal system by the tracheoesophageal venous anastomoses. The fact that the vertebroparietal venous circulation can drain 5%–10% of the blood from different regions of the body in physiological conditions (unobstructed caval and portal flow) indicates that this venous system should be considered a major component of the general venous circulation, similar to the superior and inferior caval and portal systems. This proposal has also been advanced by Batson and Herlihy.
Two names have been proposed to identify this system: *anastomotic vertebroparietal venous system* and *azygos system*. The advantage of the first term is to underline the vertebral and parietal components of this system and its anastomoses with the caval and portal circulations; it is cumbersome and contrary to the familiar terms of caval and portal system. Accordingly, we propose that the name *azygos system* be adopted in the broad sense of the term since the azygos vein is, finally, the emissary vein of the vertebroparietal circulation. Flowing into the superior vena cava, the azygos system resembles the portal system flowing into the inferior vena cava.
None of these systems is sufficiently autonomous to collect all the venous blood from its respective drainage beds. Part of each system is also drained by the anastomotic vertebroparietal system, which is itself partially drained by the other systems of venous return.

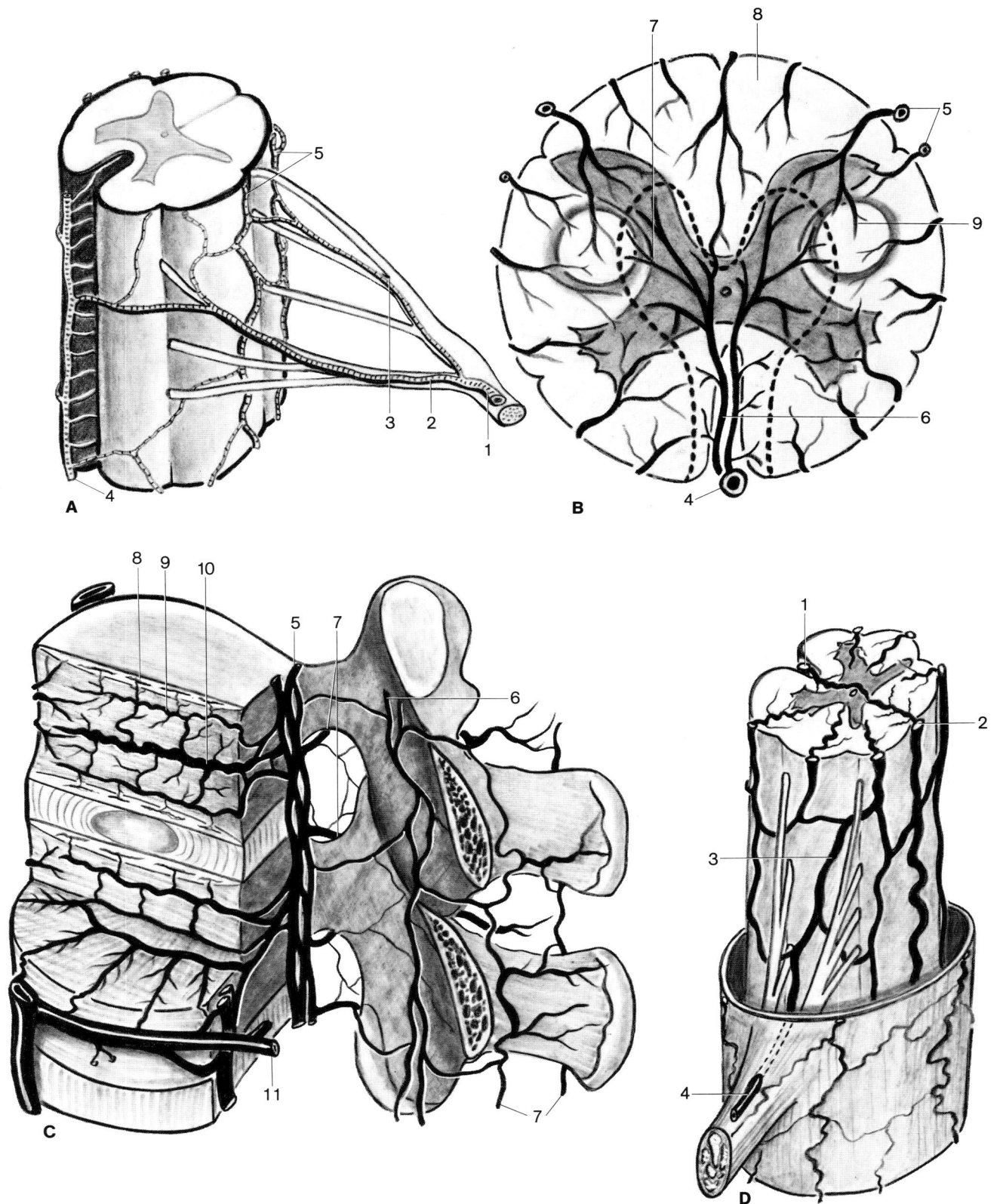

Figure 53 A–D

A The superficial spinal arteries
B The deep arteries and arterial territories of the spinal cord

C The intra- and extraspinal venous plexuses
D The spinal veins

1 ramus spinalis *2* ramus radicularius ventralis *3* ramus radicularis dorsalis *4* a. spinalis ant. *5* a. spinales post. *6* a. sulci *7* central zone *8* peripheral zone *9* tractus pyramidalis lateralis

1 v. spinalis ant. *2* v. spinalis post. *3* vv. superficiales *4* ramus spinalis *5* plexus venosi vertebrales interni ant. *6* plexus venosi vertebrales interni post. *7* plexus venosi externi post. *8* rete venosum cartilaginis vertebralis *9* rete venosum subcartilaginosum *10* vv. radiatae corporis vertebralis *11* v. intercostalis post.

V. Spinal Phlebography

Neoformations arising from the walls or the contents of the vertebral canal may leave their mark on the intraspinal venous system. Knowledge of the latter has been greatly advanced by the studies of Breschet (1928), Batson (1940), Fischgold (1952), and Theron (1976).

A. Lumbosacral Plexuses

In the lumbosacral region external and internal spinal venous plexuses can be identified. The internal plexuses form a dorsal and ventral structure with respect to the neuromeningeal formations. The ventral portion is the most developed and practically the only one visible on phlebography, and comprises a group of more or less parallel anastomotic veins running longitudinally in the vertebral canal on the inner surface of the pedicles. These veins present transverse anastomoses like the bars of a ladder, passing at the level of the middle of the vertebral bodies. The veins of the vertebral bodies join this anastomotic system anterior to the posterior longitudinal ligament. This ladderlike venous plexus leaves free spaces over the posterior and median part of the intervertebral discs. Accordingly, surgical approach to the discs in this zone does not require hemostasis. The position of these internal ventral spinal veins in the lateral recess of the vertebral canal, where most cases of discal prolapse occur, underlines the diagnostic importance of spinal phlebography. Indeed, radicular compression by a prolapsed disc amputates or partially effaces this venous column.

The ventral plexuses may be the site of pronounced hemorrhage during surgery. To avoid this problem, a correct operative position and abdominal depression should be used to collapse these veins.

Horizontal anastomoses at all spinal levels are found between the internal and external spinal venous plexuses. The anastomoses comprise two main veins in the intervertebral foramina running along the lower and upper margins of the pedicles and displaying numerous diagonal anastomoses between each other. The veins of the intervertebral foramina completely surround the spinal nerve roots, thus rendering surgical maneuvers in this zone difficult.

Finally, the external and internal plexuses are anastomosed to each other by transverse veins running more or less obliquely through the cancellous bone of the vertebral bodies. These intraosseous venous canals are the source of bleeding during partial or total excision of the vertebral bodies. Hemostasis in this zone can be achieved only by indirect methods, i.e., hemostatic compresses (Surgicel) against the dura mater or bone wax in the intraosseous canals.

B. Cervical Plexuses

Studies devoted to this region have been reported by Trolard, by Walter, by Laux, and by Louis (1965). The internal venous plexuses of the spine anastomose with the intracranial sinuses at the level of the foramen magnum. The internal venous plexuses give rise to the origin of the vertebral vein which accompanies the vertebral artery from its point of dural penetration and through the intervertebral foramina to the level of C7, where it reaches Pirogoff's venous angle. Our studies using casts demonstrated the existence of two types of vertebral vein: a well-individualized and cylindrical vein (very rare), or more often a periarterial plexiform venous network constituting the longitudinal axis of the external cervical venous plexus. Near their origin the vertebral veins anastomose the intraspinal plexuses, intracranial sinuses, and condylar mastoid, occipital, and posterior jugular veins to each other. The posterolateral atlantoaxial regions thus constitute a rich venous system of anastomoses causing major operative risks of hemorrhage. The plexiform disposition of the vertebral vein around the adventitia of the vertebral artery resembles the venous system enveloping the internal carotid artery as it passes through the cranium. This situation results from a common anatomical and perhaps physiological process involving the transosseous arteries. Similarly to other regions of the spine, the vertebral veins constitute an anastomotic system through the venous plexuses of the intervertebral foramina, which encircle the nerve roots between the internal and external spinal veins to each other. Phlebography of the cervical spine also enables identification of zones of compression due to discal prolapse or osteophytic spurs protruding into the vertebral canal or intervertebral foramina.

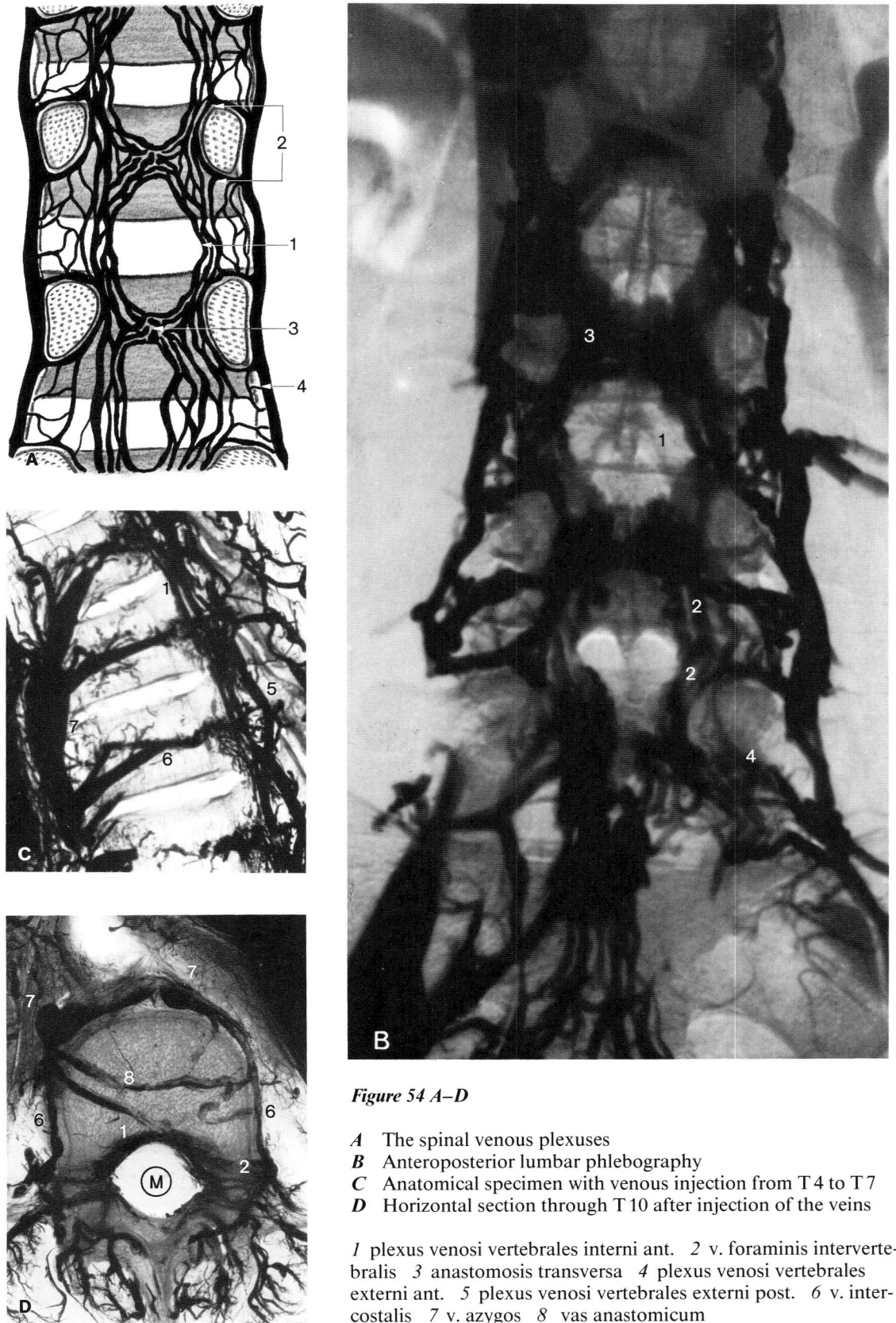

Figure 54 A–D

A The spinal venous plexuses
B Anteroposterior lumbar phlebography
C Anatomical specimen with venous injection from T 4 to T 7
D Horizontal section through T 10 after injection of the veins

1 plexus venosi vertebrales interni ant. *2* v. foraminis intervertebralis *3* anastomosis transversa *4* plexus venosi vertebrales
externi ant. *5* plexus venosi vertebrales externi post. *6* v. intercostalis *7* v. azygos *8* vas anastomicum

Part 2

Topographical Anatomy
and Operative Approaches

1 Cervical Spine

I. Posterior Region

A. Topography

1. Extraspinal Relations

The skin of the nuchal region features the presence of the hairline down to the middle region of the neck. Consequently, any surgical approach in this zone requires that the patient be shaved up to the level of the ears. The nuchal skin is rather thick and frequently displays transverse folds when the spine is erect or in extension. Distension of the skin occurs only on flexion of the cervical spine. Downward traction applied to the roots of the shoulders also tightens the skin in this region.

The muscles of the nuchal region form a large mass lying in four layers. From superficial to deep regions these are:

- First layer: trapezius
- Second layer: splenius and levator scapulae
- Third layer: semispinalis capitis and longissimus capitis
- Fourth layer: deep muscles of the neck lying directly against the spine

The neurovascular bundle of the nuchal region lies in an interstitial space between the third and fourth layers.

The *vessels* of the nuchal region run in a mainly longitudinal direction, and include five major arteries. The occipital artery runs between the mastoid process and the lateral tubercle of the atlas. The vertebral artery is exposed in this region between the transverse processes of the atlas and axis and on the posterior surface of the atlantooccipital joint. At the level of the upper margin of the atlas the vertebral artery passes through the dura mater into the vertebral canal. It should be noted that in this segment the vertebral arteries consistently lie at more than 12 mm lateral to the midline; this lateral distance must be respected when rasping the posterior arch of the atlas. The deep cervical artery, a branch of the cervicointercostal trunk arising from the subclavian artery, enters the nuchal region between the transverse processes of C7 and T1 and turns upwards along the column of the posterior articulations. Finally, the ascending cervical and descending scapular arteries are located in the lateral part of the base of the nuchal region.

The nuchal veins form longitudinal axes with numerous transverse anastomoses especially in the upper cervical region, thus constituting a veritable suboccipital venous plexus. The latter gives rise to a large descending vein at the level of the vertebral laminae, i.e., Walther's posterior jugular vein, which leaves the nuchal region under the transverse process of C7 to join the subclavian vein. The cervical azygos vein runs along the line of spinous processes, parallel to the posterior jugular vein. The deep cervical vein descends along the posterolateral part of the posterior articular columns.

The vessels very rarely interfere with surgical maneuvers extending onto the midline of the nuchal region. The anastomoses of the suboccipital plexus lying in the interlaminar spaces between C1 and C2 form one exception to this rule,

and similarly, above C1 the vertebral artery constitutes a significant lateral obstacle.

The course of the first two pairs of *cervical nerves* is entirely different from that of the other cervical pairs. The first and second cervical nerves do not exit through an intervertebral foramen in front of the posterior articulations, but rather leave the spine medial and posterior to the corresponding vertebral joints. The second cervical nerve, also known as Arnold's greater occipital nerve, is prone to injury during surgical exposure of the posterior surfaces of the arches of C1 and C2: it loops back towards the posterior surface of the occipital bone. The dorsal branches of the third through eighth spinal nerves pass through the posterior cervical region. These dorsal nerves turn lateral to the posterior articulations and then run in the muscle layer through which the vessels also pass, and thus do not hinder the median approach to the nuchal region, but may be injured when excessively deep exposure of the lateral margins of the posterior joints is attempted. Finally, lateral to the articular columns other nerve branches are found from C5 to T1, i.e., rami of the superficial cervical nerve plexus and trunks giving rise to the brachial plexus.

2. Intraspinal Relations

The posterior approach can be used to gain access to the contents of the vertebral canal and intervertebral foramina. Opening of the vertebral canal directly exposes the posterior surface of the dura mater, displaying a few veins on its surface and the surrounding epidural fat. Incision of the dura mater exposes the cervical cord and its swelling, occupying the entire volume of the dural envelope. In this region there is very little free space in which the surgeon can work between the lateral walls of the cervical canal and the spinal cord. The compact spinal nerve roots lie almost horizontally. The posterior sensory roots are exposed first and thus can be sectioned to achieve a posterior radicotomy. It should be pointed out that the medullary root of the spinal nerve runs in front of the posterior roots from C1 to C4. In the lateral recesses of the vertebral canal, superficial to the dura mater, lie the rich internal vertebral venous plexuses which may be problematic when hemostasis is attempted. Laterally, at the level of the posterior articular columns, two structures can be identified; the vertebral pedicles into which bone screws can be driven, and between the pedicles the intervertebral foramina containing the spinal nerve roots and ganglia near their external orifices. The nerve roots lie at the level of the lower half of the exposed articular pillars, while the pedicles lie at the level of the upper half of the pillars.

Flexion stretches the cervical region, thus separating the vertebral arches, opening the intervertebral foramina, and lengthening the vertebral canal. Conversely, extension has the opposite effect. These dynamic modifications must be taken into account when selecting the operative position and when performing arthrodesis.

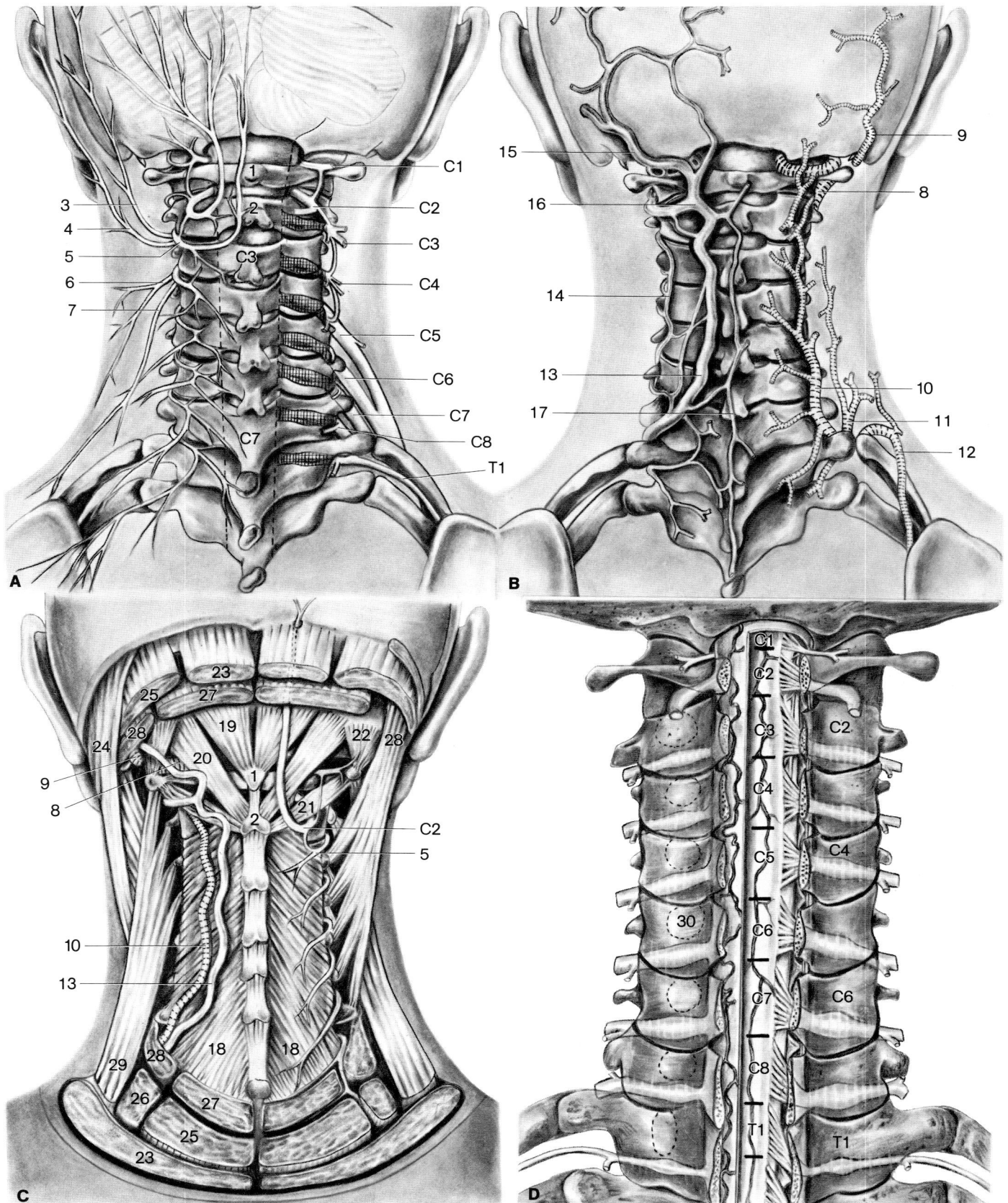

Figure 55 A–D

A Posterior neural relations of the cervical spine
B Posterior vascular relations of the cervical spine
C Posterior muscular relations of the cervical spine
D Neural relations of the vertebral canal, intervertebral foramina, and pedicles in the cervical spine

1 atlas 2 axis 3 n. occipitalis minor 4 n. auricularis magnus
5 n. ramus dorsalis C3 6 n. transversus colli 7 n. supraclaviculares
laterales; C1 n. suboccipitalis; C2 n. occipitalis major 8 a. vertebralis

9 a. occipitalis 10 a. cervicalis profunda 11 a. cervicalis ascendens
12 a. scapularis descendens 13 v. jugularis post. 14 v. cervicalis
profunda 15 v. occipitalis 16 plexus venous suboccipitalis 17 v.
azygos cervicis 18 m. transversospinalis 19 m. rectus capitis post.
minor 20 m. rectus capitis post. major 21 m. obliquus capitis inf.
22 m. obliquus capitis sup. 23 m. trapezius 24 m. sternocleidomastoideus 25 m. splenius capitis 26 m. splenius cervicis 27 m. semispinalis capitis 28 m. longissimus capitis 29 m. levator scapulae
30 pediculus arcus vertebrae

B. Operative Approaches

1. Preparation of the Patient

Surgery in the nuchal region requires that the occipital region be free of hair, and therefore shaving should extend at least to the level of the external occipital protuberance. Patients with lesions causing instability of the cervical spine must wear a plastic cervical collar (Thomas' collar) allowing the patient to be mobilized prior to surgery.

2. Anesthesia and Operative Position

General anesthesia is administered subsequent to conventional endotracheal intubation. The endotracheal tube must be securely taped around the mouth, and a curved oral cannula (Mayo tube) installed to keep the airway patent.

Surgery is performed with the patient prone, and these precautions will ensure that the endotracheal tube does not slip out of position. Induction of anesthesia is achieved with the patient supine on a wheeled stretcher next to the operating table and the patient is then turned over to lie prone on the table. The forehead is supported by a horseshoe rubber-padded headrest. Pads are placed under the sternum and iliac regions. When transferring the patient to the operating table care must be taken to turn the head and shoulders synchronously, to avoid displacement in cases of cervical trauma. The patient's feet are then fixed at the lower end of the table to avoid sliding when the table is inclined. The upper limbs should lie along the body and the tubes and intravenous material should be placed near the lower end of the table. Finally, the operator should check that the abdomen is not compressed, to ensure proper respiration and to avoid compression of the inferior caval system which can induce venous reflux into the intraspinal plexuses and thus hinder hemostasis. The sternal pad should not extend above the manubrium or below the xiphoid appendix. The iliac pads should extend under the lateral half of the iliac regions and under the antero-superior iliac spines without compressing the femoral vessels. It should also be verified that the knees are not unduly compressed against the table. The next step is to fix the head correctly in the headrest so that the cervical spine lies in the same vertical axis as the thoracolumbar spine. To allow proper opening of the posterior interlaminar spaces, the following procedure is used: With the head in the neutral position (no flexion or extension) a movement of posterior translation (sliding) is achieved by pushing the chin backwards in the direction of the occipital region. One should also check that the eyes are closed and protected from antiseptic solutions with compresses. When the correct position is achieved the head is fixed in place by circular bands of adhesive tape running over the summit of the occipital region and under the headrest. The operator should then check that the median axis of the head corresponds to the median axis of the trunk to avoid rotation of the spine. A final check is made to ensure that the endotracheal cannula is not bent and does not tend to slip out of the mouth. When in doubt, the endotracheal tube can be taped to the vertical arm of the headrest, which should be ar-

ticulated so that during surgery the cervical region can be flexed or extended if necessary. The skin of the nuchal region should be stretched free of folds by pulling the shoulders caudally; this can be achieved by using wide bands of adhesive tape placed over the shoulders and crossed over the middle of the back near the flanks. The skin is then cleansed by antiseptic solutions, care being taken to avoid trickling towards the eyes.

Operative drapes are positioned to expose the cervical region and most often one iliac region for removal of bone grafts. Three large folded towels are placed transversely, one over the head above the site of incision, one between the sites of cervical and iliac incision, and one below the iliac site to the infusion stands (to isolate the anesthesiologist's area). Two towels are placed lengthwise from the head to the gluteal region on each side and joined together by towel clips (care being taken not to tear the underlying towels). Two transparent adhesive drapes are installed over the operative sites. The clamp and wire of the coagulating apparatus and cautery knife are placed on the right side, and the suction tube and cannula on the left. The breathing device and anesthesia delivery system are placed beyond the head. Monitoring of blood pressure (taken by a cuff over the calf), pulse, and intravenous infusion is performed at the lower end of the table. The surgeon operates on the left side of the patient and the assistant on the right. Finally, the table is tilted so that the feet are lower than the head, thus decreasing venous pressure in the cervical region. The height of the table is adjusted to bring the nuchal region level with the surgeon's elbow.

3. Initial Exposure

The skin is incised on the midline, i.e., the line extending from the external occipital protuberance to the prominent spinous process of C7. Two major types of incision are used in the cervical region. The operative approach to the upper cervical spine (C1 to C2) is through an incision beginning 2 cm below the external occipital protuberance and extending to a point 2 cm below the spinous process of the axis. Access to the lower cervical spine is gained through an incision from the spinous process of the axis to that of C7. In some cases, roentgenograms are required prior to draping the operative region in order to identify the level of the lesion and to mark this site on the skin (e.g., using a small file to make a scratch mark).

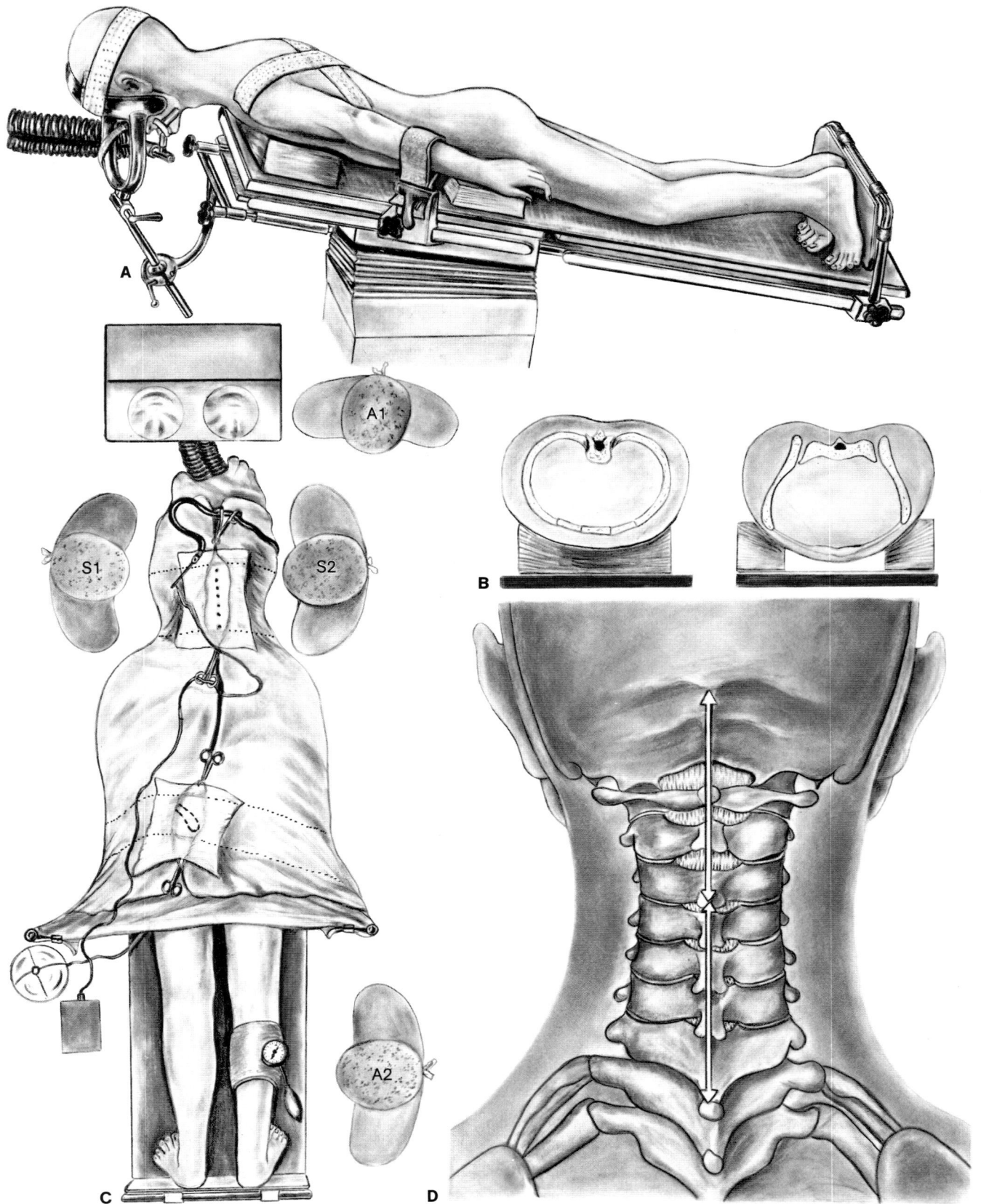

Figure 56 A–D

A Operative position used in the posterior approach to the cervical spine
B Position of the sternal and iliac pads to free the abdomen

C Overhead view of the operative position and the placing of drapes, anesthesiologists, and operators
D Skin incisions for the approach to the upper (C1 to C2) or lower (C3 to C7) cervical spine

Incision of the skin down to the superficial part of the adipose tissue is made using a plain knife. A compress soaked in iodine alcohol is used to disinfect the sudorific glands. A warm moist (well-wrung) compress is packed in the incision to stop bleeding. Hemostasis of the subdermal vessels is achieved in stepwise fashion, involving progressive exposure of the wound centimeter by centimeter, the right hand holding the sheathed coagulation clamp and the left hand the suction cannula. The intensity of the electric cautery knife should be sufficient to achieve coagulation without burning the dermis. A useful procedure is to have the assistant operator evert the skin on the side of hemostasis to expose any points of bleeding clearly. Once hemostasis has been achieved the remaining adipose tissue is incised using the cautery knife. On exposure of the aponeurotic fascia the operator should attempt to identify the midline interstitium separating the right and left nuchal muscles. Identification of this structure is facilitated by installing a Beckman orthostatic retractor from the onset to apply symmetrical tension on the cutaneous and subcutaneous margins of the incision.

4. Exposure of the Craniovertebral Junction

Subsequent to the incision of the superficial aponeurosis, the sagittal fibrous plane of the nuchal region (nuchal ligament) is incised. As the cautery knife progresses to deeper structures, the orthostatic retractor is repositioned further down in the incision to align the median sagittal plane correctly by applying tension on the lateral muscles. Normally, the procedure does not involve the section of muscle fibers, so occurrence of this signifies that the progressive incision is off track. At a depth of 2–4 cm the occipital bone at the upper end and the spine of the axis at the lower end of the operative field are reached. Once clearly identified, these bony landmarks are exposed using the cautery knife. From time to time it is necessary to achieve hemostasis of a few regional veins crossing over or running along the nuchal ligament. The bone is exposed using a middle-sized raspatory to scrape aside the muscle insertions on one side. Rasping on the occipital bone can proceed to a point 3 cm lateral to the midline and on the arch of the axis to reach, but not extend beyond the outer lateral margin of the articular pillar, which can be identified as a steplike structure. At this point in the operation, muscle fibers remain in the middle part of the operative field at the level of the posterior arch of the atlas. The tip of the cautery knife can be used to remove these muscle fibers, but if there is a risk of burning the dura mater scissors can be used to open along the midline until contact is felt with the posterior tubercle of the atlas. The raspatory can then be used again to achieve exposure to a point 12 mm lateral to the midline at least in the region of the posterior arch of the atlas. There is, however, a risk of injury to the vertebral body unless certain precautions are taken, i.e., rasping must be stopped as soon as the sharp ridge of the outer margin of the vertebral artery groove comes into view on the upper margin of the posterior arch of the atlas. The few remaining muscle fibers on the membranes which are inserted on each side of the posterior arch of the atlas are detached using fine scissors in contact with the membrane. Of course, in the region above the atlas the vertebral artery still constitutes a major risk 12 mm lateral to the midline, and below the atlas, just medial to the lateral articulation, is Arnold's greater occipital nerve, which must be left intact. The C1–C2 region is often the site of hemorrhage due to the numerous venous plexuses. Therefore, once muscle disinsertion has been achieved a warm moist compress should be packed into the vertebral groove while the operator procedes to expose the other side of the spine. If desired, the posterior arch of the atlas can be completely exposed by disinserting the supra- and subjacent membranes, bringing into view the dura mater. Similarly, the inferior margin of the spinous process of C2 can be exposed by using scissors to cut the interspinous ligament flush with the bone.

5. Exposure of the Lower Cervical Spine

In the lower cervical spine the full depth of the musculoaponeurotic layers is much less than in the upper cervical region. Transection is achieved using the electric cautery knife with progressively deeper positioning of the orthostatic retractor. The spinous processes are then exposed with the cautery knife, followed by use of a middle-sized raspatory to expose the laminae and masses of articular bone. The raspatory should be manipulated first sagittally against the flank of the spinous processes and then horizontally on the laminae and articular masses. Rasping must be stopped when the outer edge of the posterior articulations is reached. A warm moist compress is packed into each vertebral groove after muscle disinsertion. Hemostasis is required in a few zones of the muscles and interlaminar spaces. The retractor is positioned in contact with the outer edge of the articular pillars. A large curette allows completion of the exposure of the vertebral arches by removing any remaining adherent fibromuscular debris. Except in special conditions the interspinous ligaments should be preserved, since they are factors of spinal stability. Radiological identification is often required to confirm the spinal level of the exposed vertebrae.

Figure 57 A–I

A   Skin incision
B   Subdermal hemostasis
C   Aponeurotic incision
D   Muscular transection
E   Muscular disinsertion
F   Positioning of the orthostatic retractor: C1–C2 region
G   Exposure of the spinous processes
H   Muscular disinsertion
I   Exposure of the vertebral arches of C4–C6

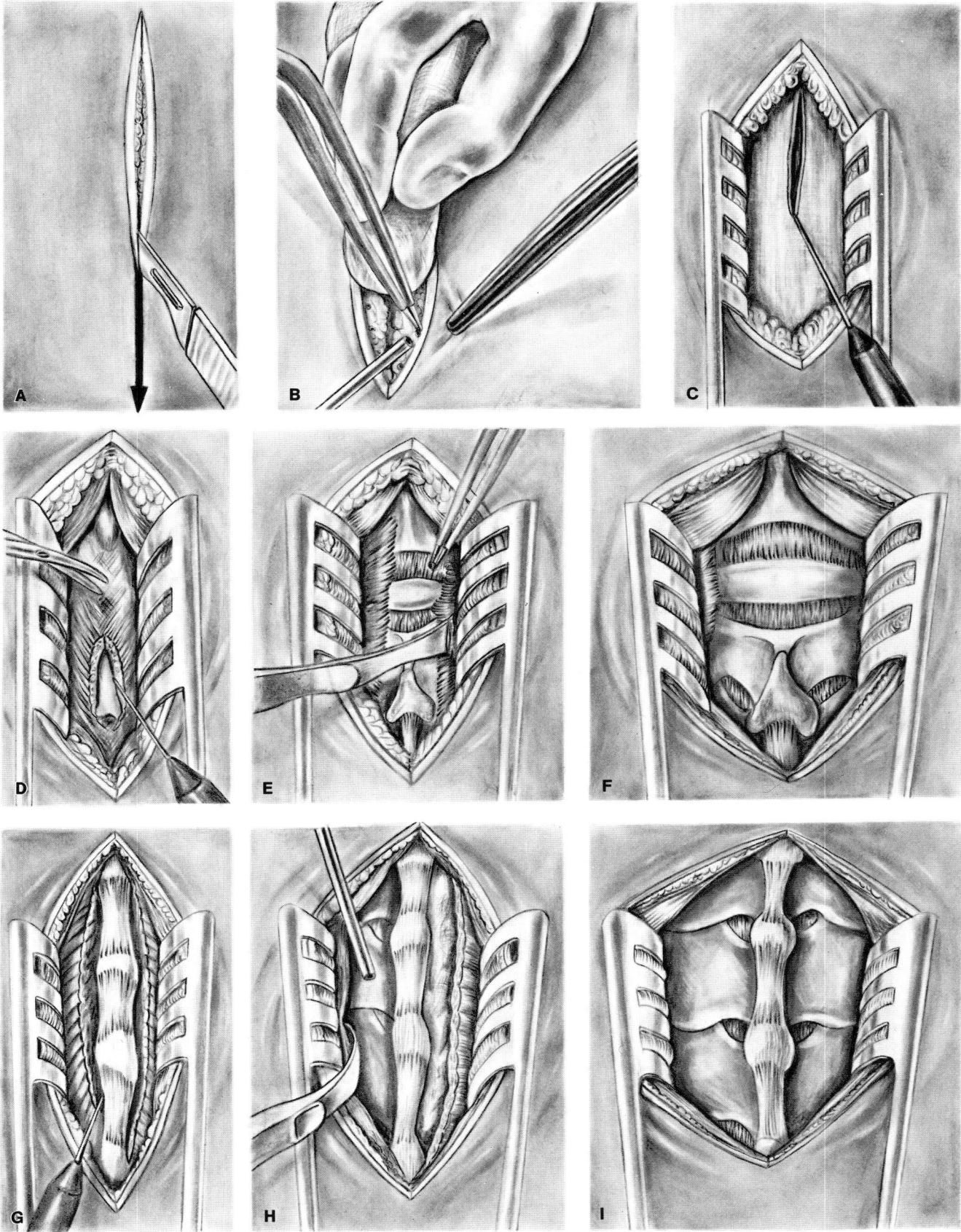

Figure 57 A–I

6. Interlaminar Cervical Approach

The interlaminar approach can be used to explore a spinal nerve root, intervertebral disc, or intervertebral foramen. It is more difficult than in the lumbar region due to the narrowness of the cervical interlaminar spaces, and enlargement of these spaces is required by removal of part of the supra- and subjacent laminae and lateral articular pillar. Once the desired interlaminar space has been verified on roentgenograms, a ligamentum flavum separator is introduced under the lower margin of the upper lamina from the base of the spinous process to the root of the articular facets. One arm of a pair of gouge forceps can be introduced through the decollement to allow removal of the lower half of the superior lamina. The removal of laminar bone should create an inverted U-shaped defect, i.e., with rectilinear walls to allow the greatest possible opening. The cut surface of the bone should be vertical and not oblique, in order not to reduce the field of exposure. The remaining part of the ligamentum flavum is then excised using a curette introduced under the upper margin of the lamina and deep surface of the posterior articulation. The tip of a scalpel can also be used to disinsert the ligamentum flavum from the upper part of the lamina. The next step is to widen the opening of the vertebral canal by resecting the upper half of the lower lamina with a rongeur. A slight increase in the field of exposure can be achieved by removing a small part of the posterior articulations, not more than one third in order not to alter the stability of the spine. Complete removal of a posterior articulation often leads to instability which would require reconstructive surgery with grafting and osteosynthesis in this region. The dural envelope with its covering of epidural fat and its few veins are thus brought into view. The veins can be coagulated if necessary. A dissector is used to retract the fat and thus expose the dural emergence of the spinal nerve root, which can be seen to enter the intervertebral foramen. Retracting the nerve root towards the midline allows access to the posterior surface of the intervertebral disc, covered on its lateral side by the anterointernal intraspinal venous plexuses, which must be coagulated if operation is to involve the posterior surface of the disc.

7. Cervical Laminectomy

Subsequent to exposure of the vertebral arches, cervical laminectomy can be achieved. The first step is to resect the spinous processes over the entire region where laminectomy is to be performed. Radiological confirmation of spinal level should be obtained. Resection is accomplished with large gouge forceps to remove the spinous processes at their base, care being taken not to bite into the laminae. Indeed this would open the vertebral canal in a single blow, with the attendant risk of injury to the dura mater. To achieve hemostasis, bone wax is applied to the cut surface of the bone using a clamp-held compress. The next step is to accomplish decollement of the ligamentum flavum, after which laminectomy can be performed. Laminectomy is begun in the lowest interlaminar space and proceeds upward. The instrument of choice is a pair of gouge forceps with long slender teeth. The lami-

nectomy should be rectangular in shape with lateral edges tangent to the articular facets and upper and lower linear cut surfaces lying horizontally. Hemostasis is achieved by applying bone wax to the cut surfaces of the laminar bone. The procedure brings into view the posterior surface of the dural envelope covered by epidural fat and a few epidural vessels. The origin of the spinal nerve roots is now exposed, and retraction of the roots towards the midline exposes the posterior surface of the vertebral bodies and intervertebral disc. Coagulation of the anterointernal intraspinal venous plexuses is required to obtain hemostasis. When opening of the dural envelope is desired, cotton tampons soaked in hot saline are applied to the site of laminectomy to avoid any trickling of blood into the subarachnoid spaces. The dura mater is then pierced in its lower region with pointed hooks, allowing the surgeon to lift up a plication of dura mater which is incised with the tip of a fine knife. The incision is continued along the posterior midline using fine scissors. The arachnoid membrane, extruded by the CSF pressure, is usually left intact. The arachnoid can then be dissociated with fine scissors, leading immediately to the expulsion of CSF. The posterior surface of the cervical swelling of the spinal cord and the posterior sensory roots of the spinal nerve are thus exposed. Retracting the spinal roots with a dissector allows visualization of the digitations of the denticulate ligament inserting laterally on the deep surface of the dura mater. Mobilization of the spinal cord requires that one or several digitations of this ligament be cut.

Figure 58 A–H

A Decollement of the ligamentum flavum
B Partial resection of a lamina
C Excision of the ligamentum flavum
D Partial resection of the opposite lamina
E Spinous resection
F Laminectomy and excision of the ligamenta flava
G Opening of the dura mater
H Exploration of the spinal cord and nerve roots

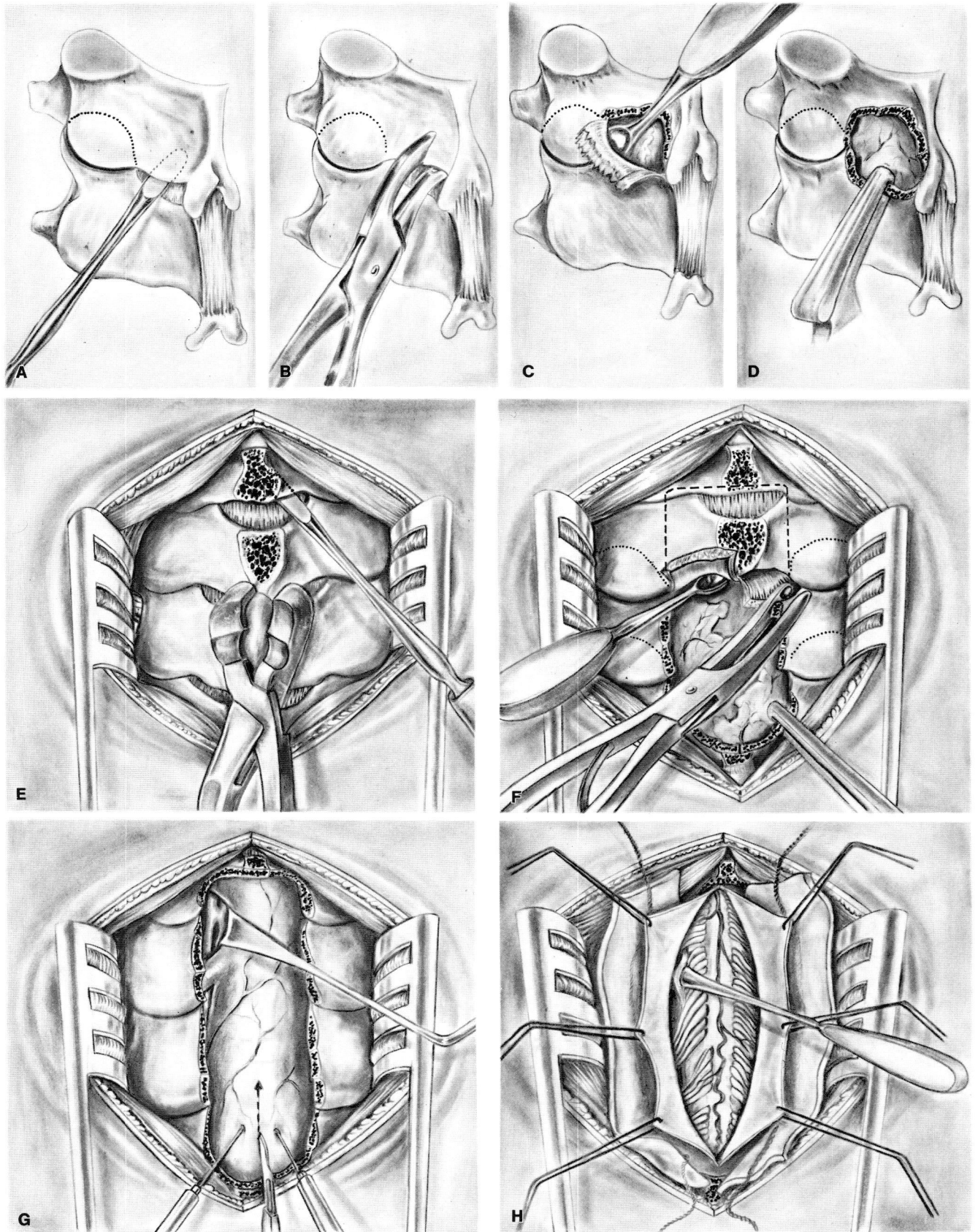

Figure 58 A–H

8. Closure

The dura mater is closed by a fine nonresorbable continuous suture using a curved small-caliber needle with a circular cross section. Subsequent to dural closure it is useful to inject pure isotonic saline into the subarachnoid space to raise the CSF pressure to near its normal value (confirmed by direct palpation of the dura mater). Surgicel is then placed on the posterior surface of the dura mater in the region of laminectomy. The surgeon must confirm the absence of CSF leakage through the sutured dura mater. We generally avoid suction drainage when hermetic dural closure and good hemostasis have been obtained. When in doubt as to the quality of hemostasis a suction drain can be installed, but it must be underlined that suction in the presence of a dural defect may lead to a drop in pressure in the subarachnoid spaces, in turn causing very serious complications. The muscles are closed in several layers owing to their thickness in this region. Care should be taken to place the sutures at reasonable intervals, e.g., 15 mm apart, and not to leave significant zones of dead space between two muscle layers, as this can lead to hematoma formation and subsequent suppuration. In the absence of laminectomy the muscle sutures are simply anchored to the supraspinous ligament. The superficial aponeurosis is then closed as a single layer using interrupted sutures. Full-thickness subcutaneous closure is achieved by interrupted sutures passing through the deep part of the dermis and the fascia covering the superficial aponeurosis in order to eliminate any dead space. Finally, the skin is closed by simple interrupted or mattress sutures. Indeed, a continuous skin suture is proscribed in this particularly mobile region, to avoid suture rupture or laceration of the skin due to movement. At the end of operation the surgeon should check for eschars on the margins of the skin incision resulting from electrocoagulation. When such lesions are observed the zones of burnt skin should be resected minimally, to avoid partial, more or less suppurative disunion.

9. Postoperative Care

When posterior cervical arthrodesis or osteosynthesis has been performed, the patient is required to wear a plastic orthopedic collar for two-and-a-half to three months, but decompressive surgery without instability or bone fusion does not necessitate this precaution. In the absence of opening of the dura mater, the patient is allowed to ambulate on the first postoperative day. However, when the dural envelope has been surgically opened, the surgeon should check that headaches are absent during the first two postoperative days, prior to allowing the patient to sit in a chair for a few minutes while verifying that dizziness does not occur. If these signs are absent the patient is allowed to ambulate thereafter.

10. Possible Complications

The operative position may lead to peroperative respiratory disturbances resulting from plication or expulsion of the endotracheal tube. Similarly, compression of the abdomen can induce serious respiratory complications. The surgeon should also check that the patient is properly secured and that progressive sliding due to the tilting of the operating table does not occur. Leaving the eyes open during surgery may lead to corneal damage. Of course, compression in the region of a cubital or peroneal nerve should also be avoided by using a correct operative position. The anesthesiologist should take appropriate measures to ensure that the patient remains under narcosis until full skin closure has been achieved, to avoid complications such as precocious expulsion of the endotracheal tube due to excess movement. The major risk of spinal surgery which must be born in mind is the creation or aggravation of a neurological lesion. Errors which may lead to this very serious complication include: false maneuvers while turning the patient prior to surgery; loosening of the headrest during operation; penetration of the raspatory into the vertebral canal through a zone of laminar fracture; slipping of instruments while performing decollement of the dura mater under the posterior arch of the atlas or during laminectomy (gouge forceps, rongeur); and occurrence of a compressive hematoma after closure resulting from poor hemostasis without drainage. Aside from the causes of sepsis common to all types of orthopedic surgery, the posterior approach to the cervical spine may lead to postoperative infection for three additional reasons: the close proximity of the hair; the thick muscle layers which after closure are prone to residual cavities and subsequent hematoma formation; and contamination of the surgical dressings by blood and food. Leakage of CSF due to a fistula is dependent on the quality of the closure of the dural envelope. The vertebral artery is prone to surgical injury, especially during procedures to achieve lateral exposure of the posterior arch of the atlas. If this complication should arise finger compression should be started immediately, followed by the compressive application of Surgicel held in place by a figure-of-eight suture anchored in the nearby fibrous and muscular tissues. A minor injury of the vertebral artery can be closed using a conventional vascular suture. Unaesthetic scar formation results from the closure of plicated skin, but a helpful way to avoid this complication is to make transverse marks on the skin prior to incision to eliminate unaligned skin segments on closure.

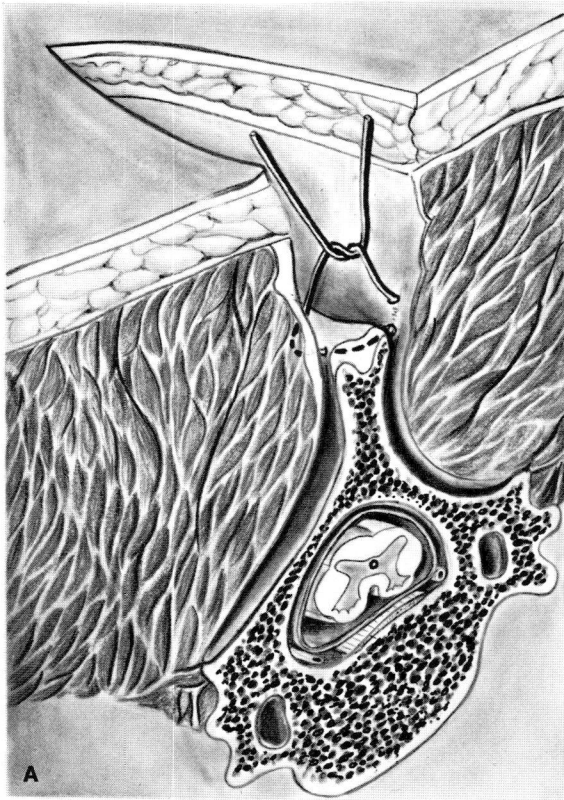

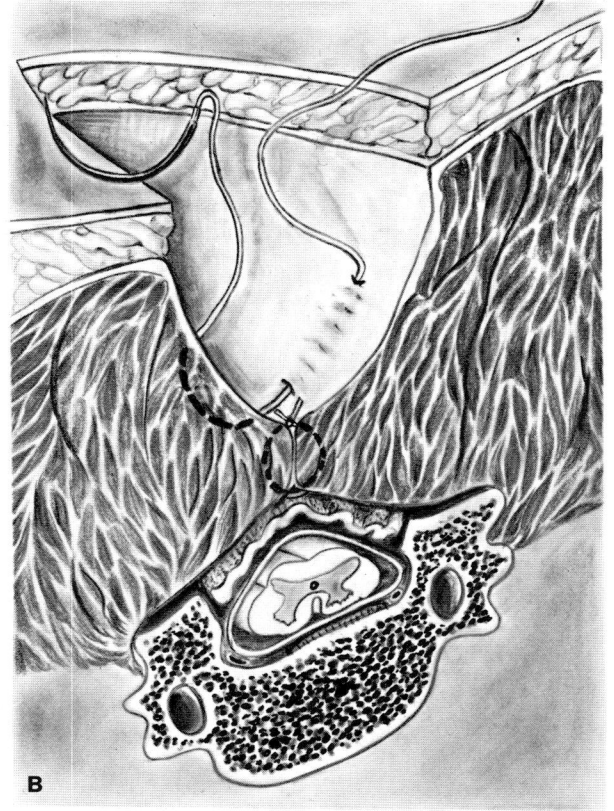

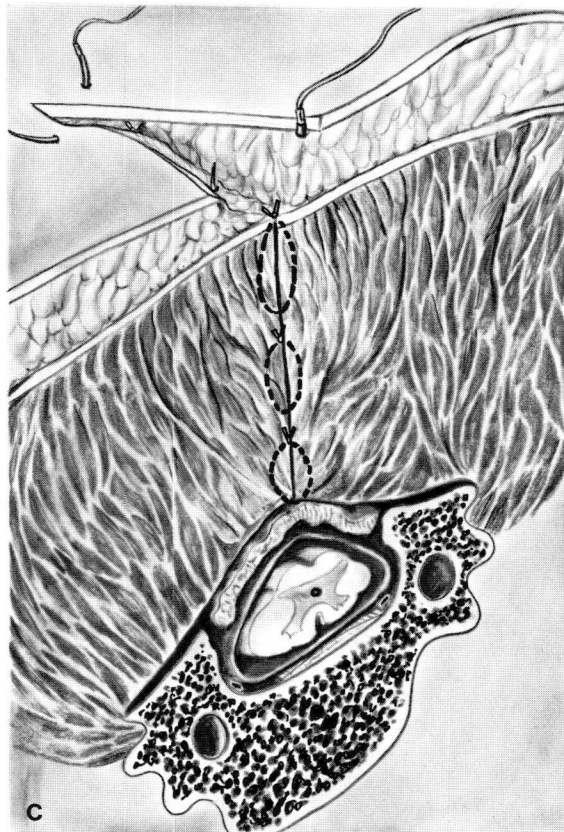

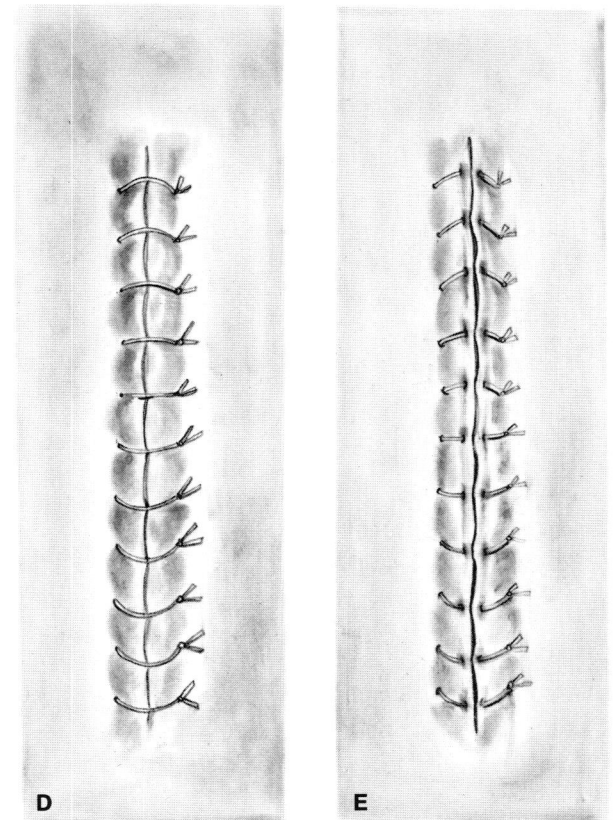

Figure 59 A–E

A   Closure of the muscle layers using the supraspinous ligaments as points of support

B   Closure of the muscle layers after laminectomy

C   Subcutaneous and cutaneous closure

D, E   Skin closure by plain interrupted or Blair Donati (mattress) sutures

II. Anterior Cervical Region

A. Craniovertebral Junction

1. Topography

The anterior surface of the cervical spine is intimately related to the facial mass above and the base of the neck below. These upper and lower regions are topographically very different and lead to separate consideration of the retrofacial craniovertebral junction and the inferior cervical spine. The *craniovertebral junction* comprises the circumference of the foramen magnum, the atlas, and axis, and the upper half of C3. This osteofibrous region forms a cubelike zone with sides on average 5 cm long. The transverse processes on the right and left lateral surfaces of the vertebrae form the boundary between the posterior and anterior cervical regions. It should be recalled that the craniovertebral junction is the site of important modifications of spinal structure, i.e., the system of three columns, discocorporeal in front and apophysoarticular behind, is transformed into a coronal system of two articular columns at the level of the atlanto-occipital junction. The body of the axis represents the crossroads of these vertebral columns. It is for this reason that the craniovertebral junction is the only spinal region where the zygapophyseal joints can be considered as part of the anterior rather than the posterior region of the spine. The unique dens axis at the top of the anterior column ensures functional specialization in the movements of rotation, and is a structure where traumatic lesions predominate. Direct access to the dens can be gained only by the transoral approach. The anterior part of the craniovertebral junction is surrounded by four topographic regions: the anterior buccal region (route of access), the posterior region of the vertebral canal, and the two lateral posterior subparotid spaces, which must be avoided during surgery.

a) The Anterior Osteoarticular Zone of the Craniovertebral Junction

This zone delimits a plane measuring 5 cm square and includes, in descending order: the basilar surface of the occipital bone (clivus) terminating at the anterior margin of the foramen magnum, and the anterior arch of the atlas with its anterior tubercle hiding the dens axis behind. Accordingly, access to the odontoid process can be gained only after traversing the anterior arch of C1. The lateral masses of the atlas lie lateral to the anterior arch and are surmounted by the occipital condyles with their intermediate articulation. Below the anterior arch of the atlas, the neck of the odontoid process forms a transverse depression occluded by fibrous and ligamentous tissue and gives insertion to the anterior longitudinal ligament. The body of the axis lies below and can be distinguished by its sagittal crest. The atlantoaxial joints are located on each side of the body of the axis, their articular interfaces slanting obliquely downward and outward. Half a centimeter below these interfaces the body of the axis narrows towards the midline due to the presence of a pronounced notch, exposing the vertebral artery laterally in the C2–C3 intertransverse space. This zone thus represents a site of operative risk. The region terminates caudally at the C2–C3 intervertebral disc and the upper half of the body of C3, continued laterally by its transverse processes protecting the vertebral arteries.

b) Anterior Relations: Buccal Cavity

The anterior region of the craniovertebral junction forms the deep posterior wall of the buccal cavity, which is about 10 cm deep. With the buccal cavity fully opened, cranial retraction of the soft palate and caudal retraction of the tongue and epiglottis directly expose the origin of the basilar surface of the occipital bone and the upper half of C3 respectively. The pharynx and prevertebral muscles are the only two layers in front of the spine in this region. The pharynx thus forms a vertical sheet stretching over the spine and extending laterally to the tonsillar regions at the level of the naso- and oropharynx. The pharyngeal wall is a three-layered structure comprising the pharyngeal mucosa, fascia, and muscles. The retropharyngeal region contains the prevertebral muscles inserting posteriorly on the spinal bone, i.e., rectus capitis anterior and lateralis, longus colli, and longus capitis.

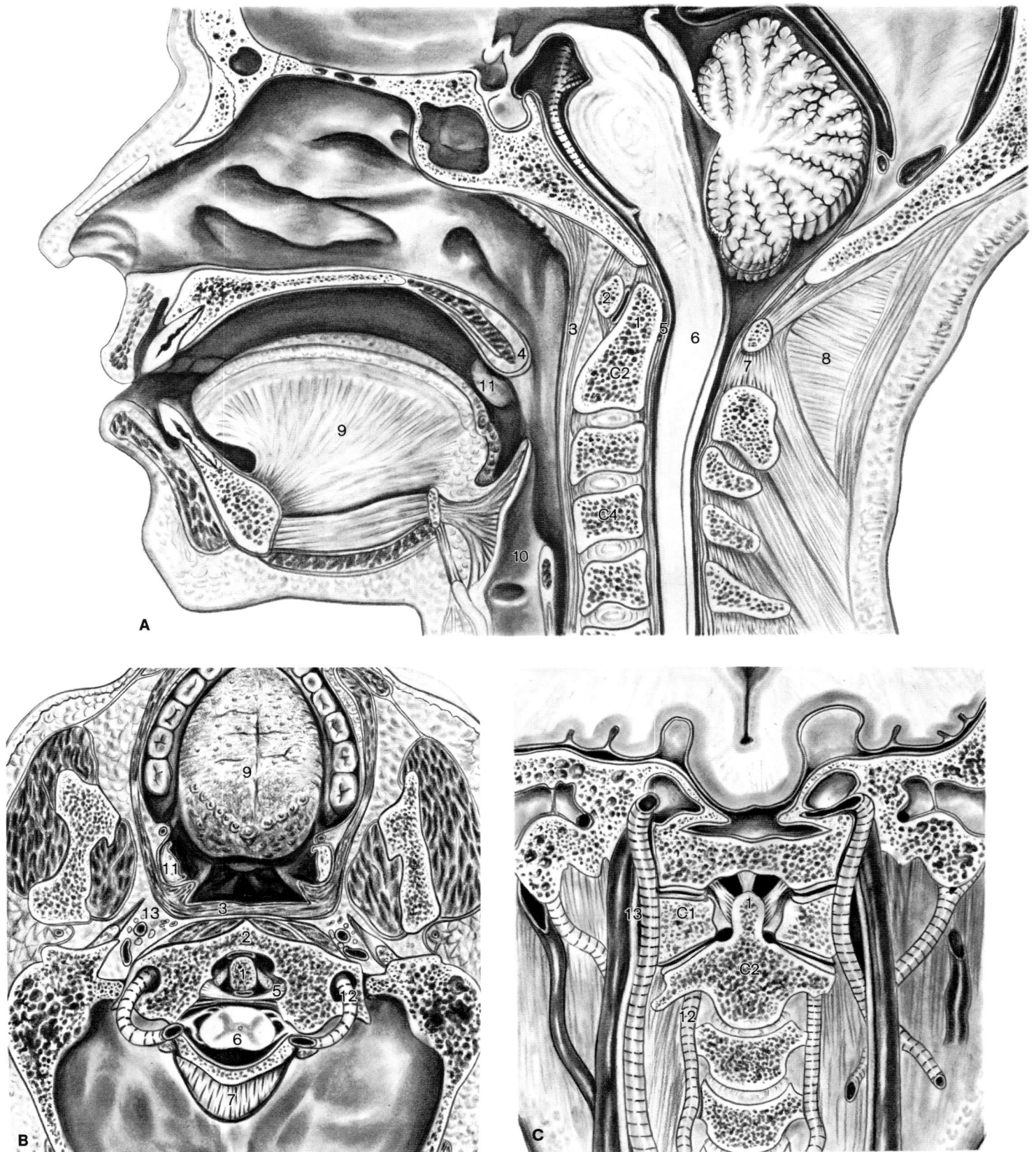

Figure 60 A–C

A Median sagittal section of the head
B Horizontal section through the atlas
C Coronal section of the head passing through the dens axis

1 dens (C2) 2 arcus ant. (C 1) 3 pharynx 4 palatum molle 5 lig. cruciforme, membrana tectoria, lig. longitudinale post. 6 medulla spinalis 7 membrana atlantoaxialis 8 lig. nuchae 9 lingua 10 larynx 11 tonsilla palatina 12 a. vertebralis 13 a. carotis interna, v. jugularis interna, n. glossopharyngeus, n. vagus, n. accessorius, n. hypoglossus, truncus sympathicus

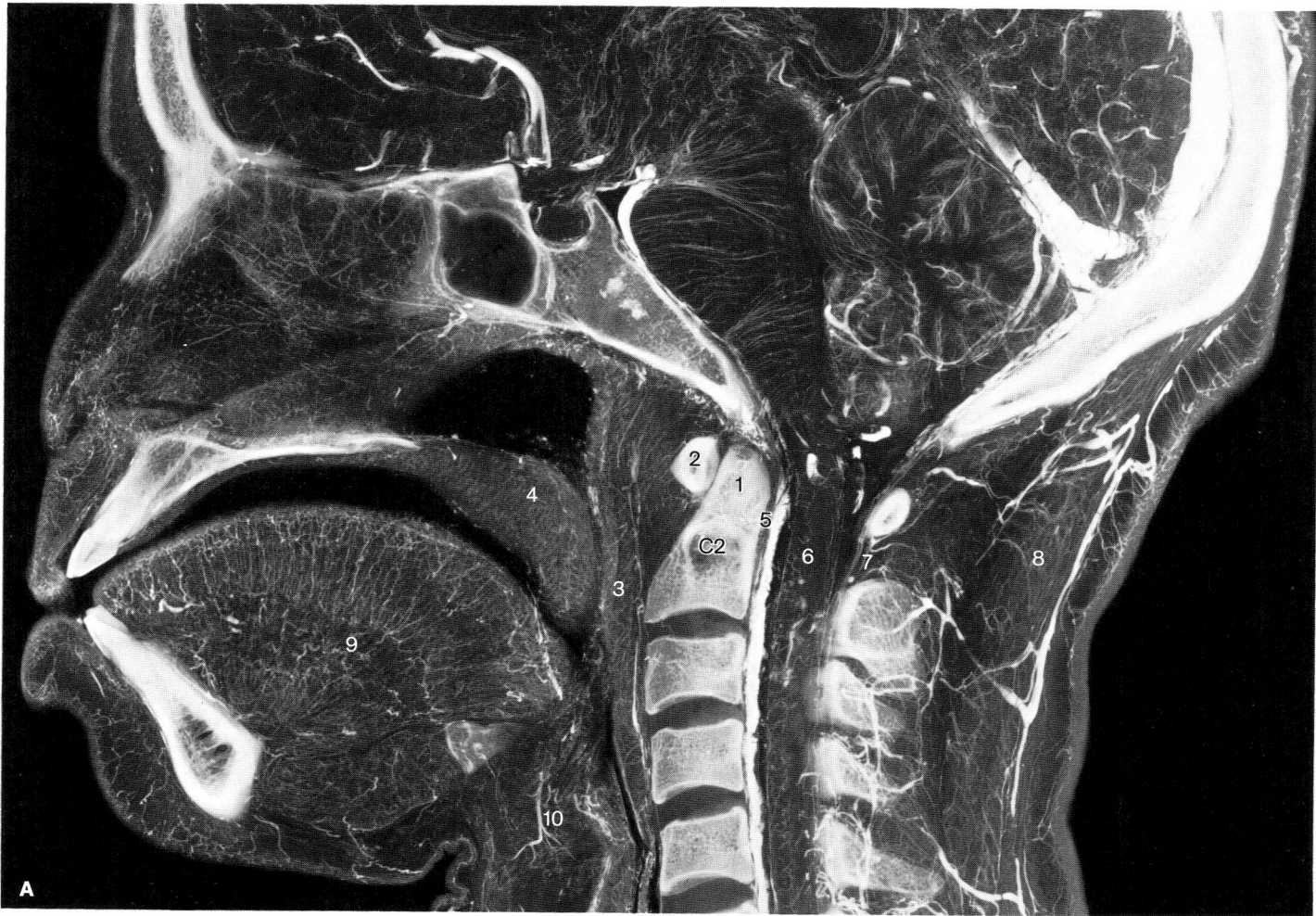

Figure 61. A Median sagittal section of the head

c) Posterior Relations: Vertebral Canal

Immediately posterior to the body and dens of the axis the vertebral canal is funnel-shaped, because the foramen magnum has a much greater diameter than the vertebral foramen of C3. The anterior wall of the vertebral canal is lined by the cruciform ligament of the axis, the membrana tectoria continuing the posterior longitudinal ligament towards the foramen magnum, and finally the dura mater separating the anterior fibrous structures from the first segment of the spinal cord. The cervical cord thus lies 3 mm behind the bony wall of the vertebral canal. This 3-mm space is sufficiently large to receive the tip of a bone screw. In cases where the cranio-vertebral junction is deformed in flexion it must be underlined that the anterior surface of the spinal cord is displaced in very close proximity to the anterior fibrous wall of the vertebral canal and is under a certain degree of tension. In these conditions the cord may be injured during an untoward operative maneuver.

d) Lateral Relations: Posterior Subparotid Space

The posterior subparotid space is located in the posteriorly open dihedral angle formed by the lateral wall of the pharynx and the prevertebral structures. Passing through this region are the internal jugular vein, the internal carotid artery, the superior cervical vegetative ganglion, and the lowest four cranial nerves. Surgical entry into this region is avoided by dissection between the prevertebral muscles and the bone, not extending more than 2 cm lateral to the midline, without exposure of the transverse processes.

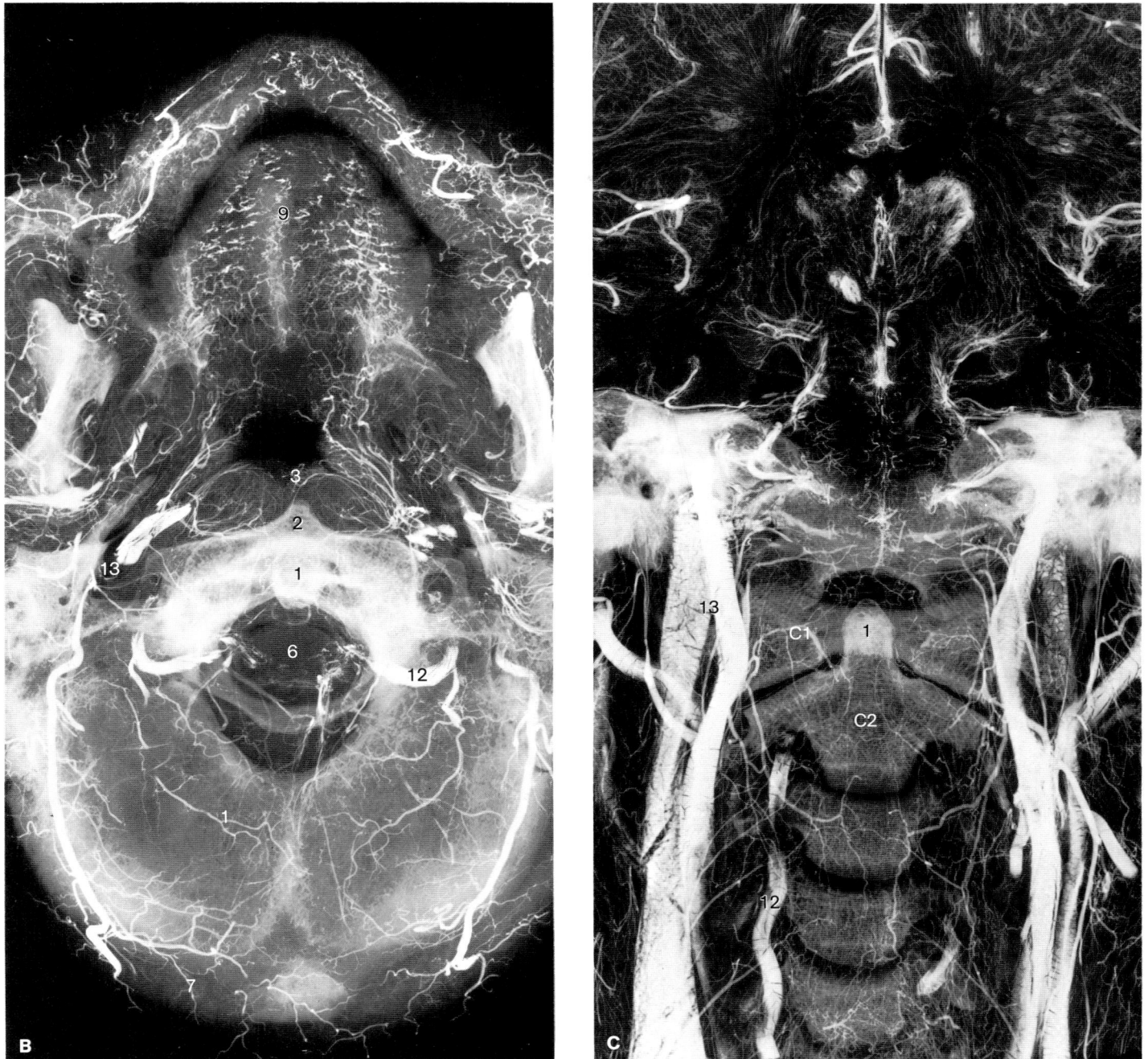

Figure 61

B Horizontal section through the atlas
C Coronal section of the head passing through the dens axis

1 dens (C2) *2* arcus ant. (C1) *3* pharynx *4* palatum molle *5* lig. cruciforme, membrana tectoria, lig. longitudinale post. *6* medulla

spinalis *7* membrana atlantoaxialis *8* lig. nuchae *9* lingua
10 larynx *11* tonsilla palatina *12* a. vertebralis *13* a. carotis interna, v. jugularis interna, n. glossopharyngeus, n. vagus, n. accessorius, n. hypoglossus, truncus sympathicus

2. Operative Approaches

a) Transoral

First referred to by Chipault (1894) and used by Le Fort (1918), the transbuccal approach was described by Southwick and Robinson (1957) and by Fang and Ong (1962), who reported a high mortality rate with this procedure. We first used this approach in 1966 without noting serious complications. Since that time we have performed transoral surgery of the spine on 19 occasions.

(1) Preparation of the Patient

During the three days prior to surgery the airway cavities in the facial region should be thoroughly disinfected. Broad spectrum parenteral antibiotics are administered. The patient should inhale an antibiotic mist four times per day and gargle with an antiseptic solution after every meal. Spinal lesions causing instability require that the patient wear a plaster or plastic orthopedic collar prior to operation.

(2) Anesthesia

Induction of anesthesia is achieved with the patient supine and after conventional endotracheal intubation. To allow full transbuccal exposure the intubation cannula is removed after tracheostomy has been performed. The region of the neck is disinfected, four surgical towels are positioned to delineate the operative field, and tracheostomy is accomplished through a midline incision of the skin and subcutaneous tissue above the sternal manubrium. A few hemostatic sutures are sometimes required after incision. A pair of closed scissors are introduced into the incision and then opened in the sagittal plane to dissect the subcutaneous tissue and superficial cervical fascia strictly on the midline in the region bounded by the sternocleidohyoid (sternohyoideus) below. Two flexible retractors are then introduced to retract the muscle bodies symmetrically. This procedure often exposes an anterior jugular vein which can be retracted without ligation. The closed scissors are introduced again to achieve sagittal dissection of the pretracheal tissue. Finger palpation is used to identify the annular midline cylinder (trachea) with the thyroid isthmus lying over its upper part. Opening and closing the scissors on each flank of the trachea prepares the space to receive the flexible retractors. When in doubt, the needle of an empty syringe is used to puncture the identified cylindrical structure, and of course air will be aspirated when it is the trachea that has been punctured. A sagittal incision is made on the trachea to open two cartilaginous rings. The lips of the tracheal opening are identified by two temporary sutures. While the anesthesiologist removes the endotracheal tube a Sjöbert's elbow-shaped rubber cannula (bent at a 45° angle) is introduced through the tracheostomy. The balloon of the cannula should be checked prior to its introduction in the trachea. When necessary the cannula can be positioned using a triple-blade tracheal retractor. The balloon is then inflated

(5 cc air) and the cannula fixed to the skin. Two temporary sutures and a light dressing are used to close the upper part of the wound. Finally, the endotracheal cannula is connected to the anesthesia apparatus.

(3) Operative Position

With the patient supine the head is positioned in slight hyperextension by angling of the headrest. The arms are placed along the body and the anesthesia equipment near the patient's feet. The eyes are kept closed and protected by dry compresses taped over the orbital regions. Thorough disinfection of the peribuccal region and buccal cavity is then begun. In the buccal cavity we use an antiseptic solution which does not attack the mucuous membranes and is safe if swallowed, e.g., Sterlane solution. Wearing surgical gloves the operator then begins thorough disinfection, applying compresses soaked in topical antiseptic to the deepest recesses of the buccal cavity, including the posterior pharyngeal wall. The cleansing procedure should be repeated several times in the ensuing 15 min. An iodide disinfectant is then used to cleanse the peribuccal region. The surgical towels are positioned to expose only the buccal cavity and the anterior part of one iliac spine for graft taking. The surgeon then changes his operative gown and disinfects his hands. He is seated on a stool so as to work directly over the buccal cavity. Roentgenograms are often necessary to verify the appropriateness of the operative position or the reduction of the osteoarticular structures of the craniovertebral junction. The two assistants stand one at each side of the patient's head.

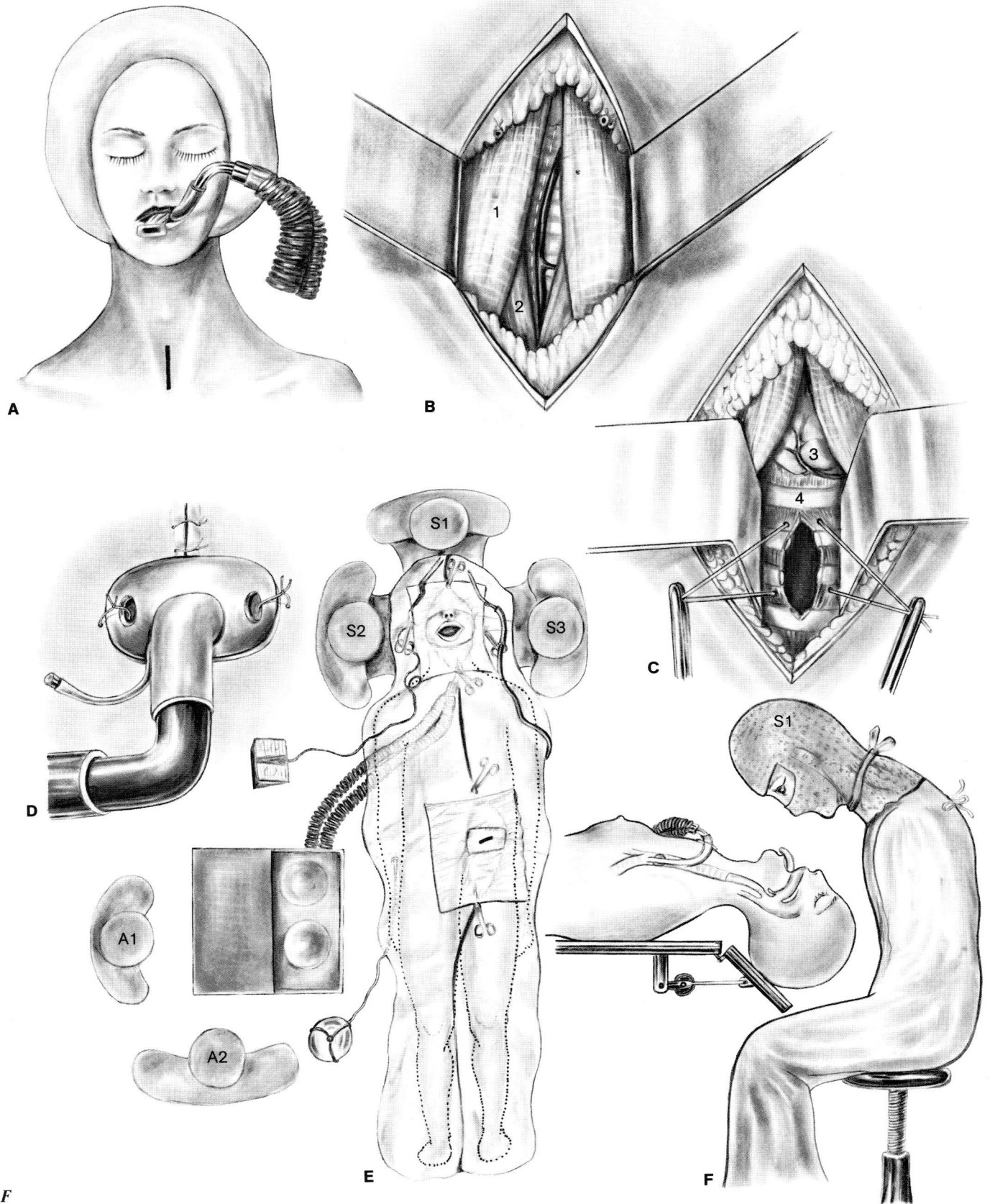

Figure 62 A–F

A   Peroral endotracheal intubation and the tracheostomy incision
B   The tracheostomy region
C   Tracheostomy
D   Introduction of Sjöbert's cannula

E   Position of the operative towels and surgical team
F   Surgeon's position

1 m. sternohyoideus   *2* m. sternothyroideus   *3* isthmus glandula thyroidea   *4* trachea

(4) Exposure of the Osteoarticular Structures

An orthostatic buccal retractor with a blade to retract the tongue is installed. The deep posterior wall of the oral cavity is thoroughly disinfected. A flexible retractor bent at a 90° angle is positioned so that its lower edge compresses the soft palate in the direction of the base of the cranium. Incision of the soft palate is not necessary. The midline region of the posterior pharyngeal wall is infiltrated down to the bone with 1% lidocaïne-epinephrine solution. A midline incision is then made with a plain knife from the upper margin of the tubercle of the atlas (palpable with the finger) to the level of C2–C3, the mean length of the incision being about 5 cm. Bony contact is sought with a raspatory to recline all the soft tissue en bloc away from the midline and flush with the bone. This procedure greatly facilitates the exposure of the anterior tubercle and lateral masses of the atlas and the body of the axis. Flexible retractors held by the assistant are modeled to retract the walls of the operative field. Hemostasis, often required on each side of the body of the axis, is achieved by electrocoagulation with aspiration. When necessary exposure of the atlas can be extended up to the lateral articulations, i. e., 2 cm lateral to the midline, but not beyond this point. Conversely, exposure at the level of the lower part of the body of the axis and upper part of C3 must not exceed 10–12 mm lateral to the midline, to avoid penetration of the intertransverse region. The middle region subjacent to the anterior arch of the atlas is a depressed area containing fibrous structures. Exposure of this area often requires the use of long fine gouge forceps. The operative field should be rinsed frequently with saline-antibiotic solution during surgery.

(5) Closure

The region is closed in two layers. The prevertebral muscles, forming the deep layer, are approximated on the midline with interrupted slow-resorbing sutures. A slender curved needle with a circular cross section is used. The pharyngeal layer is closed by interrupted sutures using nonresorbable monofilament material and a similar needle. The sutures should be moderately tightened to avoid cutting the tissue and sufficiently close-spaced (6 mm apart) to achieve a hermetic barrier between the buccal cavity and operative site. The retractors are then removed and the buccal cavity rinsed. The surgeon should check that a compress packed under the base of the tongue to avoid liquid entering the trachea has been removed. In the region of the tracheostomy the temporary sutures are removed. Retractors are then installed on each side of the trachea and the balloon of the cannula deflated, and while the Sjöbert's cannula is removed the anesthesiologist installs an endotracheal tube by the peroral route. Three or four interrupted nonresorbable monofilament sutures are required to close the trachea, using a curved, small-diameter needle. The sutures are placed mainly in the interannular regions of the trachea. Hermetic tracheal closure is mandatory, requiring a 1-mm overlapping of the lips of the incision in some cases. The superficial layers are then closed by a few slow-resorbing interrupted sutures. Finally, widely spaced interrupted sutures are used to close the skin wound and a dressing is placed over the incision. The endotracheal tube is removed when the patient is sufficiently conscious.

(6) Postoperative Care

The patient should wear a plastic orthopedic collar (Thomas' collar). Intravenous infusion of antibiotics and anti-inflammatory drugs is maintained for 24–48 h. Oral feeding with liquids and then semisolid food is started on the first postoperative day. Early ambulation is allowed. Parenteral antibiotics are continued until the end of the second postoperative week. The buccal cavity should be regularly examined during the early postoperative period. The patient is instructed to gargle with an antiseptic solution after each meal for two weeks.

(7) Possible Per- and Postoperative Complications

Aggravating the osteoarticular or neurological lesions must be avoided during manipulation of the neck when installing the patient in the operative position. During tracheostomy care must be taken not to mistake the common carotid artery for the trachea by palpation of the cartilaginous rings and needle puncture of the trachea. Introduction of Sjöbert's cannula may lead to injury of the trachea when the tracheal opening is not sufficiently retracted or when force is used. The airway may be patent for only one lung when the cannula is positioned too deeply in the trachea, so the tracheostomy should be sufficiently high (under the thyroid gland) to eliminate this complication. Poor exposure of the operative field occurs when the tongue or soft palate is not correctly retracted. Tracheal aspiration of fluid is avoided by packing a compress, identified by a thread, behind the tongue in the lower pharynx.

During operation vascular injury must be avoided, especially in the intertransverse regions on each side of the lower part of the body of C2 (vertebral arteries) and beyond the lateral masses of the atlas due to penetration of a raspatory into the subparotid space. Similarly, manipulation of the raspatory in this region more than 2 cm lateral to the midline can lead to injury of the ninth and twelfth cranial nerves with subsequent hemiparalysis of the tongue. During operation on the osteoarticular structures dangerous maneuvers in the direction of the vertebral canal must be avoided, e. g., after removal of the vertebral body due to tumor, by stopping work when the posterior fibrous structures are attained and by proscribing the use of a chisel when working in the direction of the neuraxis. Correct positioning of the head to achieve reduction, with the occipital region resting on a hard surface, is required to eliminate peroperative vertebral displacement and injury to the neural structures. The major risk of anterior surgery is postoperative infection, as evidenced by disunion of the pharyngeal wound, hyperthermia, and expulsion of the bone graft. This risk is eliminated by thorough local preparation, administration of antibiotics, absence of coagulation eschars, and the proscription of continuous and resorbable sutures of the pharyngeal wall.

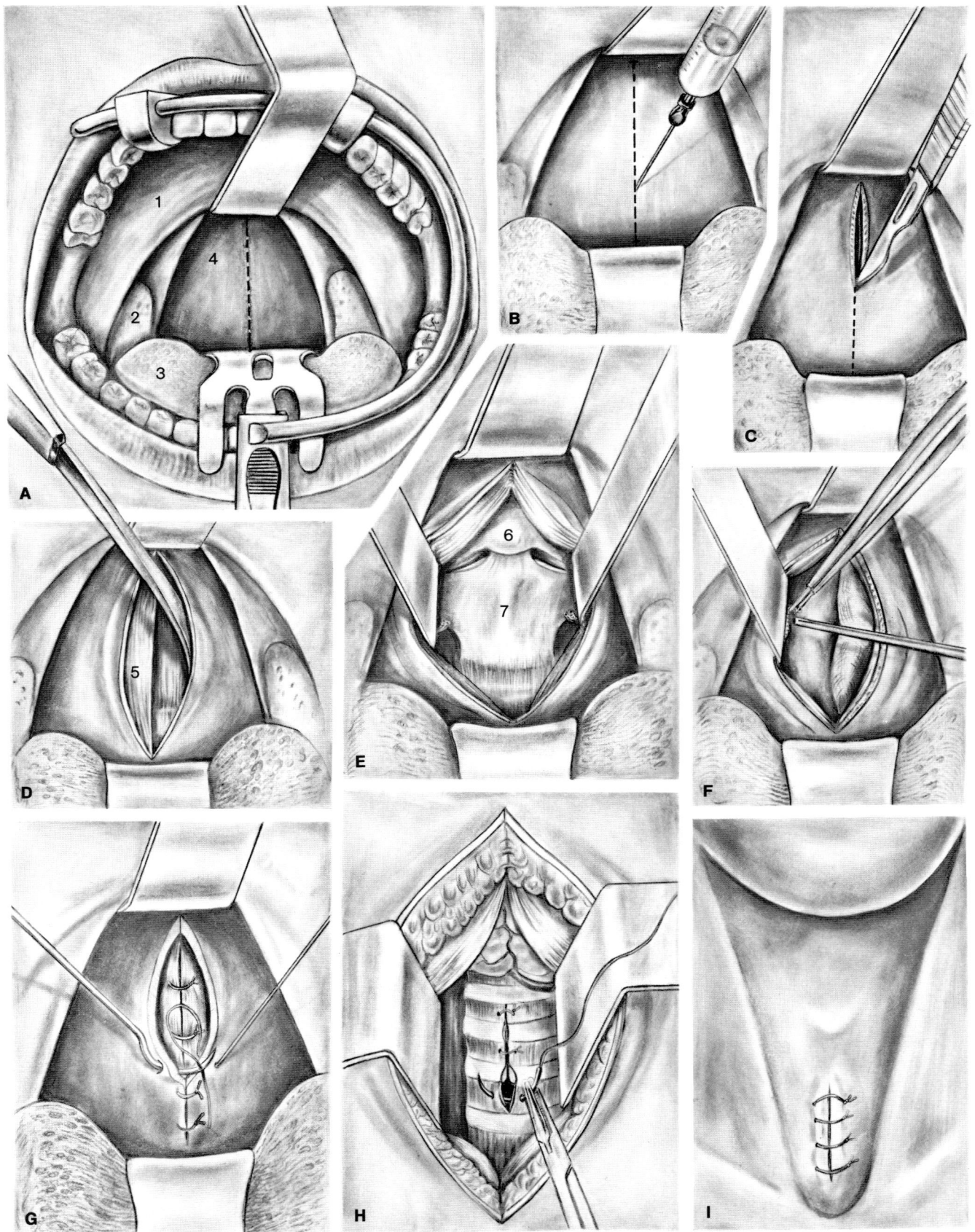

Figure 63 A–I

A   Exposure of the posterior wall of the pharynx
B   Lidocaine-epinephrine infiltration
C   Midline incision of the pharynx
D   Decollement of the prevertebral muscles
E   Exposure of the atlas and axis
F   Hemostasis

G   Two-layered closure
H   Closure of the trachea
I   Closure of the tracheostomy wound

1 velum palatinum   *2* tonsilla palatina   *3* lingua   *4* pharynx
5 m. longus colli   *6* atlas   *7* axis

b) Extrabuccal

The following section is devoted to a brief description of certain approaches we no longer use since they are less convenient and do not allow certain procedures required for bone grafting with osteosynthesis.

(1) Lateral

This approach, initially used by Jaboulay and Jonnesco to resect the superior cervical sympathetic ganglion, was described by Henry (1957). Anesthesia requires pre-, per-, and postoperative tracheostomy. The patient is positioned supine with the head in slight extension and turned to the side opposite the site of incision. The incision is begun at the tip of the mastoid process behind the ascending branch of the mandible and continued along the anterior margin of the sternocleidomastoideus to a point 2 cm below the angle of the jaw.

Once the cutaneous layers have been incised and the longissimus colli divided, the auricular branch of the superficial cervical plexus is identified and retracted and the external jugular vein ligated. The parotid gland is then retracted anteriorly and the occipital artery divided between two ligatures, thus exposing the vessels of the neck, i.e., the external carotid and internal carotid arteries and internal jugular vein. The twelfth cranial nerve can be identified as it runs over the outer surface of the carotid artery under the digastric muscle. The spinal nerve must also be identified at the upper end of the operative field, where it runs posteriorly towards the deep aspect of the sternocleidomastoideus. Using a clamp-held compress and a retractor, the neurovascular bundle is retracted forward, behind the ascending branch of the mandible, to expose the prevertebral muscles. The lateral tubercle of the atlas and the axis can then be identified. The anterior arch of the atlas and anterior surface of the axis are rasped free of the prevertebral muscles. This exposure allows only a lateral and tangential view of the craniovertebral junction. Closure is achieved after installing suction drainage. Possible complications include injury to a neurovascular structure in the posterior subparotid space and damage to the posterior surface of the pharynx.

The major drawback of the lateral approach is its very narrow exposure of the craniovertebral junction. The operative field can be enlarged by sectioning the superior insertion of the sternocleidomastoideus.

(2) Submaxillary

Access to the craniovertebral junction can also be gained by the submaxillary approach passing above or below the hyoid bone. The head is positioned as in the transbuccal approach, in hyperextension, with pre-, per-, and postoperative tracheostomy. A transverse incision may be used extending to the submaxillary regions midway between the inferior maxillary and hyoid bones. Subsequent to ligation of the anterior jugular veins the superficial cervical fascia is divided. The mylohyoideus and geniohyoideus are cut flush with the hyoid bone, divided by a median sagittal incision, and retracted,

giving access to the pharyngeal mucosa. This mucosa is opened carefully on the midline to avoid injury to the epiglottis, which is retracted using a flexible blade. A second flexible retractor is positioned to retract the tongue upwards. The posterior surface of the pharynx is thus exposed and incised as during the transoral approach. Closure is accomplished layer by layer using interrupted slow-resorbing sutures. The submaxillary approach may also be achieved through a transverse interthyroid incision with division of the subhyoid muscles and interthyroid membrane. The pharyngeal mucosa is then opened and the epiglottis and tongue reclined. Incision of the posterior pharyngeal wall is performed as in the transbuccal approach. The submaxillary approach allows access to only the axis and C3. Possible complications include disturbed phonation and deglutition, as this route passes in close proximity to the larynx. The patient may also present respiratory disturbances due to perilaryngeal edema, and therefore tracheostomy should be maintained during the postoperative period. The risks of infection are identical to those of the transoral approach.

The advantages of a well-controlled transoral approach are such that the lateral and submaxillary routes to the craniovertebral junction are of practically no interest.

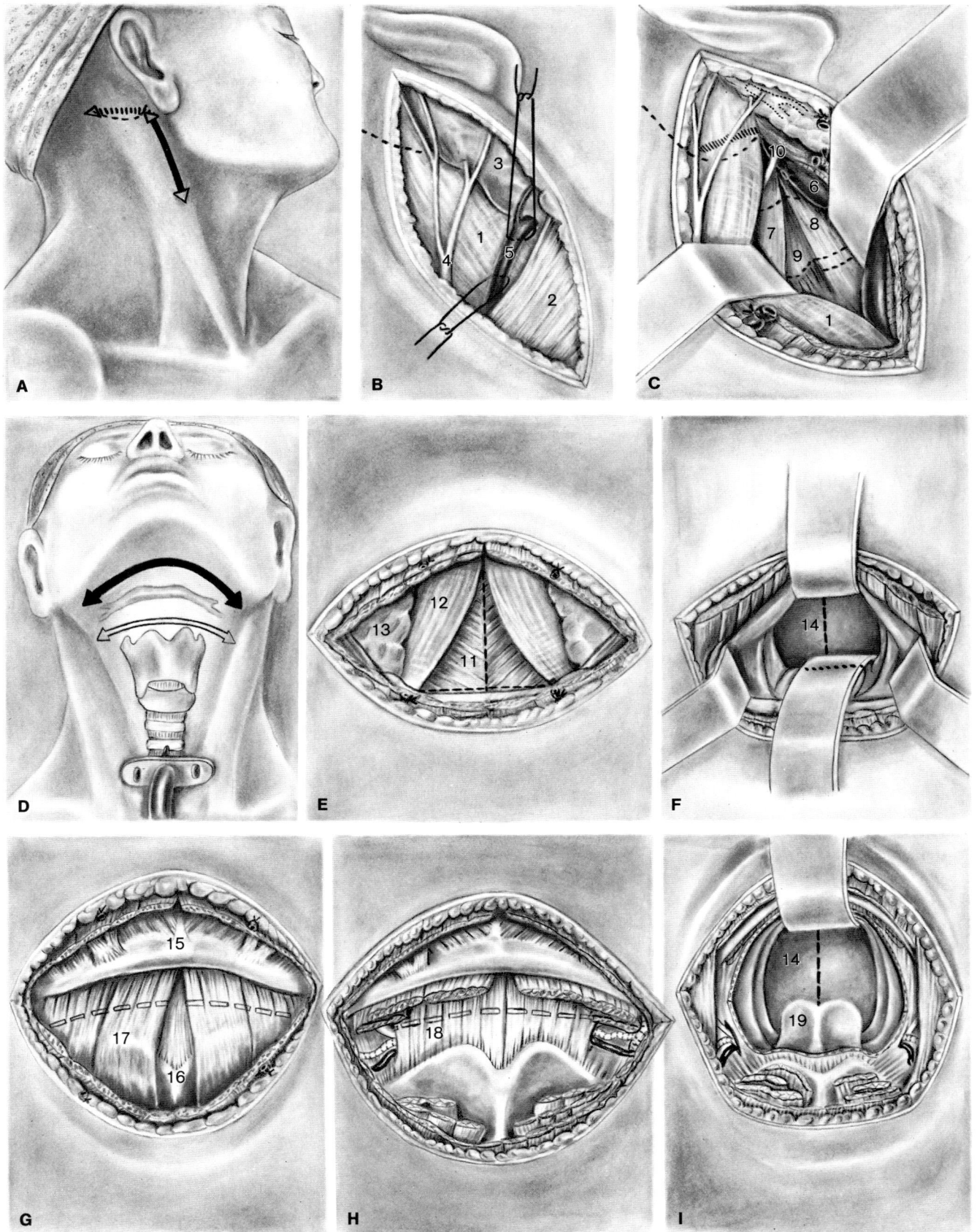

Figure 64 A–I

A–C   Retromaxillary approach to C1 and C2
D–F   Subhyoid approach to C1, C2, and C3
G–I   Interthyroid approach to C2, C3, and C4

7 m. scalenus   *8* m. longus capitis   *9* processus transversus C2
10 n. accessorius   *11* m. mylohyoideus   *12* m. digastricus venter ant.
13 n. glandula submandibularis   *14* pharynx   *15* os hyoideum
16 prominentia laryngea   *17* m. sternohyoideus   *18* membrana thyro-
hyoidea   *19* epiglottis

1 m. sternocleidomastoideus   *2* m. cutaneus colli   *3* glandula parotis
4 n. auricularis magnus   *5* v. jugularis externa   *6* v. jugularis interna

B. Lower Cervical Spine

Transverse Section Through C7. This section clearly shows the anterior relations of the lower cervical spine and the possible routes of surgical access to this region. Access is more superficial anteriorly than posteriorly despite the axial position of the vertebrae. The anterior approach allows exposure of those parts of the vertebrae located in front of the posterior articular pillars, i. e., the intervertebral foramina, anterior wall of the vertebral canal, transverse processes, vertebral bodies, and intervertebral discs. The prevertebral muscles and the scaleni muscles anteriorly cover the bony structures. The deep cervical fascia, also known as the lamina prevertebralis, is applied to the vertebrae and axial muscles. Three regions and groups of organs can be described anterior to the spine: the visceral axis of the neck, the vascular bundle, and the cervical and brachial nerve plexuses.

The *anterior triangle* of the neck is bounded by the two sternocleidomastoideus muscles, the sternum, and the mandible. The triangle contains the supra- and subhyoid muscles and the viscera of the neck, i. e., the pharynx and esophagus posteriorly and the larynx and trachea with the overlying thyroid gland anteriorly. The parathyroid glands and the recurrent and superior laryngeal nerves are also located in this median visceral region. The middle cervical fascia gives rise to the visceral sheath surrounding the median visceral region of the neck. This middle fascial layer is also referred to as the lamina pretrachealis.

The *vascular bundle* of the neck, corresponding to the sternocleidomastoid region, lies on the right and left flanks of the visceral axis of the neck. From the superficial to deep parts the following structures are found: the platysma and sternocleidomastoideus, the internal jugular vein, the common, internal, and external carotid arteries, the pneumogastric nerve (tenth cranial nerve), and lymph nodes. The vascular structures are contained within a common sheath connected to the visceral sheath of the neck and the lamina prevertebralis. The vascular bundle supplies and drains the visceral axis.

The *posterior triangle* of the neck, also called the supraclavicular region, is bounded laterally by the anterior margin of the trapezius and the posterior margin of the sternocleidomastoideus, and below by the clavicle. The superficial part of the triangle comprises the latissimus colli and the superficial cervical fascia (also covering the other neck regions). A thick adipocellular layer lies below, covering the scaleni muscles and the branches of the superficial cervical and brachial plexuses lying between the anterior and middle scaleni muscles. This lateral region is thus located at the level of the transverse processes.

Three anterior approaches to the cervical spine were first cited by Chipault (1894). These approaches are distinguished according to their plane of incision:

Presternocleidomastoid. This approach to the anterior surface of the cervical spine (Robinson 1955) passes between the lateral surface of the visceral axis of the neck and the medial margin of the sternocleidomastoideus and vascular bundle. Two variants can be described according to the route of passage through the fascial layers. The classical variant involves opening the sheath of the sternocleidomastoideus and incision of the vascular sheath. The second variant, used by us, comprises the dissection of the lamina pretrachealis in order to pass directly against the subhyoid muscle fibers without opening the vascular sheath. Finally, access is gained to the retropharyngeal space in front of the prevertebral fascia. This approach can be used to expose the right or left side of the cervical spine.

Anterolateral. The first steps of this approach (Verbiest 1961; Jung 1963) are identical to those described above, i.e., passage between the visceral axis of the neck and the vascular bundle medial to the sternocleidomastoideus. However, once the inner margin of the carotid artery has been passed, the approach is directed towards the transverse processes rather than the median corporeal region of the spine. Accordingly, the anterior part of the transverse foramina is resected to mobilize the vertebral artery and allow direct access to the intervertebral foramina. This is an excellent approach when surgery involves the intervertebral foramina directly, but associated operative procedures such as osteosynthesis cannot be performed.

Retrosternocleidomastoid Lateral. This approach has practically been abandoned. The route of access passes through the supraclavicular depression behind the posterior margin of the sternocleidomastoideus and then anterior to the scaleni muscles and phrenic nerve, i.e., behind the vascular bundle of the neck. Access is gained to the intervertebral foramina or the anterolateral surface of the vertebral bodies and intervertebral discs, and the spinal nerves and vertebral artery can also be exposed. However, only unilateral spinal access is achieved, and furthermore operative maneuvers are highly tangential with respect to the greater axis of the spine, thus not allowing anterior decompression of the vertebral canal or osteosynthesis of the vertebral bodies.

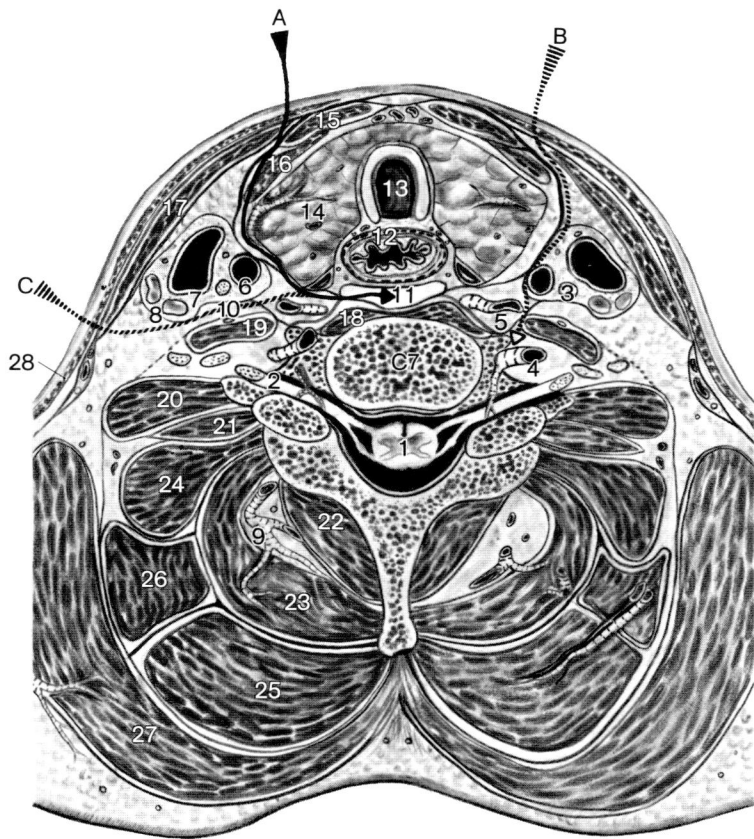

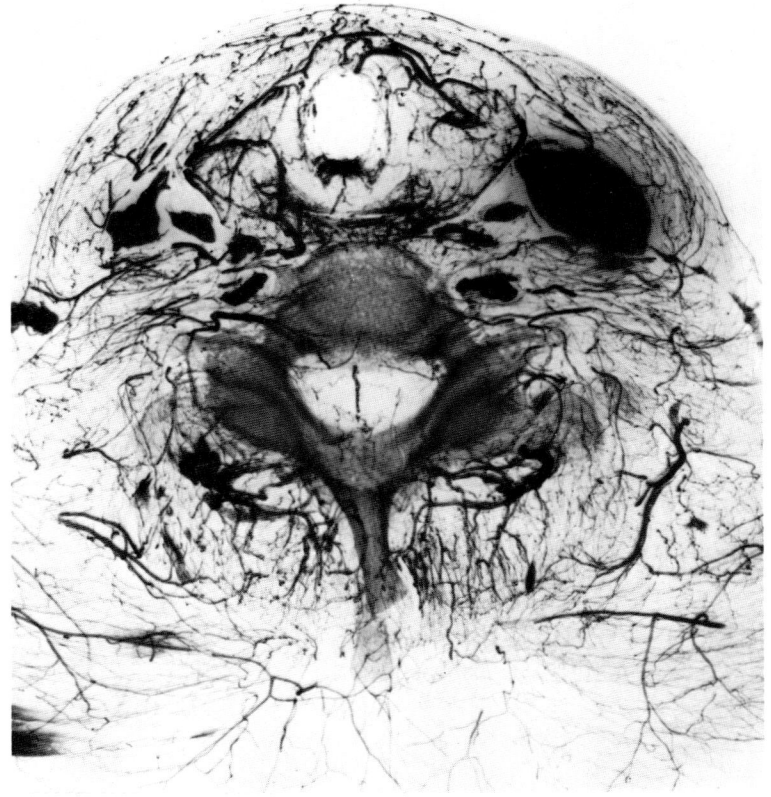

Figure 65

Transverse section through C7: diagram and radiography after opacification of arteries

1 medulla spinalis   *2* n. spinalis   *3* n. vagus   *4* a. vertebralis
5 a. thyroidea inf.   *6* a. carotis interna   *7* v. jugularis interna   *8* nodi lymphatici cervicales   *9* a. cervicalis profunda   *10* n. phrenicus

11 regio retropharyngea   *12* esophagus   *13* trachea   *14* glandula thyroidea   *15* m. sternohyoideus   *16* m. sternothyroideus
17 m. sternocleidomastoideus   *18* m. longus colli   *19* m. scalenus ant.
20 m. scalenus medius   *21* m. scalenus post.   *22* m. transversospinalis
23 m. semispinalis capitis   *24* m. levator scapulae   *25* m. splenius capitis   *26* m. splenius cervicis   *27* m. trapezius   *28* m. platysma or cutaneus colli

1. Topography

a) Landmarks and Layers of the Neck

(1) Landmarks

The shape of the neck varies according to the individual, especially to stoutness. However, according to Richet the length of the neck is practically constant in all individuals. The bony frame of the neck comprises the clavicle, the lower margin of the mandible, and the mastoid bone. The anterior and posterior margins of the sternocleidomastoideus are also easy to identify. Identification of the hyoid bone below the mandible permits determination of the level of C4. The cricoid cartilage lies at the level of the C6–C7 intervertebral disc. It should be kept in mind that T1 and T2 extend above the level of the sternal manubrium. In certain subjects with very sloping shoulders and an inclined first rib, T3 may lie in the cervical region. The external jugular vein is easily identified by compressing the supraclavicular region. Finally, the surgeon should be familiar with the horizontal skin folds of the neck allowing aesthetic transverse incisions.

(2) Layers

The platysma muscle lies immediately under the skin, its fibers running obliquely downward and backward from the lower margin of the mandible to the clavicle. It extends barely above the angle of the mandible. Owing to its role in facial expression, the platysma must be identified and reconstituted by sutures. Cutaneous neurovascular bundles pass through the muscle. Deep to the platysma the superficial cervical fascia lines the full circumference of the neck up to the superior and inferior bony margins, forming a full sheath around the external and anterior jugular veins and sternocleidomastoideus muscle. The fat pad of the neck, interposed between the platysma muscle and the superficial fascia, varies in thickness according to the individual and is separated from the superficial cervical fascia by its proper fascia superficialis. Indeed, blunt dissection (with a clamp-held compress) can be used to separate the skin, platysma, and fat pad from the superficial cervical fascia, thus transforming a horizontal incision into a vertical operative field. This decollement requires the sectioning of only a few fine vascular bundles. Removal of the superficial cervical fascia allows clear identification of three regions: the anterior triangle, the sternocleidomastoid region, and the posterior triangle of the neck. At the level of the supraclavicular region, between the posterior margin of the sternocleidomastoideus and the anterior margin of the trapezius, the external jugular vein can be identified above a fold of fascia. Branches of the supraclavicular nerve arising from the cervical plexus also pass through this region. The sternocleidomastoid region thus delimits a rectangular area bounded by the inferior sternal and clavicular bundles of the muscle (with a triangular slit between the muscle bundles) and the superior mastoid and occipital muscle bundles. Rotation of the head to one side stretches the muscle on the opposite side and relaxes the muscle on the same side. Neurovascular structures pass through the region of the sternocleidomastoideus: the external jugular vein, running from the angle of the mandible towards the posterior triangle of the neck, and three branches of the superficial cervical plexus, from bottom to top the transverse nerve of the neck (transverse cervical branch), the greater auricular nerve (auricular branch), and the lesser occipital nerve (mastoid branch). Finally, the parotid gland partially extends over the anterior margin of the mastoid muscle bundle. Owing to this neural arrangement, the anterior margin of the sternocleidomastoideus can easily be dissected without injury to the nerves, whereas the posterior margin of the muscle is punctuated by the emergence of the nerves. In the region of the anterior triangle of the neck the anterior jugular veins and a few arterioles run in a vertical direction, whereas the terminal rami of the transverse nerve of the neck traverse horizontally. On the whole, the rami of the superficial cervical plexus run first deep to the fascia and then in a fascial fold, finally emerging through the fascia to reach the skin.

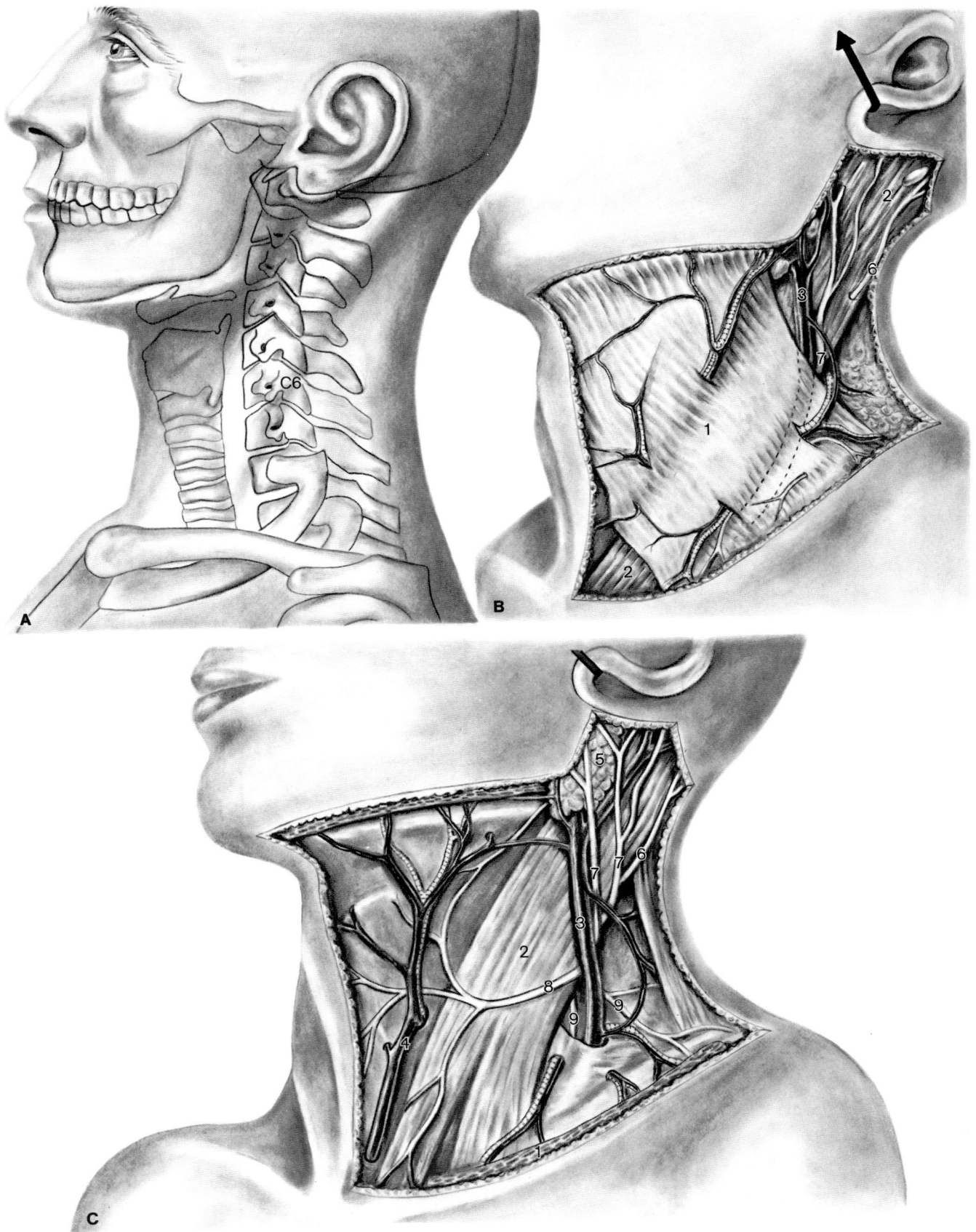

Figure 66 A–C

A   Cutaneous projection of the bony landmarks of the neck
B   Subcutaneous layer of the neck
C   Subplatysmal layer of the neck

1 m. cutaneus colli platysma   *2* m. sternocleidomastoideus   *3* v.
jugularis externa   *4* v. jugularis ant.   *5* glandula parotis   *6* n. occipitalis minor   *7* n. auricularis magnus   *8* n. transversus colli   *9* n. supraclaviculares

b) Neurovascular Bundle of the Neck

The neurovascular bundle of the neck comprises the carotid arteries medially, the internal jugular vein laterally, and the pneumogastric nerve posteriorly. It is normally covered by the sternocleidomastoideus regardless of the position of the head, and accordingly pronounced lateral retraction of the muscle is required to expose the structures of the neurovascular bundle. Furthermore, the connective tissue sheath surrounding the bundle must be opened to achieve exposure.

The *common carotid artery* forms the medial margin of the neurovascular bundle, running first obliquely upward and outward and then vertically in front of the cervical transverse processes just lateral to the trachea, esophagus, pharynx, and larynx. The carotid bifurcation, giving rise to the external and internal carotid arteries, is situated 1 cm above the upper margin of the thyroid cartilage. The carotid sinus, located at the dilated part of the common carotid artery, contains the highly sensitive intracarotid baroceptors, and thus local anesthetics can be infiltrated into the subadventitial tissue of the common carotid and its sinus to avoid changes of blood pressure due to manipulation with retractors in this region. The external carotid artery is at its origin anterior and medial to the internal carotid artery, then runs lateral to it. Only the external carotid artery gives off branches in the cervical region: the superior thyroid artery, arising very close to the origin of the external carotid; the lingual and ascending pharyngeal arteries, arising 1 cm higher; the facial and occipital branches, 5 mm higher again; and finally the posterior auricular artery.

The *internal jugular vein* lies lateral and superficial to the arteries, its outer surface covered by a network of fat and lymphatic tissues. It receives numerous tributaries homologous to most of the collateral branches of the external carotid artery. These veins draining the facial, lingual, and thyroid regions frequently fuse to form a common venous trunk, crossing over the outer part of the common carotid artery, which is referred to as Farabeuf's thyrolinguofacial trunk. In some cases a middle thyroid vein crosses over the common carotid artery below the common venous trunk.

The *pneumogastric or vagus nerve* (tenth cranial nerve) lies in the neurovascular bundle in the posterior dihedral angle between the carotid artery and internal jugular vein, and gives off rami to the heart which run along the common carotid artery. The neurovascular bundle is traversed by two surgically important nerves, the superior laryngeal and the hypoglossal. The superior laryngeal nerve arises from the lower part of the plexiform ganglion of the tenth cranial nerve, runs anterior to the prevertebral region and medial to the jugulocarotid bundle, and emerges below the origin of the lingual artery. Near the tip of the greater horn of the hyoid bone the nerve divides to form superior and inferior terminal branches, which penetrate into the larynx through the thyrohyoid and cricothyroid membranes respectively. The superior laryngeal nerve carries essentially sensory impulses form the larynx and base of the tongue and transmits motor impulses to the cricothyroid muscle. The hypoglossal nerve, innervating the muscles of the tongue, enters the upper part of the anterior cervical region, where it passes behind the carotid arteries and then runs along their outer surface and medial to the internal jugular vein. It often passes under a small sternocleidomastoid branch of the external carotid artery and then runs along the lower margin of the posterior belly of the digastric muscle, describing a curve with superior concavity above the greater horn of the hyoid bone; it finally disappears towards the base of the tongue in the region medial to the tendon of the stylohyoid muscle. The hypoglossal nerve gives off a descending branch where it passes behind the external carotid artery. This branch runs in the anterior dihedral angle between the common carotid artery and internal jugular vein, describing a loop near the lower middle part of the vein, and then ascends toward nerve roots C2 and C3. The descending branch of the hypoglossal nerve gives off motor rami to the subhyoid muscles.

The vascular axis of the neck is traversed by three groups of muscles: the sternothyroid muscle below; the intermediate tendon of the omohyoid muscle, attached to the middle cervical fascia; and the digastric muscle, slung over the upper part of the vascular bundle.

Surgical access to the underlying prevertebral region requires the ligation of one or several venous or arterial collaterals of the vascular bundle in order to allow anterior and medial retraction of the visceral axis of the neck. It should be noted that rotation of the head tends to displace the upper carotid region towards the midline. Consequently, during the anterior approach to the upper cervical spine the head should be positioned looking directly forward or with slight rotation to the side of approach, in order to expose the anterior surface of the spine clearly with respect to the neurovascular bundle of the neck.

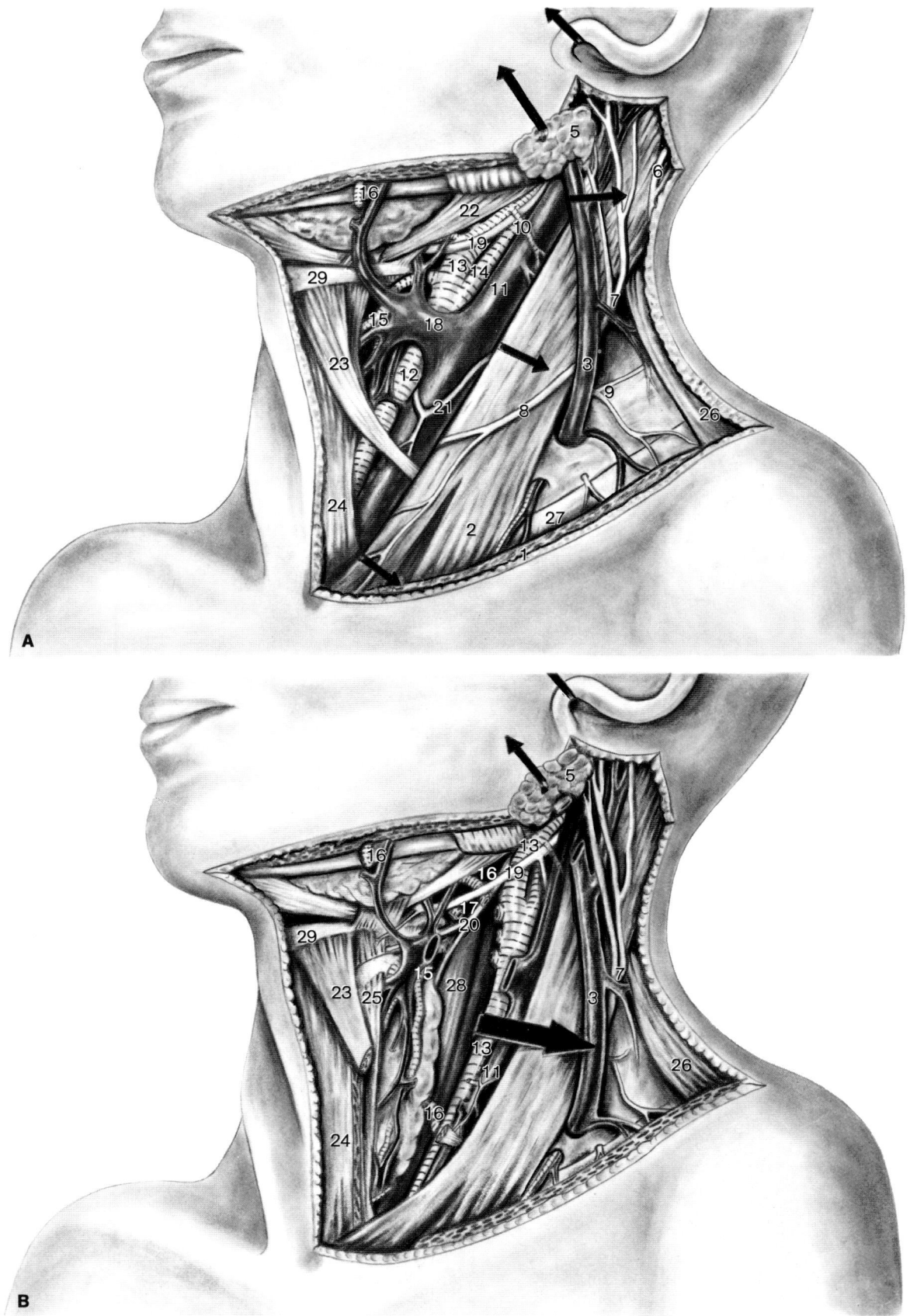

Figure 67 A, B

A The jugulocarotid region
B The median visceral region of the neck

1 m. cutaneus colli, platysma *2* m. sternocleidomastoideus
3 v. jugularis externa *5* glandula parotis *6* n. occipitalis minor *7* n. auricularis magnus *8* n. transversus colli *9* n. supraclaviculares
10 ramus sternocleidomastoideus *11* v. jugularis interna *12* a. carotis communis *13* a. corotis externa *14* a. carotis interna *15* a. thyroidea sup. *16* a. facialis *17* a. lingualis *18* v. facialis, lingualis, thyroidea *19* n. hypoglossus *20* n. laryngeus sup. *21* ansa cervicalis *22* m. digastricus venter post. *23* m. omohyoideus *24* m. sternohyoideus *25* m. thyrohyoideus *26* m. trapezius *27* clavicula *28* pharynx *29* os hyoideum

c) Spinal Axis

Retraction of the visceral and neurovascular axes of the neck exposes the spinal axis, displaying an anterior discocorporeal region, the lateral zone of the intervertebral and transverse foramina, and the anterior surface of the vertebral canal.

(1) Anterior Discocorporeal Region

The anterior surface of the vertebral bodies and intervertebral discs of the lower cervical spine lies on the midline in a cephalocaudal plane displaying anterior convexity. In fact, this approach allows access to the anterior tubercle of the atlas above and the first two or three thoracic vertebrae below. Identification of the numerical correspondence of the vertebrae requires the identification of the anterior tubercle of C6 (Chassaignac's tubercle). The prevertebral muscles i.e., longus colli, longissimus capitis, and rectus capitis anterior, lie over the lateral parts of the vertebral bodies. The scaleni muscles, lying more laterally, do not belong to this region. The vessels of this region are the branches of the right and left subclavian arteries (vertebral arteries and thyrocervical trunks). The vertebral arteries, the first branches of the subclavian arteries, ascend vertically in the dihedral angle formed by the longissimus colli and anterior scalenus muscles and then enter the sixth transverse foramina to continue upwards towards the foramen magnum. The vertebral arteries are normally hidden by the prevertebral muscles and the transverse processes. During operation the intertransverse segments of the arteries are exposed at the level of the intervertebral discs. The vertebral arteries give rise to transverse arterioles running over the middle part of the vertebral bodies. The thyrocervical trunk gives rise to the ascending cervical artery, anterior to the anterior scalenus, and the inferior thyroid artery, which passes at some distance in front of the prevertebral muscles. A vertical arterial branch arising from either the inferior thyroid artery or the thyrocervical trunk runs anterior to the lateral part of the vertebral bodies and anastomoses with the transverse branches of the vertebral arteries. Hemostasis of these small arterioles is required during operation. Relations with the nervous structures in this region include the cervical sympathetic trunk, lying in a fold of the prevertebral fascia anterior to the prevertebral muscles. Lying more laterally, the phrenic nerve runs in the fascia covering the anterior scalenus muscle. The branches of the brachial plexus lie lateral to the transverse processes.

(2) Intervertebral and Transverse Foramina

The cervical intervertebral foramina are continued by the grooves of the transverse processes, transforming the foramina into 15-mm long canals. The deep part of these canals is formed by the posterior articular pillars and their medial wall by the vertebral unci, which close the intervertebral spaces. The intervertebral foramina thus open anteriorly with a lateral and slightly downward slant. They contain five different structures. Horizontally, the large spinal nerves form the pos-

terior and inferior part of the intervertebral canals, whereas the vertebral arteries, running vertically and lying anterior to the spinal nerves, constitute the anterior and medial contents. Radiculomedullary arteries arising from the posteromedial surface of the vertebral arteries pass through the intervertebral foramina to supply the spinal nerves, dura mater, lateral walls of the vertebral canal, and spinal cord. These arterial branches must not be injured during surgery. Netlike vegetative fibers (Franck's nerve) run along the vertebral artery giving off rami to the spinal nerves. Finally, numerous veins occupying the spaces between the preceding structures form veritable venous plexuses along the vertebral arteries and spinal nerves. Hemostasis of these veins is sometimes difficult to achieve, and their presence may hinder operative dissection in the intervertebral foramina.

(3) Vertebral Canal

The anterior part of the vertebral canal can be considered part of the anterior cervical region when the vertebral bodies and intervertebral discs have been resected. The different layers forming the anterior wall of the canal comprise the posterior surface of the vertebral bodies and intervertebral discs, the posterior longitudinal ligament, the anterior surface of the dural envelope, and numerous intervening blood vessels. The latter include the arterioles arising from the radiculomedullary arteries and running anterior to the anterior longitudinal ligament, followed by the veins and longitudinal anterointernal intraspinal venous plexuses running in the lateral recesses of the vertebral canal in front of the emergence of the spinal nerve roots. The transverse anastomoses of these plexuses traverse the posterior longitudinal ligament to lie near the posterior surface of the vertebral bodies, where hemostasis of these veins must be accomplished. Exposure of the anterior surface of the dural envelope requires that the anterior longitudinal ligament be sectioned, preferably on the midline to avoid injury to the lateral plexuses. Finally, deep to the dura mater the anterior surface of the spinal cord may be the site of compression, especially of the anterior spinal artery.

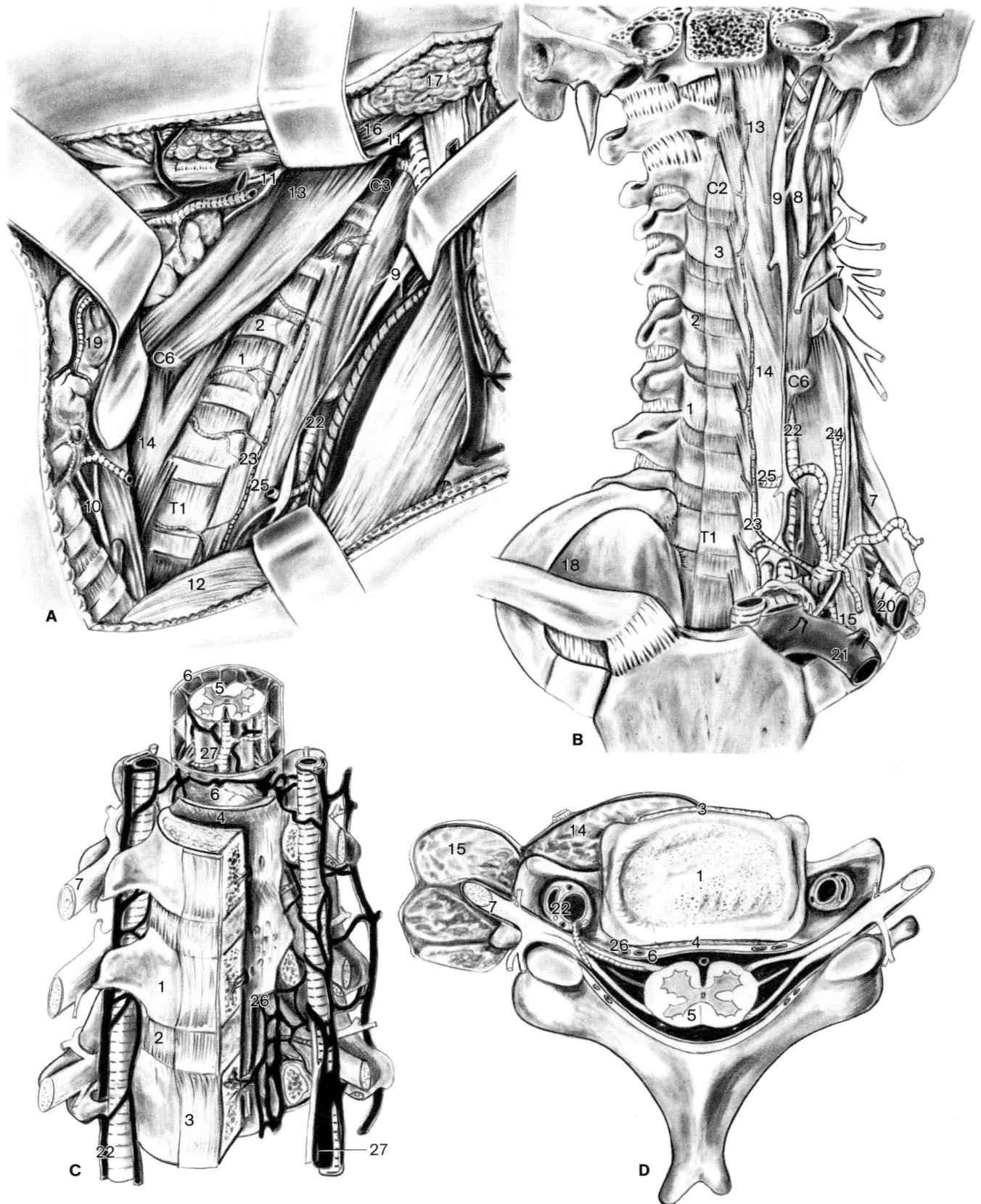

Figure 68 A–D

A   Left anterior approach to the inferior cervical spine
B   Prevertebral region
C   Intrinsic relations of the inferior cervical spine
D   Horizontal section of the spine through C6

1 corpus vertebrae 2 discus intervertebralis 3 lig. longitudinale ant.
4 lig. longitudinale post. 5 medulla spinalis 6 dura mater spinalis
7 n. spinalis 8 n. vagus, ganglion inf. 9 ganglion cervicale sup.

10 n. laryngeus recurrens 11 n. hypoglossus 12 m. sternocleidomastoideus 13 m. longus capitis 14 m. longus colli 15 m. scalenus
ant. 16 m. digastricus 17 glandula parotis 18 pleura parietalis
19 glandula thyroidea 20 a. subclavia 21 v. subclavia 22 a. vertebralis 23 ramus vertebralis trunci thyrocervicalis 24 a. cervicalis
ascendens 25 a. thyroidea inf. 26 plexus venosi vertebralis
interni ant. 27 v. vertebralis

d) Variations of the Vertebral Arteries

Knowledge of the anatomical variations of the vertebral arteries is of prime importance owing to the risks of injuring these vessesl during anterior surgery of the cervical spine. The statistical data given below were reported by Argenson, Francke, Papasian (1979). The vertebral artery is divided into two surgical segments in the cervical region. The pretransverse segment (V1) is that part of the artery between its origin and point of penetration in the transverse foramen. The transverse segment (V2) extends from the point of entry in the transverse foramen to the C2–C3 intertransverse space.

Number and Caliber. The mean caliber of the vertebral arteries is 4.5 mm. Symmetry of the vertebral arteries with respect to caliber is found in 40.8% of cases. The right vertebral artery is dominant in 35.8% of cases and the left in 23.4%. Finally, it is important to know that one vertebral artery is lacking in 2.5% of cases and that the incidence of unilateral hypoplasia (caliber less than 2 mm) is 9.3%.

Origin. The vertebral artery is commonly the first collateral branch of the subclavian artery. The most frequent variations in the site of origin are the following: the left vertebral artery arising directly from the aorta (3.9%), or from the common carotid artery; trifurcation of the brachiocephalic trunk (1.1%); and bifid origin of one vertebral artery.

Pretransverse Segment. The vertebral arteries usually enter the spine through the transverse foramina of C6. The V1 segment lies in a triangle bounded inferiorly by the prescalenic segment of the subclavian artery and laterally by the longus colli and anterior scalenus, and in this triangle enters into relation with the pleural dome, the vertebral veins, and the stellar ganglion, the latter thus being divided into pre- and retroarterial portions. On the left the thoracic duct runs medial and then anterior to the vertebral artery. The length of V1 varies according to the level of its entry in the transverse foramen. In 90% of cases the artery enters the spine at C6, whereas in the remaining 10% penetration of the spine is at C5, C7, exceptionally C3, or C4. It is thus necessary to identify the presence of ectopic spinal penetration when surgery involves freeing of the vertebral artery.

Transverse Segment. The V2 segment of the vertebral arteries extends from the transverse foramen of C6 to the C2–C3 intertransverse space. It is alternately transosseous (passing through the transverse foramen) and free (intertransverse). The vertebral artery passes through the anteromedial part of the transverse foramen in contact with the anterior root of the transverse process, which is about 2.6 mm thick. The V2 segment is practically rectilinear but in rare cases may display a few loops, thus constituting an additional risk of surgical injury. Each vertebral artery is accompanied by its veins which most often resemble a veritable vertebrotransverse venous sinus, as described by us in 1962 based on the initial studies by Trolard (1868) and Laux (1949). Hemostasis in the region of these periarterial venous networks may therefore be problematic. The V2 segment relates especially to neural structures: a vegetative nerve running along the artery and the spinal nerve roots lying behind and below the artery in their intervertebral foramina.

Branches and Distribution. As the vertebral arteries course through the cervical region they give off many branches of varying caliber. Most of these branches supply the pre- and laterovertebral muscles while others enter the intervertebral foramina (spinal arteries) to supply the radiculomedullary structures. The largest-caliber spinal arteries enter the C5–C6 and C6–C7 intervertebral foramina, but it should be underlined that smaller spinal arteries exist at all levels. During surgery it is very important to identify and protect these arteries. Indeed, the neural areas supplied by the vertebral arteries include the cervical spinal cord and nerve roots, the brain stem, the cerebellum, and the occipital lobes. Injury to the vertebral artery can thus induce severe complications in this vast region of supply. Bilateral damage of the vertebral arteries theoretically has a fatal outcome unless retrograde repermeation occurs through the internal carotid arteries.

Figure 69 A–J

A Lateral view of the left vertebral artery from its origin to its point of entry into the vertebral canal
B Distribution of the vertebral arteries to the cervical spinal cord and medulla oblongata
C–F Variant types of vertebral artery penetration of the transverse foramina
G Hypoplasia of the vertebral artery
H An arterial loop
I, J Variant origins of the vertebral arteries

1 a. subclavia *2* a. vertebralis *3* truncus costocervicalis *4* a. carotis communis *5* a. spinalis ant. *6* a. basilaris *7* ramus spinalis

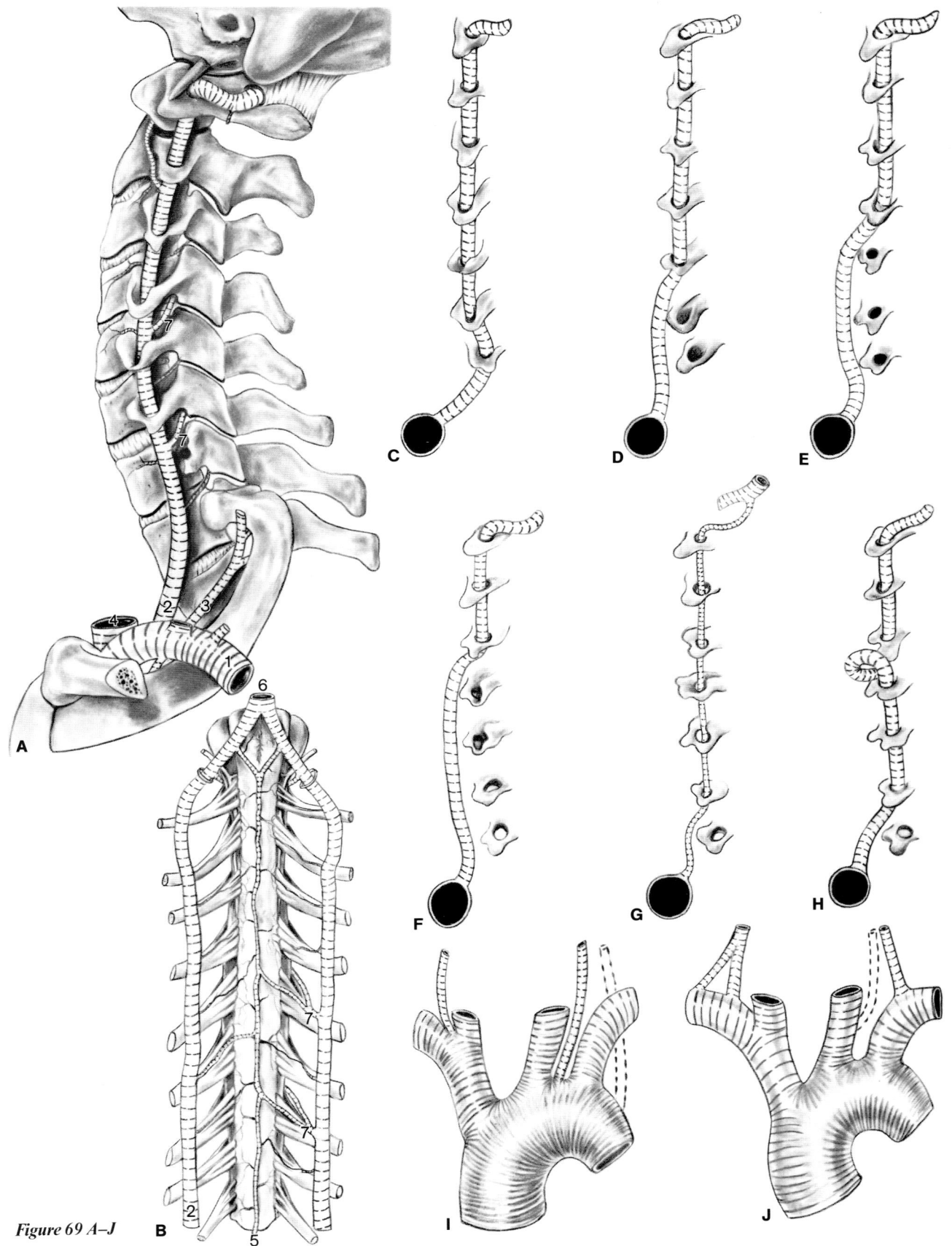

Figure 69 A–J

2. Anterior Approach

a) Preparation and Anesthesia

This approach does not generally require any special preparation of the patient. However, in cases of deformity due to trauma, orthopedic reduction without anesthesia is performed with the patient in a scoliosis frame on the day before or a few hours before operation. Reduction is monitored under the image intensifier. A plastic orthopedic collar allows maintenance of reduction until surgery is begun. Induction of anesthesia is achieved conventionally with endotracheal intubation. The head is positioned in slight posterior deflection to avoid flexion displacement in cases of traumatic lesion. Of course, as in all types of spinal surgery, the operating room is equipped with an automatic breathing device, appropriate material for cardiovascular monitoring, and an image intensifier equipped with a memory circuit.

b) Operative Position

The patient lies strictly supine with a cushion placed under the shoulders to allow full exposure of the anterior cervical region. The head should be positioned in zero rotation or turned to the side opposite the incision, i.e., facing to the right, bearing in mind that over-rotation of the head stretches the sternocleidomastoideus on the side opposite rotation, whereas the neutral position relaxes the muscle. The table is tilted downwards at the feet to drain the territory of the superior vena cava. The arms are placed along the body with the elbows resting on soft cushions to avoid compression of the cubital nerves. Finally, the feet are fixed to the operating table to ensure that the patient cannot slide down the table during surgery.

c) Identification of the Site of Incision

It is helpful to identify the site of skin incision prior to draping the operative field. This can be done using a coloring solution or by making a scratch mark on the skin with a small file. The bony frame of the neck, anterior margin of the sternocleidomastoideus, external jugular vein, and horizontal skin folds of the neck are identified. It is also helpful to identify the site of bone lesions with respect to the skin, using the image intensifier. When radiological monitoring is not available the following clinical guidelines may be used: incision of the upper third of the neck for lesions at C3 to C4, the middle third for lesions at C5 to C6, and the lower third for lesions at C7 to T1.

d) Preparation of the Operative Fields

The anesthesia apparatus is positioned beyond the patient's head, the infusion material near the feet. Two operative fields are then prepared: the cervical region and one anterior iliac region for taking bone-grafting material. Five large double-thickness towels (2 m × 1.5 m) are then placed in position. One towel is draped transversely over the head extending down to the angle of the mandible, a second is placed horizontally over the trunk from the sternal manubrium to the top of the left iliac crest, and a third is draped from the left anterosuperior iliac spine to the lower end of the table. The last two towels are then draped lengthwise, one on each side from the cervical region to the iliac crest. We recommend the left-sided approach, especially for spinal lesions below C6, because of the topographical differences between the left and right recurrent laryngeal nerves. Indeed, on the right side the loop of the recurrent laryngeal nerve is situated higher (from the right subclavian artery to the inferior pole of the thyroid gland), thus representing an obstacle to surgical incision in the lower operative field. Conversely, on the left side the recurrent laryngeal nerve, with its loop lying below the aorta, remains in contact with the visceral axis of the neck and is thus less prone to surgical injury. Removal of bone from the iliac crest is easier to achieve on the same side as the operator, i.e., the left. The site of bone removal is the anterior third of the iliac crest 2–3 cm posterior to the anterosuperior iliac spine. Four towel clips are used to maintain the lengthwise towels on each side of the two operative fields. After each operative step the electric cautery knife is attached to the towel clip to the right of the surgeon and the suction tube is fixed to the towel clip on the left (the reverse for left-handed surgeons). A transparent adhesive drape is placed over the skin to be incised.

e) Possible Complications

When preoperative reduction cannot be achieved it may be necessary to employ cervical traction using a head sling. Sliding of the subscapular pad towards the neck region tends to close and deepen the cervical operative field. Improper fixation of the feet to the operating table can lead to the patient sliding downward, thus modifying the position of the operative towels. The elbows must be correctly protected against compression to avoid postoperative cubital paralysis. Finally, poor radiological identification may considerably hinder the operative procedures.

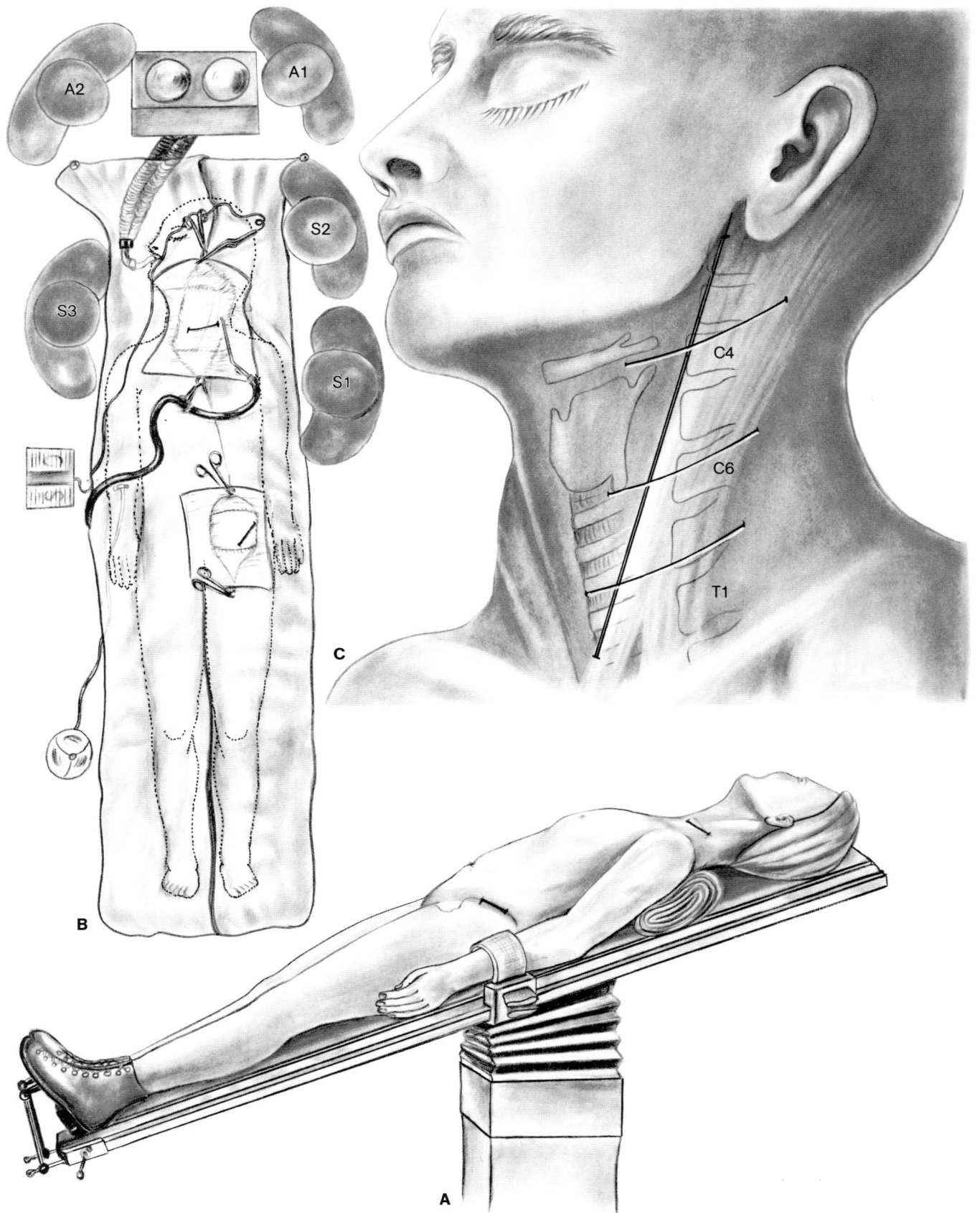

Figure 70 A–C

A   Operative position with a cushion under the shoulders, downward tilting of the operating table, and fixation of the feet to the table

B   Position of the operative fields with a transparent adhesive drape over the left cervical region and iliac crest. Note the position of the surgeons (S1, S2, S3) and the anesthesiologists (A1, A2)

C   Cutaneous landmarks and either longitudinal skin incision along the anterior margin of the sternocleidomastoideus or horizontal incision in a skin fold

f) Initial Exposure

Either a vertical or a horizontal incision can be used. The vertical incision along the anterior margin of the sternocleidomastoideus allows a wide exposure of the cervical spine in cases where more than three vertebrae must be exposed. The aesthetic horizontal incision in a transverse skin fold is made straddling the sternocleidomastoideus for 7–8 cm, and can be used when the operative approach requires exposure of only two to three vertebrae or one or two intervertebral discs. The external jugular vein must first be identified to avoid injury to it when making the transverse incision. The skin and subcutaneous tissue are incised with a plain knife to expose the fibers of the platysma muscle. Hemostasis of the subdermal vessels is achieved by electrocoagulation, using a very fine tipped cautery clamp in the right hand and a suction cannula in the left hand. The intensity of electrocoagulation must be adjusted so as not to burn the skin. The platysma is then transected with a plain knife, either in the same direction as the skin incision or parallel to its muscle fibers (after decollement of the skin and subcutaneous tissue from the muscle body).

g) Identification of the Vasculovisceral Axis

Transection of the platysma exposes the superficial cervical fascia, which is opened by blunt dissection using clamp-held compresses. When a vertical skin incision has been made the fascia is dissected in the same direction as the incision, but when a horizontal skin incision is used the cranial and caudal lips of the wound must be retracted by blunt dissection in order to expose a vertical field of fascia over the anterior margin of the sternocleidomastoideus. This procedure leads to minor bleeding of the small perforating vessels running through the fascia to the overlying tissues, but hemostasis is achieved by electrocoagulation. Flexible retractors, one at the top and one at the bottom of the horizontal incision, are manipulated by the assistant to achieve a vertical skin opening 7–8 cm long. The next step is the dissection of the fascia followed by the identification of the correct route between the visceral axis of the neck and the jugulocarotid vascular bundle. Blunt fascial dissection is begun half a centimeter superficial to the anterior margin of the sternocleidomastoideus by applying pressure against the subhyoid muscles. The fascia stretches and then gives way to expose the pretracheal (middle cervical) fascia surrounding the subhyoid muscles. The pretracheal fascia is also opened by blunt dissection, bringing the omohyoid or sternothyroid muscle directly into view. The operator than checks by palpation that the carotid artery, lying deep to the anterior margin of the sternocleidomastoideus, is situated well lateral to the fascial opening. Force must never be applied to the vascular bundle. In cases where the omohyoid obstructs the center of the operative field, the ventral belly of the muscle can be divided between two moderately tight ligatures placed half a centimeter apart. One curved needle holder is placed under the muscle to raise up the latter while a second needle holder is used to pass the suture material. The muscle is then tied off and divided. In cases where the muscle is sufficiently loose to allow its displacement to the lower edge of the operative field, division is not necessary. The clamp-held compresses are then manipulated to expose the lateral margin of the thyroid gland which is practically camouflaged by the sternothyroid muscle. Blunt dissection allows rapid passage deep to the visceral structures of the neck to reach the level of the pharynx and esophagus. At this point in the operation the hard anterior surface of the cervical spine is felt. When such is the case, it is certain that the correct plane of incision has been used. Two flexible retractors are then introduced, one retracting the visceral axis towards the midline, the other displacing the sternocleidomastoideus and the vascular bundle towards the lateral margin of the operative field. The upper and lower parts of the vasculovisceral axis remain to be exposed. Indeed, retraction brings into view fascial sheets which are remnants of the fascia between the viscera and vessels of the neck. These fascial structures are then partially dissociated by blunt dissection allowing by transparency the visualization of the structures contained within. Scissors can also be introduced in the closed position and then cautiously opened to isolate fibrous bands spanning the fascia. The contents of these bands are identified by palpation or by sight, isolated by two curved fine needle holders, and tied off and divided. The vasculovisceral structures must be clearly exposed in all parts of the operative field.

h) Vascular Ligation

To obtain clear exposure of the operative field it is necessary to section the vessels running between the visceral and vascular axes of the neck. The most superficial vessels are veins. In the lower part of the neck the inferior thyroid vein (inconsistently present) may require sectioning. In the upper cervical region either the large common venous trunk (Farabeuf's trunk) or one of its afferents to the internal jugular vein may also require sectioning. The afferents are the superior thyroid, facial, and lingual veins. The arteries lie deep to the veins. In the lower neck the inferior thyroid artery may traverse the operative field below the level of the carotid tubercle of C6 (Chassaignac's tubercle). This artery is sufficiently long and sinuous to allow either its retraction towards the lower part of the operative field or its section between two ligatures. In the upper cervical region the first collateral branch of the external carotid artery (superior thyroid artery), sometimes the second branch (lingual artery), and exceptionally the third branch (facial artery) may require sectioning.

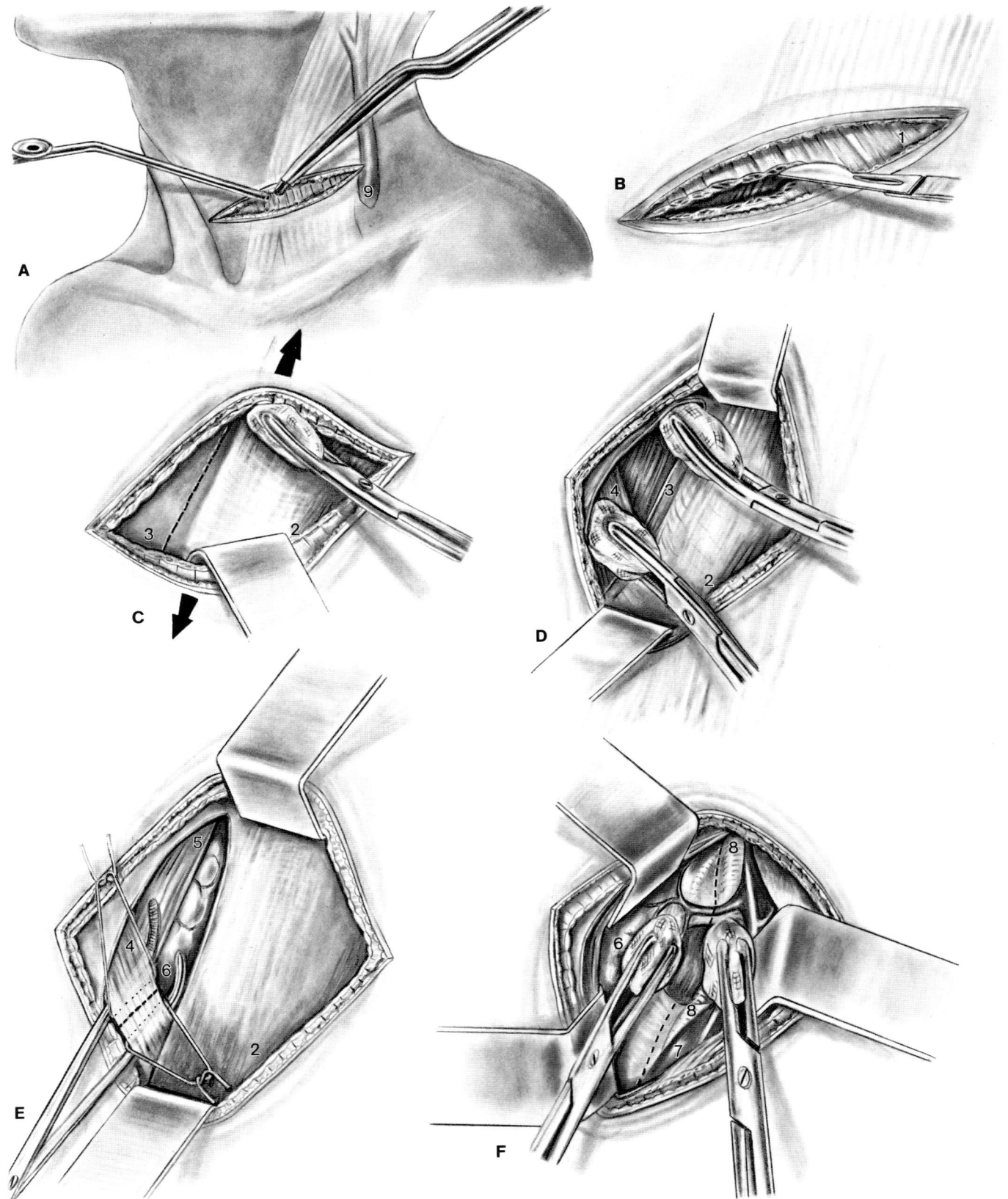

Figure 71 A–F

A   Left transverse skin incision straddling the anterior margin of the sternocleidomastoideus

B   Incision of the platysma muscle

C   Decollement of the superficial layers from the superficial cervical fascia

D   Dissection of the superficial and pretracheal fascia lying over the subhyoid muscles anterior to the sternocleidomastoideus

E   Exposure of the omohyoid muscle and its transection between two ligatures

F   Exposure of the intervasculovisceral space by blunt dissection

1 platysma   *2* m. sternocleidomastoideus   *3* fascia superficialis
4 m. omohyoideus   *5* m. sternothyroideus   *6* glandula thyroidea
7 v. jugularis interna   *8* a. carotis communis   *9* v. jugularis externa

i) Nerves to be Conserved

The anterior approach to the lower cervical spine is in close relation to many nerves which must be conserved to avoid permanent sequelae. The hypoglossal nerve (twelfth cranial nerve) may be visible in the operative field as it runs along the lower margin of the digastric muscle just above the greater horn of the hyoid bone, and is exposed when the approach involves the upper third of the neck, especially C4 and C3 and even C2. The loop of the hypoglossal nerve joining the cervical plexus can almost always be identified in the region where it descends anterior to the internal jugular vein to give off motor rami to the subhyoid muscles. In some cases one of these rami must be cut to allow proper operative exposure. The superior laryngeal nerve must also be conserved. It appears in the operative field below the lingual artery at the level of the greater horn of the hyoid bone and practically in contact with the prevertebral muscles, and must be identified and protected. Finally the phrenic nerve, under the laterally retracted vascular bundle, and in the outermost part of the operative field the roots of the cervical and brachial plexuses, may be brought into view.

j) Exposure of the Cervical Vertebrae

The vascular bundle and visceral axis of the neck are separated using either a Cloward orthostatic retractor, or preferably narrow- and flexible-bladed retractors modeled to fit the neck structures exactly. It is often helpful to model the visceral retractor into a Z shape, hooking its tip on the transverse processes with its large curve passing over the visceral axis without excess traction towards the midline. The anterior surface of the cervical spine is exposed by blunt dissection, followed by a strictly midline incision using the electric cautery knife. The bone is exposed by rasping free the right and left lips of the incision out to the lateral margins of the vertebral bodies and intervertebral discs. Beyond the vertebral bodies the anterior surface of the transverse processes may be rasped, but only in their region flush with the upper half of the vertebral body. The raspatory must not enter the intertransverse spaces, i. e., the region flush with the discs and lower half of the vertebral bodies. The retractors are then repositioned to retract the prevertebral muscles out to the transverse processes. Hemostasis is achieved by electrocoagulation or by applying bone wax to the vertebral bodies. Bleeding can also be arrested by packing a warm compress into place for a few minutes. At this point in the operation a metal clip can be installed to verify the level of the lesion under the image intensifier.

k) Closure

Closure is a simple procedure. Suction drainage is required, and when transected the omohyoid is approximated by a figure-of-eight suture, the platysma by interrupted sutures. Skin closure is achieved with moderately tight interrupted sutures.

l) Postoperative Care

When arthrodesis has been performed, the patient is required to wear an orthopedic collar immediately after surgery and for a period of 2–3 months, but an orthopedic device is not necessary when only simple decompression has been carried out. Suction drainage is maintained for at least 48 h. The patient is allowed to ambulate the day after surgery. The sutures are removed on about the tenth postoperative day.

m) Possible Complications

Complications may be of visceral, vascular, or neural origin. Visceral complications include respiratory disturbances resulting from excess tracheal traction leading to postoperative edema. Although we have never encountered this problem, postoperative tracheostomy would be required. Perforation of the pharynx or the esophagus may arise when dissection or retraction is too forceful. Blunt dissection with clamp-held compresses and the use of flexible-bladed retractors should avoid these complications. The most common vascular complication is postoperative hemorrhage due to release of a ligature. In such cases, the resulting hematoma causing respiratory distress requires emergency surgical intervention. Injury to the different nerves in the cervical region may also occur. Stretching of the right recurrent laryngeal nerve leads to bitonal speech, and a lesion of the superior laryngeal nerve modifies speech tone. Trauma to the twelfth cranial nerve causes hemiparalysis of the tongue, and denervation of the subhyoid muscles or nonreconstitution of the omohyoid may lead to difficulties in swallowing.

Figure 72 A–F

A   Hemostasis of the inferior thyroid artery and middle thyroid vein
B   Hemostasis of Farabeuf's venous trunk and the superior thyroid artery
C   Exposure of the anterior surface of the spine and midline incision
D   Decollement of the prevertebral muscles with the raspatory
E   Exposure of the transverse and intertransverse regions
F   Two-layered closure of the superficial structures, platysma, and skin, with suction drainage

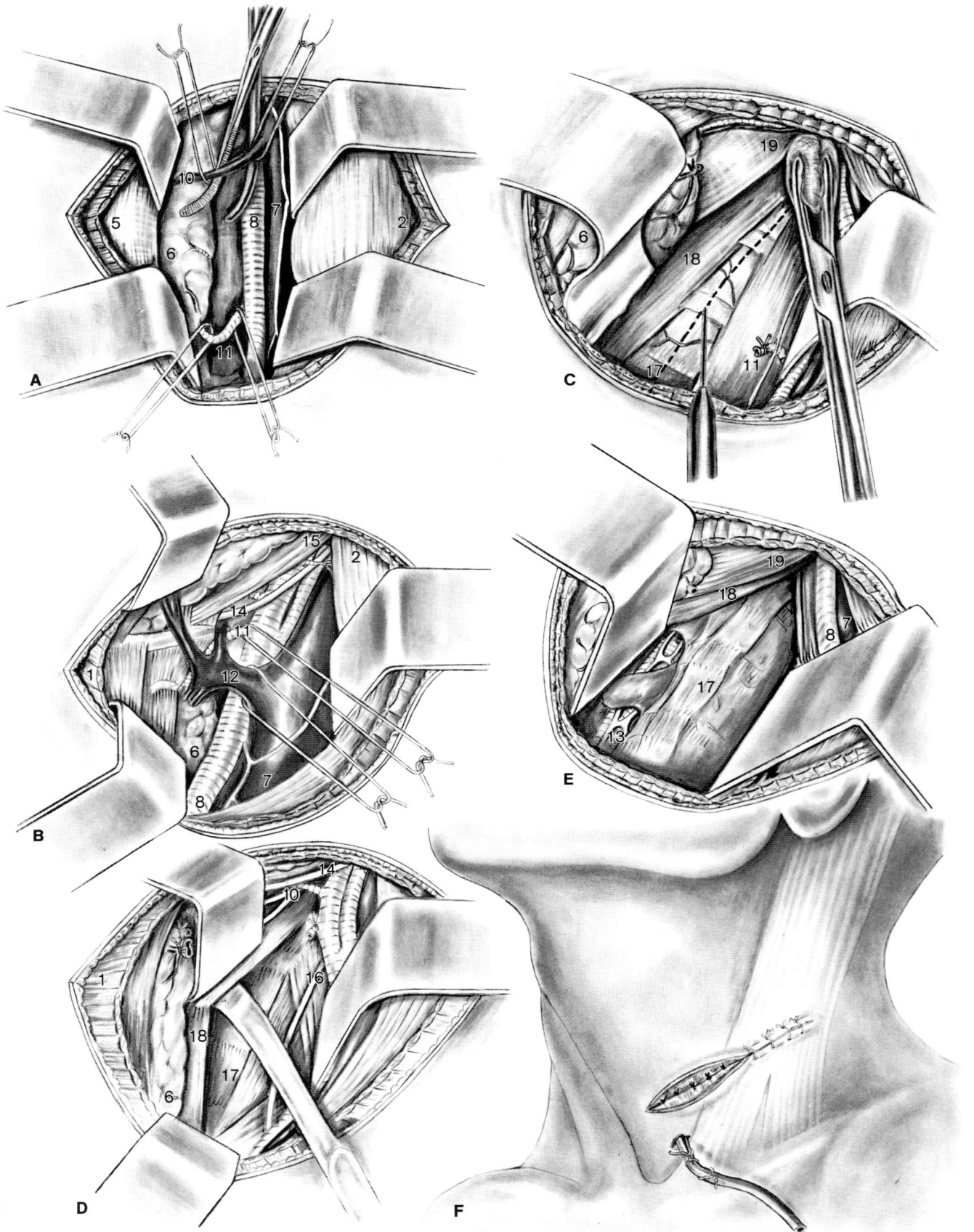

Figure *72 A–F*

1 platysma 2 m. sternocleidomastoideus 5 m. sternothyroideus
6 glandula thyroidea 7 v. jugularis interna 8 a. carotis communis
10 n. laryngeus sup. 11 a. thyroidea sup. 12 vv. facialis, lingualis

thyroidea sup. 13 v. and a. vertebralis 14 n. hypoglossus
15 m. digastricus 16 truncus sympathicus 17 lig. longitudinale
ant. corpus vertebrae 18 m. longus colli 19 m. constrictor pharyngis

2 Thoracic Spine

I. Thoracic Regions

The thoracic spine features the insertion of the ribs on its transverse processes and participates with the sternum in the formation of the thoracic cage. It is the posterior pillar of the thorax and is subdivided by the ribs into two parts, the posterior extrathoracic and anterior intrathoracic regions.

A. Posterior Region

The posterior region of the thoracic spine is situated behind the rib cage and thus posterior to the transverse processes, forming a regional entity with topographical particularities. It is a relatively superficial region lying deep to a thick muscle layer. Posterior access can be gained to the vertebral arches, but access to the vertebral canal and intervertebral foramina and their contents requires laminectomy. Accordingly, only a single posterior operative approach will be described.

B. Anterior Region

This region comprises the vertebral bodies, intervertebral discs, and rib heads. The anterior part of the vertebral canal can also be included in this region since it is accessible after median rachiotomy. Although the entire thoracic spine participates in the formation of the thoracic cage, the anterior region of this spinal segment does not belong topographically only to the thorax. Indeed, the obliquity of the thoracic inlet and outlet is such that the extremities of the thoracic spine can be considered as parts of the boundary zones of the neck above and abdomen below. Consequently, three sectors can be described in the anterior region.

1. Superior Sector (T2 to T4)

As previously discussed, T1 is clearly part of the lower cervical region, but T2 to T4 lie below the oblique plane of the thoracic inlet, posterior to the sternal manubrium. Furthermore, the scapular girdle laterally blocks access to these three vertebrae. Thus exposure of T2 to T4 can be achieved by only three approaches; caudal extension of a cervical approach, cervical extension of a transthoracic approach, or specifically the approach via the manubrium by sternotomy, which we will describe.

2. Middle Sector (T4 to T10)

This sector is very deeply situated and access to it obligatorily involves penetration of the thorax and posterior mediastinum. Indeed, the presence of the scapular girdle at the level of the upper half of the thoracic cage creates three topographical sectors: the anterior third, with the region of the pectoralis major; the middle axillary region, where the intercostal spaces lie very superficially; and the posterior third between the spine and scapula, where the scapular muscles constitute an additional layer to be traversed. Thus three types of approach to the anterior middle thoracic sector can be described; the strictly anterior, the lateral, and the posterolateral.

3. Inferior Sector (T10 to L2)

The last two thoracic vertebrae and the first two lumbar vertebrae constitute a topographical unit, the thoracolumbar junction. The presence of the thoracic outlet obturated by the diaphragm creates the thoracoabdominal region, where access to the vertebral bodies and intervertebral discs can be achieved only by mobilizing the posterior diaphragmatic crura. Given the large circumference of the thoracic outlet, three sectors of access to the thoracolumbar junction can be described: an anterior sector, at the level of the anterior part of the costal arches and at the limit of the abdominal wall; a frankly lateral sector, with access through the intercostal spaces; and a posterolateral route, at the level of the posterior arch of the ribs.

The one easy route of access to the posterior thoracic spine thus contrasts sharply with the complexity and multiplicity of the nine separate approaches to the anterior thoracic spine.

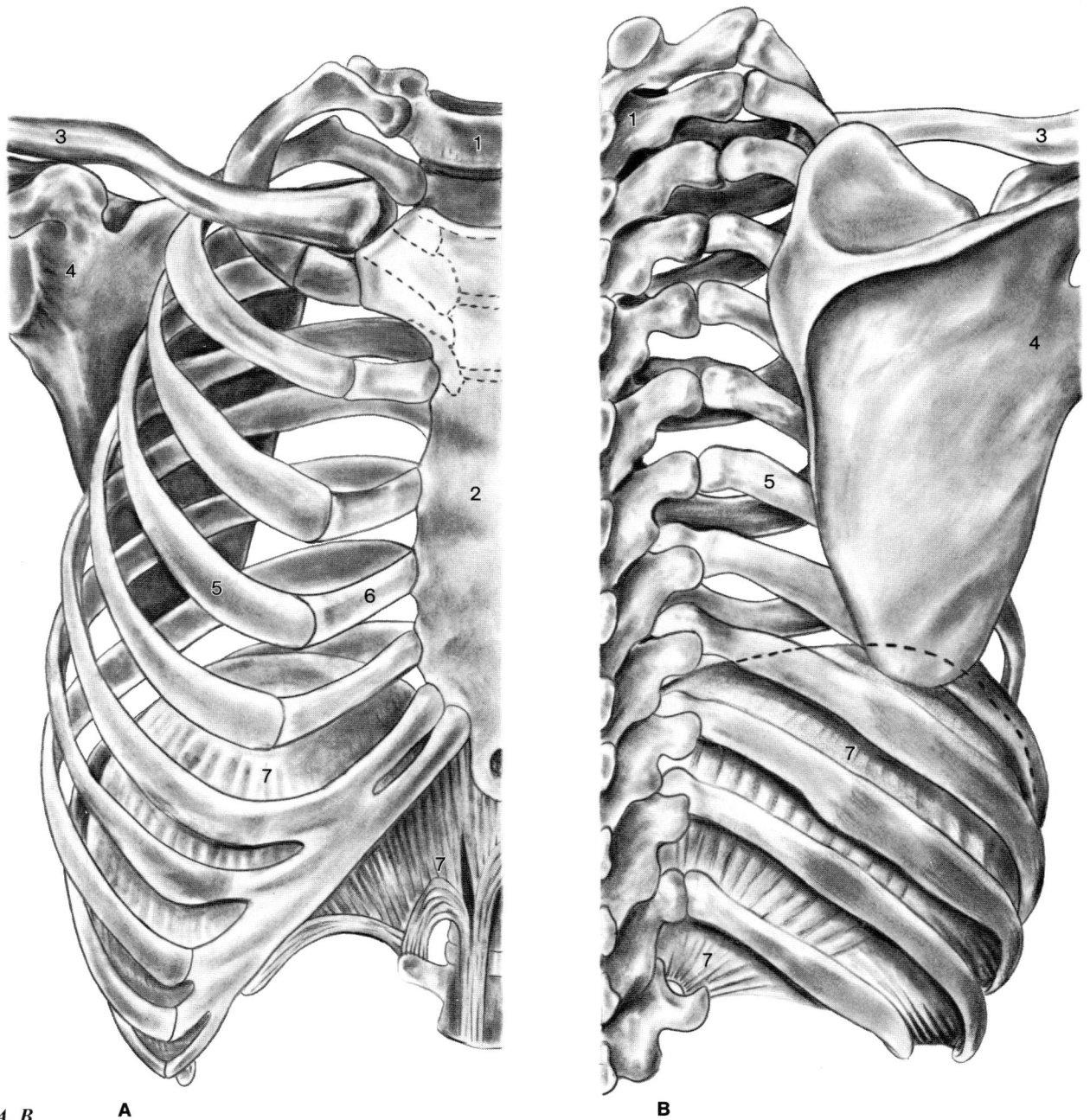

Figure 73 A, B

A   Anterior aspect of the right hemithorax
B   Posterior aspect of the right hemithorax

1 vertebrae thoracicae   2 sternum   3 clavicula   4 scapula   5 costae
6 cartilago costalis   7 diaphragma

II. Posterior Region

A. Topography

The different layers of the posterior thoracic region that must be traversed to gain access to the vertebral grooves, vertebral canal, and intervertebral foramina are described below.

1. Superficial Landmarks and Skin of the Back

The thoracic spine forms the median axis of the dorsal region from the base of the neck to the lumbar region. The main cutaneous landmark is the crest of the spinous processes, which is generally linear and convex except in cases of static anomalies with lateral deviation (scoliosis) or hollow back (lordosis). Numerical correspondence of the vertebrae is essentially identified by the spinous process of C7 (vertebra proeminens) and that of T12, which lies immediately below the posterior arch of the twelfth rib and can often be palpated. The dorsal skin is very thick and perfectly mobile over the subjacent structures. The skin is lined by a fat pad and a superficial fascia deep to the pad. Deep to the superficial fascia lies a layer of subcutaneous tissue through which pass vascular and superficial neural rami.

2. Musculofascial Layers

After traversing the skin and fat, only the large musculofascial masses of the back hinder access to the vertebral grooves on each side of the spinous processes. The muscles form three layers according to the direction of their constituent fibers: a superficial layer of flat muscles with practically transverse fibers (latissimus dorsi, trapezius, rhomboideus, serratus posterior superior); the vertical spinal muscles with longitudinal fibers (iliocostalis, longissimus, spinalis thoracis, spinalis cervicis); and the oblique spinal muscles whose deep fibers stretch between the spinous and transverse processes (transversospinalis). This muscle region is characterized by the absence of a surgically useful plane of incision between the muscle groups and by the presence of uninterrupted insertions over the entire bony and ligamentous layer of the spine. Accordingly, there is only one correct route of access to the posterior thoracic spine, i.e., disinsertion of the entire muscle mass, from the crest of the spinous processes to the transverse processes.

3. Region of the Vertebral Grooves

Disinsertion of the muscles allows access to the two surfaces of the spinous processes, the laminae, the articular processes, the transverse processes, and the posterior arch of the ribs. The inferior articular process must be identified below the root of the transverse processes, since it enables determination of the site of the zygapophyseal articulation. Inscribing a circle 8–10 mm in diameter in the rounded right angle of the inferior articular process corresponds to the site of the posterior joint. The isthmic region, concave downward and outward, lies between the zygapophyseal articulation and the base of the transverse process. The neurovascular bundle containing the dorsal rami of the spinal vascular and neural branches lies at the level of the isthmic region. The neurovascular pedicles are subdivided by the lateral costotransverse ligaments into medial and lateral segments: the medial segment runs along the laminae and enters the intermuscular interstices near the spinous processes, while the lateral segment lies in the muscle layers flush with the costotransverse joints. This isthmic region must thus be conserved to avoid injury to the nervous and vascular supply to the groups of muscles. When vascular sectioning is required, hemostasis must be achieved.

4. Vertebral Canal

To gain access to the vertebral canal laminectomy with conservation of the zygapophyseal joints must be performed, thus exposing the contents of the vertebral canal, including the epidural fat, traversed by a few epidural veins and arterioles, and the dural envelope. Opening of the dura mater exposes the thoracolumbar spinal cord and the corresponding nerve roots. The denticulate ligament, lying between the points of emergence of the ventral and dorsal nerve roots, is inserted on the deep surface of the dura mater. In this thoracic part of the vertebral canal displacement of the dural envelope and spinal cord to allow exposure of the posterior aspect of the vertebral bodies and intervertebral discs is more difficult than in other regions, owing to the narrowness of the canal relative to the volume of its contents. The bulky anterointernal intraspinal venous plexuses also hinder access to the anterior structures. In the thoracic region the myelomeres (n) lie at the level of the vertebral laminae ($n - 1$). The first two lumbar myelomeres lie behind the laminae of T11 and the third and fourth lumbar myelomeres lie anterior to the laminae of T12.

5. Intervertebral Foramina

Access to the intervertebral foramina can be gained by resection of the articular processes. The site of a given intervertebral foramen can be identified with respect to the vertebral arch by determining the level of the vertebral pedicle, which is 10–12 mm high. The upper third of the pedicle extends over the inferior articular process. The position of the thoracic spinal nerves varies according to the spinal level. In the upper third of the thoracic spine the spinal nerves run in an ascending retrograde direction in the upper part of the intervertebral foramina, and in the middle thoracic spine they display a transverse horizontal direction through the middle of their corresponding intervertebral foramina. Finally, the spinal nerves in the lower thoracic spine run obliquely downward and diagonally through the intervertebral foramina. Knowledge of these topographical features is necessary to achieve osteosynthesis involving the vertebral pedicles without injuring the spinal nerves.

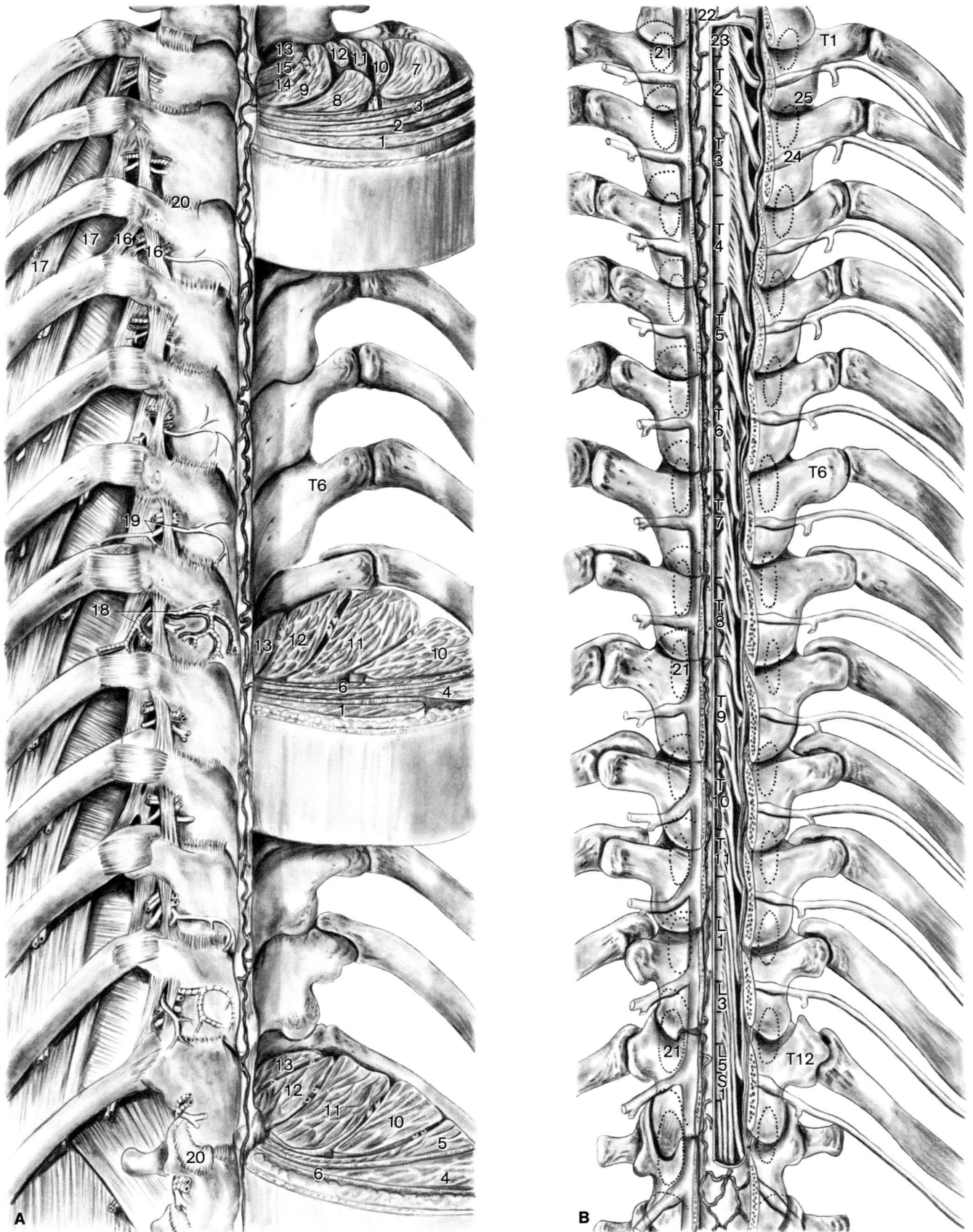

Figure 74 A, B

A   External anatomy of posterior aspect of thoracic spine
B   Internal anatomy of posterior aspect of thoracic spine

1 m. trapezius   *2* m. rhomboideus   *3* m. serratus post. sup.   *4* m. latissimus dorsi   *5* m. serratus post. inf.   *6* fascia thoracolumbalis *7* angulus sup. scapulae   *8* m. splenius cervicis   *9* m. splenius capitis *10* m. iliocostalis   *11* m. longissimus   *12* m. spinalis thoracis   *13* m. transversospinalis   *14* m. semispinalis capitis   *15* m. semispinalis cervicis   *16* lig. costotransversaria   *17* mm. intercostales   *18* a. intercostalis: ramus dorsalis   *19* n. thoracicus: ramus dorsalis   *20* articulationes zygapophyseales   *21* pediculus arcus vertebrae   *22* dura mater spinalis   *23* medulla spinalis   *24* n. thoracicus   *25* lig. denticulatum

B. Posterior Approach

1. Preparation and Anesthesia

Displaced fractures require orthopedic reduction in a scoliosis frame prior to operation to facilitate surgical procedures. When roentgenography is not available in the operating room X-ray identification of the lesional level can be achieved preoperatively, e.g., by using paper clips taped along the ridge of spinous processes as landmarks. The skin of the back and buttocks is shaved on the morning of operation. In cases of pronounced static anomalies peroperative vertebral traction should be used: the feet are fixed to the table and traction is applied to the head by a leather headpiece wired to a tackle block fixed to a wire half-circle attached to the operating table. Anesthesia is induced with the patient intubated and lying supine on a wheeled stretcher beside the operating table. Care should be taken to confirm that the endotracheal tube creates a hermetic seal and is securely taped to the peribuccal region. Cardiovascular monitoring is performed throughout the operation.

2. Operative Position and Field

The patient is turned over to lie prone on the operating table with the head supported by a headrest, the eyes occluded, and the intubation cannula securely fixed in place. The sternum and the lateral inguinal and iliac regions are supported: either large rubber pads (15 cm high) or an adjustable support frame can be used. The abdomen and neck must be free of compression and properly suspended. The arms are placed on supports lying along the sides of the thorax, care being taken to ensure that the cubital groove rests on a soft spongy pad. Small pads can also be placed under the insteps and a harness used to hold the thighs. Disinfection of the skin should begin at the base of the nuchal region and extend down to the gluteal folds and lateral parts of the buttocks. One large double-thickness towel is placed over the head and shoulders and a second over the buttocks and lower limbs. Two further towels are then folded and placed laterally to create a triangular operative field widely exposing the iliac crests for graft taking. An adhesive drape is then taped over the entire operative field. The electric cautery knife (on the right for right-handed surgeons) and suction cannula are placed one at each side of the operative field. A right-handed surgeon places himself to the left of the patient.

3. Skin Incisions

Two incisions are frequently required: the vertebral incision and an iliac incision for removal of graft material.

a) Vertebral

The procedure of choice is a median sagittal incision along the crest of the spinous processes. The incision should extend the length of one vertebra above and below the field to be exposed. The spinous processes cannot be considered reliable landmarks to identify the exact position of the vertebrae requiring operation. Either preoperative X-ray with metal points of reference or peroperative verification under the image intensifier is mandatory to identify correctly the level of the spinal lesion, which is then marked on the skin with a dye solution or scratch mark.

b) Iliac

Removal of iliac bone-graft material requires exposure of the posterior third of the external iliac fossa, beginning in the region of the posterosuperior iliac spina. Three types of incision can be used. The most convenient approach is to incise along a line extending the arciform iliac crest. However, the disadvantage of this incision is the possibility of sectionning the cutaneous nerve fibers and disinserting too great on area of gluteal muscle, often leading to permanent muscular disinsertion and pain on walking. A second approach is to make an aesthetic horizontal incision beginning at the level of the posterosuperior iliac spina, but this incision also leads to excess disinsertion of muscle fibers and does not allow full exposure of the iliac crest. Our preference is for an oblique incision perpendicular to the iliac crest 4 cm lateral to the anterosuperior iliac spine, 8 cm long and extending 2 cm above the iliac crest. This incision does not damage the cutaneous nerve fibers, as it runs parallel to the nerve branches of roots T12 and L1 innervating the gluteal region. Furthermore, access can be gained to the iliac bone without muscle transection, since the incision is parallel to the muscle fibers. Finally, the continuity between the gluteal and lumbar fasciae is retained by disinserting them from the iliac crest on each side of the incision.

4. Possible Complications

The patient may present severe *respiratory disturbances* and shock due to the ejection of a poorly secured endotracheal tube, or in the obese to the incorrect position of the thoracic and iliac pads. Emergency treatment requires the placing of a transparent adhesive drape over the operative field, turning the patient supine, and rapidly reestablishing airway patency.

Movement of the patient due to insufficient anesthesia or precocious return to consciousness may lead to displacement of the different points of body support, complicating further surgical procedures. Accordingly, it is imperative that the patient be properly secured to the operating table.

Neural compression involving the cubital nerves in the elbow region or the femorocutaneous nerves in the region of the anterosuperior iliac spines can result from the lack of a sufficiently soft support surface.

The operation itself may be complicated by an *error of identification of the correct spinal level* when pre- or peroperative X-ray monitoring is not performed. Finally, *edema of the face* and *irritation of the conjunctiva* may result from poor facial position during surgery and the absence of full eye closure.

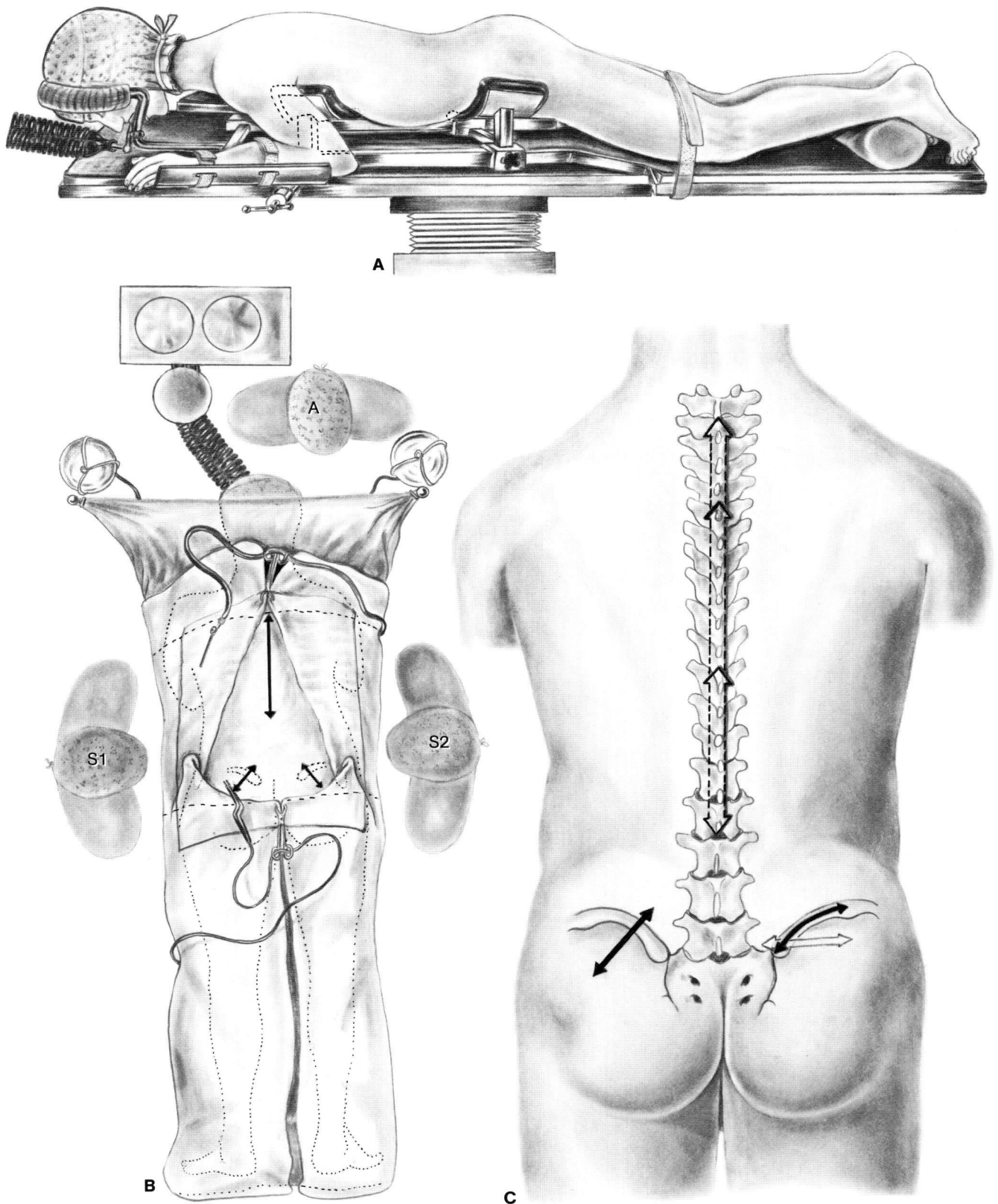

Figure 75 A–C

A   The operative position, with the patient lying prone after
    endotracheal intubation, the head supported by a headrest, and
    pads under the sternum and external inguinal and iliac regions. The
    neck and abdomen are freely suspended. The lower limbs are
    secured and the elbows protected in the region of the cubital nerves

B   Overhead view of the operative position and field. Note the position
    of the operative team; anesthesiologists (A), surgeon (S1), and
    assistant (S2)

C   The lines of cutaneous incision. Over the spine a strictly median
    sagittal incision is made along the spinous crest as indicated by pre-
    or peroperative radiological identification of the spinal lesion. The
    iliac incisions for taking bone grafts may be arciform or horizontal
    on the right (not recommended), or oblique on the left with
    conservation of cutaneous innervation and avoidance of painful
    disinsertion of the gluteal muscles (preferred approach)

5. Initial Exposure

In cases where a long incision is required, the skin should be incised in (10–12-cm) segments to facialitate hemostasis. Incision is made using a plain knife down to the layer of fat. Hemostasis is progressively achieved by compression, using a rolled, warm, moist, and well-wrung compress. The incision is exposed centimeter by centimeter to allow coagulation of all the subdermal vessels with the electric cautery knife, which should be adjusted so as not to burn the skin. The subcutaneous and adipose tissues are then incised down to the fascia using the cautery knife.

6. Fibromuscular Disinsertion

The muscle fibers are exposed by incising the fascia with the electric cautery knife, using one of two techniques. When laminectomy is to be performed, the fascia is incised exactly on the midline by working along the left and right flanks of the spinous processes. When laminectomy is not required, the fascia is opened on each side of the spinous processes to leave a fibrous band inserted on the bone. Toothed dissecting forceps, held in the left hand, are used to identify the crest of spinous processes to allow manipulation of the cautery knife in the correct direction. The spinal muscles are then successively disinserted on each side of the spinous processes, using a large raspatory or a large periosteal rasp, which must not be capable of being introduced between two laminae or transverse processes. The instrument is used first along the vertical flank of the spinous processes, then in the region of the laminae, and finally upward along the inclined surface of the transverse processes. Rasping must not extend beyond the tip of the latter. After exposure of each 5-cm long zone, hemostasis is achieved by packing a warm moist compress in accordion fashion as far as the transverse processes. When surgery does not involve the transverse processes, rasping should be stopped at their base and at the lateral margin of the articular capsules, in order not to section the dorsal neurovascular bundles located midway between the transverse process and articular facets. In children, subperiosteal muscle disinsertion is performed by rasping at the tip of the spinous processes to achieve subperiosteal decollement which is less hemorrhagic. Hemostatic compresses are packed in place using a large curette to prevent the instrument slipping into the interlaminar or intertransverse spaces. In cases of fracture of the posterior arches, the surgical maneuvers must be performed with utmost caution. Rasping is begun in the healthy zones above and below the lesion to allow identification of the deep part of the vertebral arches, and only after these zones have been exposed is very cautious rasping in the region of the fractured vertebral arches started, without forcing.

7. Exposure of the Vertebral Arches

The moist compresses are removed from the vertebral grooves and an orthostatic retractor (usually a Beckman retractor) installed at each end of the operative field. Hemostasis is completed with the aspiration cannula held in the left hand and the electrocoagulation device in the right hand. Clear exposure of the bony structures requires the removal of all remaining muscle debris using a very large curette, followed by rinsing with warm saline-antibiotic solution.

8. Possible Complications

The most common problem is *difficult hemostasis,* which may arise when the initial incision is too long, thus creating numerous simultaneous sites of bleeding. In other cases, abdominal compression due to improper positioning of the support pads leads to venous congestion. Finally, correct hemostasis of the superficial layers must be achieved to prevent blood trickling down to the deeper layers and hindering the hemostasis there. In short, proper hemostasis requires a progressive technique to avoid overwhelming bleeding from numerous sites.

A frequent risk is the *slipping of an instrument* off track. The use of a narrow raspatory or slender instruments to pack the compresses into place may result in the instrument slipping into an interlaminar space, a zone of fracture of the vertebral arch, or an intertransverse space. Instrumental penetration of the vertebral canal can induce severe neurological lesions, and passage between two transverse processes can lead to hemothorax. When the latter complication arises, thoracic suction drainage is begun and the intertransverse space is opened widely to allow hemostasis of a parietal vessel.

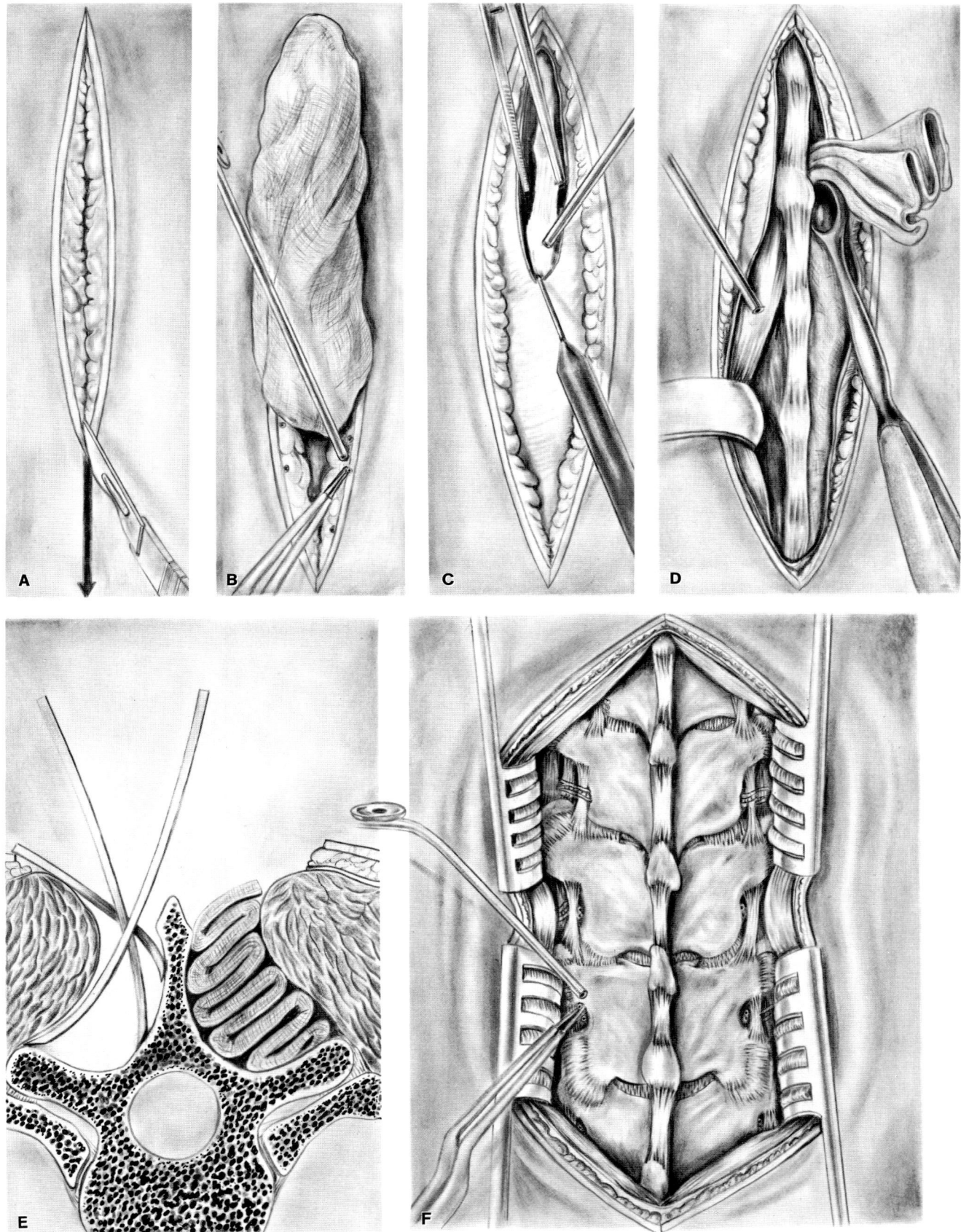

Figure 76 A–F

A   Skin incision with the plain knife
B   Hemostasis of the subdermal layers using a warm compress,
    aspiration, and electrocoagulation
C   Section of the fascia of the spinal muscles on the spinous crest
D   Disinsertion of the spinal muscles from the vertebral arches
    followed by packing of warm moist compresses in the vertebral
    grooves to achieve hemostasis

E   Section showing on the *left* the manipulation of the raspatory to
    disinsert the muscles from the spinous processes and then the
    transverse processes. On the *right*, accordion packing of warm moist
    compresses to obtain hemostasis
F   Exposure of the vertebral arches subsequent to installation of the
    orthostatic retractors and completion of hemostasis, especially in
    the regions of the dorsospinal bundles near the isthmic zones

9. Laminectomy

Exploration of the vertebral canal requires laminectomy. The procedure is begun using very large gouge forceps to resect the spinous processes down to their base without biting into the laminae from the onset, to avoid sudden opening of the vertebral canal and injury to the dura mater. Bone wax is applied to the cut surface of the spinous processes to achieve hemostasis. The ligamenta flava are disinserted from the lower margin of the laminae with a narrow raspatory to allow the subsequent introduction of slender gouge forceps. Resection of the laminae is begun in their caudal segment with work progressing cranially using the slender curved bone forceps directed to cut obliquely into the right and left sides of the laminae. Laminectomy should not extend laterally beyond the origin of the articular processes, in order to conserve the posterior articulations. The cut surface of the laminar bone must be vertical, to avoid progressively narrowing the operative field, and laminectomy should extend clearly above the level of the lesions to be explored. Resection of the remaining fragments of the ligamentum flavum is achieved by incision of the ligament on the midline followed by its lateral disinsertion towards the intervertebral foramina with a curette. Hemostasis of the bone is achieved with bone wax. Cotton tampons are then placed along the margins of the laminectomy in order to prevent the blood trickling into the vertebral canal. During laminectomy the operative field should be rinsed several times with warm saline.

10. Exploration of the Epidural Space

A blunt-tipped dissector is used to displace the epidural fat laterally, followed by hemostasis of the clearly exposed epidural vessels. The dissector can then be manipulated to retract the dural envelope cautiously and expose the emergence of the spinal nerve roots, the posterior surface of the vertebral bodies and intervertebral discs, and the origin of the intervertebral foramina. This procedure risks tearing the anterolateral venous plexuses, which must be conserved or coagulated.

11. Intradural Exploration

When exploration of the intradural structures is to be performed, moist cotton tampons should be positioned on each side and at each end of the dural envelope to avoid intradural bleeding leading to irritation of the neural structures in the same way as a meningeal hemorrhage. Opening of the dural envelope is prepared by using two small hooked instruments to grasp a transverse fold near the caudal end of the dura mater. The plication is then partially incised with a scalpel and the opening enlarged on the midline using fine scissors, working in the cranial direction. Frequently only the dura mater is opened in this way, the arachnoidea remaining intact and bulging under the CSF pressure. In such cases, the operator needs to break open the arachnoidea along the entire dural opening with a blunt instrument. Stay sutures are then in-stalled on the right and left lips of the dural wound to maintain proper exposure. A blunt-tipped dissector can be used to explore the dural emergence of the spinal nerve roots, the denticulate ligament lying between the nerve roots, and especially the posterior and lateral surfaces of the spinal cord. The posterior approach allows an easy selective sensitive radicotomy. It must be borne in mind that the neural structures, especially the spinal cord, are very fragile and that the spaces between the spinal cord and dura mater are very narrow. Surgical maneuvers in this region must be performed with utmost caution to avoid irreversible neurological damage.

12. Possible Complications

Injury to the dura mater from the gouge forceps during laminectomy may arise when excessive resection of the spinous processes or laminae is performed. Dural injury in itself is not serious if the spinal nerve roots remain intact; the wound requires only simple closure by continuous or interrupted nonresorbable sutures.

Off-track instrumental maneuvers may lead to spinal cord trauma and possibly permanent neurological damage. All operative manipulations in this region must therefore be perfectly controlled.

Untoward hemorrhage considerably hinders the operative procedures, and may result from poorly achieved progressive hemostasis during the operative approach or excessive intra-abdominal pressure due to improper positioning of the abdominal pads or incomplete anesthesia. Bleeding can be interrupted by installing moist cotton tampons along the lateral recesses of the vertebral canal. In such cases, exposure is achieved by momentarily retracting the cotton tampons in the desired zone.

Fracture of the articular processes may arise per- or postoperatively when excessively wide laminectomy has been performed, and can lead to very bothersome painful instability.

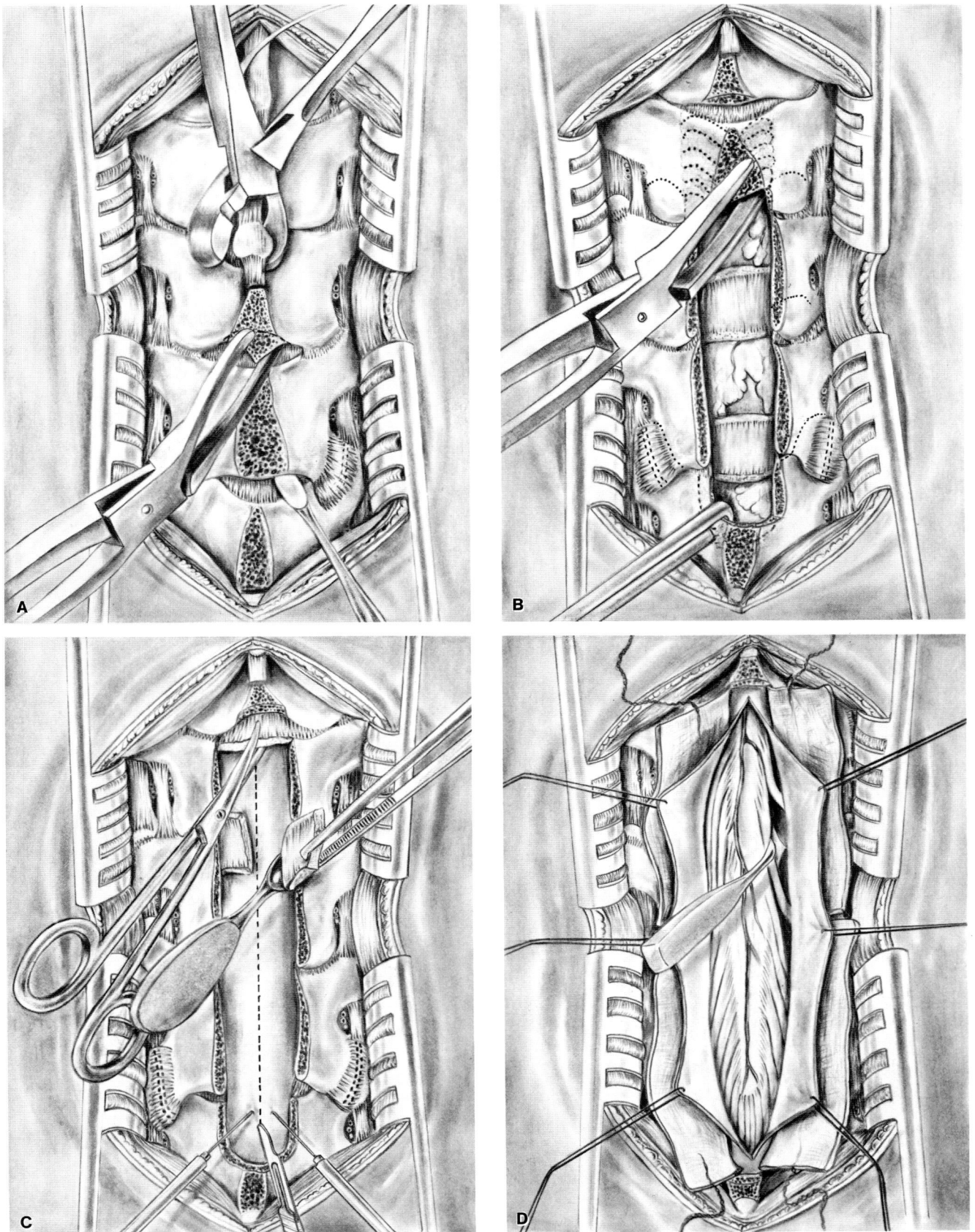

Figure 77 A–D

A Resection of the spinous processes and decollement of the ligamenta flava

B Resection of the laminae using gouge forceps and rongeur with conservation of the posterior joints

C Removal of the remaining parts of the ligamenta flava and opening of the dura mater

D Exploration of the spinal nerve roots and cord with the dura mater opened

13. Meningeal Closure

The entire operative field is liberally rinsed with saline and the dural stay sutures removed. Dural closure is achieved using a continuous nonresorbable atraumatic suture (double or triple zero) with a curved vascular-type needle. The CSF pressure in the subarachnoid space is reestablished by transdural puncture and injection of saline solution. The CSF pressure level can easily be estimated by digital palpation of the dural envelope, thus eliminating the risk of cerebellar herniation through the foramen magnum and allowing early ambulation. The quality of hemostasis, especially in the region of the anterointernal venous plexuses, is then verified. When coagulation hemostasis is insufficient, Surgicel can be placed in the lateral recesses of the vertebral canal over the entire length of the region of laminectomy on the right and left sides. Suction drainage should be avoided in cases of dural opening, since it carries a risk of rapid CSF depletion.

14. Musculofascial Closure

Parietal closure differs slightly according to whether or not laminectomy has been performed. In the absence of laminectomy the muscle layer is closed with U-shaped sutures passing through the interspinous spaces. The fascia is then closed with the same type of interrupted sutures passing through the crest of spinous processes to approximate the right and left margins of the fascia. When laminectomy has been performed, closure of the muscle layer is accomplished by full-thickness moderately tightened interrupted sutures. The fascia is then closed using plain nonresorbable or very slow resorbing interrupted sutures. Fascial closure with a continuous suture is proscribed due to the attendant risk of disunion or hematoma formation.

15. Skin Closure

Subcutaneous closure is achieved by full-thickness slow-resorbing interrupted sutures passing through the subdermal region down to the tissue layer covering the fascia. This type of closure eliminates any dead spaces which could lead to hematoma and subsequent infection. Skin closure is achieved by plain or mattress-type interrupted sutures to allow good skin approximation, since the patient will lie on the wound, submitting it to sliding and stretching forces. An intradermal continuous suture with the aim of cosmetic skin closure can be used only in cases of extensive arthrodesis, e.g., Harrington's operation for scoliosis. Indeed, continuous sutures must be avoided in mobile regions due to the risk of rupture and wound disunion. When the patient is to wear a plaster brace in the early postoperative period, slow-resorbing rather than nonresorbable skin sutures are indicated, thus obviating suture removal. The operation is terminated by placing a thick hermetic dressing over the wound.

16. Postoperative Care and Possible Complications

Early ambulation, on the day after surgery, is allowed when arthrodesis or dural opening has not been performed. In cases of extensive spinal fusion (Harrington's operation) the patient is allowed to rise on the fourth or fifth postoperative day while wearing a plaster corset brace. When the dural envelope has been opened ambulation is started on the third postoperative day if headache and dizziness are absent. Before allowing the patient to stand a test is made with the patient seated for a few minutes.

A *hematoma* may form in the region of the dorsal incisions if hemostasis is insufficient or closure has left dead spaces between the different tissue layers. When this complication arises the hematoma should be evacuated and a compressive dressing applied. Recurrence of hematoma requires reintervention to close the different layers in the region. *Blood loss* through a suction drain can be controlled by periodic clamping of the drain for a few hours. In cases of *postoperative infection* we recommend that the wound be opened down to the infected layer followed by excision of the necrotic or soiled tissue and installation of a filiform silk-gut drain. Closure is then effected with full-thickness nonresorbable sutures, which should be sufficiently spaced to allow evacuation. The sutures are left in place for three weeks and the drain removed when full evacuation has been achieved. *Postoperative meningitis* requires parenteral antibiotherapy with an appropriate drug passing the blood-brain barrier coupled with intrathecal injection by lumbar puncture.

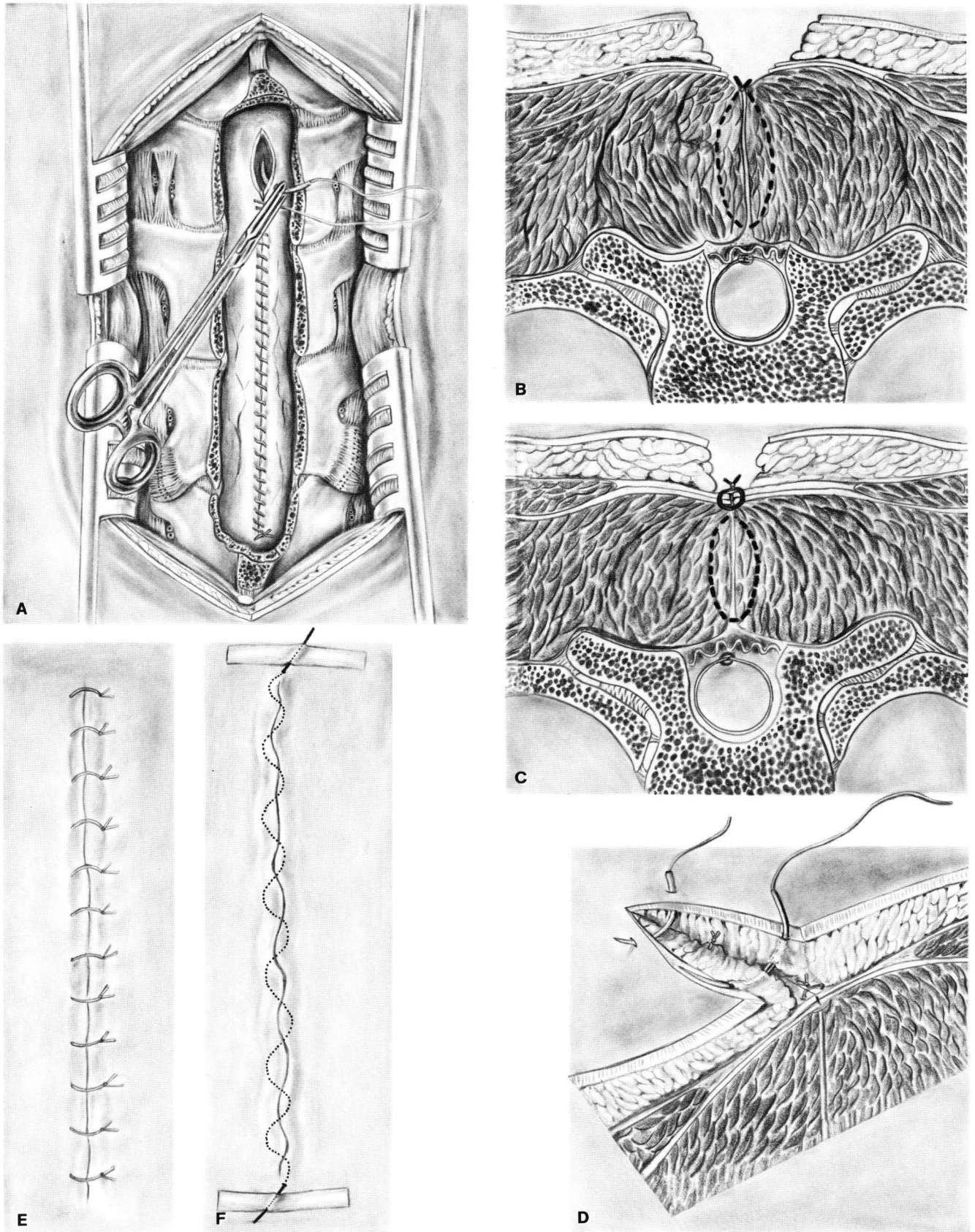

Figure 78 A–F

A   Closure of the dura mater with a continuous nonresorbable suture
B   Closure of the spinal muscles in one layer with interrupted sutures
    over a sheet of Surgicel
C   Suture of the thoracic fascia

D   Suture of the subcutaneous tissue without leaving dead space
E   Skin closure with interrupted sutures
F   Skin closure with an intradermal continuous suture

III. Anterior Region

A. Cervicothoracic Junction (T2 to T4)

1. Topography

The cervicothoracic junction is a deep spinal region lying between the inferior cervical region, accessible by cervicotomy, and the middle thoracic region, accessible by thoracotomy. Direct access to the cervicothoracic junction requires traversing of the sternal manubrium and retraction of the greater mediastinal vessels.

a) Sternocostal Wall

Three layers can be described from the superficial to the deep regions of the sternocostal wall. The superficial skin layer is thick and of reduced mobility. The fibrocellular tissue of this layer joins the intermediate fascia to the pectoral muscles. Numerous vessels running through this layer cross the midline. The middle layer is the sternum, with its wide thick manubrium facing T2, T3, and T4. The manubrium and body of the sternum are joined at the sternal angle (Louis' angle) which is a landmark for the second costal cartilage. The xiphoid process extends the sternal body inferiorly and lies slightly deep to the latter. The jugular notch represents the upper limit of this middle layer, and laterally the costal cartilages form the margins of the anterior ends of the intercostal spaces. The deep layer of the sternocostal wall is represented in its upper third by the insertions of the sternohyoideus and sternothyroideus muscles and in its lower two thirds by the triangularis sterni (transversus thoracis). These muscles and the intercostal spaces are lined by the endothoracic fascia.

b) Retrosternal Fibroserous Layer

This layer is the most superficial part of the anterior mediastinum. The thyroid fossa lies above, but may enter this region behind the sternum in cases of goiter. The thymic fossa is large in children, but in adults it is reduced to an adipose remnant covered anteriorly by a deep fascial layer originating from the lamina pretrachealis (middle cervical fascia) and the superior sternopericardial ligament. It is limited posteriorly by the thyropericardial fascia and laterally by the internal thoracic vessels (internal mammary vessels), and contains the brachiocephalic veins and pericardium. The pericardium extends downwards from the thymic fossa at the level of the lower half of the sternum. Laterally, the anterior costomediastinal recesses of the pleura expose a triangular region along the sternal manubrium down to the level of the second intercostal space, where the two pleural recesses overlap. Retraction of these recesses is thus necessary to gain access to this region.

c) Pretracheal Neurovascular Structures

Access to the vertebrae in this region requires the traversing of a veritable lattice work of vessels and nerves, some of which must be ligated or mobilized during the anterior approach to the cervicothoracic junction. The *veins* of this region comprise the left brachiocephalic vein, running obliquely from the left sternoclavicular joint to the second costal cartilage on the right, and the right brachiocephalic vein running vertically along the right margin of the manubrium. The *arterial structures* include the aortic arch, lying behind the left half of the sternum from the third through first intercostal spaces. The right brachiocephalic trunk (hidden behind the right brachiocephalic vein) lies along the right flank of the trachea, and the left internal carotid artery at the level of the left half of the manubrium and left flank of the trachea. Finally, the left subclavian artery lies posterior to the preceding vessel on the left side of the trachea. These large vessels give rise to the following collateral branches: the internal thoracic arteries (internal mammary arteries), lying 1 cm lateral to the lateral sternal margins; the pericardial and thymic arterial branches, lying on the midline below the left brachiocephalic vein; and the median and superior pedicle of the arteria thyroidea ima, supplying the thyroid gland.

The *neural structures* traversing this region which must be conserved during surgery are the vagus and phrenic nerves. The right vagus (tenth cranial, pneumogastric) nerve runs anterior to the origin of the right subclavian artery, where it gives off the loop of the inferior laryngeal (recurrent) nerve, and then leaves the region near the right flank of the trachea. The left vagus nerve runs along the lateral margin of the left common carotid artery and then passes anterior to the aorta, where it gives rise to the left inferior laryngeal nerve, which runs upward behind the aorta in the left tracheoesophageal angle. The right and left phrenic nerves, displaying practically symmetrical courses, lie more laterally against the mediastinal surface of the pleura. The right phrenic nerve runs along the superior vena cava and the left nerve passes anterior to the aortic arch. Numerous rami from the sympathetic plexuses and vagus nerves form the cardiac nervous plexuses anterior to the great vessels and aorta. Finally, it should be noted that the anterior mediastinal lymphatic ducts lie amid these neurovascular structures.

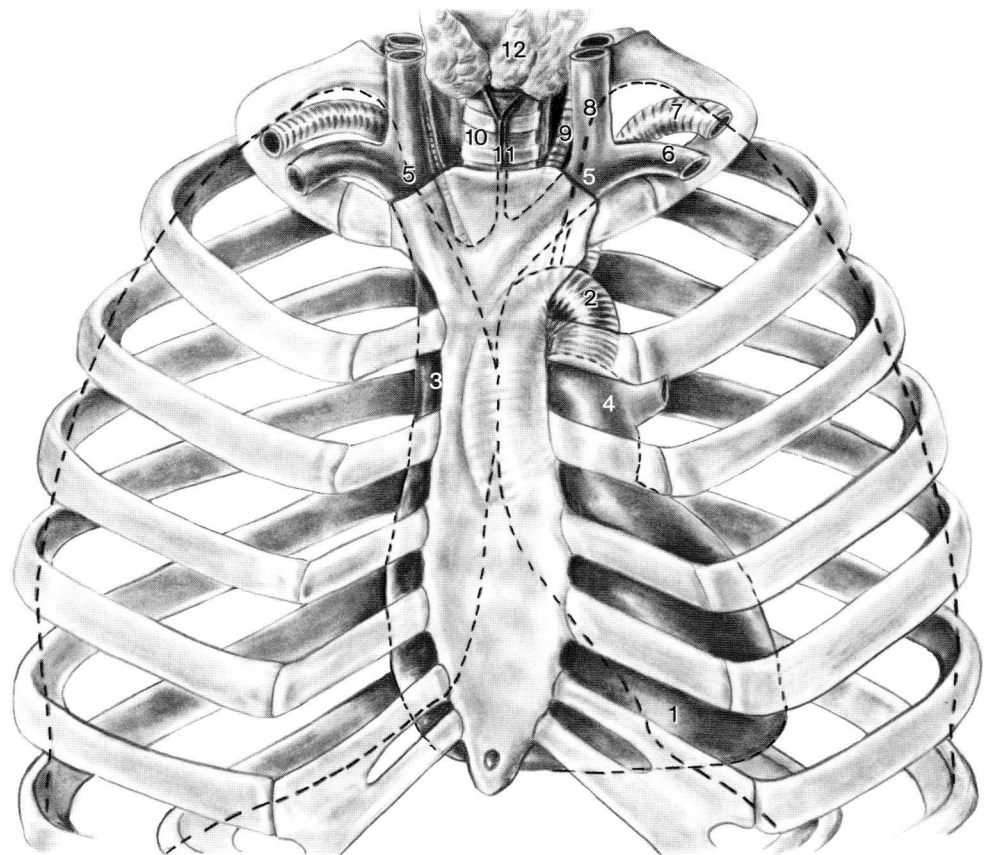

A

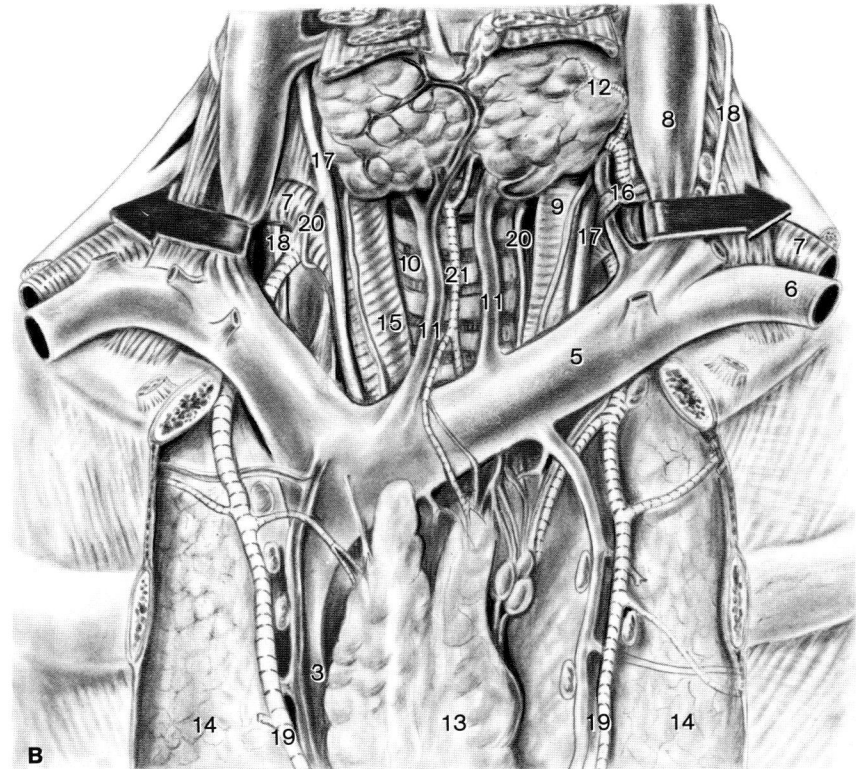

B

Figure 79 A, B

A   The cervicothoracic junction with its anterior relations as seen by transparency through the thoracic cage

B   The neurovascular and fibroserous structures of the cervicothoracic junction after resection of the sternum

1 cor *2* aorta *3* v. cava sup. *4* truncus pulmonalis *5* vv. brachiocephalicae *6* v. subclavia *7* a. subclavia *8* v. jugularis interna *9* a. carotis communis *10* trachea *11* v. thyroidea inf. *12* glandula thyroidea *13* thymus *14* pulmo *15* truncus brachiocephalicus *16* ductus thoracicus *17* n. vagus *18* n. phrenicus *19* a. and v. thoracicae internae *20* n. laryngeus inf. *21* a. thyroidea ima

d) Visceral Structures

The median visceral axis comprises the trachea and esophagus. The trachea can be identified during operation by the presence of the cartilaginous rings and when in doubt by the aspiration of air on needle puncture. The trachea as it descends is slightly deviated to the right by the aorta and then separates from the thyroid gland to pass behind the aortic arch where it divides to form the right and left main bronchi at the level of T5. Lymph nodes run along both surfaces of the trachea, which can easily be mobilized using a retractor. The esophagus lies posteriorly and extends laterally beyond the left margin of the trachea, and is attached to it by fibromuscular tracts. The left inferior laryngeal nerve runs anterior to the left margin of the esophagus, and care must be taken not to stretch it when retracting the esophagus. The visceral axis must be mobilized towards the right and not the left to avoid trauma to the loop of the right inferior laryngeal nerve.

e) Prevertebral Neurovascular Structures

Numerous collateral vessels, sometimes requiring ligation, are located anterior to the upper thoracic vertebrae (T2 to T5), i.e., above the aortic arch. Branches of the thyrocervical arterial trunk run toward the anterior surface of the bodies of T2 and T3, the ascending branch running along the longus colli and the descending branch anastomosing with the superior intercostal arteries, sometimes represented by the costocervical trunk. Distal to the cervicalis profunda this trunk gives off the intercostalis suprema, which runs toward the first intercostal space and usually anastomoses with the subjacent intercostal artery. In other cases, the superior intercostal arteries correspond to the second, third, and fourth intercostal arteries on the right and left sides, which run obliquely downward from their origin on the aorta to T4–T5. Exposure of the anterior surface of the upper thoracic spine should thus be accomplished on the midline to avoid the sectioning of a large number of these arteries supplying the spinal cord. Indeed, transverse sectioning at the level of T3–T4 may result in the interruption of four to six of these arteries with the attending risk of ischemic paraplegia. The veins accompanying the arteries of this region include the thyrocervical and costocervical venous trunks and the intercostal veins, which in part give rise to the right superior intercostal vein and the accessory hemiazygos vein. The translucid thoracic duct runs upward along the left anterior flank of T3 and T4, deviates anteriorly with respect to the spine to pass above the left sublavian artery, and finally runs toward the confluence of the left brachiocephalic venous trunks and the left subclavian vein. The duct may thus be injured during the anterior approach to the cervicothoracic junction, and as opening can lead to severe complications ligation is recommended in such cases. Finally, the sympathetic trunk extending down from the cervicothoracic or stellar ganglion surrounds the origin of the vertebral artery immediately above a small supra- and retropleural fossa. The sympathetic trunk lies anterior to the intercostal vessels and just lateral to the heads of the ribs.

f) Vertebrae

The upper thoracic vertebrae articulate with the heads of the ribs. The first rib articulates with T1 below the C7–T1 intervertebral disc, whereas the subjacent costovertebral joints lie flush with the corresponding discs. The heads of the ribs can thus be used as landmarks to identify the numerical correspondence of the discs. The longus colli muscles cover the anterolateral surfaces of the vertebral bodies, leaving a narrowly exposed anterior region down to T3, and must thus be rasped laterally from the bone to expose the vertebral bodies. Furthermore, the narrow, thick common anterior vertebral ligament must be cut at this level to gain access to the discs and vertebral bodies.

Figure 80 A–C

A Exposure of the anterior surface of the cervicothoracic junction after median sternotomy, section of the left brachiocephalic venous trunk, and displacement of the visceral axis of the neck towards the right

B Anterior aspect of the cervicothoracic junction and the prevertebral neurovascular structures. The muscles and sympathetic trunk are shown only on the right

C Horizontal section of the trunk passing through T3

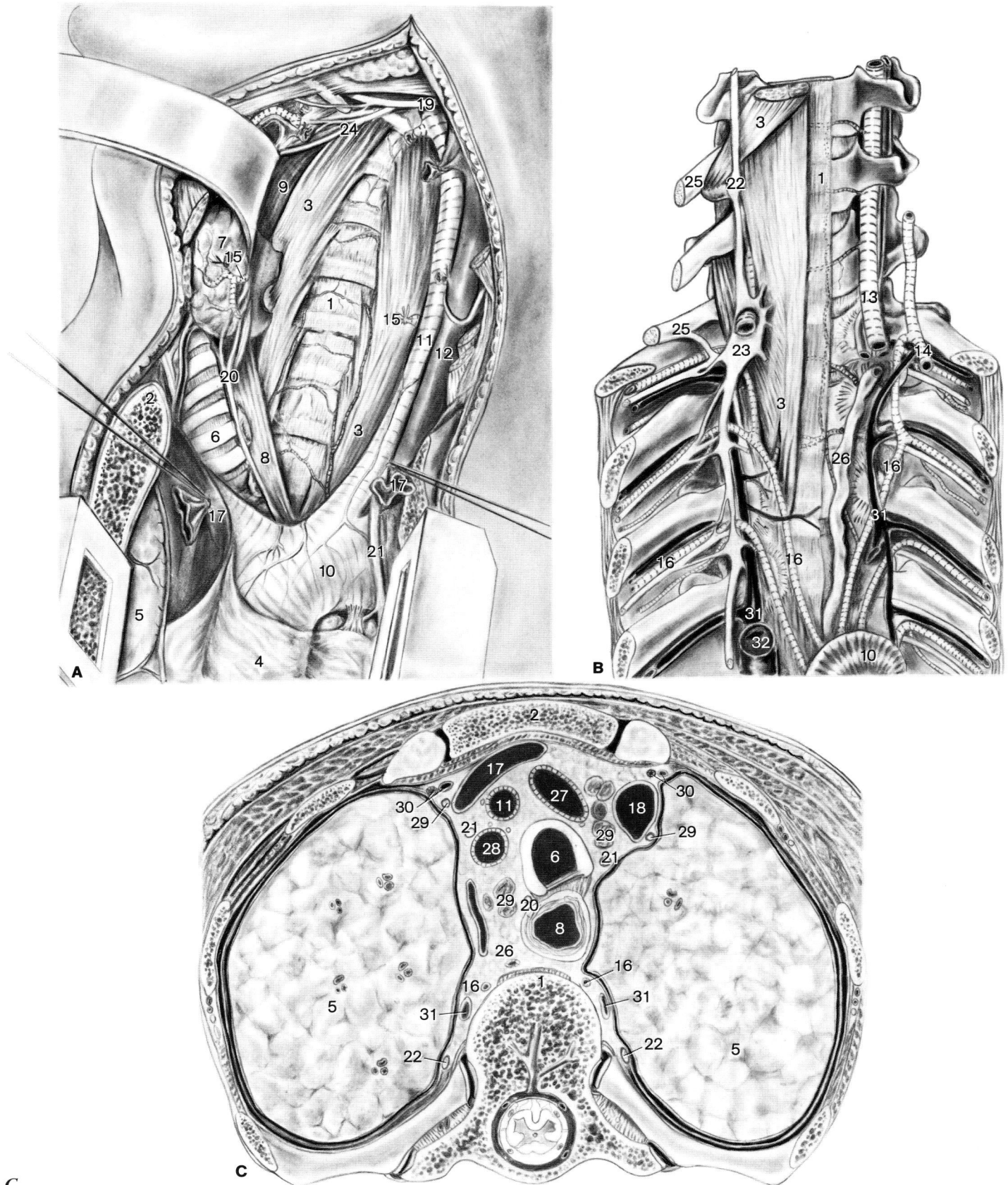

Figure 80 A–C

1 columna vertebralis 2 sternum 3 m. longus capitis and m. longus colli 4 pericardium 5 lobus sup. pulmonis 6 trachea 7 glandula thyroidea 8 oesophagus 9 pharynx 10 aorta 11 a. carotis communis 12 v. jugularis interna 13 a. vertebralis 14 truncus costocervicalis 15 a. thyroidea inf. 16 a. intercostales post. 17 v. brachiocephalicae sinistra 18 v. brachiocephalicae dextra

19 n. hypoglossus 20 n. laryngeus recurrens 21 n. vagus 22 truncus sympathicus 23 ganglion cervicothoracicum stellatum 24 n. laryngeus sup. 25 radices plexus brachialis 26 ductus thoracicus 27 truncus brachiocephalicus 28 a. subclavia 29 n. phrenicus 30 a. thoracica interna 31 v. intercostalis sup. dextra, v. hemiazygos accessoria 32 v. azygos

2. Cardiovascular Variations

The surgery of cardiovascular malformations is obviously beyond the scope of this book. Nevertheless, surgical procedures in the anterosuperior part of the mediastinum require the knowledge of certain essential anomalies, which if overlooked may result in untoward vascular ligation with a catastrophic outcome.

Situs Inversus. The symmetrical inversion of the thoracic viscera leads to the inversion of the position of the great supracardiac vessels, i.e., the aortic arch running to the right, the pulmonary artery on the left, and the vena cava running along the left margin of the aortic arch.

Coarctation of the Aorta Proximal to a Patent Ductus Arteriosus. In this anomaly a shunt persists between the descending aorta and the pulmonary artery. Aside from the arterial hyperpressure in the vessels arising from the aortic arch, this malformation interferes very little with thoracic spinal surgery.

Coarctation of the Aorta Distal to the Ductus Arteriosus. In this case the arterial ligament remains collapsed without the presence of an aortopulmonary shunt.

Duplication of the Aortic Arch. This rather curious anomaly creates an arterial loop around the visceral axis of the neck (trachea and esophagus) and considerably hinders its surgical mobilization. The duplication must not be mistaken for a large vein which may be ligated and divided.

The Retroesophageal Right Sublavian Artery. In this case the right subclavian artery arises from the left side of the thoracic aorta and then runs behind the esophagus to reach the right upper limb. Untoward ligation of the artery to allow mobilization of the visceral axis of the neck must be avoided.

Anomalous Origin of the Left Common Carotid Artery. An exceptional finding is the left common carotid artery arising from a trunk common with the right brachiocephalic trunk, rather than directly from the aortic arch. This malformation is not surgically problematic if care is taken not to confuse the anomalous artery with a left brachiocephalic venous trunk in the pretracheal position. Ligation of the artery may induce severe brain damage.

Anomalous Termination of the Superior Vena Cava. This topographical inversion, an exceptional finding, corresponds to the superior vena cava lying on the left of the aorta and left atrium and terminating directly in the coronary sinus. The superior vena cava should not be mistaken for a left brachiocephalic venous trunk and ligated: only the right brachiocephalic venous trunk should be ligated.

Duplication of the Superior Vena Cava. In some cases two superior venae cavae may be found. One lies on the right in the normal anatomic position but does not receive the left brachiocephalic venous trunk, and the other, representing a ver- tical left brachiocephalic trunk, passes to the left of the aorta and left atrium to terminate directly in the coronary sinus. This anomaly should not hinder operation since midline vascular ligation is not required to approach the cervicothoracic junction.

Anomalous Pulmonary Venous Return. This exceptional anomaly is represented by the termination of the left brachiocephalic venous trunk in the left atrium, and the resulting interatrial shunt leads to overloading of the right atrium. Ligation of the brachiocephalic trunk on the midline can induce venous stasis of the left hemifacial region.

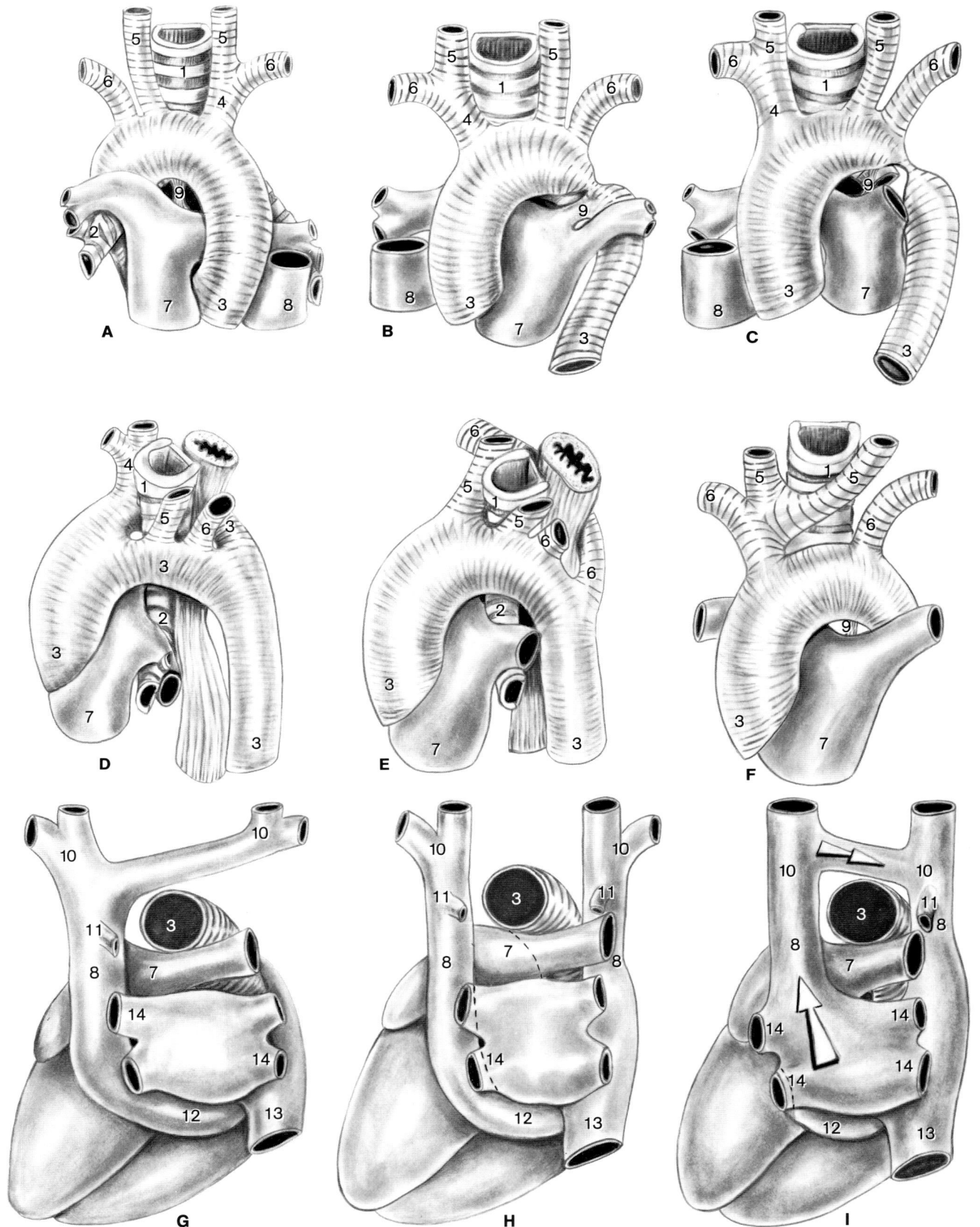

Figure 81 A–I

A   Situs inversus
B   Coarctation of the aorta proximal to the ductus arteriosus
C   Coarctation of the aorta distal to the ductus arteriosus
D   Duplication of the aortic arch
E   Retroesophageal right subclavian artery
F   Left common carotid artery arising from the brachiocephalic trunk
G   Left superior vena cava terminating directly in the coronary sinus

H   Duplication of the superior vena cava
I   Total anomalous pulmonary venous return

1 trachea 2 bronchus principalis 3 aorta 4 truncus brachiocephalicus 5 a. carotis communis 6 a. subclavia 7 truncus
pulmonalis 8 v. cava sup. 9 lig. arteriosum; ductus arteriosus
10 v. brachiocephalica 11 v. azygos 12 sinus coronarius 13 v. cava
inf. 14 v. pulmonalis

3. Trans-sternal Approach: Cervicosternotomy

This operative approach, proposed by J. Cauchoix, J. P. Binet, and J. Evrard (1957) allows direct access to the cervicothoracic junction, but is technically difficult and time consuming. Many surgeons frequently prefer to use either an enlarged cervical approach with retrosternal dissection of a transthoracic route extending up to the pleural dome.

Operative Position and Anesthesia. With the patient lying supine, the head is turned to the right and a cushion placed under the shoulders to create slight extension of the neck. The operator stands on the patient's left with the two assistants on the right. Conventional endotracheal intubation is installed, care being taken to ensure a tight endotracheal seal and nonselective airway patency.

Incision. The incision is relatively long, with a midline portion extending the full length of the sternum and 4–5 cm below the xiphoid process. The second, cervical portion is made for 6–8 cm along the anterior margin of the left sternocleidomastoideus. The incision is made through the skin and adipose tissue down to the presternal and cervical fasciae.

Cervical Stage of Operation. The superficial cervical fascia is opened to allow identification of the subhyoid muscles. The left omohyoideus, sternohyoideus and sternothyroideus are tied off and divided in their region near the sternal notch. The left jugulocarotid bundle can then be easily retracted along with the sternocleidomastoideus without opening the fascial sheath of the bundle. Clamp-held compresses are used to expose the anterior surface of the lower cervical spine with its overlying prevertebral muscles. In some cases, the left inferior thyroid artery must be ligated and sectioned. Blunt dissection is used to expose the visceral axis of the neck and thyroid gland and to identify the position of the left recurrent laryngeal nerve in the tracheoesophageal angle. The visceral axis is then retracted towards the right side. The nerve must not be stretched by vigorous traction during operation, as this may lead to postoperative vocal bitonality.

Thoracic Stage of Operation. The presternal fascia is incised down to the periosteum using the electric cautery knife, and hemostasis of the many transected transverse vessels is performed. Work is next begun on the xiphoid process, which must be freed of all its abdominal fascial insertions. Round-tipped scissors are used to retract the peritoneal serosa from behind the xiphoid process. The next step is to perform a median section of the sternum by one of two techniques. The first uses an oscillating saw, similar to that employed to open a plaster cast. The second technique involves first passing a finger- or clamp-held compress between the posterior surface of the sternum and mediastinal viscera, followed by sternotomy beginning at the top of the bone and working downward. With each tap of the hammer on the chisel the posterior surface of the sternum is more deeply exposed. Hemostasis of the cut sternal bone should be achieved with hot saline and Surgicel, as bone wax is a factor of pseudarthrosis during sternal consolidation. An orthostatic retractor is introduced in the sternal fissure, and clamp-held compresses are used to retract the two pleural recesses towards the right and left in order to expose the anterior surface of the pericardial envelope and the great supracardiac vessels. The left brachiocephalic venous trunk is identified and sectioned between two solid double ligatures. In some cases exposure requires the section of the very small venous tributaries above or below the venous trunk. The visceral axis of the neck is retracted laterally down to the upper margin of the aortic arch, exposing the anterior surface of the spine down to the level of T4. The cautery knife is used to open the prevertebral fascia on the midline, and the prevertebral muscles are rasped aside to expose the lateral surfaces of the vertebral bodies. It is sometimes necessary to mobilize or ligate the superior intercostal vessels, but the horizontal section of several intercostal arteries (particularly numerous above the aortic arch) must be avoided. A cautious procedure is to make an oblique incision in front of the spine between the right and left intercostal arteries.

Closure. Closure is carried out after installing double suction drainage: one drain in the deep part of the cervical region, one in the retrosternal region near the xiphoid process. The subhyoid muscles are approximated using figure-of-eight sutures, and the superficial layers closed with interrupted sutures. Postoperative care includes regular monitoring of the suction drains with frequent tube changes until all flow has ceased on the third or fourth postoperative day. The sternotomy should be reviewed for 2–4 months, since in some cases sternal fusion is slow and painful. Early ambulation is allowed except in cases of special spinal contraindications.

Possible Complications. The major complication is the rupture of vascular ligatures leading to cervical or retrosternal hematoma and asphyxiation, requiring emergency reintervention to achieve hemostasis. Pseudarthrosis of the sternum may arise when the sternal sutures have not been correctly tightened or when bone wax has been placed along the regions of future sternal fusion.

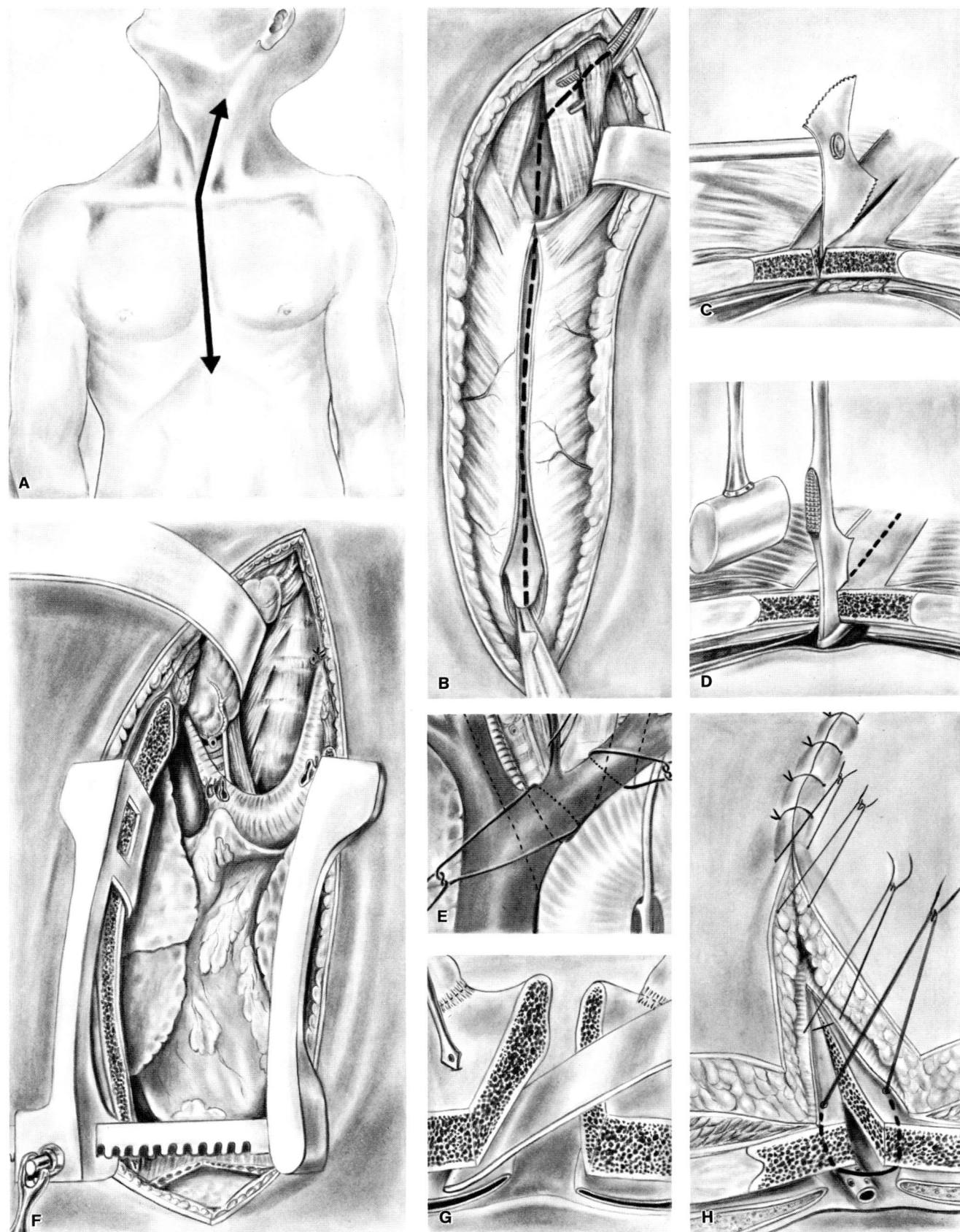

Figure 82 A–H

A   Operative position with the head turned to the right showing the sternal and cervical incisions

B   Incision of the superficial layers; exposure of the xiphoid process and transection of the left subhyoid muscles

C   Sternotomy using the oscillating saw

D   Sternotomy using a sternotome

E   Identification and section of the left brachiocephalic venous trunk between two ligatures

F   The full operative field after installing the orthostatic retractor and retraction of the visceral axis of the neck towards the right side. Exposure of the cervicothoracic spine

G   Closure with perforation of the cut sternal walls and protection by a flexible retractor

H   Parietal closure of the sternotomy using nonresorbable sutures followed by closure of the presternal fascia, the subcutaneous layer, and the skin, with suction drainage

B. Middle Thoracic Spine (T4 to T10)

1. Topography

a) Anterolateral Thoracic Wall

The anterolateral thoracic wall covers each hemithorax when the subject is viewed face on. The region is bounded by the clavicle above, the sternum on the midline, the common costal cartilage below, and the mid axillary line laterally.

(1) Cutaneous and Mammary Layer

Owing to the great mobility of the skin in this region an incision may easily be displaced with respect to the rib cage. The breast extends from the third to the seventh rib, and the nipple must of course be conserved in both sexes. The bony landmarks of this region include the sternal angle lying at the level of the second costal cartilage. The submammary fold identifies the site of skin incision. The subcutaneous and adipose tissue as well as the mammary gland can easily be mobilized en bloc over the fascia covering the pectoral muscles.

(2) Superficial Muscle Layer

This layer comprises the pectoral muscles, the serratus anterior, and the superior digitations of the abdominal muscles. The pectoralis major is a powerful fleshy muscle with tendinous extremities and is made up of three parts, the clavicular, sternocostal, and abdominal muscle bodies. The abdominal muscle body inserts on the fascial sheath of the rectus abdominis. The terminal tendon inserts on the greater tubercle of the humerus and displays a U-shaped section, since the inferior pectoral fibers turn around the tendon to insert on its deep surface. The pectoralis minor extends from the tip of the coracoid process to the second, third, fourth, and fifth ribs. Both pectoral muscles are innervated by ventral thoracic rami of the brachial plexus, which pass under the clavicle and thus are not exposed to injury during thoracic surgery. The serratus anterior originates on the spinal margin of the scapula, passes over the anterolateral wall of the thorax, and inserts on the anterior arch of the first nine ribs. It receives its motor supply from the long thoracic nerve lying in the posterior part of the axillary region. In the lower part of the superficial muscle layer the insertions of the oblique abdominal muscle fibers blend with those of the serratus anterior.

Three essential neurovascular bundles can be described in this region. The first is made up of the supraclavicular branches of the superficial cervical plexus and the superficial cervical vessels passing anterior to the clavicle, and the second comprises the anterior branches of the intercostal nerves and blood vessels lying 1–2 cm lateral to the sternum. Finally, the branches of the external thoracic vessels and the lateral branches of the intercostal nerves enter this region at the level of the anterior axillary line. In the course of surgery the transection of these vessels requires numerous sites of hemostasis.

(3) Intercostal Region

This region, forming the posterior limit of the anterolateral thoracic wall, is the boundary of the thoracic cavity, and comprises the anterior arch of the ribs with their costal cartilage extending to the lateral margin of the sternum, thus forming the anterior part of the intercostal spaces. The costal cartilaginous segments joining the ribs and sternum are 4–5 cm long. The cartilage can easily be sectioned and closure obtained by simple sutures. Identification of the cartilaginous segments is achieved using the clavicle and sternum as landmarks. The first costal cartilage is located precisely under the internal end of the clavicle, but the second lies at the level of the sternal angle. Knowing this, the other cartilaginous segments can be identified: the third, fourth, and fifth insert on the lateral margin of the body of the sternum, and the sixth and seventh on the base of the xiphoid process. The anterior part of the intercostal spaces is relatively wide (about 2 cm) and is deeply concave superiorly. The contents of the intercostal spaces form five layers:

- The layer formed by the external intercostal muscle, running obliquely downward and forward and not extending beyond the lateral part of the costal cartilage.
- The external fibrocellular layer.
- The middle intercostal muscle, extending over the anterior half of the intercostal space up to the sternum.
- The middle intermuscular cellular tissue, in which the costal grooves contain the intercostal pedicles running vertically with the vein above and the nerve below.
- The deep muscle layer comprising the internal intercostal muscle, which does not fully span the intercostal space and is limited on its deep surface by the endothoracic fascia and the parietal pleura.

The internal thoracic vascular pedicles (internal mammary artery and vein) lie in the deep anterior part of the intercostal spaces, 10–15 mm lateral to the lateral margin of the sternum. The opening of the intercostal space should thus not extend medially beyond this 15-mm limit if ligation of the vascular pedicle is to be avoided. These vessels run towards the lower half of the sternum between the digitations of the triangularis sterni and the deep wall of the intercostal spaces.

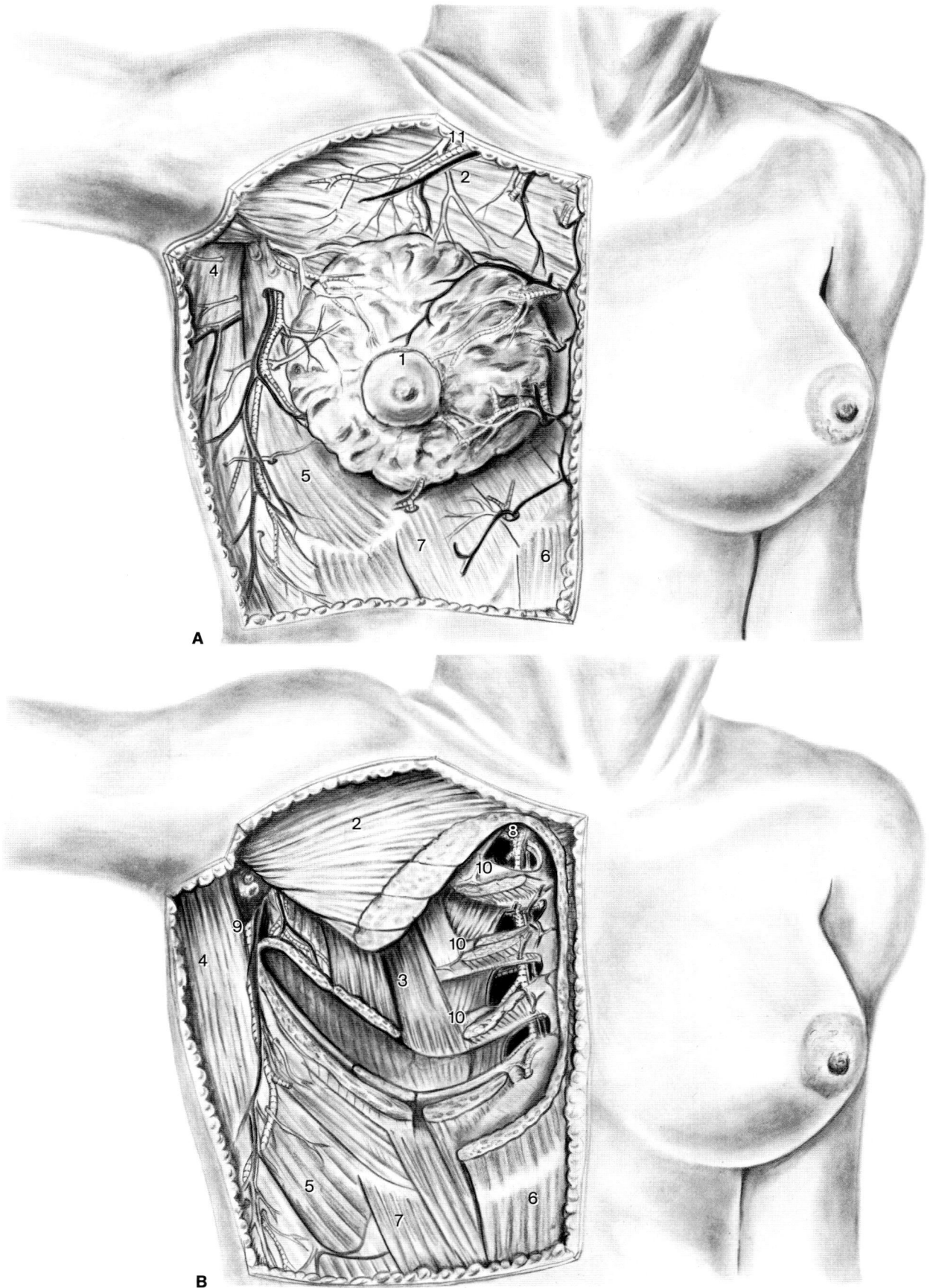

Figure 83 A, B

A   Anterior aspect of the thorax with the superficial layer removed on the left

B   Anterior aspect of the thorax after removal of the mammary gland and a window opening of the intercostal spaces

1 mamma   *2* m. pectoralis major   *3* m. pectoralis minor   *4* m. latissimus dorsi   *5* m. serratus ant.   *6* m. rectus abdominis   *7* m. obliquus externus abdominis   *8* a. and v. thoracica interna   *9* a. and v. thoracica externa   *10* costae   *11* n. supraclavicularis, a. and v. cervicalis superficialis

b) Lateral Thoracic Wall

Exposure of the lateral thoracic wall requires the abduction-elevation of the upper limb to open the axillary region forming the summit of the lateral wall. Access to the thoracic cavity is gained by traversing three parietal layers.

(1) Superficial Cutaneoadipose Layer

The skin of this region bears hair and is slightly adherent to the deeper layers in the region of the axillary fossa. The palpable margins of the axilla are represented by the pectoralis major anteriorly and the latissimus dorsi posteriorly. The angle formed between these two muscles permits identification of the anterior and posterior axillary lines: the midaxillary line bisects the angle. The costal arches are easily palpable in the lower axillary region.

(2) Muscular and Neurovascular Layer

Removal of the subcutaneous and adipose tissues exposes the muscular structures forming three vertical bands. The pectoralis major, with the pectoralis minor lying deep to it, occupies the anterior part of this region. The most distal fibers of the pectoralis major blend into the sheath of the rectus abdominis muscles. The posterior muscle band is formed by the latissimus dorsi, camouflaging the axillary margin of the scapula. A small depression lies between these two prominent muscles, and the wall of this depressed zone corresponds to the digitations of the serratus anterior flattened against the intercostal spaces. The anterior and inferior insertions of this muscle blend with those of the obliquus externus abdominis. The uppermost digitations of the serratus anterior, hidden by the deep surface of the pectoral muscles, insert on the anterior costal arches. At the top of the middle axillary band lies the origin of the internal muscles of the arm: the coracobrachialis muscle and a short portion of the biceps and triceps brachii. The neurovascular axillary bundle, containing the vein, artery, and nerves of the upper limb, lies between these brachial muscles. Only the collateral branches of this bundle supplying the thorax are involved in the approach through the lateral thoracic wall: the external or lateral thoracic pedicle, just posterior to the pectoralis major, and the lateral cutaneous rami of the intercostal nerves, which lie more posteriorly and emerge through the intercostal spaces to give off an anterior and posterior branch to the subcutaneous and cutaneous tissues. Posterior to the emergence of these sensory nerves lies the thoracodorsal vascular bundle, arising from the subscapular vascular bundle. The artery and vein descend vertically in the middle part of the axillary region, the vein anastomosing with the superficial abdominal veins to form the greater thoracoepigastric anastomotic vein. The long thoracic nerve lies posterior to the thoracodorsal vascular bundle under the anterior margin of the latissimus dorsi, and should be conserved so as not to alter the respiratory function of the serratus anterior muscle. Finally the subscapular vascular bundle, hidden under the latissimus dorsi, leaves the region near the tip of the scapula. It should be noted that aside from the abundant adipose tissue enveloping the contents of the axillary region, numerous axillary lymph nodes lie along the venous structures.

(3) Deep Costal and Intercostal Layer

The lateral part of the costal arches, and the intercostal spaces slanting obliquely downward and forward, lie below the insertions of the superficial parietal muscles. The five layers forming the intercostal space have been described above, i.e., the three (external, middle, and internal) intercostal muscle layers and the two layers of cellular tissue with the neurovascular bundle lying under the costal groove between the internal and middle intercostal muscles. In craniocaudal order this neurovascular bundle comprises the vein, artery, and nerve, each of which gives off an inferior branch which runs along the lower margin of the intercostal space. The deep wall of the intercostal layer is formed by the endothoracic fascia lined by the parietal pleura. The lateral transthoracic approach allows access to the first six intercostal spaces, especially the fourth and fifth. Opening of the fifth intercostal space with section of the fifth costal cartilage, to widen the operative field anteriorly, allows access to the thoracic cavity.

(4) Lateral Aspect of the Thoracic Cavity

Anterolateral thoracotomy allows clear exposure of the thoracic cavity with the diaphragmatic cupula below and the spine in the deep posterior region with the overlying intercostal bundles, azygos vein, and mediastinal pleura. Exposure of the spine requires the anterior retraction of the right lung. This approach allows easy access to T4 through T10. At the limits of the operative field T2, T3, T11, and T12 can be exposed only exceptionally.

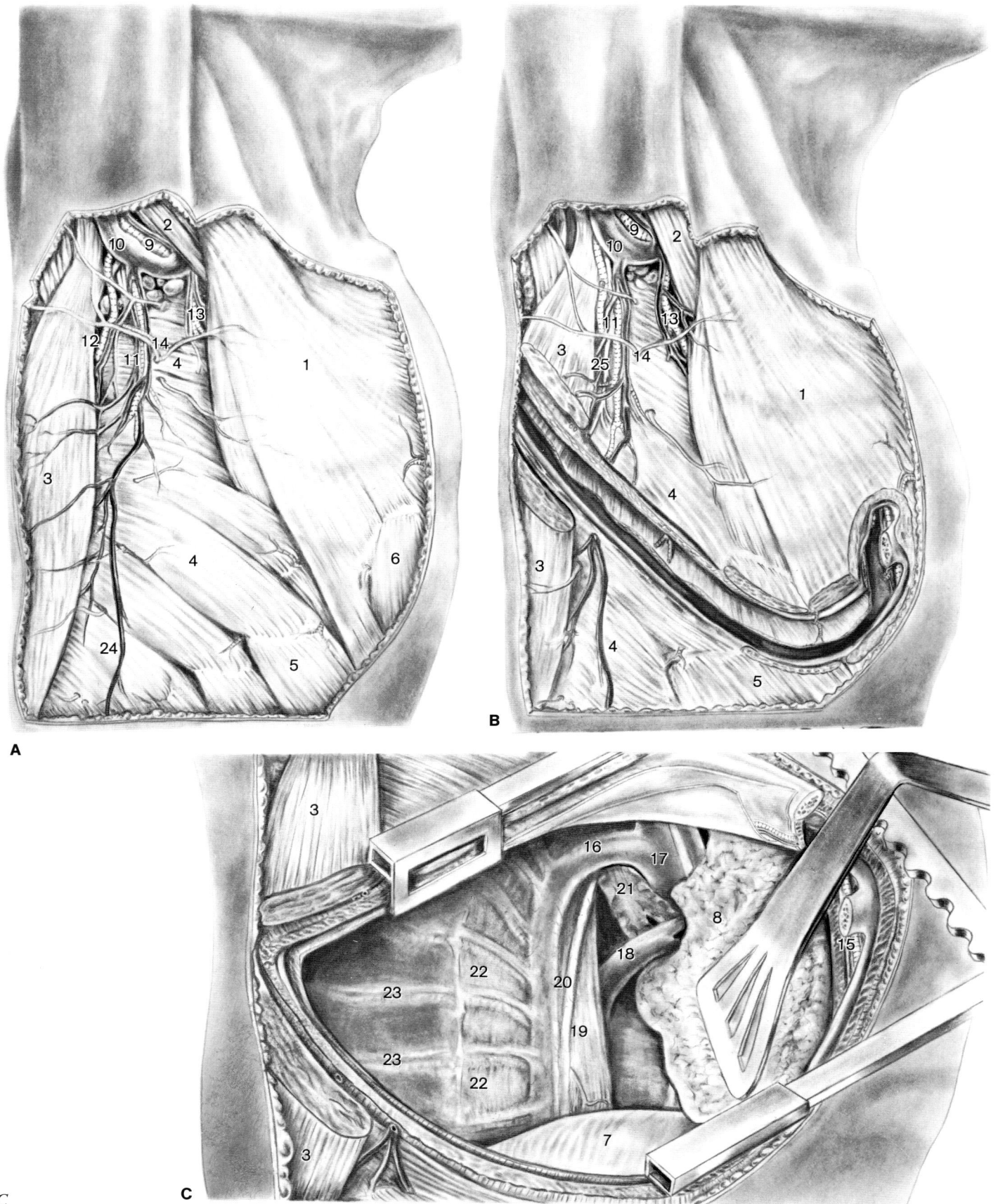

Figure 84 A–C

A   Lateral aspect of the thoracic wall
B   Lateral view through the fifth intercostal space after thoracotomy
C   Transpleural anterolateral thoracotomy showing the lateral aspect of the spine and mediastinum

1 m. pectoralis major 2 m. coracobrachialis 3 m. latissimus dorsi
4 m. serratus ant. 5 m. obliquus externus abdominis 6 m. rectus abdominis 7 diaphragma 8 pulmo 9 a. axillaris 10 v. axillaris
11 a. thoracodorsalis 12 a. subscapularis 13 a. and v. thoracica externa 14 rami cutanei laterales nervosum intercostalium 15 a. and v. thoracica interna 16 v. azygos 17 v. cava sup. 18 v. pulmonalis
19 oesophagus 20 n. vagus 21 bronchus principalis dexter
22 columna vertebralis 23 v., a., and n. intercostalis 24 v. thoraco-epigastrica 25 n. thoracicus longus

c) Posterior Thoracic Wall

Access to the thoracic cavity is limited by the three layers of the posterior thoracic wall.

(1) Superficial Cutaneoadipose Layer

The skin of the posterior region of the thorax is very thick and mobile over the underlying layers. Palpable landmarks are essentially the crest of spinous processes and the spine of the scapula. The accessible region of the posterior thoracic wall lies between the spinous processes and the spinal margin of the scapula. This region is obviously enlarged by applying anterior traction to the shoulder. The posterior costal arches cannot be numerically identified by manual palpation.

(2) Middle Muscular and Neurovascular Layer

The spinal muscles and those of the scapular girdle form a large mass spread between the spine and scapula. Three main layers can be identified. The superficial layer is formed by large flat muscle bodies, i.e., the trapezius forming the upper medial two thirds and the latissimus dorsi forming the lower lateral third. The space between these muscles forms, with the spinal margin of the scapula, a triangular zone exposing the underlying layer, which comprises the rhomboideus major and minor extending from the spinal margin of the scapula to the spinous processes. The deep layer is formed by the muscles originating on the spinous processes and inserting on the transverse processes and posterior angle of the ribs. These muscles (the longissimus thoracis lying medial to the iliocostalis) form a 6–8-cm wide band on each side of the midline. Both muscles insert on all the subjacent bony structures, thus rendering their surgical disinsertion a laborious procedure. The serratus posterior superior, extending between the superior angle of the scapula and the spinous processes of the cervicothoracic junction continues the middle muscular layer in the cranial direction. The scapula and the supraspinatus, infraspinatus, and teres minor and major muscles lie lateral to the middle muscular layer. A vascular bundle enters the superior part of this region, including the posterior scapular artery and vein running along the spinal margin of the scapula below the rhomboideus muscles. The terminal branches of the inferior scapular artery and veins enter the region lateral to the lower tip of the scapula. Finally, the posterior collateral rami of the intercostal nerves and blood vessels traverse the different muscle layers near the tip of the transverse processes to reach the skin.

(3) Deep Costal and Intercostal Region

The deep wall of this region is formed by the rib cage. The ribs and intercostal spaces are slanted markedly downward and outward. The different layers forming the intercostal space comprise the external intercostal muscle with the levatores costarum lying superficial to it, followed by the external fibrocellular layer constituting the posterior external intercostal membrane. The upper part of this membrane forms an envelope around the intercostal neurovascular bundle running under the costal groove. The deeper internal intercostal layer does not extend to the spine, but is lined on its deep surface by the endothoracic fascia and parietal pleura. Owing to the presence of the endothoracic fascia, decollement of the parietal pleura from the deep surface of the intercostal spaces and ribs is relatively easy to achieve during operation, and this maneuver is thus very useful when the posterior retropleural approach is used. The intercostal spaces are limited near the spine by the costotransverse joints and intertransverse spaces, the latter being obturated by the superior costotransverse and the intertransverse ligaments. Mobilization of the ribs during the posterior approach thus requires the disarticulation of the costotransverse and costovertebral joints in the region of the heads of the ribs.

(4) Thoracic Cavity

Access to the thoracic cavity can be gained through the posterior segment of the intercostal space or through a gap obtained by the resection of the posterior arch of several ribs. Such access, then, is achieved by either the subpleural or the transpleural route. Regardless of the route employed, this approach allows exposure of only one lateral surface of the vertebral bodies covered by the intercostal neurovascular bundles. Identification of a vertebral lesion and orientation of the operative approach are based on the fact that the head of a given rib lies at the level of the intervertebral disc suprajacent to the vertebra numerically corresponding to the rib. The rib thus represents a reliable landmark for the disc.

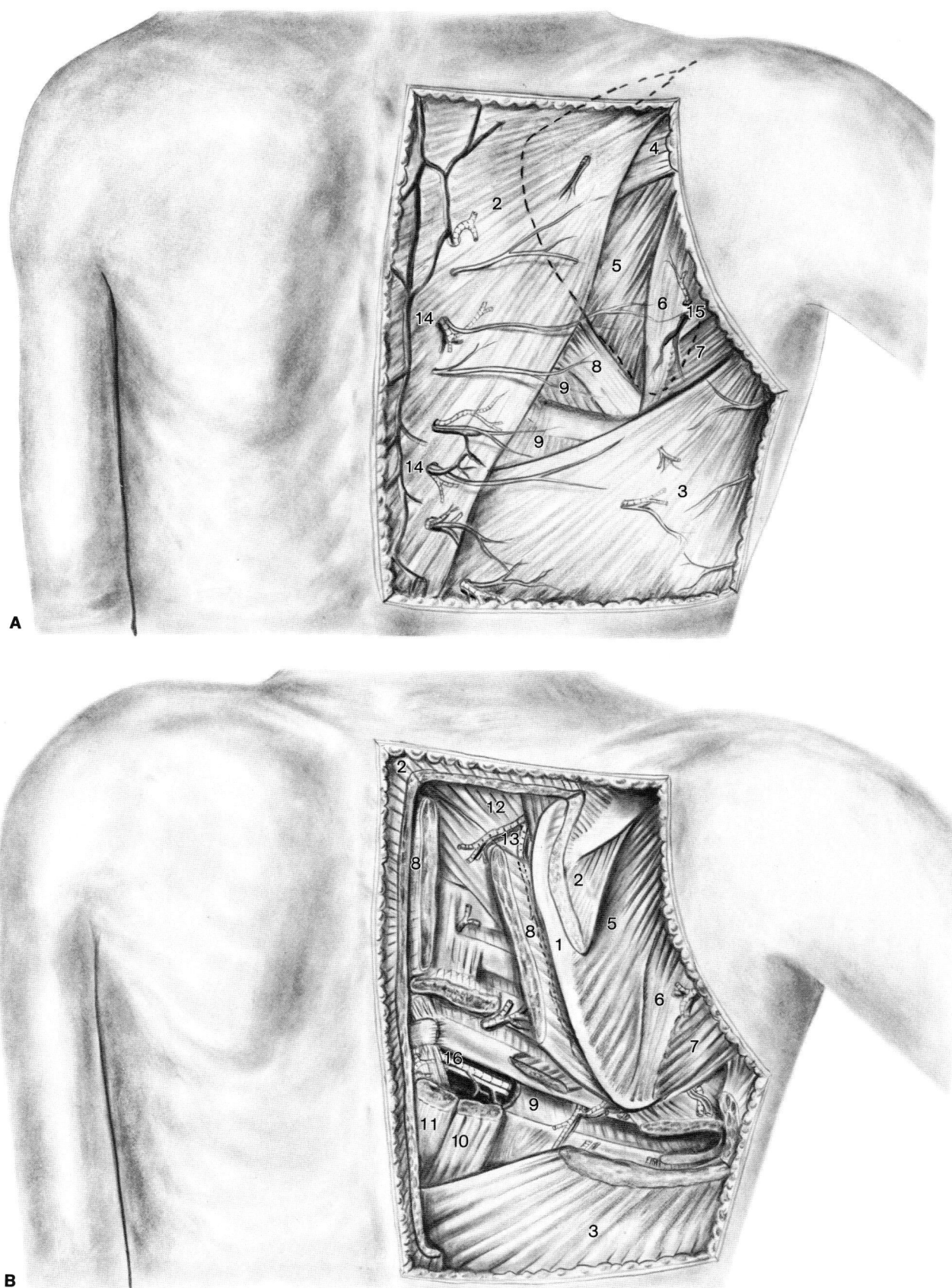

Figure 85 A, B

A   Posterior aspect of the thoracic wall showing the cutaneous region on the left and the underlying layers on the right

B   Posterior aspect of the thoracic wall with a window opening exposing the scapula and intercostal spaces

1 scapula *2* m. trapezius *3* m. latissimus dorsi *4* m. deltoideus *5* m. infraspinatus *6* m. teres minor *7* m. teres major *8* m. rhomboideus major *9* m. intercostalis *10* m. iliocostalis *11* m. longissimus thoracis *12* m. rhomboideus minor *13* a. and v. suprascapularis *14* ramus cutaneus rami dorsi nn. thoracici; rami dorsales aa. and vv. intercostales post. *15* rami a. and v. thoracicae externae *16* a. and v. intercostales post. and n. thoracicus

d) Mediastinum

The anatomical relations of the thoracic spine within the thoracic cavity are considered below with respect to the approach via the right and left pleural cavities.

(1) Approach Via the Right Pleural Cavity

The *thoracic spine* forms the posterior limit of the mediastinum. On the midline of the thoracic cage, it is concave in front of the costal insertions. Exposure of the thoracic spine requires retraction of the lung and diaphragmatic cupula and opening of the mediastinal pleura.

The *right lung* is thus collapsed and retracted anteriorly and medially to allow visualization of the spine.

The *diaphragmatic cupula* also forms a large obstacle in the inferior part of the thoracic cage. The obstacle is reduced by applying pressure to the cupula with a retractor.

The costovertebral joints can be seen by transparency through the *parietal pleura* lining the intercostal spaces. Opening of the parietal pleura at the level of the costovertebral joints allows exposure of the mediastinal structures. Three mediastinal sectors can be described with respect to the arch of the azygos vein:

The *supra-azygos sector* corresponds to T2 and T3. The right brachiocephalic venous trunk lies in the anterior part of this sector, with the internal thoracic artery running anterior to it and the phrenic nerve running along its right flank. The brachiocephalic artery and the trachea, with the right vagus nerve passing in front of them, lie in the posterior part of the sector. Finally the esophagus, lying in contact with the spine, represents the most posterior structure of the sector. A vascular latticework is located between the spine and esophagus, comprising the second through fourth intercostal arteries running obliquely and accompanied by their corresponding veins. The sympathetic ganglions lie just lateral to the heads of the ribs.

The *sector of the azygos arch* lies at the level of T4. The azygos arch runs in the posteroanterior direction from the spine towards the posterior surface of the superior vena cava. Along its course the left flank of the azygos arch crosses over the esophagus, the right vagus nerve, the tracheal bifurcation, and the brachiocephalic artery. The intercostal veins of the upper intercostal spaces on the right join the superoposterior angle of the azygos arch.

The *infra-azygos sector* extends from T4 to T10–T11. From anterior to posterior, this sector contains the right pulmonary hilus, the right atrium with its overlying pericardium, the esophagus flanked by the right vagus nerve, and the azygos vein lying along the junction of the right anterior and lateral surfaces of the thoracic spine. The metameric intercostal vascular bundles, comprising an artery and one or two accompanying veins, lie between the azygos vein and the intercostal spaces. Only the intercostal arteries arising from the thoracic aorta are found on the spinal midline, i.e., to the left of the azygos vein. Finally, the sympathetic ganglions and splanchnic nerves descend between the azygos vein and the costovertebral joints. The mediastinal viscera are surrounded by loose connective tissue allowing relatively easy operative dissection.

(2) Approach by the Left Pleural Cavity

Exposure of the left flank of the thoracic spine requires that the *left lung* be collapsed and retracted.

The left cupula of the *diaphragm* must be retracted downward to allow the best possible exposure of the inferior operative field.

Exposure of the mediastinal viscera and spine is achieved by opening of the *mediastinal pleura* where it joins the costal pleura at the level of the costovertebral joints. Three mediastinal sectors can be described with respect to the aortic arch:

The *supra-aortic sector* lies at the level of T2 and T3. From anterior to posterior, the following structures are found: the internal thoracic vascular bundle, the branchiocephalic venous trunk with the left phrenic nerve running along its left flank, the left common carotid artery with the left vagus nerve running along its left flank, the left subclavian artery, the thoracic duct, and the esophagus.

The *sector of the aortic arch* lies at the level of T4. The aortic arch is easily identified by its volume and pulsatility. From anterior to posterior, the aortic arch enters into relation with the phrenic nerve, the vagus nerve, the loop of the left recurrent laryngeal nerve, and the left superior intercostal arteries running obliquely along the lateral surface of the spine. The upper intercostal veins anastomose to form the accessory hemiazygos vein.

The *infra-aortic sector* contains the left lung and hilus and the left ventricle and atrium with their overlying pericardium. Posterior to the heart, the esophagus is visible with the left vagus nerve running along its left anterior surface. The descending thoracic aorta covers the anterior surface of the spine. The intercostal arteries arise from the posterior aspect of the aorta with the upper arteries running obliquely upward, the middle arteries running horizontally, and the lower pairs running slightly downward. The intercostal vascular bundles lie against the flank of the spine, with the hemiazygos and accessory hemiazygos veins lying over their left surface. Both of these veins anastomose with the azygos vein by passing posterior to the thoracic aorta, generally at the level of T6–T7. The sympathetic ganglions and splanchnic nerves lie anterior to the heads of the ribs.

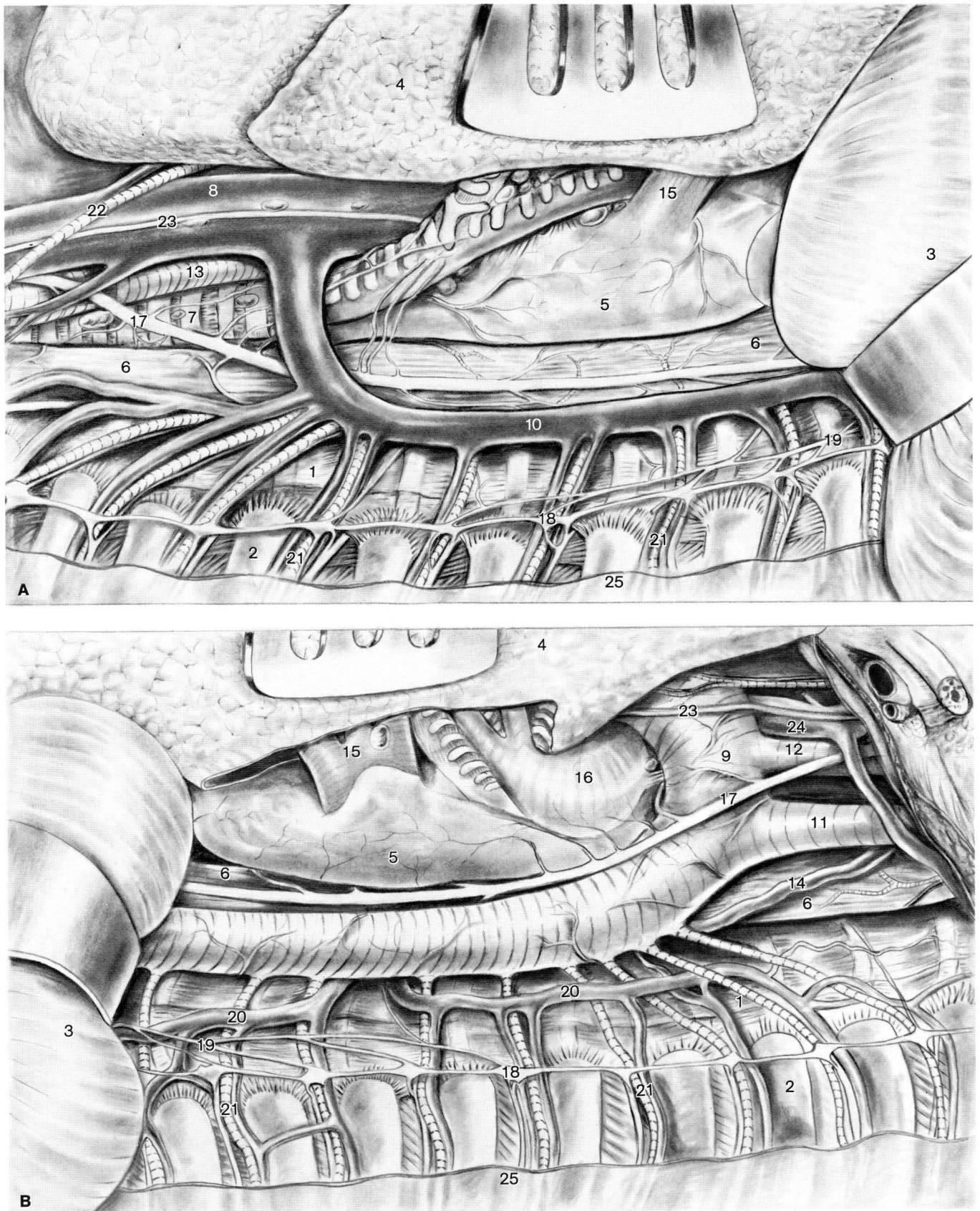

Figure 86 A, B

A The mediastinum viewed from the right in a recumbent subject
B The mediastinum viewed from the left in a recumbent subject

1 fourth vertebra thoracica *2* fourth costa *3* diaphragma *4* pulmo
5 cor pericardium *6* oesophagus *7* trachea *8* v. cava sup. *9* aorta
10 v. azygos *11* a. subclavia *12* a. carotis communis *13* truncus
brachiocephalicus *14* ductus thoracicus *15* v. pulmonalis
16 a. pulmonalis sinistra *17* n. vagus *18* truncus sympathicus
19 n. splanchnicus major *20* v. hemiazygos accessoria *21* v., a., and
n. intercostalis *22* a. thoracica interna *23* n. phrenicus *24* v. brachiocephalica *25* pleura costalis

e) Thoracic Spine

Retraction of the mediastinal viscera by the approach through the right or left pleural cavity exposes the anterior surface of the spine with the overlying collateral vessels of the aorta, the azygos vein, the thoracic duct, and the sympathetic nervous trunks. Access to the structures contained within the intervertebral foramina and vertebral canal can be gained by trepanation of the thoracic spine, i.e., rachiotomy.

The *azygos vein* originates anterior to the twelfth thoracic vertebra from the confluence of two tributaries, a medial tributary from the inferior vena cava and a lateral tributary formed by the anastomosis of the twelfth intercostal and ascending lumbar veins. From its site of origin the azygos vein runs upwards along the right lateral flank of the spine to the level of T4, where it leaves the spine and runs in a posteroanterior direction above the left pulmonary hilus, finally joining the posterior surface of the superior vena cava. In its course the azygos vein receives the hemiazygos vein on its left flank and the intercostal veins on its right flank.

The *hemiazygos vein* is formed by the confluence of three tributary veins, and runs upward along the left flank of the spine to the T6–T7 level, where it crosses the midline behind the thoracic aorta to join the azygos vein. The lowest intercostal veins anastomose with the left flank of the hemiazygos vein.

The *accessory hemiazygos vein,* formed by the confluence of the upper intercostal veins, descends along the left flank of the thoracic spine to T6–T7, where it crosses the spine to join the azygos vein.

The *thoracic duct* enters the inframediastinal region posterior to the aorta, and runs upward and toward the spinal midline to the level of T4, above which it progressively diverges to the left of the spine to enter the cervical region.
The intercostal arteries arise from the posterior surface of the aorta slightly to the left of the midline. The four to six uppermost intercostal arteries run in a retrograde direction from T4 towards the suprajacent vertebrae and thus run almost vertically or very obliquely over the anterior surface of the spine. Conservation of these arteries requires an oblique or vertical operative approach to the spine. The middle intercostal arteries run in a practically transverse direction anterior to the spine, and the lower intercostal arteries from T9 to T12 in some cases run obliquely downward anterior to the spine.

The *sympathetic nervous trunks* run along the flanks of the thoracic spine and lie in the lateral external position with respect to the heads of the ribs in the upper half of the spine and in the lateral internal position with respect to those in the lower half of the spine. The splanchnic nerves enter the thoracic region at the level of T6 and run downward medial to the sympathetic trunks.

The *anterior surface* of the spine is covered by the anterior longitudinal ligament, which adheres strongly to the intervertebral discs. To expose the anterior surface of the spine it is easier to work in front of the ligament rather than to attempt its disinsertion.

The *intervertebral foramina* lie at the level of the rib heads and intervertebral discs. Anterior trepanation of the foramina exposes their contents; the intercostal nerve, the spinal ganglion, and the veins of the foramina. A superior and an inferior vein run in contact with the vertebral pedicles and numerous other veins run diagonally through the foramina. The spinal arteries arising from the intercostal arteries penetrate through the foramina to supply the neuromeningeal structures of the spine. The intercostal nerves run in a retrograde direction through the upper foramina in close proximity to the lower margin of the upper vertebral pedicle of each foramen. Conversely, in the middle and lower foramina the intercostal nerves run either transversely through the middle of the foramen or descend obliquely towards its lower pedicular margin.

The *vertebral canal,* from anterior to posterior, contains the posterior longitudinal ligament and the anterointernal intraspinal venous plexuses. The latter have a longitudinal column in the lateral recesses of the vertebral canal and transverse anastomoses running over the posterior and medial surface of the vertebral bodies. In the zone flush with the intervertebral discs, the absence of venous structures delimits a median avascular region. Opening of the dura mater exposes the thoracic spinal cord, displaying the anterior spinal artery on the midline and the metameric emergence of the radicular nerve rootlets which form the intercostal nerves.
The denticulate ligament can be seen from each side of the spinal cord between the emergence of the anterior motor and posterior sensory radicular nerve rootlets. Finally, it should be pointed out that the sympathetic trunks give off their communicating rami to the intercostal nerves subsequent to the emergence of the latter from the intervertebral foramina.

Figure 87 A–D

A   Anterior aspect of the thoracic spine after removal of the major mediastinal structures. Three sectors can be described: a superior sector at T1 to T2, between the pleural domes; a middle sector from T3 to T10, where an opening has been made to expose the contents of the intervertebral foramina and vertebral canal; and an inframediastinal sector, hidden behind the posterior vertical part of the diaphragm
B   Horizontal section of the mediastinum and thoracic spine through T4 at the level of the aortic arch and azygos arch
C   Horizontal section of the thoracic spine and posterior mediastinum passing through T7
D   Horizontal section of the thoracic spine passing through the T9–T10 intervertebral disc

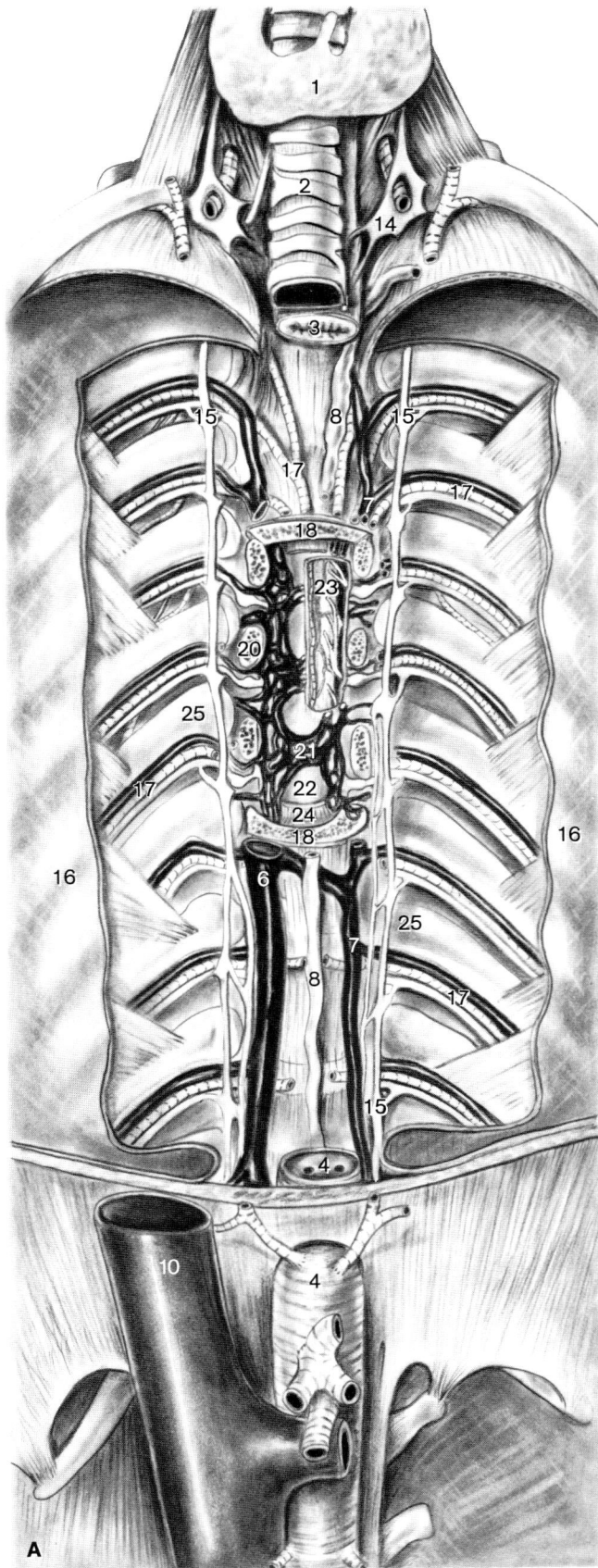

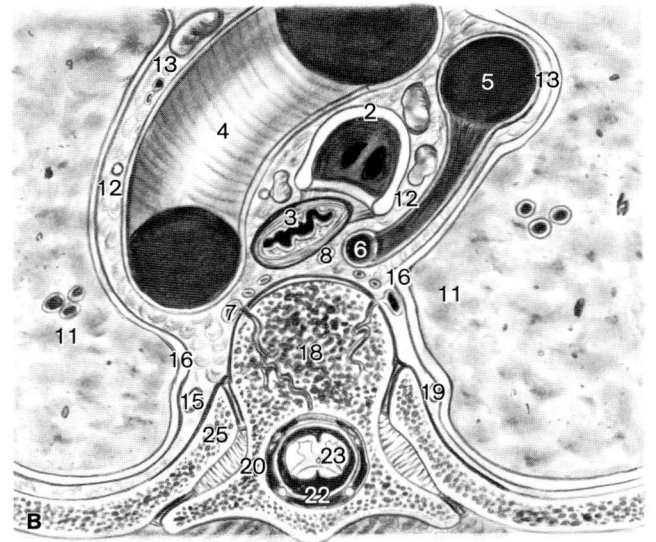

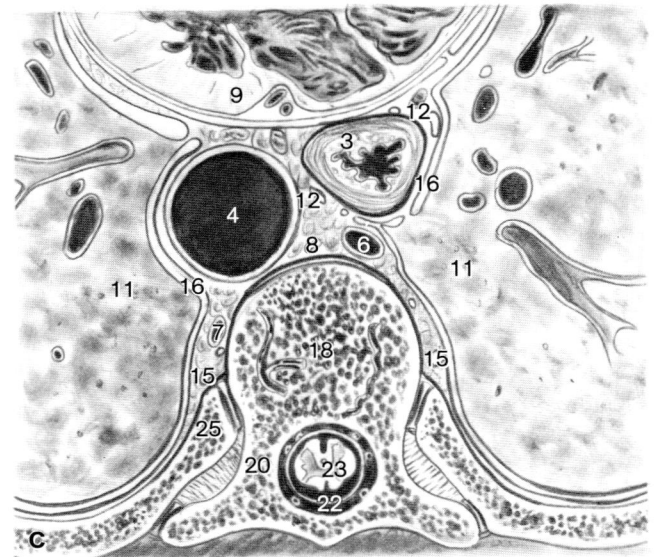

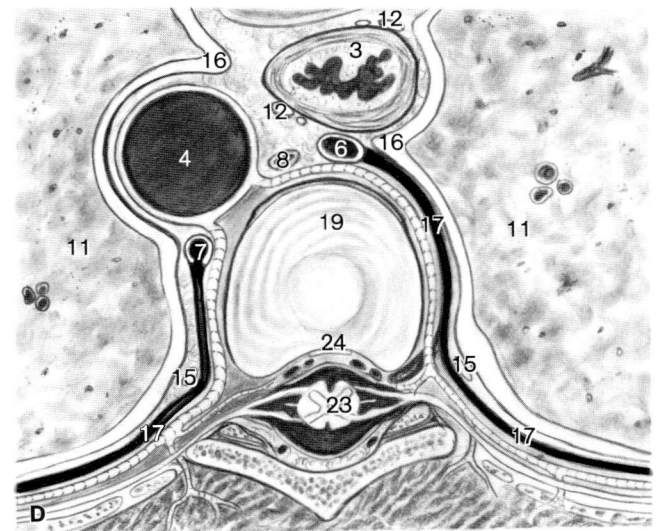

Figure 87 A–D

1 glanda thyroidea 2 trachea 3 oesophagus 4 aorta 5 v. cava sup.
6 v. azygos 7 v. hemiazygos accessoria 8 ductus thoracicus 9 cor
10 v. cava inf. 11 pulmo 12 n. vagus 13 n. phrenicus 14 ganglion
stellatum 15 truncus sympathicus 16 pleura 17 a., v., and n.
intercostalis 18 corpus vertebrae 19 discus intervertebralis
20 pediculus arcus vertebrae 21 plexus venosi vertebrales interni
22 duramater 23 medulla spinalis 24 lig. longitudinale post.
25 caput costae

f) Variations of the Azygos Venous System

The topography of the azygos venous system displays a relatively pronounced degree of variability. The surgeon who is aware of the possible variations gains in precision and security: he can achieve economical hemostasis and conserve proper azygos return in the presence of an anomaly of the inferior vena cava. Numerous classical studies have been published in this domain. The numerical date given below are derived from our studies in collaboration with R. M. Ouiminga based on the venous injection of plastic material in over 100 West African cadavers (Dakar, 1969). Multiple investigations during surgery in European subjects have confirmed that the topographical types found in Europeans and Africans are strictly identical, although the relative frequency of each type varies according to the population. One topographical variety which is by far the most frequent will be described as typical, followed by the less frequent varieties of azygos venous return.

(1) Type 1: Typical Azygos Venous Return (55.2%)

Regardless of race, the azygos system can be classically described as comprising three structures; the azygos vein (greater azygos vein), the hemiazygos (left inferior hemiazygos), and the accessory hemiazygos (left superior hemiazygos). The azygos vein is formed by the confluence of two tributaries. The internal tributary arises in the abdominal region from the posterior surface of the inferior vena cava near the upper lumbar vertebrae, and along with the splanchnic nerve traverses the abdomen through the diaphragmatic hiatus lying slightly lateral to the right crus to penetrate the inframediastinal space, where it joins the external tributary. The external tributary is formed by the confluence of the twelfth intercostal and ascending lumbar (lumbar azygos) veins which enter the inframediastinal space after passing under the psoas arcade. The external and internal tributaries join at the level of the upper half of the right anterolateral flank of the twelfth thoracic vertebra. The azygos vein runs upward along the spine to the level of T5 to T3, according to the individual (most often T4). The ascending part of the azygos lies a mean distance of 13.2 mm lateral to the spinal midline (range 9.3–19.9 mm). At its point of origin the mean caliber of the vein is 3.8 mm. The second segment of the azygos vein is the horizontal arch lying at the level of T4, which joins the posterior surface of the superior vena cava after passing above the right pulmonary hilus. The mean caliber of the terminal azygos vein is 8.5 mm. On its right flank up to the arch the azygos vein receives the right intercostal veins, of which the uppermost are often grouped together to form a common venous trunk known as the right superior intercostal vein. On its left flank in the middle thoracic region (T6 to T9) it receives the hemiazygos veins.

The hemiazygos vein, originating at the level of the middle or lower third of T12, is formed by the confluence of two medial and one lateral venous tributaries. The medial tributaries are constituted by an anastomosis with the left renal vein, passing through the same diaphragmatic orifice as the greater splanchnic nerve, and the lateral tributary arises from the confluence of the left twelfth intercostal vein and the left ascending lumbar vein. At its origin the hemiazygos vein has a mean diameter of 3.4 mm. It runs upward along the left anterolateral flank of the spine and then turns to the left to join the azygos vein anterior to the middle thoracic region between T5 and T11 (most frequently at the level of T9). The mean terminal diameter of the hemiazygos vein is 5.4 mm. It receives on its left flank the left inferior intercostal veins corresponding to the vertebrae over which it has passed.

The accessory hemiazygos vein runs downward along the left anterolateral aspect of the spine. The tributaries of this vein are the left upper intercostal veins, in cases where these do not meet to form a single venous trunk known as the left superior intercostal vein, which when present anastomoses directly to the left brachiocephalic vein. The accessory hemiazygos also receives the other middle intercostal veins from T3 to T8–T9. The accessory hemiazygos turns to the right to join the azygos vein between T4 and T11 (most often at the level of T6 or T7). It is on average 2 mm in diameter at its origin and 2.8 mm at its end, and is thus markedly more slender than the other two azygos trunks.

The azygos venous system is consistently found in the prearterial position with respect to the intercostal arteries. The descending thoracic aorta partially camouflages the hemiazygos veins, and the thoracic duct runs posterior to the aorta halfway between the azygos and hemiazygos veins. Exposure of the anterior surface of the spine should thus be achieved by sectioning the vessels between the azygos and hemiazygos veins, where ligation of a very limited number of intercostal arteries is required. Indeed, an operative approach lateral to the azygos system would also require the ligation of the intercostal veins, whose course over the vertebral bodies varies from oblique to horizontal. The only reliable landmark for identifying these veins is their position between the rib heads next to the intercostal artery lying in the depression of the lateral surface of the vertebral bodies anterior to the intervertebral foramina.

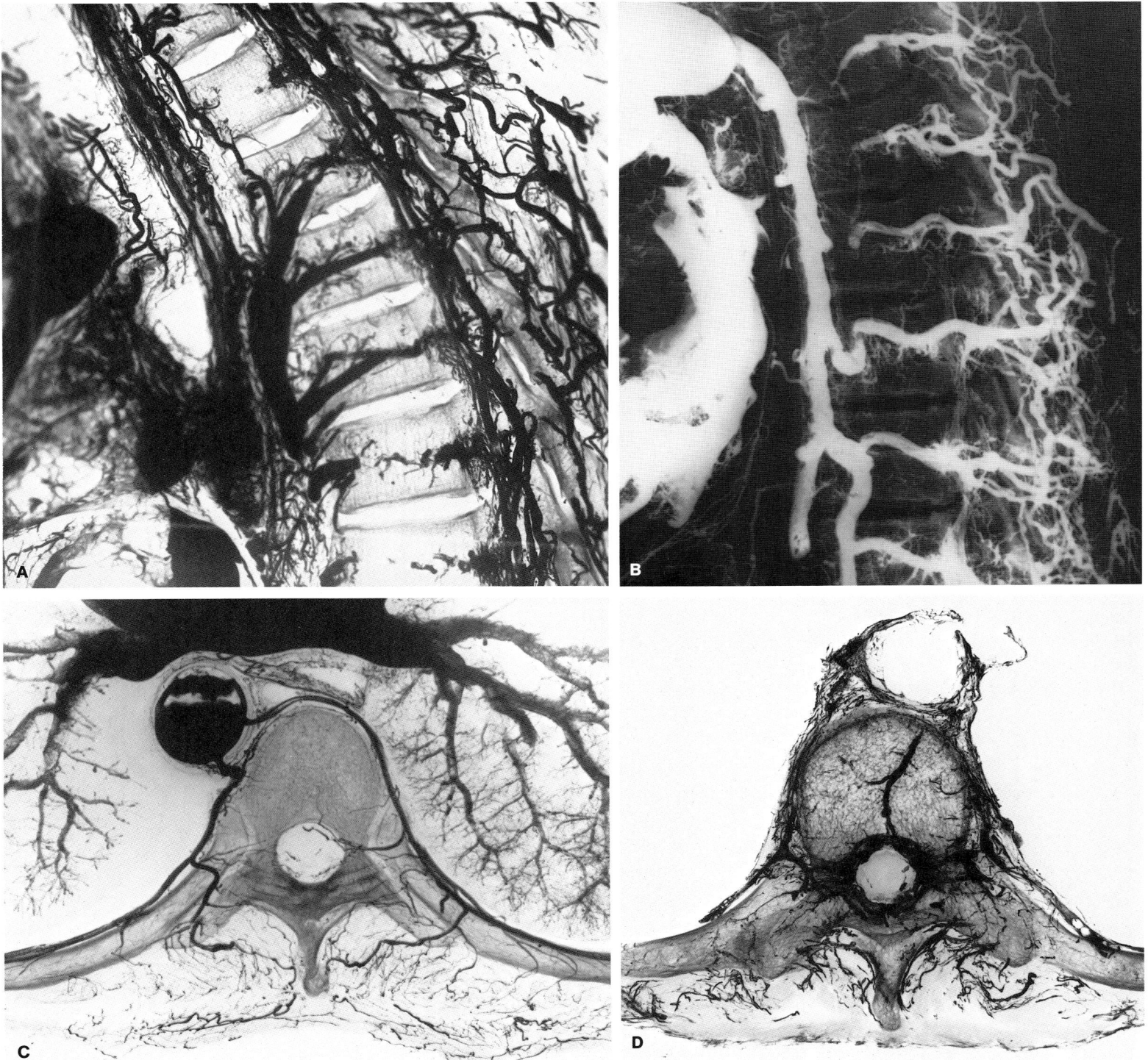

Figure 88 A–D

A Roentgenogram of the accessory hemiazygos vein subsequent to venous injection of contrast material

B Anatomical specimen with opacification of the azygos vein from T9–T4

C Horizontal section at the level of T7 after injection of the arterial system to demonstrate the aorta and intercostal arteries

D Horizontal section through T7 after opacification of the venous system to show the intra- and extraspinal venous plexuses

(2) Type 2 (27.8%)

In this case the hemiazygos vein is reduced to a very short trunk which joins the azygos vein at the level of T10. The suprajacent veins form small trunks anastomosing directly with the azygos vein and without constituting a true accessory hemiazygos vein. Accordingly, in this type of azygos return the longitudinal venous trunk is lacking along the left flank of the spine.

(3) Type 3 (9.2%)

The hemiazygos vein is absent in this case. The twelfth left intercostal vein joins the inferior vena cava directly, and the other intercostal veins anastomose directly with the azygos vein. The accessory hemiazygos vein persists. Access to the lower left flank of the thoracic spine thus requires common ligation of the intercostal veins and arteries at each vertebral level.

(4) Type 4 (1.3%)

In this case the azygos system is reduced to a median azygos vein, which receives on its flanks the upper pairs of lumbar veins followed by the right and left intercostal veins. The operative approach to the spine allows preservation of the midline venous axis but requires the ligation of the intercostal arteries and veins on one flank of the spine. The right and left superior intercostal veins anastomose with the arch of the azygos vein.

(5) Type 5 (1.3%)

This type features a symmetrical azygos system with two azygos veins, one joining the inferior vena cava on the right, the other joining the brachiocephalic venous trunk on the left. In this case the spinal midline is free of venous structures.

(6) Type 6 (1.3%)

In this type of venous return the symmetrical azygos and hemiazygos veins are separate down to the level of T7, where they fuse on the left flank of the spine to form a single paramedian venous axis, which receives the intercostal and lumbar veins on the right and left sides. At the level of T11 the azygos and accessory hemiazygos veins display their typical topographical positions. Consequently, the inferior part of the azygos veins is lacking from T7 to T11.

(7) Type 7 (1.3%)

In this case the azygos vein originates in the lumbar region near L3 and runs upward along the left flank of the spine to terminate with its arch in the typical position. The azygos vein

thus receives the lumbar veins on both flanks but the intercostal veins only on its right flank. The hemiazygos and accessory hemiazygos veins join to form a common trunk anastomosing with the azygos vein at the level of T7.

(8) Type 8 (1.3%)

This type features a common azygos vein and a hypertrophic accessory hemiazygos vein descending to the T10 level, thus eliminating the hemiazygos vein. The left inferior intercostal veins join the azygos or accessory hemiazygos vein directly.

(9) Type 9 (1.3%)

This type is represented by a major anomaly previously described by Brodelius. The absence of the suprahepatic part of the inferior vena cava is compensated by an oversized azygos vein carrying blood from the drainage bed of the inferior vena cava to the superior vena cava, and the intercostal veins are generally dilated and varicose. During surgery, this anomaly requires the preservation of the azygos venous axis in order not to hinder the venous return from the regions normally drained by the inferior vena cava. The exaggerated caliber of the azygos vein and its right intercostal tributaries should lead to suspicion of this anomaly and to operative mobilization and not ligation of the azygos vein.

Figure 89 A–H

A The hemiazygos vein joining the azygos vein at T10. Note the absence of the accessory hemiazygos vein (Type 2; 27.8%)
B Absence of the hemiazygos vein (Type 3; 9.2%)
C Sagittal median azygos vein with absence of the hemiazygos vein (Type 4; 1.3%)
D Presence of two symmetrical azygos veins (Type 5; 1.3%)
E A bayonetlike azygos vein running over the lower left and upper right thoracic spine (Type 6; 1.3%)
F Origin of the azygos vein in the lumbar region with fusion of the two hemiazygos veins (Type 7; 1.3%)
G Absence of the hemiazygos vein with hypertrophy of the accessory hemiazygos vein (Type 8; 1.3%)
H Absence of the suprahepatic part of the inferior vena cava, compensated by an enlarged azygos vein (Type 9; 1.3%)

1 v. cava sup. *2* v. brachiocephalica dextra *3* v. brachiocephalica sinistra *4* v. cava inf. *5* vv. renales *6* vv. hepaticae *7* arcus v. azygos *8* v. azygos *9* v. hemiazygos *10* v. hemiazygos accessoria

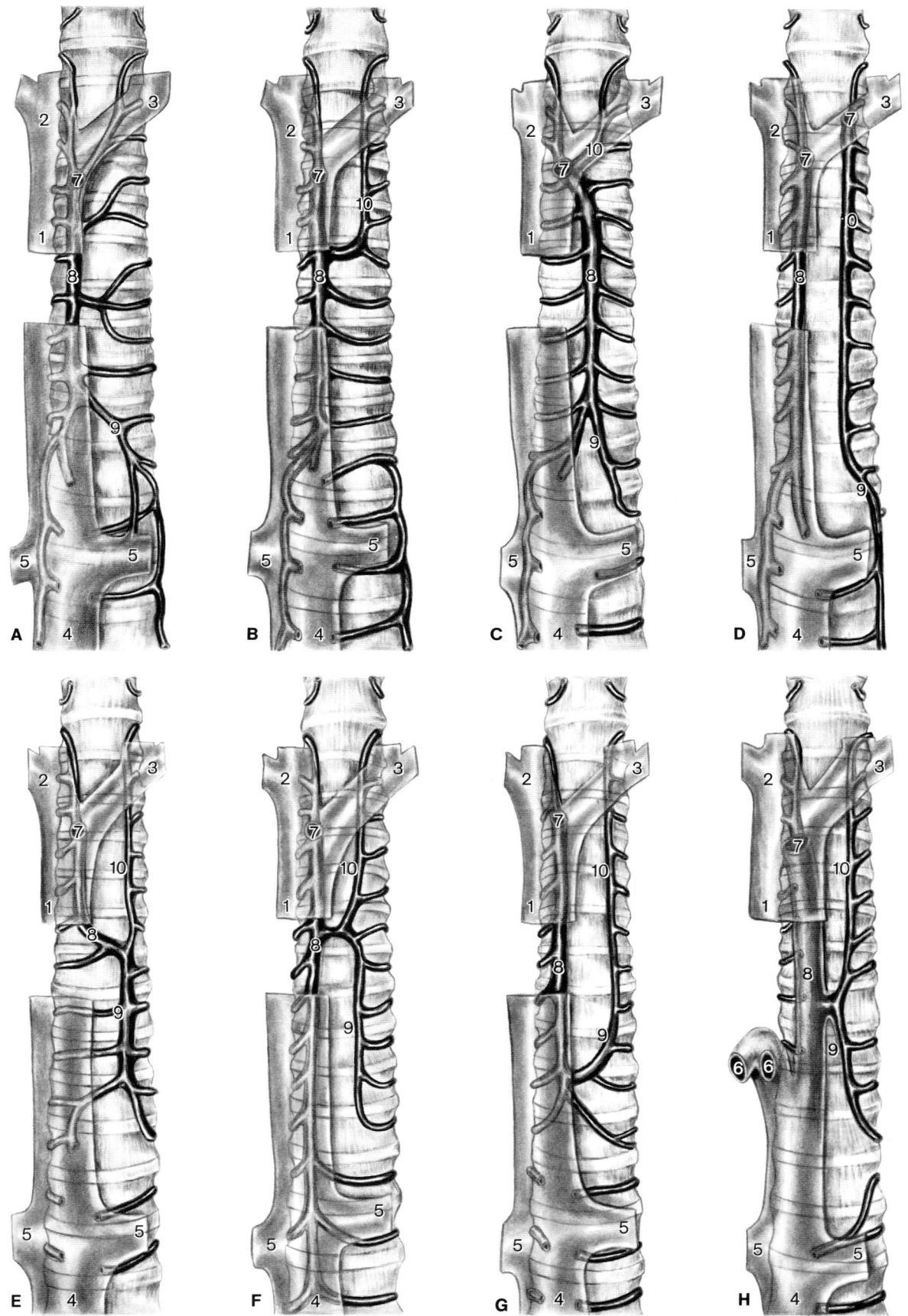

Figure 89 A–H

g) Other Venous and Arterial Variations

(1) Lumbar Veins

In the most frequent topographical type the lumbar veins display a classical metameric position, running horizontally just below the middle of the concave part of the vertebral bodies to join the juxtamedian posterior surface of the inferior vena cava, and anastomose with the vertical axis of the ascending lumbar vein at the level of the intervertebral foramina. Operative dissection should not be carried out in this zone, to avoid hemorrhage and neurological injury. The other topographical varieties of lumbar venous return include the division of the lumbar vein into two branches prior to its terminal anastomosis. In other cases two contiguous lumbar veins may be joined together by a vertical anastomosis lying over the intervertebral disc. In a few cases two ascending lumbar veins fuse to form a common trunk a few millimeters prior to joining the inferior vena cava, and in such cases the veins run obliquely over the vertebral bodies and sometimes over a disc. The most curious topographical venous distribution is that of a median lumbar azygos system originating in the lumbar region and forming a median retrocaval venous axis receiving the right and left lumbar veins, which thus do not join the inferior vena cava directly. Finally, mention should be given to the anastomosis of the first and second lumbar veins with the medial tributary of the hemiazygos and left renal veins to form the renoazygolumbar anastomotic trunk.

(2) Parietal Thoracic and Lumbar Arteries

It is important that the surgeon be familiar with the topographical variations of the parietal collaterals of the aorta lying over the thoracic and lumbar vertebrae, as such knowledge helps hemostasis of these vessels during exposure of the vertebral bodies. The arterial topography varies according to the spinal sectors. At the level of T1 to T3 the anterior surface of the vertebral bodies is generally free of overlying intercostal arteries. The most frequent variation is the presence of vertically descending right and left arterioles originating from the inferior thyroid or vertebral artery and sometimes anastomosing with the second or third intercostal artery. The operative approach to these vertebrae thus requires the ligation and section of these small arteries.

Form T3 to T5 the intercostal arteries run almost vertically over the vertebral bodies. The third through sixth intercostal arteries arise as a group from the posterior surface of the origin of the thoracic aorta at the level of T4–T5 and ascend almost vertically with a very slight lateral slant, thus running over several intervertebral discs and vertebral bodies prior to reaching the lower margin of their corresponding ribs. This greatly hinders the surgical exposure of the vertebral bodies and may lead to the risk of untoward arterial ligation and subsequent medullary ischemia. It is thus recommended that only one intercostal branch be ligated, since the remaining branches can be mobilized to expose the anterior surface of the vertebrae.

From T6 to T10 the intercostal arteries are generally arranged in a metameric recurrent fashion. Their origin is on each side of the posterior aortic midline followed by a short vertically ascending segment, i.e., opposite to the direction of aortic blood flow. They then run horizontally from the flank of the aorta below the level of the middle of their corresponding vertebral bodies to reach the intervertebral foramen. Each of these intercostal arteries thus arises at the level of the intervertebral disc subjacent to its corresponding vertebra, so the discs are free of overlying arteries in this spinal region. Identification of the intercostal artery is thus achieved on the aortic flank at a point halfway between two neighboring discs. Rupture of an arterial ligature is not problematic in this region, since the remaining part of the intercostal artery posterior to the aorta can be ligated near the lower disc.

From T10 to L2 the intercostal and lumbar arteries display an essentially horizontal metameric distribution. They arise on each side of the posterior aortic midline and then run in a frankly horizontal direction over the middle of the corresponding vertebral bodies. Ligation should thus be made halfway between two intervertebral discs, leaving intact a short retroaortic segment of the intercostal arteries which can be ligated if the initial suture gives way.

The metameric lumbar arteries from L2 to L4 often run in a descending direction, arising on each side of the posterior aortic midline at the level of the intervertebral disc just above their numerically corresponding vertebrae and then running vertically downward behind the aorta and finally horizontally towards the middle of the vertebral bodies before entering the intervertebral foramina. Ligation of these lumbar arteries should thus be made lateral to the aorta midway between two neighboring discs and lateral to the vertebral body, leaving a sufficiently long arterial stump to allow religation of the artery on the posterior surface of the aorta when necessary.

Aside from these typical topographical varieties, minor right or left variations involving only one or two parietal arteries may be found. For example, the right metameric parietal artery may run downward while its metameric homologue on the left runs upward. In such cases the origin of the homologous arteries on the posterior surface of the aorta may be separated by as much as one vertebral body.

Sometimes the anterolateral surfaces of a vertebral body are not traversed by a parietal artery: in this situation the suprajacent artery forms a single common trunk giving rise to an intercostal artery which then runs upward 1 cm anterior to the vertebral pedicles to reach its intervertebral foramen. In other cases the homologous pair of parietal arteries arises from a common retroaortic trunk which then bifurcates on the aortic midline or near one aortic flank to give off right and left branches. Finally, in cases where the aortic bifurcation is located cranial to its typical position the lumbar arteries do not arise from the posterior surface of the aorta, but from the middle sacral artery, which runs over the midline of the lowest lumbar vertebrae.

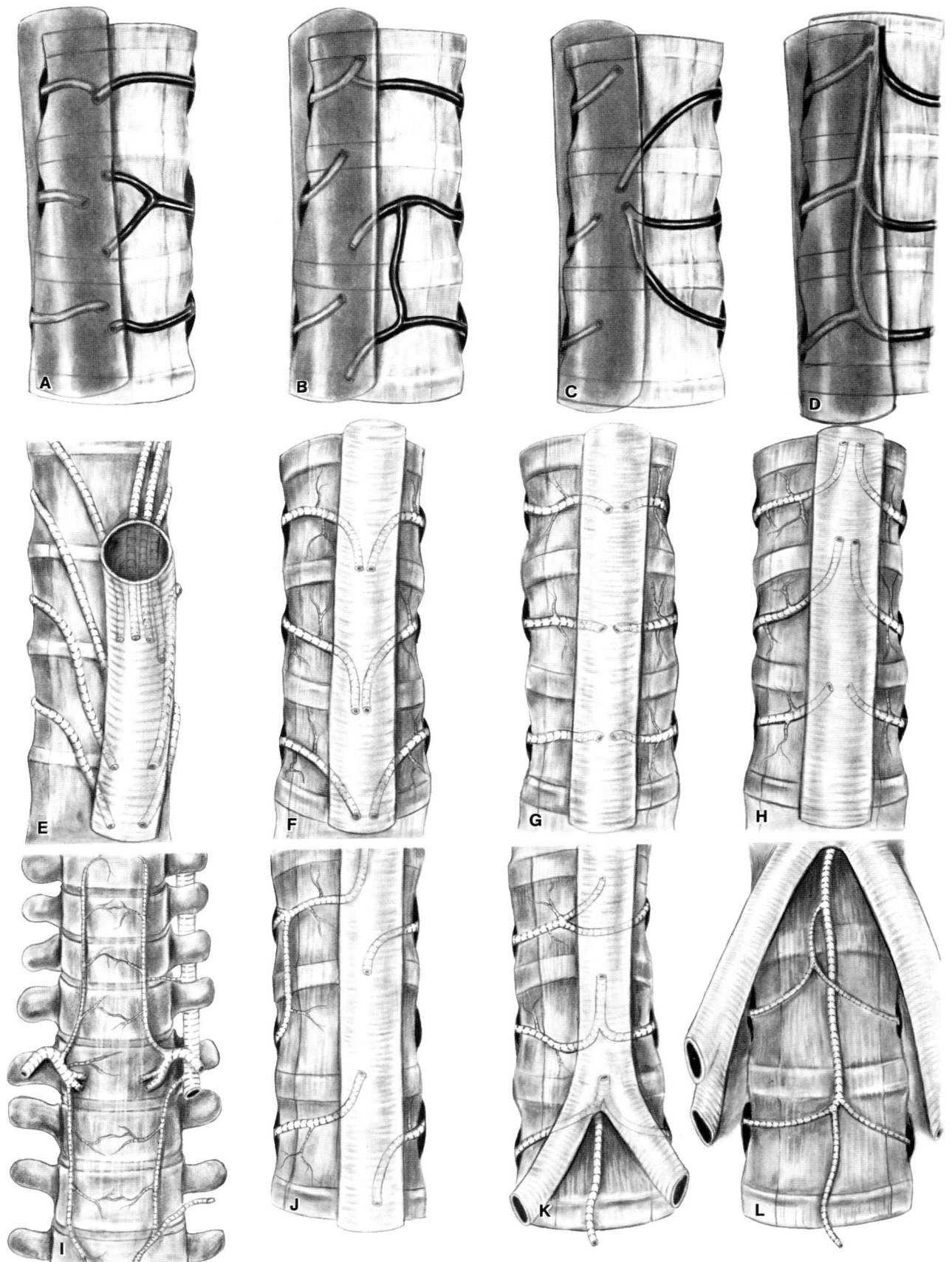

Figure 90 A–L

A–D   Topographical variations of the lumbar veins

E–L   Topographical variations of the parietal arteries lying over the thoracic and lumbar vertebral bodies

h) Variations of the Parietal Aortic Collaterals

(1) Frequency of the Topographical Variations

The first pair of intercostal arteries do not usually run over the vertebrae, since they arises directly from the cervicointercostal trunk (on the right in 95%, on the left in 90% of cases) or from a common trunk with the second intercostal artery (right 3%, left 4%). They arise directly from the aorta to run vertically upward over the vertebral bodies only in exceptional cases (right 1%, left 6%). In 62% of subjects the second intercostal artery arises from the aorta and thus runs vertically over the vertebrae, and in the remaining cases arises from the cervicointercostal trunk, the inferior thyroid artery, or a common trunk with the third intercostal artery.

The fact that the parietal arteries arising from the aorta can run in an ascending recurrent, horizontal, or descending direction probably results from the differential rate of growth of the aorta and spine. The ascending recurrent variety specially involves the upper intercostal arteries, although this type of course is also found, albeit with decreasing frequency, for the other parietal arteries: the third intercostal artery (100%), the tenth intercostal artery (57%), and the fourth lumbar artery (7%). Similarly, a descending course of the parietal arteries increases in frequency from the sixth intercostal artery (1%) to the first lumbar artery (53%) and finally the fifth lumbar artery (100%). Conversely, the frequency distribution of the strictly horizontal metameric course resembles a parabolic curve from the fourth intercostal to the fourth lumbar artery, with maximum occurrence (42%) at the 12. intercostal artery. In our experience, based on examination of 100 spines, we found a common trunk giving rise to two homologous parietal arteries in 17 cases, a common trunk giving off two contiguous arteries on one side in 32 cases, and an asymmetrical origin of two homologous arteries in 44 cases.

(2) Number and Dimensions of the Parietal Aortic Arteries

The aorta gives rise to ten right intercostal arteries in 51% of cases and eleven left intercostal arteries in 44.4% of cases. The presence of twelve intercostal arteries is a relatively rare finding (2.1% on the right, 4% on the left). In 1% of subjects only six or seven right and left intercostal arteries are present. With respect to the lumbar arteries, the most common variation is the presence of four arteries (74.2% on the right, 70.7% on the left). In a few cases three (20%–22%) or five (5%–7%) lumbar arteries may be noted.

The caliber of the parietal arteries increases in craniocaudal fashion. Accordingly, in postmortem specimens the upper intercostal arteries have a mean diameter of 1.1 mm whereas that of the lower lumbar arteries is 1.5 mm. An exception to the rule is the twelfth intercostal artery, displaying a mean diameter of 1.1 mm.

The length of the parietal arteries decreases from the first intercostal artery (mean length 42 mm) to the tenth intercostal artery (34 mm on the right, 27 mm on the left), and then increases down to the fourth lumbar artery (41.6 mm on the right, 40.7 mm on the left).

The intervals between the aortic site of origin of the parietal vessels vary from the second intercostal to the fourth lumbar artery: 5–7 mm between the second and third intercostal arteries, increasing to 18–22 mm between the eleventh and twelfth intercostal arteries, and then decreasing in the region of the first to fourth lumbar arteries from 24–17 mm.

(3) Venous Relations of the Parietal Aortic Arteries

In the great majority of cases the satellite veins run along the cranial margin of the parietal arteries, and usually cross them anteriorly. However, in a few cases the parietal arteries, running horizontally, pass anterior to the longitudinal venous trunks. Despite the intimate contact between the parietal arteries and veins, they can easily be separated to achieve hemostasis. Although the arteries and veins are sometimes at some distance from each other near the midline region of the vertebral bodies, they are consistently in contact with each other by means of metameric bundles anterior to their point of penetration into the intervertebral foramen, i.e., below the middle of the lateral surfaces of the vertebral bodies.

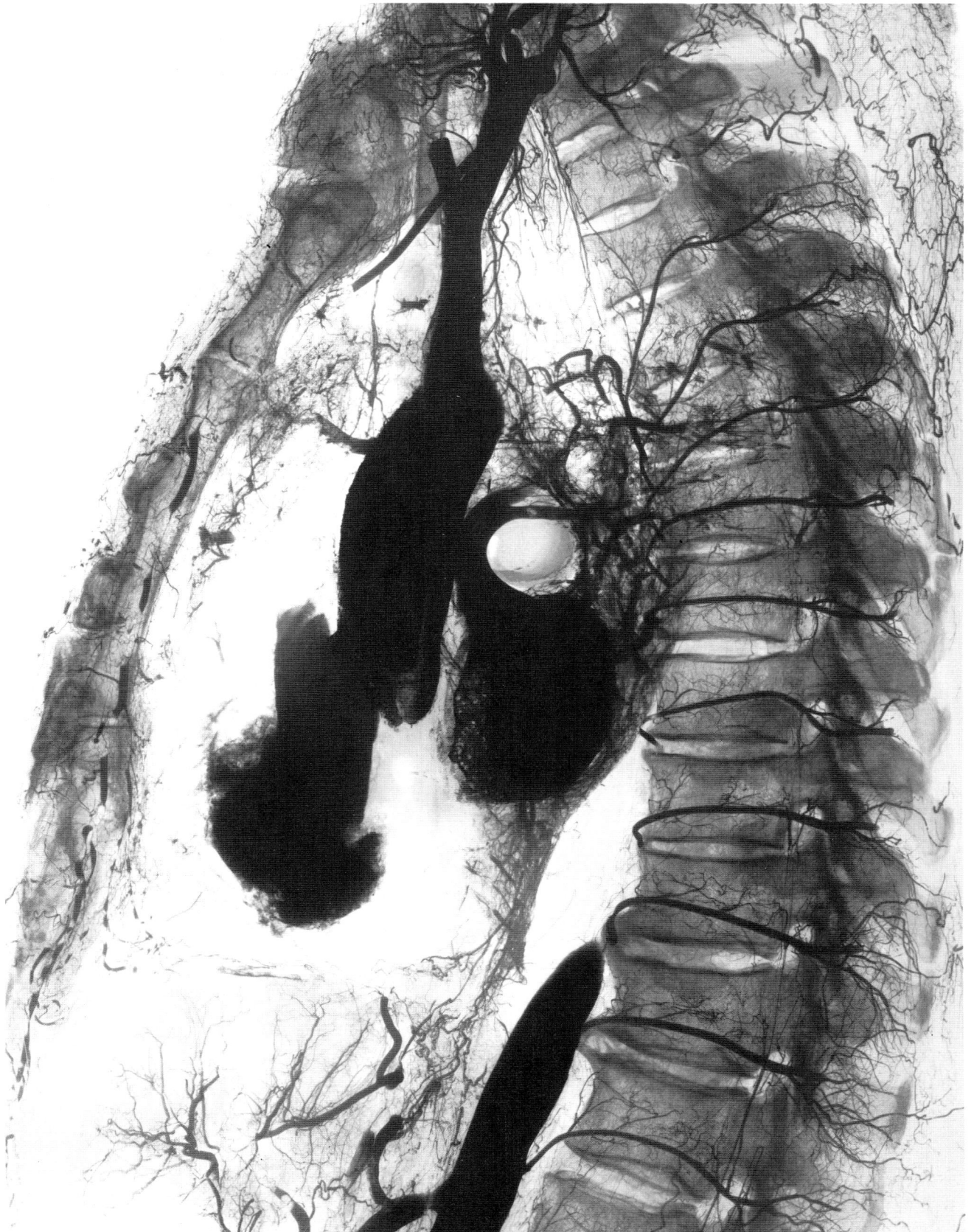

Figure 91. Median sagittal section of the thorax after arterial injection of contrast material

2. Anterior Transpleural Approach

a) Preparation and Anesthesia

In patients with respiratory insufficiency, preparation for the transpleural approach requires that respiratory function testing be carried out, followed by appropriate breathing exercises when necessary. In cases of bronchitis the patient can be prepared by antibiotic inhalation therapy. On the morning of operation the thorax is prepared by thoroughly shaving the right axillary region. Anesthesia obviously requires automatic respiratory assistance and hermetic endotracheal intubation allowing patency of both main bronchi. It must be borne in mind that during operation the right lung is collapsed, and thus functionally excluded, to allow exposure of the spine. Monitoring of blood gas levels may be required during operation.

b) Operative Position

The patient is placed supine on the operating table with the left upper limb lying along the trunk. The right upper limb is positioned so that the forearm lies horizontally over the mandible, i.e., the shoulder and elbow are placed at a 90° angle. The right limb should be securely attached to a flexible metal arch. The right limb must not drop towards the head during operation, as this may lead to elongation of the brachial plexus. Preparation of the operative field requires thorough disinfection of the skin from the right clavicle to the right chondral margin and from the sternum to the posterior axillary line. Operative draping is installed to isolate the anesthesiologist at the patient's head from the surgical field at the thorax. The surgeon and first assistant work on the patient's right, and the second assistant on the left. It is often necessary to prepare a second operative field, usually the right fibular region, for the removal of bone-graft material. For a right-handed surgeon the suction cannula is placed to the left of the operative field and the coagulation apparatus to the right.

c) Incision

An arcuate incision with superior concavity is made upward from under the breast, and should extend laterally to the mid-axillary line and medially to the right lateral margin of the sternum. This operative approach requires the section of two or three segments of costal cartilage between the second and fifth ribs. The most frequently employed and useful variation is that allowing access to the spinal sector from T4 to T10, which requires that the fourth and fifth segments of costal cartilage be sectioned. In such cases the skin incision should follow the anterior arch of the fourth rib precisely down to the fourth costal cartilage and then extend 2–3 cm upward, toward the third costal cartilage. This type of incision can easily be achieved in men, but in women it is necessary to make the incision in the submammary fold and to displace the breast upward, thus allowing subsequent exposure of the anterior arch of the fourth rib. When operation requires the exposure of a more cranial spinal segment, e.g., T3 to T9, the second and third segments of costal cartilage are sectioned to allow access through the third intercostal space. Access to a more caudal region (T6 to T11) requires the section of the fourth and fifth segments of costal cartilage through an incision running along the anterior arch of the fifth rib and the fifth costal cartilage. Identification of the intercostal spaces is achieved by using as a landmark the sternal angle (Louis' angle), situated at the junction of the manubrium, body of the sternum, and second costal cartilage. The space lying immediately below the sternal angle is the second intercostal space. In difficult cases, anteroposterior roentgenograms of the thorax allow identification of the appropriate intercostal space whose anterior region radiographically projects over the site of the spinal lesion. The skin is incised with a plain knife and the wound disinfected with iodine alcohol. A moist compress is then packed over the incision. Next, the compress is lifted up centimeter by centimeter to allow progressive hemostasis of the sites of subdermal hemorrhage. The subcutaneous tissue is then sectioned down to the superficial thoracic fascia using the electric cautery knife.

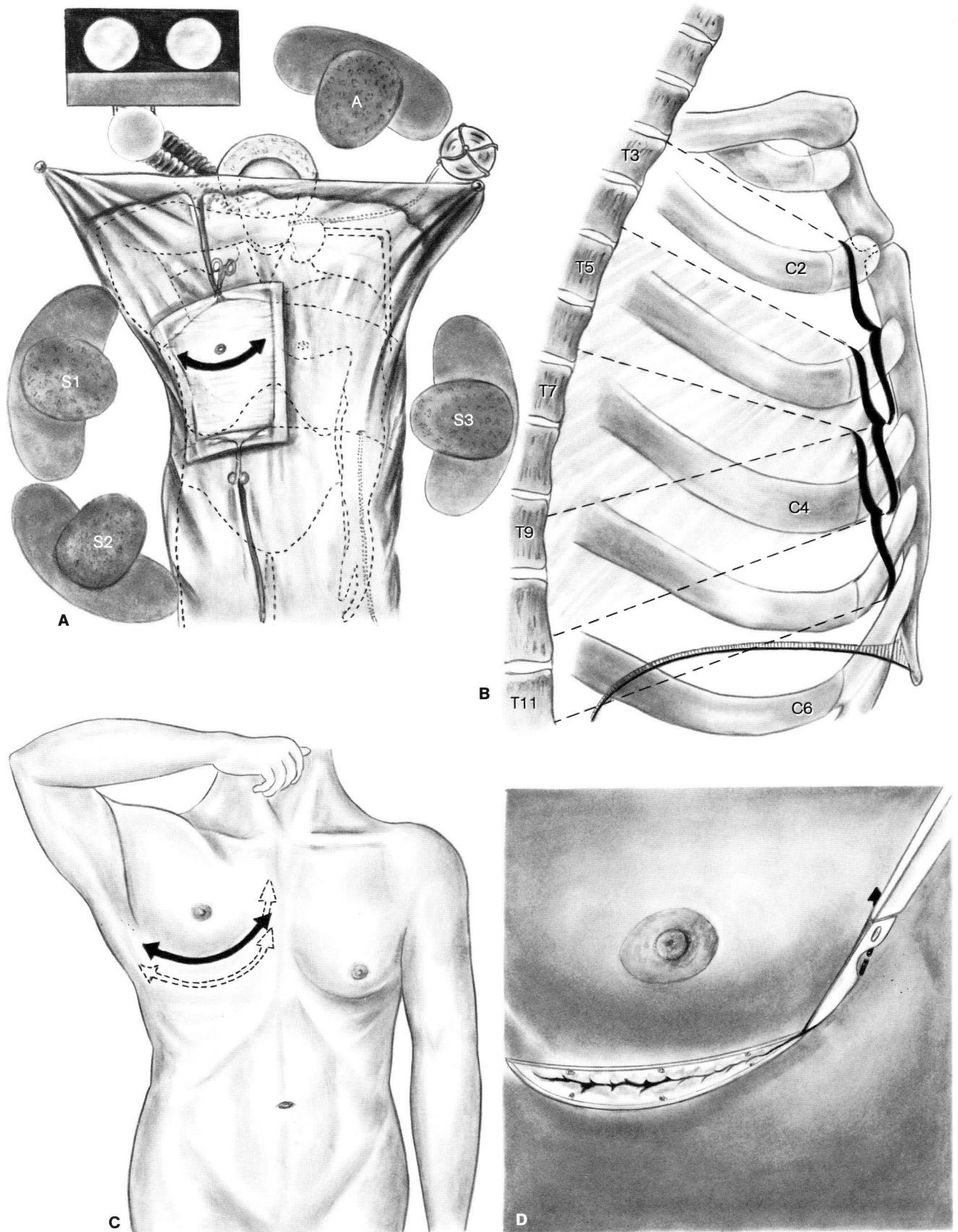

Figure 92 A–D

A Overhead view of the operative position and surgical team
B The correlations between the costal cartilaginous segments to be sectioned and the different regions of the thoracic spine
C Different types of skin incision according to the spinal segment to be exposed
D Submammary skin incision using the plain knife

d) Parietal Exposure

Retraction of the cutaneous and adipose tissues of the incision exposes the fascia superficialis of the thorax and the underlying muscle fibers of the pectoralis major. Transection of the latter is achieved in the region lying flush with the fourth rib, using the electric cautery knife. Transection should extend laterally to include the anterior fibers or the serratus anterior. Hemostasis of the cut muscle surfaces is progressively achieved by electrocoagulation. Retraction of the muscle fibers exposes the fourth rib and costal cartilage. Near the medial margin of the operative field dissection in contact with the cartilage is stopped and work is directed upward parallel to the lateral sternal margin up to and above the suprajacent (third) costal cartilage. Section of the rib is prepared by tracing a line on the middle part of the fourth rib using the tip of the cautery knife. The periosteum and the pericostal fibrous tissue are then rasped free from the upper half of the rib, a few points of hemostasis being achieved by electrocoagulation. A raspatory with a central notch is then manipulated from the lateral to the medial part of the upper margin of the fourth rib to disinsert the fibromuscular structures from the intercostal space. Rasping must be stopped 12–13 mm lateral to the medial margin of the body of the sternum, so as not to injure the internal thoracic vascular bundle (internal mammary vessels). This technique of disinsertion of the intercostal muscles allows direct opening of the pleural cavity. The third intercostal cartilage is then exposed by rasping along its upper and lower margins to reveal the pleural cavity. The structures of the intercostal space can then be tied off en bloc and sectioned between two ligatures at a point 13 mm lateral to the sternum. The next step is to pass a large needle holder under the second and third segments of costal cartilage and to section them 13 mm lateral to the sternum with the plain knife. When injury to the internal thoracic vessels occurs, one should not hesitate to ligate and divide the bleeders. An orthostatic retractor is then installed with the mechanism facing the axillary region. The section of the two segments of costal cartilage allows wide exposure between the fourth and fifth ribs without fracturing them. Such exposure is generally sufficient, although in some cases the section of an additional upper or lower costal cartilage may be necessary. The pulmonary parenchyma bulging through the thoracotomy is thus brought into view. The mobility of the lung with respect to the parietal pleura is verified, and if pleural adhesions are found the pleura must be freed progressively. This is accomplished by exposing the adhesions using clamp-held compresses and by retracting the lung from the parietal pleura using a flexible retractor to stretch the adhesions, which are then cut with fine scissors flush with the parietal pleura. The scissors should not be manipulated directly against the lung, since this may lead to puncture and subsequent pneumothorax. The adhesions should be removed up to the region of the mediastinal pleura, i.e., around the pulmonary hilus. Partial pulmonary exposure will not allow proper exposure and surgical maneuvers of the spine, the entire right pleural cavity must be freed. The lung is manually collapsed, protected by a warm moist compress, and retracted towards the midline with large flexible pulmonary retractors.

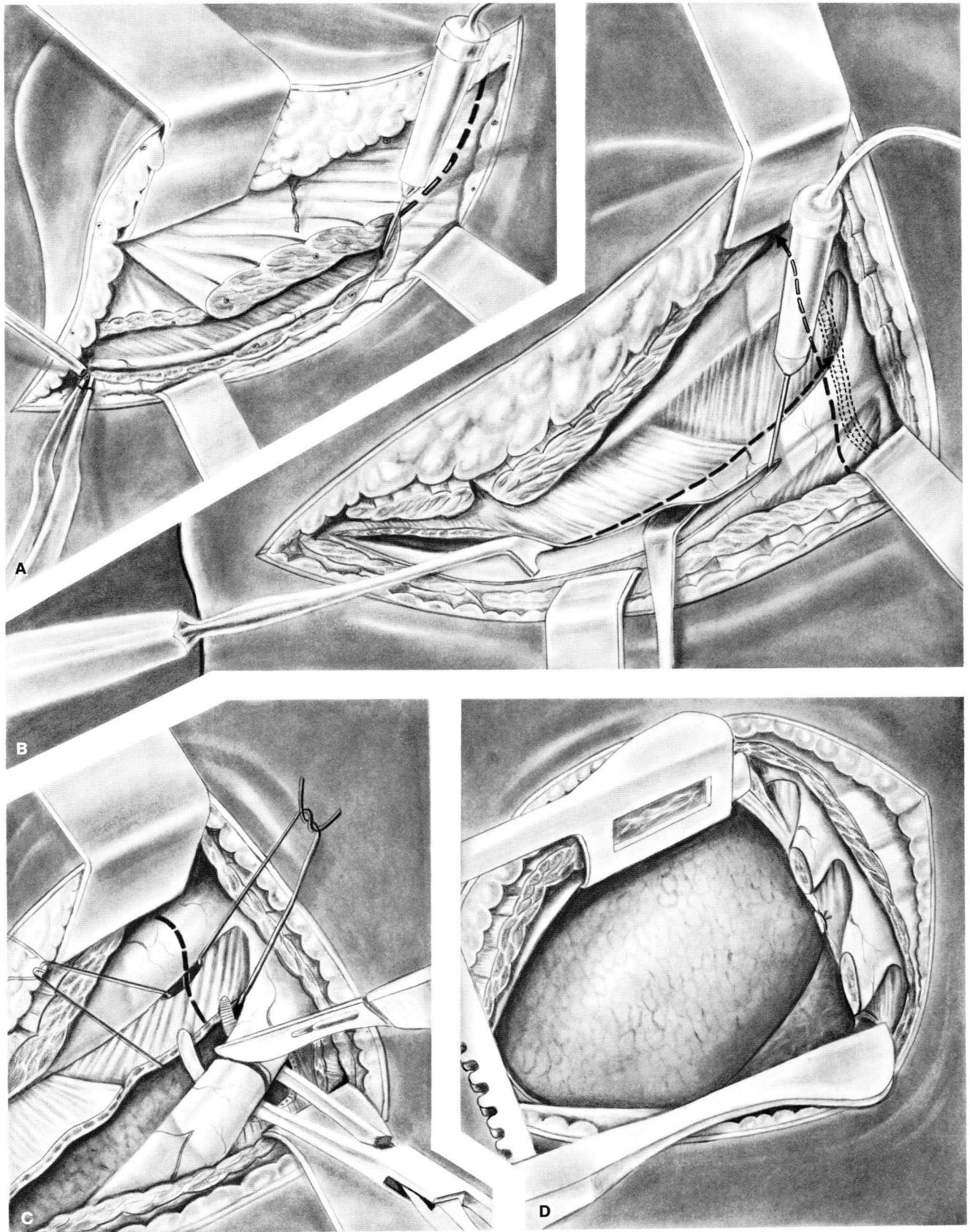

Figure 93 A–D

A Section of the superficial muscle layers (pectoralis major and serratus anterior) flush with the fourth rib

B Transection of the intercostal muscles along the upper margin of the fourth rib with preservation of the internal mammary vessels

C Section of the third and fourth costal cartilages 13 mm lateral to the sternum

D Position of the orthostatic thoracic retractor and verification of the mobility of the pulmonary parenchyma with respect to the parietal pleura

e) Exposure of the Anterior Surface of the Thoracic Spine

With the right lung retracted towards the midline, a large flexible retractor is positioned to expose the right anterolateral surface of the spine with the overlying mediastinal pleura. The diaphragmatic cupula must be displaced downward to allow full exposure, and this is achieved with a flexible retractor held in place by two Steinmann pins inserted through the pleura into a vertebral body. The pins must be positioned in an avascular part of the vertebra. The azygos vein is then identified under the transparent pleura in the region anterior to the right costal heads. The pleura is sectioned along the left margin of the azygos vein, the incision extending the full length of the vertebral region to be exposed. The intercostal arteries are thus brought into view in the region where they are practically devoid of accompanying veins. The hemiazygos veins join the left margin of the azygos vein at a point between T6 and T9. The spinal approach by section of the intercostal vascular bundles on the right flank of the azygos vein would require the interruption of many vessels, since in this region each intercostal artery is accompanied by one or two veins. The intercostal arteries are isolated one by one using a long slender needle holder and then divided between two ligatures or preferably two clips, one placed lateral to and the other between the arms of the needle holder. The vessel is then cut with long fine scissors. Of course, only a necessary minimum of arteries should be interrupted. Theoretically the approach to a single intervertebral disc does not require vascular section, and furthermore the excision of several thoracic discs can be achieved without interruption of the intercostal arteries. The flexible retractor placed anterior to the spine is then positioned to reflect the superomedial lip of the mediastinal pleural opening. A long curved raspatory is used to retract the tissues lying over the anterior longitudinal ligament to progressively expose the left flank of the spine. Use of this plane of incision does not carry a risk of injury to the intercostal vessels or thoracic duct, since these structures, more or less adherent to the posterior surface of the aorta, are reflected by the flexible retractor. The right lateral flank of the vertebral bodies is also exposed by rasping, thus displacing the azygos vein towards the rib heads. Hemostasis is required to arrest the bleeding of the fine branches of the intercostal bundles supplying or draining the region of the vertebral bodies and anterior longitudinal ligament. It is sometimes helpful to place Surgicel anterior to the rib heads and intervertebral foramina lying deep to the pleural opening. Exposure of the thoracic spine can be terminated by installing a counter-angled flexible retractor along the spinal margin opposite the side of approach, i.e., on the left. The second curve of the retractor can thus be used to maintain the mediastinal viscera free of the operative field. The flexible retractor is held in place by a Steinmann pin fixed to the two ends of the orthostatic retractor. At this stage the surgeon should check that the herart has not been excessively displaced and that the superior or inferior vena cava is not obstructed by torsion resulting from the displacement of the heart. If these complications are noted, the mediastinal retractor should be relaxed.

This approach allows the best possible anterior exposure of the thoracic vertebrae. It is very useful, and often mandatory, to expose the anterior part of the vertebral lesions in order to allow full excision from the right to left. This approach also allows median vertebral excision when necessary to gain direct access to the vertebral canal. Furthermore, bone grafting and installation of screw plates should be as close as possible to the midline.

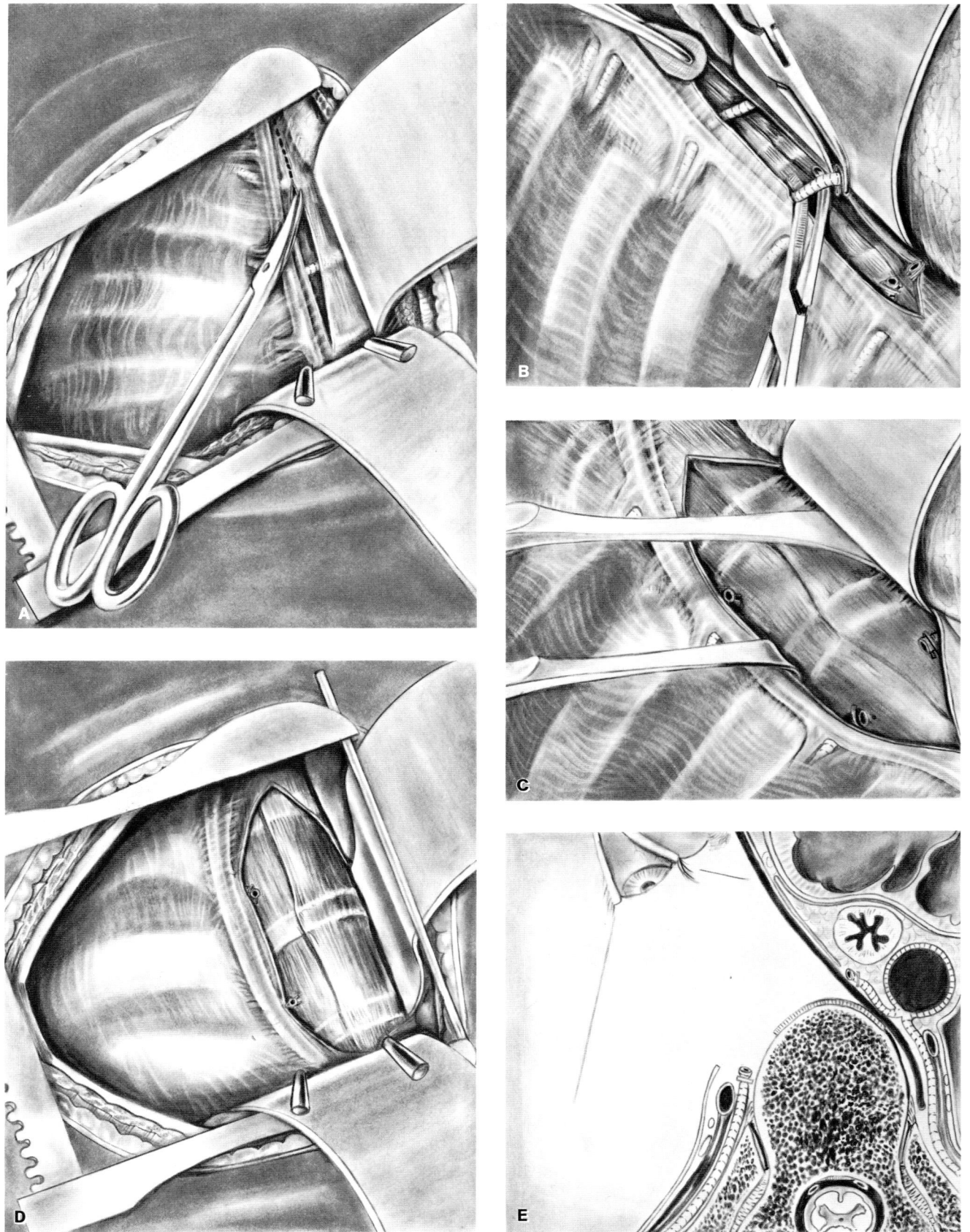

Figure 94 A–E

A   Opening of the mediastinal pleura and positioning of the flexible retractors

B   Hemostasis of the intercostal vessels using clips

C   Exposure of the anterior and lateral surfaces of the spine with the raspatory

D   Installation of the controlateral retractor held in place by a horizontally positioned Steinmann pin

E   Horizontal section showing the position of the controlateral retractor and the field of vision in close proximity to the midline of the spine

f) Special Cases

When the thoracic approach requires exposure at the level of T3 and T4, the operation is considerably hindered by the presence of a latticework of dense vessels running obliquely (almost vertically) anterior to the vertebral bodies. Hemostasis should involve only the azygos vein and its arch in order to avoid the risk of sectionning many of the intercostal arteries supplying the spinal cord. An appropriate procedure is to incise the mediastinal pleura in an oblique and almost vertical direction between two arteries, coupled with ligation of the arch of the azygos vein. This offers much less risk to the spinal cord, since the numerous venous anastomoses within the spine continue to allow correct azygos drainage. In cases of long-standing inflammatory lesions of the thoracic spine, e.g., sequelae of Pott's disease, the technique of spinal exposure should be modified. Such cases require that the fibrous lesions be sectioned on the right anterolateral flank of the spine, anterior to the rib heads, and on the left side of the azygos vein which is almost always visible. The difficulty of this procedure rests in the impossibility of visualizing the position of the intercostal vascular bundles by transparency. The operator must therefore use the cautery knife to incise down through the entire depth of the abnormal fibrous tissue centimeter by centimeter until contact is felt with spinal bone. Every 2.5 cm the incision causes hemorrhage of an arteriole, which should rapidly be clamped using a long hemostat. Hemostasis is then achieved by coagulating the clamped vessel directly. This method is consistently effective and rapid and should thus be preferred to an apparently more secure but time-consuming technique, i.e., placing of two rows of transfixing sutures on each side of the incised fibrous tissue. The cut margins of the fibrous mass are then freed by rasping in direct contact with the bone without trying to identify the anterior longitudinal ligament, which is enveloped by the fibrous tissue. In short, the exposure of the thoracic vertebrae using the rasp differs according to the presence or absence of inflammatory lesions. In the absence of inflammation the proper plane of incision lies anterior to the anterior longitudinal ligament. Conversely, the presence of inflammatory sequelae requires that exposure be achieved by rasping in direct contact with the spinal bone deep to the anterior longitudinal ligament.

g) Parietal Closure

At the end of the operation the mediastinal pleura can be closed with one continuous or a few interrupted sutures, although this procedure is not absolutely necessary. However, proper hemostasis must be achieved. Closure is prepared by reinflating the right lung by applying positive pressure to the airway until full pulmonary expansion occurs. If a few pulmonary sectors remain collapsed, i.e., black and flat, the involved region should be delicately manipulated between the fingers during positive pressure until full inflation ensues. Indeed, if closure is made without full expansion of the lung complications such as atelectasis may occur. Two rigid drains 6–8 mm in diameter and perforated at one end are then installed. The lower drain is positioned first, on the midaxillary line through the seventh or eighth intercostal space, with its tip directed toward the posterior groove of the pleural cavity to evacuate the fluid that collects in this region when the patient is supine. The second drain, to evacuate air, is installed through the anterior part of the second or third intercostal space to lie over the pulmonary parenchyma. The drains should be securely fixed to the skin near their site of entry to avoid postoperative expulsion. Parietal closure is begun by reconstruction of the costal cartilage by figure-of-eight sutures of nonresorbable material mounted on an atraumatic curved needle yielding a true "osteosynthesis" of the cartilage with properly aligned consolidation. The intercostal space is then closed by two or three full-thickness sutures on each side of the two exposed ribs. Care should be taken to place these sutures perpendicular to the ribs, to avoid a shearing effect when the sutures are tightened. The intercostal space is thus closed with the lower margin of the intercostal muscles practically in contact with the lower rib. It is not necessary to place a continuous suture on the intercostal muscles. Only the gaping anterior end of the intercostal space requires closure with a few transfixing sutures to attach the intercostal muscles to the upper margin of the fourth costal cartilage. Tight closure of the operative field is then achieved by using continuous sutures to approximate the superficial muscles. Finally, the subcutaneous tissue and skin are closed as two separate layers using continuous sutures. At the end of the operation the anesthesiologist should apply positive pulmonary pressure to evacuate any remaining fluid and eliminate residual air pockets prior to clamping the thoracic drains.

h) Postoperative Care

Pulmonary inflation is monitored by auscultation of the thorax, which should normally reveal the presence of vesicular respiration of equal intensity on both sides. The patient is placed supine in bed and the two thoracic drains are joined by a Y tube, connected to the suction device under mild negative pressure (not more than 50 cm H_2O), and finally unclamped. Pulmonary inflation and inspiratory function must be checked several times daily, and chest X-rays should be made at the bedside once a day. When respiratory complications are absent the drains can usually be removed on or after the fourth postoperative day. This is achieved by clamping and then removing the drains one after the other while the patient performs Valsalva's maneuver, forced expiration against the closed glottis. Purse-string closure of the drainage orifices is not necessary; the wounds require only a simple dressing with petroleum jelly compresses.

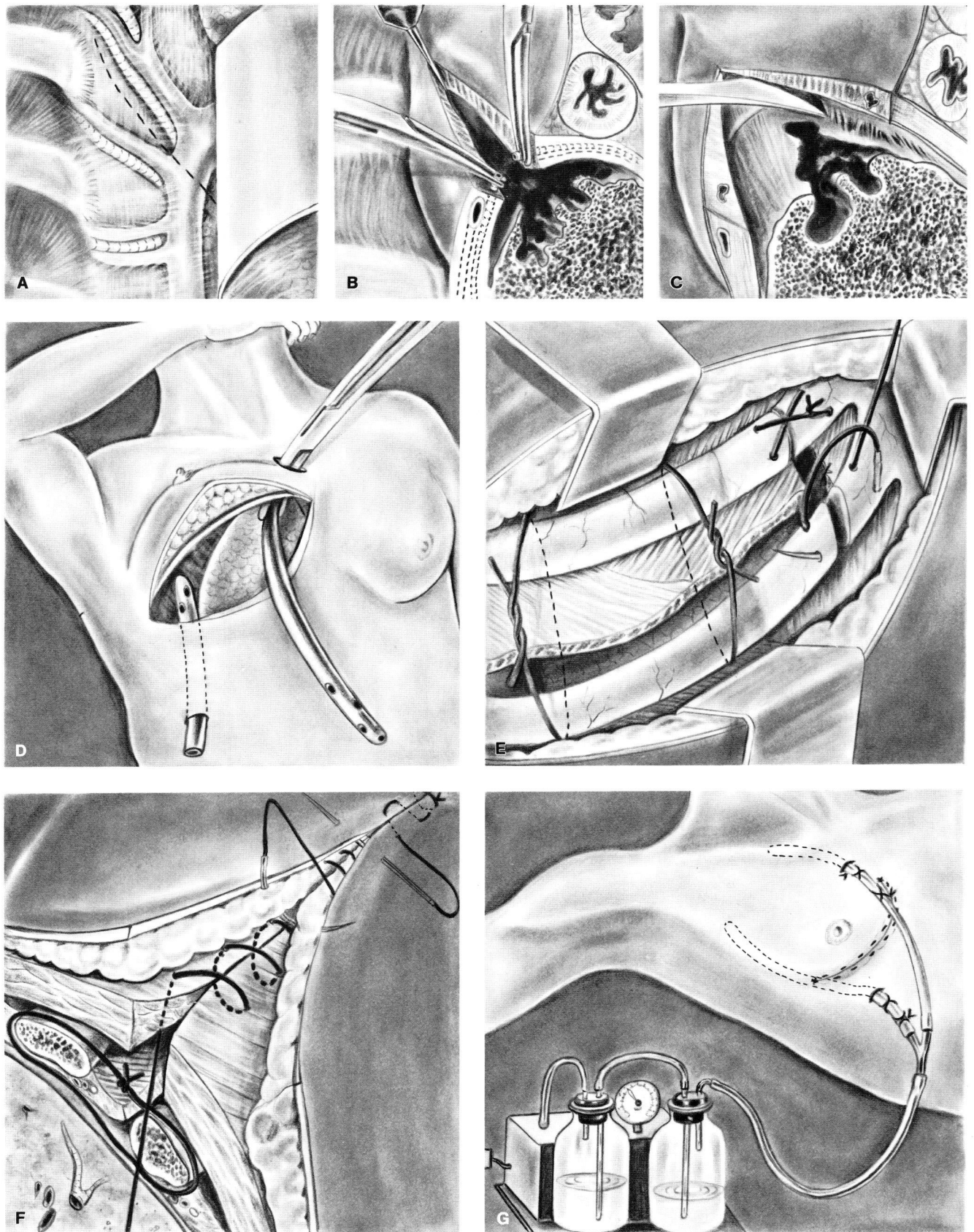

Figure 95 A–G

A   The route of passage between the intercostal vessels in the region of the arch of the azygos vein

B, C   The dissection, hemostasis, and exposure in contact with the spinal bone in cases of fibro-inflammatory lesions

D   Installation of the two thoracic drains

E   Parietal closure by reconstruction of the costal cartilage and approximation of the ribs

F   The three-layered closure by continuous sutures

G   Thoracic suction drainage

i) Possible Complications

During operation a frequent complication is the hemorrhage of an intercostal vessel. Hemostasis can be achieved by applying pressure to the site of bleeding with a clamp-held compress followed by clamping with a hemostat. One should also avoid excess torsion of the caval veins resulting from overdisplacement of the heart to the left side. Postoperative complications include hemorrhage as evidenced by the aspiration of bloody fluid through the thoracic drains. In such cases hemostasis requires reintervention. The most frequent complication is pulmonary atelectasis due to poor inflation of the lung at the end of operation. The quality and the patency of the thoracic suction drains should be closely monitored. When obstruction is present an endoscopist may be required to perform tracheobronchal clearance. Recurrence of pneumothorax or pulmonary effusion after removal of the drains can be remedied by installation of a new drain under local anesthesia.

3. Anterolateral Transpleural Approach

a) Operative Position

Lateral thoracotomy is classically performed in the laterosupine position. Approach from the right is obviously preferable, the absence of the aortic arch and thoracic aorta facilitating access to the vertebrae. The patient is thus placed in the left laterosupine position. The left lower limb is flexed to a 90° angle at the knee to prevent the patient rolling, and the right lower limb is fully extended. The pelvis is maintained in place by pads supporting the pubis and sacrum. The left axillary region is elevated by cushion to avoid compression of the intravenous infusion running through the left upper limb. The right upper limb is flexed to 90° at the shoulder and elbow to allow full exposure of the axillary region. The right forearm is maintained in place by a metal arch passing above the patient's chin. The elbow must not drop onto the head, since this may lead to elongation of the brachial plexus. Lateral flexion of the neck is avoided by placing a cushion under the patient's head. Prior to incision the axilla is shaved and the entire right hemithorax thoroughly disinfected.

b) Parietal Exposure

The skin incision is made obliquely along the arch of the appropriate rib from the latissimus dorsi to the lower margin of the pectoralis major. Incision of the skin and thick adipose layer in this region exposes the external thoracic (external mammary) artery accompanied by its satellite veins, and these vessels are ligated and divided. The perforating branches of the intercostal nerves should be preserved. The underlying muscle layers, including part of the latissimus dorsi and lower margin of the pectoralis major, are then transected with the electric cautery knife. The digitations of the serratus anterior are transected flush with the fifth rib. Periosal decollement is prepared by tracing a longitudinal line on the rib with the cautery knife. A raspatory is then used to expose the upper margin of the rib and disinsert the intercostal muscles, thereby opening the pleural cavity.

c) Exposure of the Spine

Installation of the orthostatic retractor allows moderately wide exposure: full exposure can be achieved by extending the incision anteriorly and posteriorly. The lung must be freed of any pleural adhesions to allow pulmonary deflation below and in front of the hilus. The adhesions are removed using a clamp-held compress applied with force against the parietal pleura, not against the pulmonary parenchyma. The remaining pedicular adhesions are sectioned against the parietal pleura using fine scissors. Care must be taken not to injury the pulmonary parenchyma, since this may lead to a fistula and subsequent pneumothorax. The mediastinum and thoracic spine can be seen at the deep wall of the thoracic cavity in front of the heads of the ribs. The mediastinal pleura is opened anterior to the rib heads, thus exposing the parietal intercostal vessels, which must be ligated sparingly. The section of the practically vertical segment of the superior intercostal arteries can be avoided by dissecting parallel to them, followed by ligation and division of the azygos arch. Work can then proceed anterior and to the right of the azygos vein. After achieving hemostasis, the anterior and right lateral surfaces of the spine are rasped in front of the anterior longitudinal ligament. A flexible retractor is modeled to press against the anterior surface of the spine, held in place by Steinmann pins to maintain good exposure in the region of the mediastinal pleura. Regardless of the quality of exposure, this approach allows clear visualization of only the right aspect of the spine with tangential visualization of the anterior surface. Trepanation of the vertebral bodies to gain access to the vertebral canal can only be achieved in an oblique direction.

d) Parietal Closure

After achieving proper hemostasis the mediastinal pleura can either be closed by a few interrupted sutures or left open. Inflation of the lung is accomplished by applying positive pressure during inspiration. Two pencil-thick rigid suction drains are installed, one through the lower intercostal space on the midaxillary line with its tip directed towards the posterior groove of the pleural cavity, the other above the operative field through one of the upper intercostal spaces with its tip lying over the pulmonary parenchyma. The intercostal space is closed without reinserting the intercostal muscles on the lower rib. Only two or three full-thickness sutures from one side of the space to the other are required to achieve full closure.

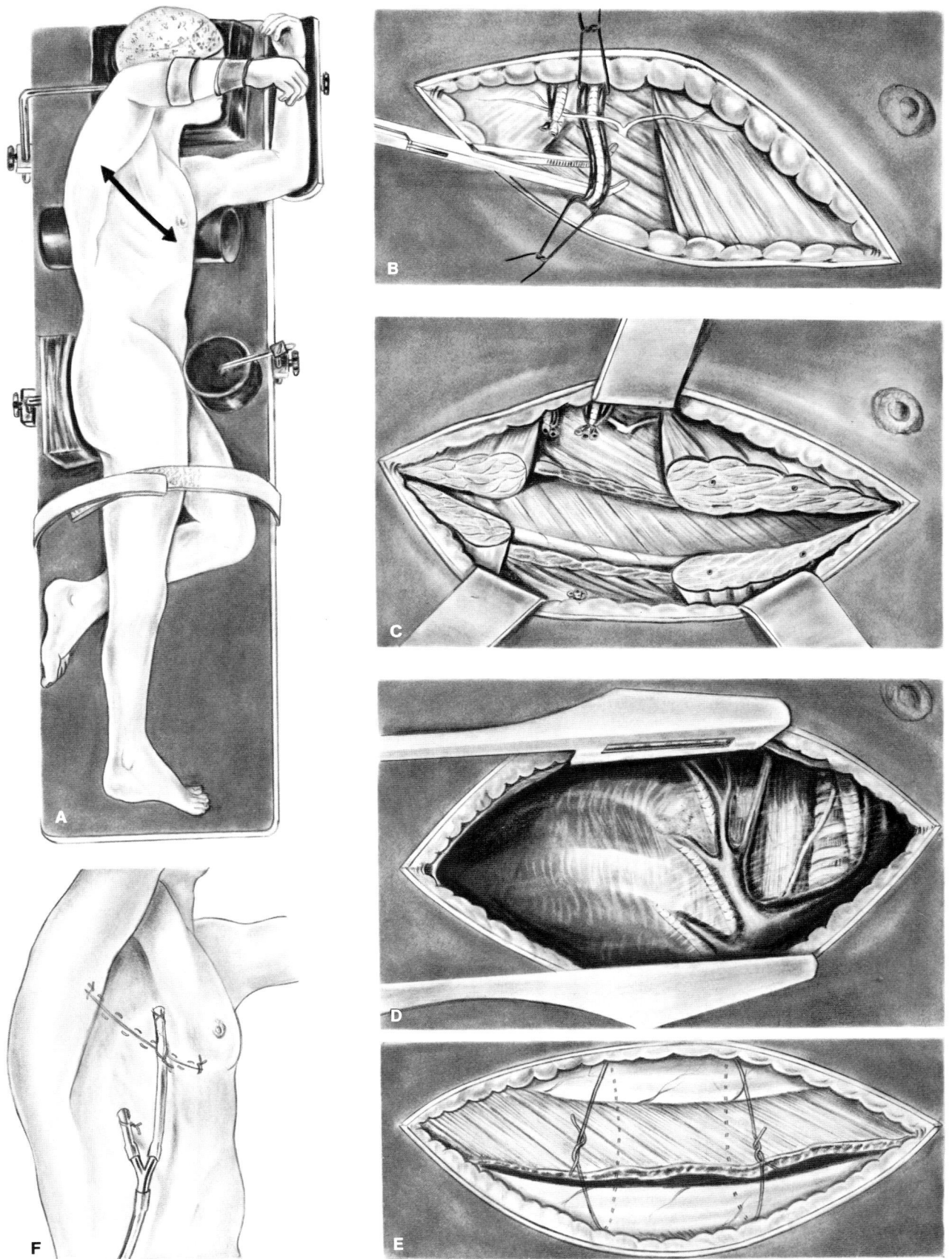

Figure 96 A–F

A Overhead view of the left laterosupine position
B The oblique axillary incision with hemostasis of the external thoracic vessels
C Section of the muscle layers: latissimus dorsi, pectoralis major, and serratus anterior
D Exposure of the mediastinum, thoracic spine, and intercostal vessels
E Closure of the intercostal space with full-thickness sutures
F Twin thoracic suction drainage

The superficial layers are closed by continuous suture of the muscles, subcutaneous tissue, and skin. Finally, the thoracic drains are fixed to the skin without making a purse-string closure. At the end of the operation the lung is reinflated by the following technique: The drains are opened while positive inspiratory pressure is applied and are then clamped when the pressure is released. This maneuver is repeated until the lung becomes fully expanded, and the two drains are then joined by a Y tube and suction applied at a negative pressure of about 50 cm H_2O.

4. Posterolateral Transpleural Approach

a) Operative Position and Anesthesia

The patient is anesthetized in the supine position with endotracheal intubation, and then placed in the left laterosupine position to allow right thoracotomy. This approach is preferable, as the thoracic aorta does not then constitute an obstacle. The left lower limb is flexed under the extended right lower limb to improve stability. The left upper limb is flexed to 90° at the elbow with the hand facing the head to allow intravenous infusion. The upper right limb is suspended over the head, care being taken to avoid stretching of the shoulder region. Pads are placed against the pubis and sternum and the thighs taped to the table to fix the patient securely in position. Obstruction to intravenous infusion of the left upper limb is avoided by placing a cushion under the thorax slightly below the level of the axillary region.

b) Landmarks and Incision

Identification of the fifth rib is necessary as the approach through the thorax is made in its bed. One can proceed in the caudocranial direction by first identifying the twelfth rib, whose length is confirmed by X-ray. The tip of the scapula, lying over the fifth rib, is a very useful landmark. The incision begins halfway between the scapula and the spinous crest one hand's breadth above the tip of the scapula. The incision is then extended as a superiorly concave curve passing forwards around the tip of the scapula to the anterior axillary line. The incision terminates two fingers below and lateral to the nipple in men and the submammary fold in women.

c) Dissection of the Superficial Layers

The plain knife is placed perpendicular to the skin to make the initial incision. Hemostasis of the subdermal and underlying subcutaneous tissue is then achieved. The electric cautery knife is used to transect the superficial muscle layer, comprising the trapezius posteriorly and the latissimus dorsi anteriorly separated by a thin fascia. The cut edge of the muscles also requires hemostasis of a few bleeding sites. The next layer to be transected is that of the rhomboideus and serratus anterior muscles. The rhomboideus is incised in the center of the muscle body near the tip of the scapula, thus allowing access to the more anterior serratus anterior muscle, which is then sectioned. Hemostasis of several small vascular bundles is required. After transection of this muscle layer, the tip of the scapula can be tilted forwards to expose the entire length of the fifth rib.

d) Resection of the Fifth Rib

The costal diaphysis is freed from the costovertebral joint up to the anterior angle of the rib. The rib is rasped along its upper, lower, and finally its medial surface, and sectioned at both ends. The posterior site of section lies at the costal tubercle, near the tip of the transverse processes, and the anterior site at two fingers from the costal cartilage. The pleura is then opened with scissors and an orthostatic retractor installed.

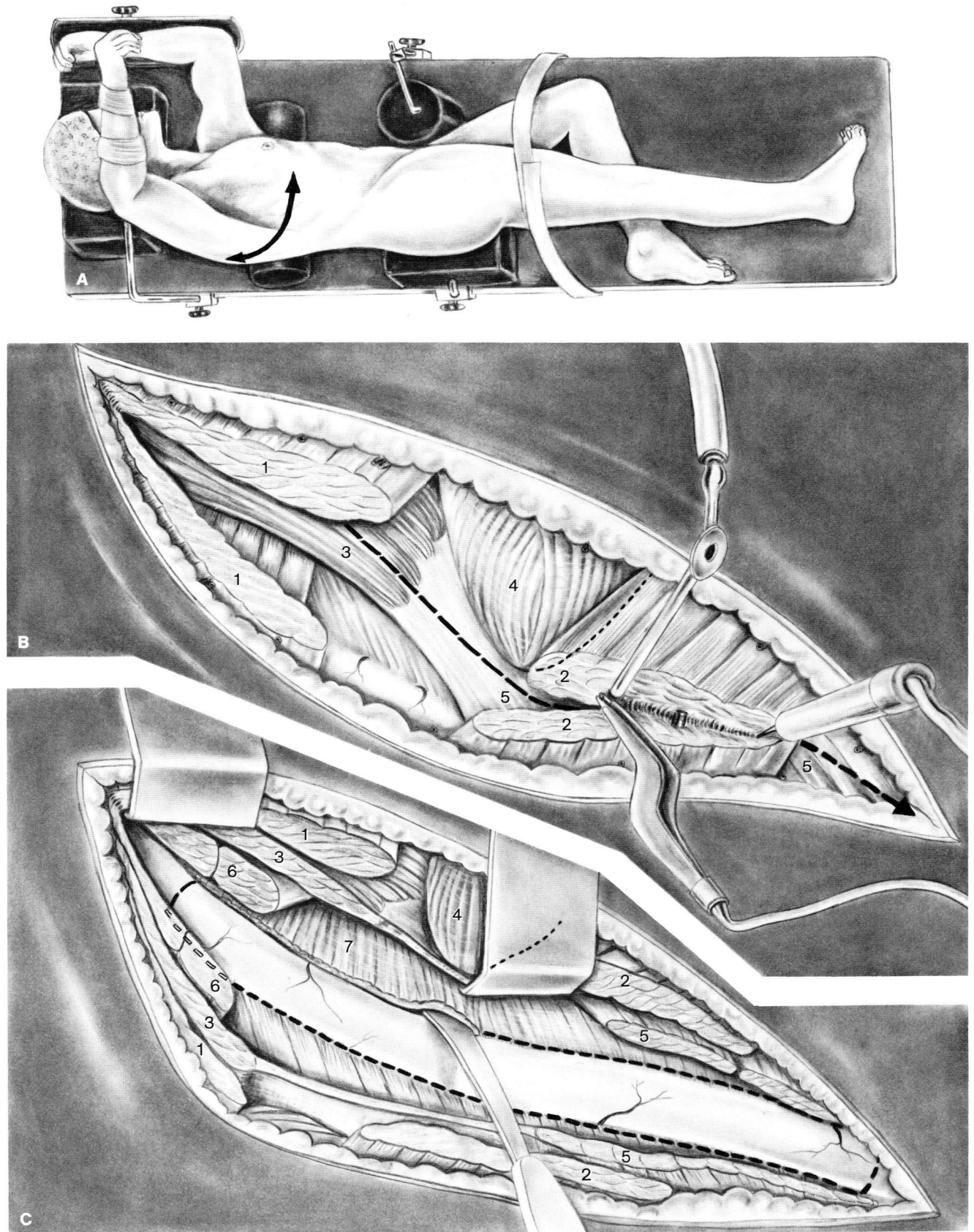

Figure 97 A–C

A Overhead view showing the left laterosupine operative position. Note the curved incision passing around the tip of the scapula and along the fifth rib

B Transection of the superficial layers comprising the trapezius and latissimus dorsi. Preparation of the rhomboideus-serratus anterior incision

C Resection of the fifth rib subsequent to rasping the upper and lower margins and medial surface of the rib

1 m. trapezius *2* m. latissimus dorsi *3* m. rhomboideus major *4* m. infraspinatus *5* m. serratus ant. *6* m. erector spinae *7* mm. intercostales externi

e) Exposure of the Spine

The orthostatic retractor is opened gradually to avoid fracture of a rib. Avoidance of fracture requires that the entire length of the costal diaphysis be freed, that the costal cartilage retain its capacity to undergo torsion, and that the ribs be sufficiently mobile at the level of the costovertebral joints. Adhesions between the visceral and parietal pleural sheaths must be removed, and this is accomplished by blunt dissection with clamp-held compresses, followed by cutting the adhesions flush with the parietal and not the visceral pleura. The right lung is then collapsed, protected by a moist surgical towel, and retracted toward the mediastinum with a large flexible retractor, exposing the spine with the overlying mediastinal pleura. The latter is incised and the azygos vein identified. As in anterior thoracotomy, hemostasis of the parietal vessels anterior to the azygos vein is achieved, followed by exposure of the anterior surface of the spine by using the raspatory anterior to the anterior longitudinal ligament. A counterangled flexible retractor is then installed in front of the spine to retract the mediastinal viscera towards the midline: care must be taken to avoid torsion of the superior vena cava. The azygos vein is retracted towards the rib heads using the raspatory. Wide exposure of the operative field is maintained by planting two or three Steinmann pins in the vertebral bodies at the limit of the area exposed.

f) Parietal Closure

Closure is begun only after perfect hemostasis has been achieved with clips, coagulation, and Surgicel. Closure of the mediastinal pleura is not absolutely necessary. Two thoracic drains are installed: the tip of the posteroinferior drain is placed in the laterovertebral groove to allow evacuation of fluid, and the drain emerges through an intercostal space subjacent to the skin incision; the second, air-evacuating drain is placed over the pulmonary parenchyma, and exits through the anterior part of an intercostal space lying above the site of skin incision. The right lung must be fully inflated prior to closure. After removal of the orthostatic retractor, a Bailey instrument can be used to pull the ribs closer to each other. Several sutures are then installed to close the space between the ribs delimiting the operative field. Large-caliber slow-resorbing sutures should be used, placed perpendicular to the long axis of the rib, and passing through the lips of the intercostal muscles freed by the costal resection. The pericostal sutures should be positioned before the ribs are pulled toward each other with the Bailey instrument, and tied down afterwards. The considerably retracted muscle layers must now be approximated: this is achieved with slow-resorbing continuous sutures. A suture is placed in the serratus anterior at the level of the tip of the scapula, and extended to the right and left of the rhomboideus and serratus anterior. Closure of the overlying layer comprising the latissimus dorsi and trapezius is accomplished by first placing an interrupted suture on the posterior margin of the latissimus dorsi, and then making two continuous sutures, one closing the latissimus dorsi and the other closing the trapezius. A subcutaneous continuous suture passing through the subdermal tissue is made, and finally the skin is closed with a fine continuous suture or with sterile adhesive strips.

g) Postoperative Care

At the end of the operation the two drains are joined by a Y tube and mild suction (about 50 cm H$_2$O) is applied. Proper inflation of the lung is confirmed by auscultation in the operating room and by thoracic X-ray as soon as the patient leaves the operating room. The patient usually remains in the supine position, which slightly hinders respiration. This underlines the importance of appropriate suction drainage and full lung inflation. The drains can usually be removed on or about the fourth postoperative day.

h) Possible Complications

As in all types of thoracotomy with opening of the pleura, the most common complications involve the respiratory apparatus, e.g., pneumo- and hemothorax. Poor functioning of the drains or suction apparatus is frequently encountered. Total or partial atelectasis of the right lung may also occur: prophylactic measures to avoid this include proper reinflation of the lung before closure. Bronchial congestion should be avoided during operation, but if it occurs bronchoaspiration may be required postoperatively.

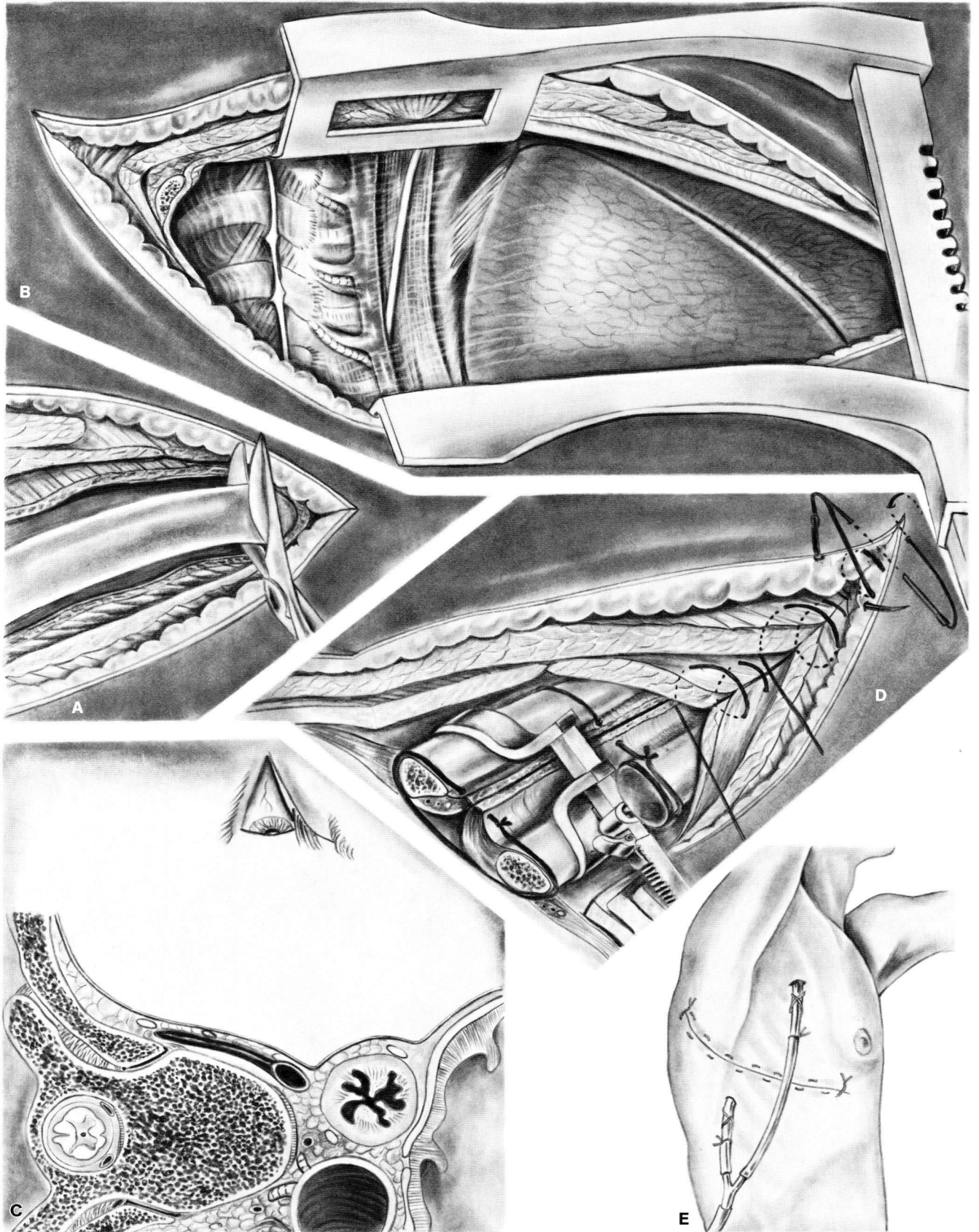

Figure 98 A–E

A Resection of the anterior part of the rib
B Position of the retractor to expose the vertebral lesions after collapsing of the right lung
C Transverse section showing the field of vision with the postero-lateral transpleural approach. Note that essentially the lateral aspect of the vertebrae is viewed

D Different steps to close the thoracotomy after pulling the ribs together and installing several layers of continuous sutures
E Full closure with twin thoracic suction drains

5. Posterolateral Retropleural Approach

a) Anesthesia and Operative Position

The patient is anesthetized in the supine position with tracheal intubation and then placed in the left laterosupine position to allow right thoracotomy. Stability is increased by flexing the left lower limb to a 90° angle at the knee while the overlying right lower limb is placed in extension. A pad is placed under the thorax caudal to the axillary region to avoid compression of the vessels of the left upper limb, which is positioned near the head with the elbow flexed at 90°. The right upper limb can either be left to lie free over the left arm or fixed to a vertical support. A cushion is placed under the head to maintain alignment of the spine. Finally, the pelvic region is held in place by pads against the pubis and sacrum and adhesive tape over the thighs.

b) Landmarks and Skin Incision

The surgeon operates in the seated position, facing the dorsal surface of the patient, and first identifies the crest of the spinous processes and the spinal margin of the scapula. The site of the vertebral lesions is identified in relation to the presence of gibbosity or by X-ray. It is of utmost importance that the level of the lesion be correctly identified by locating the two or three ribs lying at the level of the lesion, since these ribs will be resected.

Access to the vertebrae from T1 to T10 is gained through a linear paravertebral incision three or four fingers lateral to the spinous processes, i.e., between the scapula and spine. The center of the incision should lie over the central part of the lesions identified radiologically. When operation involves the lower thoracic vertebrae (T10 to T12) the lower end of the incision should be curved to run along the twelfth rib.

c) Transection of the Superficial Layers

Once the skin has been opened, the subcutaneous tissue is incised with the electric cautery knife and hemostasis of the subdermal and adipose vessels is achieved by electrocoagulation. The next step is the transection of the superficial muscle layer (trapezius), followed by hemostasis of the cut surface of the muscle. The procedure is continued by the transection of the underlying layer, comprising the rhomboideus major and minor. These muscles retract subsequent to their transection, thus bringing into view the costal region. The ribs are then exposed by rasping the costal insertions of the spinal muscles towards the spine. Hemostasis is accomplished by electrocoagulation and aspiration.

d) Costal Resection

The first step is to expose the posterior angle of the three or four ribs lying over the spinal site of lesion. Exposure should extend to and include the transverse processes. Rasping of the bone induces periosteal hemorrhage which is controlled by appropriate means of hemostasis. The operative field is then fully exposed by installing a Beckman orthostatic retractor or an angled retractor. Exposure of the ribs and transverse processes is accomplished using either a slightly curved raspatory or a sharp curette. The risk of pleural perforation is greatly reduced when the curette is used, since its round convex end affords better protection than the raspatory. The curette is first manipulated along the upper and lower margins of the ribs and transverse processes and then along the medial surface of the rib, in constant contact with the bone in order to displace the pleura. Subsequent to the exposure of each rib, a warm moist compress is packed into the exposed region to achieve hemostasis and to allow work on the other ribs in a perfectly clear operative field. The exposed ribs are then sectioned at a point 8–10 cm from the costotransverse articulation.

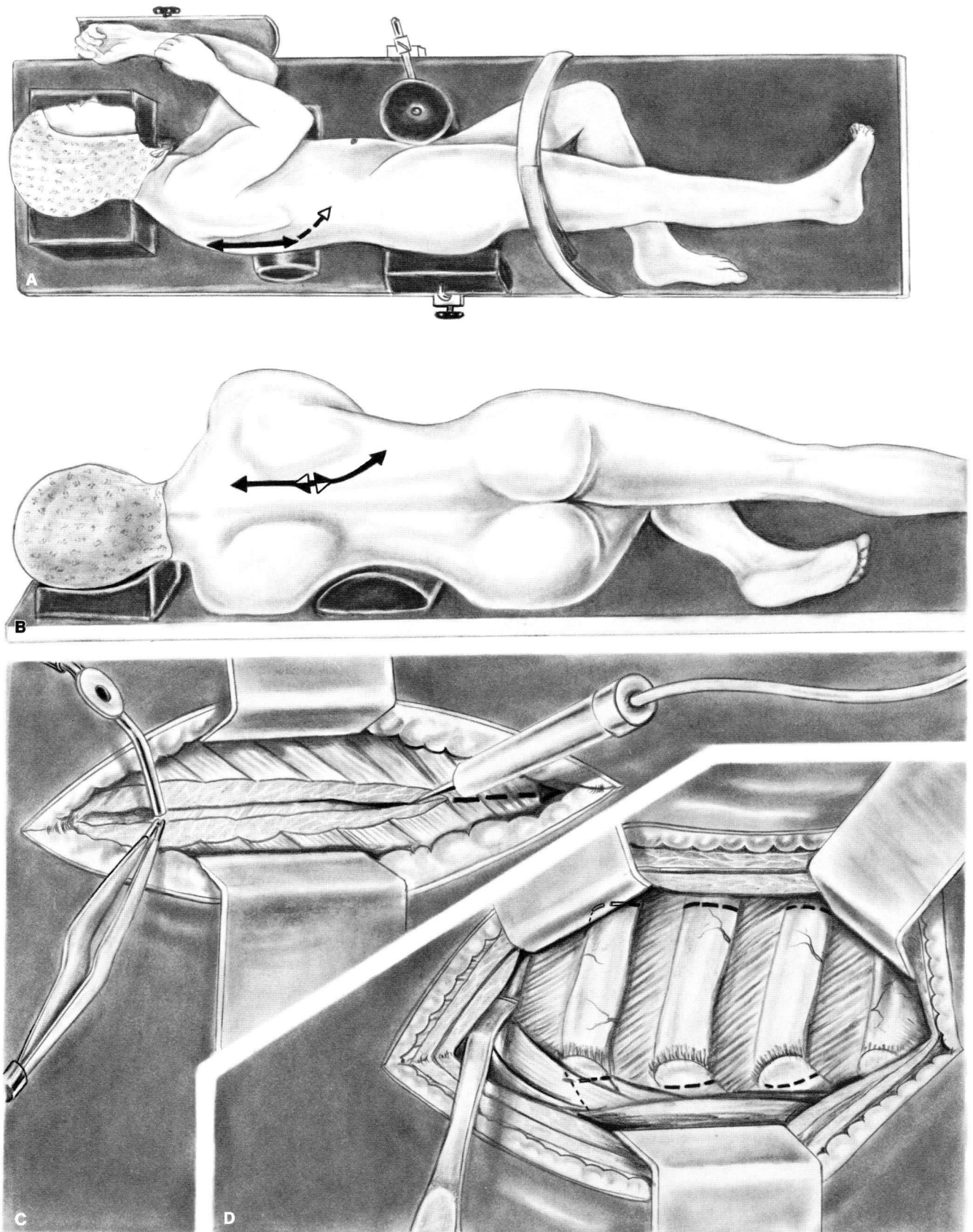

Figure 99 A–D

A   Overhead view of the left laterosupine operative position
B   The site of incision between the scapula and spine, three to four
    fingers lateral to the spinous processes. Radiological landmarks
    are mandatory

C   Transection of the superficial layers formed by the trapezius,
    rhomboideus, and erector spinae muscles
D   Exposure of the posterior costal arches and costotransverse articula-
    tions. Installation of a retractor and hemostasis

The cut end of the rib is grasped with a pair of small toothed forceps in order slightly to separate the rib from the pleura. Disarticulation of the costotransverse and costovertebral joints is prepared by the decollement of the parietal pleura from the medial surface of the rib until contact is felt with the head of the rib. The transverse process is sectioned 1 cm from its tip to free the rib from the costotransverse joint. The surgeon selects a middle-sized curette, whose opening should be large enough to receive the rib head, and slides it along the rib to engage the head. A few oscillatory movements are applied to the instrument to disinsert the stellate ligament (ligamentum capitis costae radiatum), and the resected costal arch is finally extracted using the toothed forceps. The resection procedure is then applied to the remaining two or three ribs to be excised. The contents of two or three intercostal spaces, i.e., muscles, vessels, and intercostal nerve, are thus fully free in the operative field. The decollement of the parietal pleura is continued, using clamp-held compresses to expose the spine and prevertebral vessels. When necessary, the operative field can be enlarged by the ligation and transection of the structures of one intercostal space.

e) Exposure of the Spine

The bulging intervertebral discs and depressed vertebral bodies are identified on the right lateral aspect of the spine. The intercostal bundles lying in this region must be sectioned to allow full spinal exposure, so one to three bundles are isolated by passing a needle holder under each one which is then clipped off and sectioned. A long curved raspatory, which should be manipulated in contact with the anterior longitudinal ligament, is used to expose the vertebral bodies and the discs by displacing the prevertebral structures towards the midline. A flexible retractor is then modeled to engage the anterior surface of the spine and retract the parietal pleura and thoracic structures upward. The right posterolateral approach allows easy access to only the right lateral surface of the spine. Anterolateral decompression can be achieved by opening the vertebral canal at the level of the intervertebral foramina, subsequent to identification of the intercostal nerves, but this route of access to the vertebral canal leads to marked hemorrhage. It is thus preferable to achieve decompression by the anterior approach, obviating the surgical maneuvers in the intervertebral foramina.

f) Closure

When the operation is concluded, removal of the flexible retractor and installation of extrapleural suction drainage allow the pleura to return to normal position. The muscles are closed in two layers with hemostatic continuous sutures. The subcutaneous tissue and skin are then closed with continuous and interrupted sutures respectively.

g) Postoperative Care and Possible Complications

Postoperative care in cases of retropleural surgery is simple, since respiratory disturbances and hemorrhage are generally absent. The suction drain should be monitored, and can be removed after two days if all flow of bloody aspirate has stopped. The most common complication is the opening of the pleura during operation. In cases where the peural wound is small, it can be closed by a continuous suture while positive pulmonary pressure is applied to evacuate the intrapleural air completely, thus obviating postoperative thoracic suction drainage. However, in cases of a more extensive pleural wound, where the continuous suture does not allow hermetic closure, a suction drain should be installed in the pleural cavity through a supra- or subjacent intercostal space. Another possible problem is difficulty in exposing the right lateral surface of the spine due to the presence of inflammatory adhesions. In such cases, the operator should seek instrumental contact with the vertebral bone by fully incising the inflammatory tissue while progressively accomplishing hemostasis.

Figure 100 A–J

A   Decollement of the parietal pleura from the medial surface of the rib

B   Horizontal section showing the procedure to expose the rib using the curette

C   Manual identification of the rib head near the spine

D   With the pleura protected by a warm moist compress, the rib is sectioned 10 cm from the spine subsequent to resection of the tip of the transverse process

E   Disinsertion of the costotransverse ligaments using a straight chisel

F   The curette is used to free the head of the rib

G   Exposure of the right lateral surface of the spine by clipping and dividing the intercostal vessels

H   Exposure of the right anterolateral aspect of the spine with the raspatory manipulated anterior to the anterior longitudinal ligament

I   Tangential lateral view of the spine obtained with the posterolateral retropleural approach

J   The different layers of closure with extrapleural suction drainage

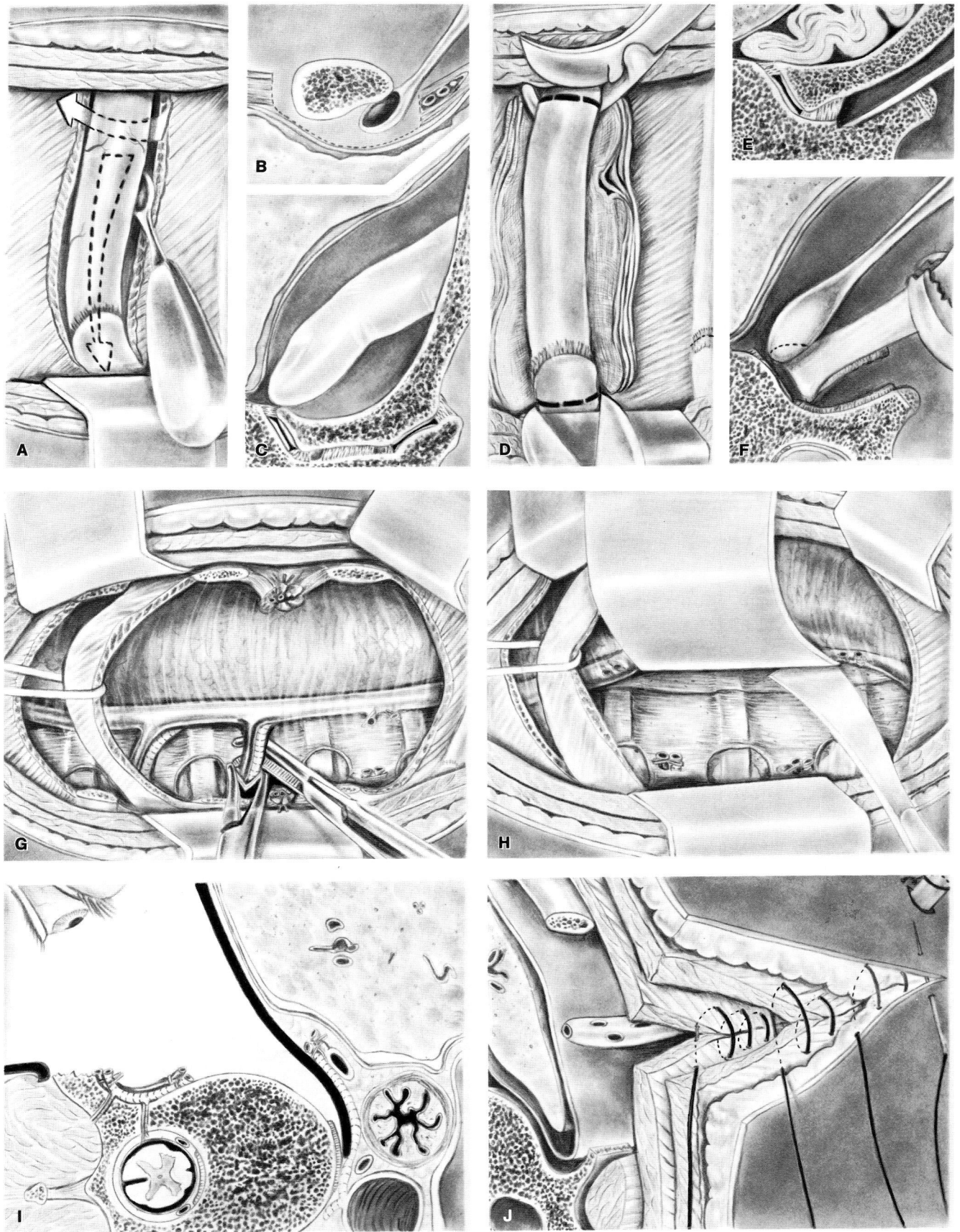

Figure 100 A–J

C. Thoracolumbar Junction (T10 to L2)

1. Topography

The thoracolumbar junction is formed by the lower three thoracic and upper two lumbar vertebrae, and constitutes a veritable crossroads with respect to the anatomy, function, and relations of the spine. Analysis of spinal anatomy shows that the vertebrae of this region progress morphologically from the thoracic to the lumbar type, while the physiological spinal curvature changes. The posterior region of the thoracolumbar junction resembles that of the other spinal sectors in that it lies superficially and can easily be approached deep to the spinal muscles. Conversely, access to the anterior discocorporeal region is complex due to its deep position posterior to the thoracic and abdominal viscera. It is thus useful to describe the parietal and visceral relations of the anterior region of the thoracolumbar spine in order to underline both the difficulties and possibilities of the operative approach to this region. The posterior, anterior, and lateral relations of the thoracolumbar junction are described below.

a) Posterior Relations

Examination of the posterior aspect of the thoracolumbar spine shows that it lies entirely below the diaphragmatic cupulae and the centrum tendineum, which is located at the level of T9–T10. The thoracolumbar region thus relates to the inframediastinal space, which lies between the vertical posterior part of the diaphragm out to the crura and the anterior surface of the spine and contains the thoracic aorta, the thoracic duct, the nerves running between the thorax and abdomen (the splanchnic and intercostal nerves and the laterovertebral plexus), and the azygos system with its tributary veins. Lateral to the spine, the costodiaphragmatic sinus contains the parietal pleura, whose lower margin lies horizontally at the level of T11–T12. The pulmonary parenchyma terminates 5 cm above the lower limit of the sinus. The resulting free zone between the lung and parietal pleura is referred to as Fontan's space. The retroperitoneal region of the abdominal cavity lies anterior to the diaphragm. The renal fossae flank the thoracolumbar junction on each side from the eleventh rib to the transverse process of L3. The left kidney extends a mean distance of 2 cm above the right kidney.

b) Anterior Relations

From the anterior aspect the thoracolumbar junction is deeply camouflaged by the abdominal viscera lying anterior to the posterior wall of the diaphragm, which covers the spine from the T9–T10 intervertebral disc to the body of T12. The prevertebral segment of the abdomen corresponds to the celiac region. The abdominal esophagus and the stomach occupy the left lateral part of the celiac region, and the liver and its hilus occupy the right anterior part. The body of the pancreas runs upward to the level of the body of L1. The strictly anterior approach to the thoracolumbar junction would require the traversing of a manifestly overdense region comprising not only the viscera, but also their neurovascular bundles, i.e., the celiac trunk with its splenic, gastric, and hepatic arterial collaterals surrounded by the various ganglions and rami of the solar plexus. Accordingly, the strictly anterior route is not a reasonable approach to the thoracolumbar spine.

c) Right Lateral Relations

The right flank of the thoracolumbar junction is also camouflaged by the right cupula and the right part of the crura of the diaphragm. The pleural cavity lies between the diaphragmatic cupula and the costal wall. The lower margin of the pleural cavity lies 10 cm from the spinous processes at the level of the tenth rib, and right lateral access to the thoracolumbar junction thus requires the opening of the pleural cavity or the retraction of the pleural sinus. The abdominal viscera lying below the diaphragmatic cupula and superficial to the spine are the right lobe of the liver, the right kidney posterior to the liver and the hepatic flexure of the colon and duodenopancreatic block. Right lateral access to the thoracolumbar junction requires that these viscera be displaced forward to expose the lateral aspect of the spine.

d) Left Lateral Relations

When viewed from the left the thoracolumbar spine is covered by the left cupula and the left part of the crura of the diaphragm. The pleural cavity, lying between the diaphragm and spine, descends to the level of the tenth rib 10 cm from the spinous processes. As on the right, the left lateral approach requires that the pleural cavity be opened or the pleural sinus and its contents displaced forward. Exposure of the thoracolumbar junction also necessitates the disinsertion and retraction or section of the diaphragm. Below the diaphragmatic cupula, the thoracolumbar spine is camouflaged by the spleen, the left kidney, the fundus of the stomach, the tail of the pancreas, and the splenic flexure of the colon. The left lateral approach requires the forward displacement of these viscera to expose the spine.

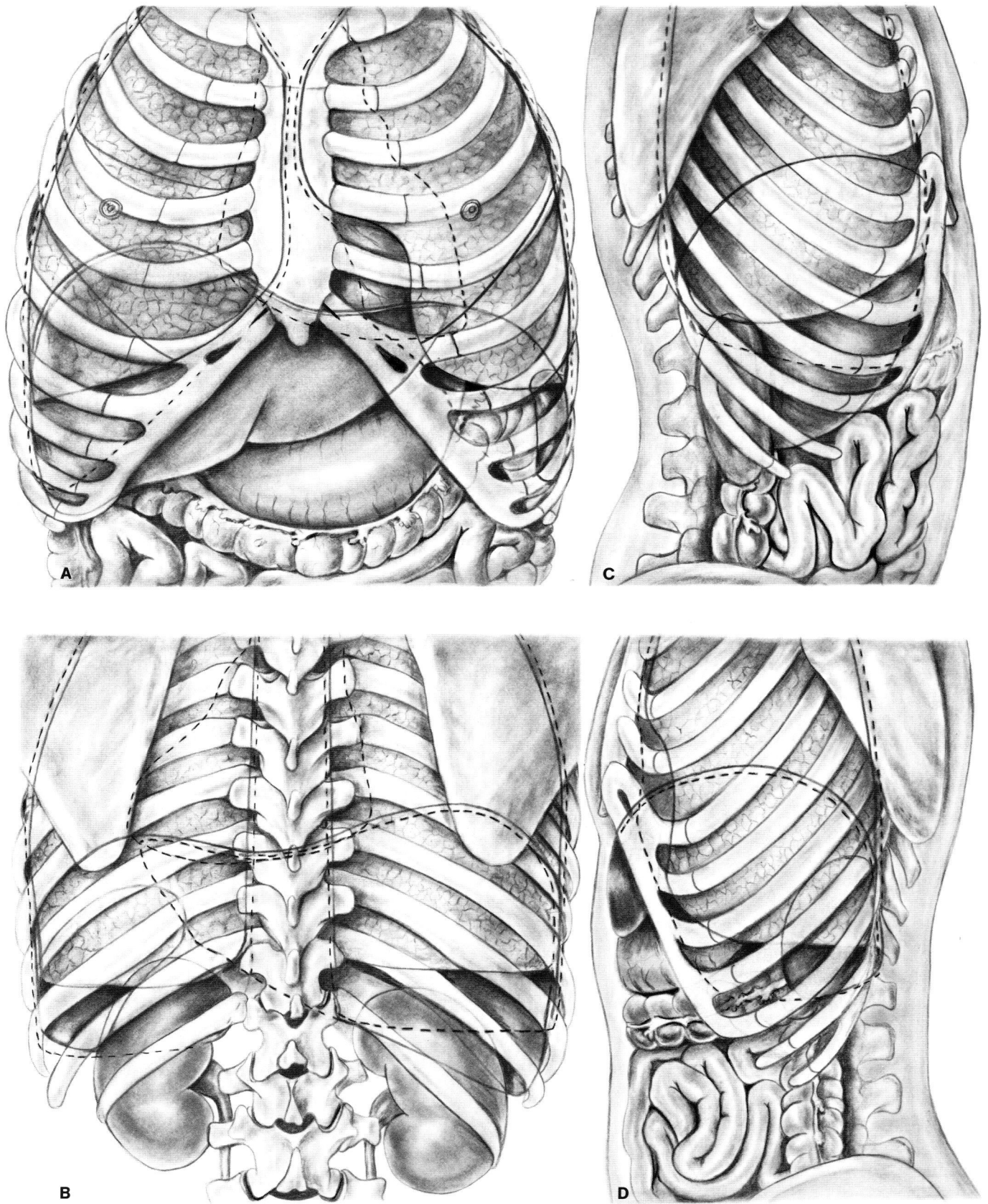

Figure 101 A–D

A   Anterior view of the parietal and visceral relations of the thoraco-
    lumbar junction
B   Posterior view of the parietal and visceral relations of the thoraco-
    lumbar junction

C   Right lateral relations of the thoracolumbar junction
D   Left lateral relations of the thoracolumbar junction

e) Anterolateral Abdominal Wall

The operative approach to the thoracolumbar junction requires knowledge of the anterolateral abdominal wall lying between the xiphoid process and umbilicus. The skin of this region is thick, in males covered by hair, and is marked by the profile of the different abdominal muscles, especially the rectus abdominis. The subcutaneous region contains more or less abundant fat tissue, according to the individual. The thoracoepigastric veins form an important venous network here from the root of the lower limb (great saphenous vein) to the axillary region, representing a system of intercaval anastomosis. Via the umbilicus, this network also communicates with the portal venous system. Bundles of arteries and nerves traverse the subcutaneous tissue to supply the skin, i.e., lateral bundles passing lateral to the rectus muscles and anterior bundles passing flush with the sheath of the rectus muscles. Two groups of muscles form the anterior abdominal wall; the anterior rectus group, and the lateral group comprising the obliquus externus and internus and the transversus.

(1) Rectus Abdominis Muscle

The rectus abdominis extends from the xiphoid process to the pubis on each side of the abdominal midline, and is enveloped in a sheath and separated from its homologue by the linea alba. It is long, flat, and relatively wide (about three fingers), and originates on the anterior surface of the xiphoid process and the crest and symphysis of the pubis to insert on the cartilaginous segments of the fifth through seventh ribs. Three or more tendinous bands segment the muscle and fuse it to the anterior part of its sheath, which is formed by anterior and posterior sheets. The anterior sheet is formed by the fascia of the obliquus externus abdominis, the anterior fold of the fascia of the obliquus internus (adherent to the rectus abdominis except in the suprapubic region), and the fascia of the transversus abdominis (in the region extending from a few centimeters below the umbilicus to the pubis). The posterior sheet is composed of musculofascial tissue running from the xiphoid process to a few centimeters below the umbilicus, where it is interrupted by an arcuate line. Caudal to this line, the posterior sheet is formed by the medial fibers and the fascia of the transversus abdominis muscle. The posterior fold of the fascia of the obliquus internus muscle lies anterior and adherent to the preceding structures. Below the arcuate line the sheath of the rectus muscle is interrupted only by the fascia transversalis, which lines the entire deep surface of the anterolateral abdominal wall. The anastomotic superior and inferior epigastric arteries run vertically through the rectus abdominis and its sheath. The superior epigastric artery, branching medially from the internal thoracic (internal mammary) artery, penetrates the sheath of the rectus abdominis lateral to the xiphoid process. The inferior epigastric artery, a branch of the external iliac artery, penetrates the sheath of the rectus abdominis below the arcuate line. The lateral margin of the sheath forms a semilunar line penetrated by the motor nerves of the rectus abdominis, i.e., the seventh through twelfth intercostal nerves.

Accordingly, an incision made along this semilunar line leads to denervation of the rectus abdominis.

(2) Obliquus Externus Muscle

The obliquus externus is the most superficial of the three muscles forming the anterolateral abdominal wall. Several fleshy bands of the obliquus externus insert on the lateral surface of the lower eight ribs and blend with those of the serratus anterior and latissimus dorsi muscles, frequently fusing with the external intercostal muscles. The fibers of the obliquus externus run obliquely downward and medially to the iliac crest and join the lateral margin of the fascia, which arises 2–3 cm from the lateral margin of the rectus abdominis and participates in the formation of the rectus sheath.

(3) Obliquus Internus Muscle

The obliquus internus originates from the thoracolumbar fascia inserting on the lumbar transverse processes, the iliac crest, and the fascia iliaca. Its fibers run obliquely upward and medially to join the fascia inserting above on the arches of the lower ribs and medially on the rectus sheath. The obliquus internus blends directly with the internal intercostal muscles of the lower intercostal spaces.

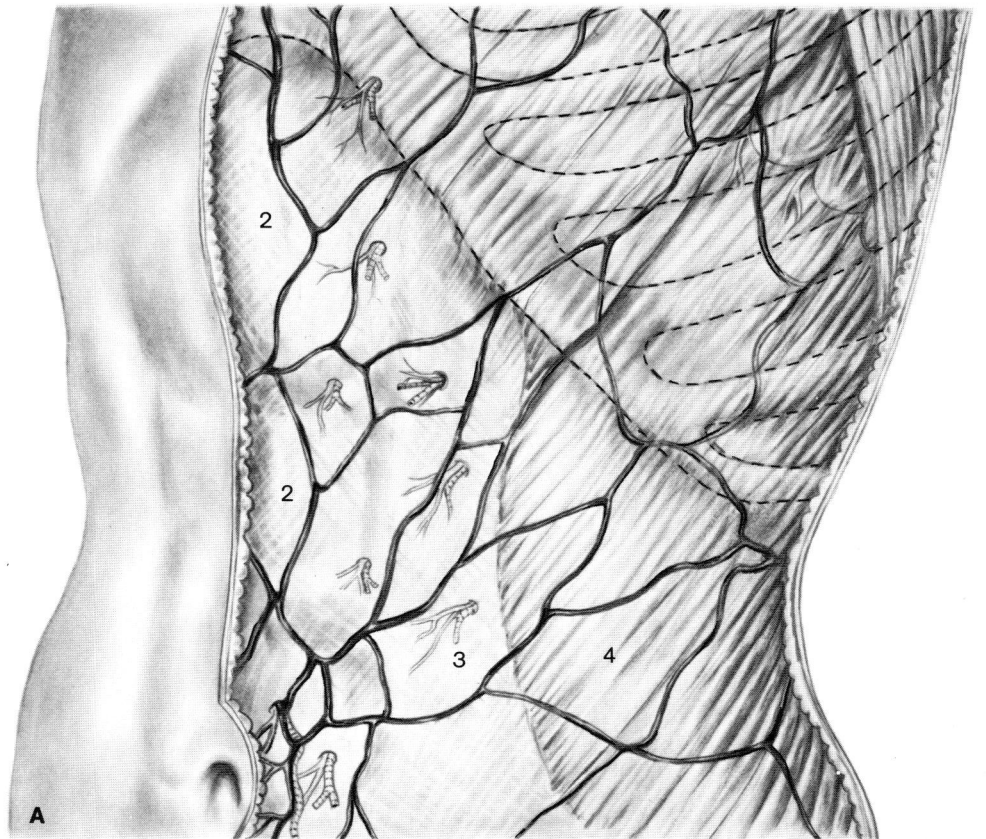

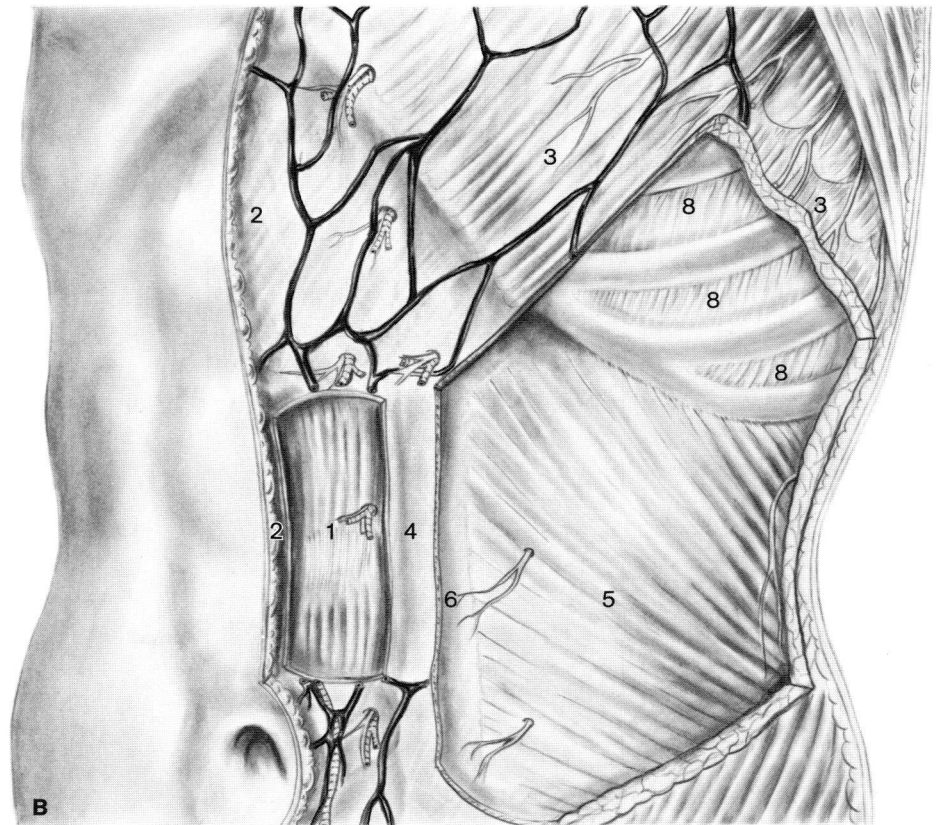

Figure 102 A, B

A   Superficial layer of the anterior thoraco abdominal region

B   Middle layer of the anterior thoracoabdominal region

1 m. rectus abdominis *2* vagina m. recti abdominis (lamina ant.) *3* m. obliquus externus abdominis *4* aponeurosis m. obliqui abdominis externi *5* m. obliquus internus abdominis *6* aponeurosis m. obliqui interni abdominis *8* mm. intercostales externi

(4) Transversus Abdominis Muscle

The tranversus abdominis originates on the fascia iliaca, the internal lip of the iliac crest, the thoracolumbar fascia, and the medial surface of the cartilaginous segments of the lower six ribs, where its fibers blend with those of the diaphragm. The fibers run in a mainly horizontal direction except for the lower fibers, which run obliquely downward. The uppermost fibers disappear behind the rectus sheath, whereas the middle and lower fibers are continued by an aponeurosis which passes behind the rectus muscles to participate in the formation of the posterior lamina of the rectus sheath and then terminates to form the arcuate line a few centimeters below the umbilicus. Caudal to the arcuate line the aponeurosis of the transversus passes anterior to the rectus abdominis to form part of the anterior lamina of the rectus sheath.

(5) Neurovascular Bundles

At the level of the anterolateral muscles of the abdomen, neurovascular bundles run in the interstitial space between the transversus and obliquus internus muscles. These bundles arise from the lower five intercostal spaces and the subcostal region (twelfth bundle). Their course is such that the bundle of the ninth intercostal space reaches the abdominal midline a few centimeters above the umbilicus, that of the tenth intercostal space reaches the umbilicus, that of the eleventh space reaches the midline between the umbilicus and pubis, and the subcostal bundle reaches the inguinal region. The first lumbar nerve gives rise to the iliohypogastric and ilioinguinal nerves, which run from the posteroinferior part of the anterolateral abdominal muscles toward the external inguinal region and carry mainly sensory impulses. The lateral (musculophrenic) branch of the internal thoracic (internal mammary) artery lies behind the cartilaginous segment common to the seventh through tenth ribs, and anastomoses with the intercostal arteries. Section of a costal arch requires the ligation of this artery and its accompanying vein. Traversing the anterolateral abdominal muscles therefore requires an oblique incision parallel to the neurovascular bundles or a route of access with dissection but not transection of the muscle fibers.

(6) Fascia Transversalis and Peritoneum

Dissection of the transversus abdominis muscle exposes the delicate fascia transversalis, separated from the peritoneum by a fat pad varying in thickness according to the individual. Decollement of the peritoneum from the fascia transversalis is relatively easy to achieve and represents a useful plane of incision to displace the abdominal viscera without opening the overlying serous envelope. A few vessels running through the superficial part of the peritoneum distinguish it from the fascia transversalis. Decollement of the lateral and posterior parts of the peritoneum is easily accomplished, but near the diaphragmatic cupulae the peritoneum is tightly adherent. Accordingly, surgical decollement of the peritoneal serosa must be avoided in the region of the centrum tendineum, tear-

ing the serosa would lead to expulsion of the abdominal viscera due to the intra-abdominal pressure. Retraction of the peritoneal envelope toward the midline exposes the inferior surface of the diaphragmatic cupula and the branches of the inferior phrenic vascular bundle. The posterior wall of the abdomen in this region is in continuity with the quadratus lumborum and iliopsoas muscles. The parietal operative field can be enlarged by sectioning the common costal cartilage and opening the intercostal spaces. The musculophrenic vascular bundle and the diaphragmatic crura lie behind the common costal cartilage. The internal intercostal muscles terminate on the diaphragmatic crura: dissection of the muscles and transection of the crura allow penetration of the pleural cavity to gain access to the superior surface of the cupulae. At this stage of parietal dissection the cupula can be freed completely and thus grasped between two fingers by the displacement of the peritoneum and the retraction of the lung (suppression of the pleural vacuum).

(7) Diaphragm

The diaphragm is a large, flat, radiate muscle composed of fleshy and tendinous fibers. By inserting on the lumbar vertebrae, the tip of the lower six ribs, and the xiphoid process it separates the thoracic and abdominal cavities. It forms a transverse septum elevated at the right and left cupulae and notched posteriorly over the spine. The right cupula extends up to the level of the anterior part of the fourth intercostal space, but the left cupula does not reach further than the anterior part of the fifth intercostal space. Essentially a respiratory muscle, the diaphragm contracts against the intra-abdominal structures and thus descends towards the abdominal cavity to increase intra-abdominal and decrease intrathoracic pressure during inspiration. Reciprocal phenomena occur during expiration. The muscle fibers of the diaphragm are of the digastric type, and display a peripheral costosternotransverse insertion, an intermediate insertion on the cloverleaf centrum tendineum, and a second peripheral insertion lateral to the centrum tendineum. Accordingly, the diaphragmatic muscle fibers radiate out from the centrum tendineum. The peripheral insertions of the diaphragm can be classified as sternal, costal, and lumbar. The sternal part of the diaphragm inserts on the posterior surface of the xiphoid process. The costal segment inserts on the medial surface of the lower six segments of costal cartilage and the lower four ribs. The fibers blend with those of the costal origin of the transversus abdominis.

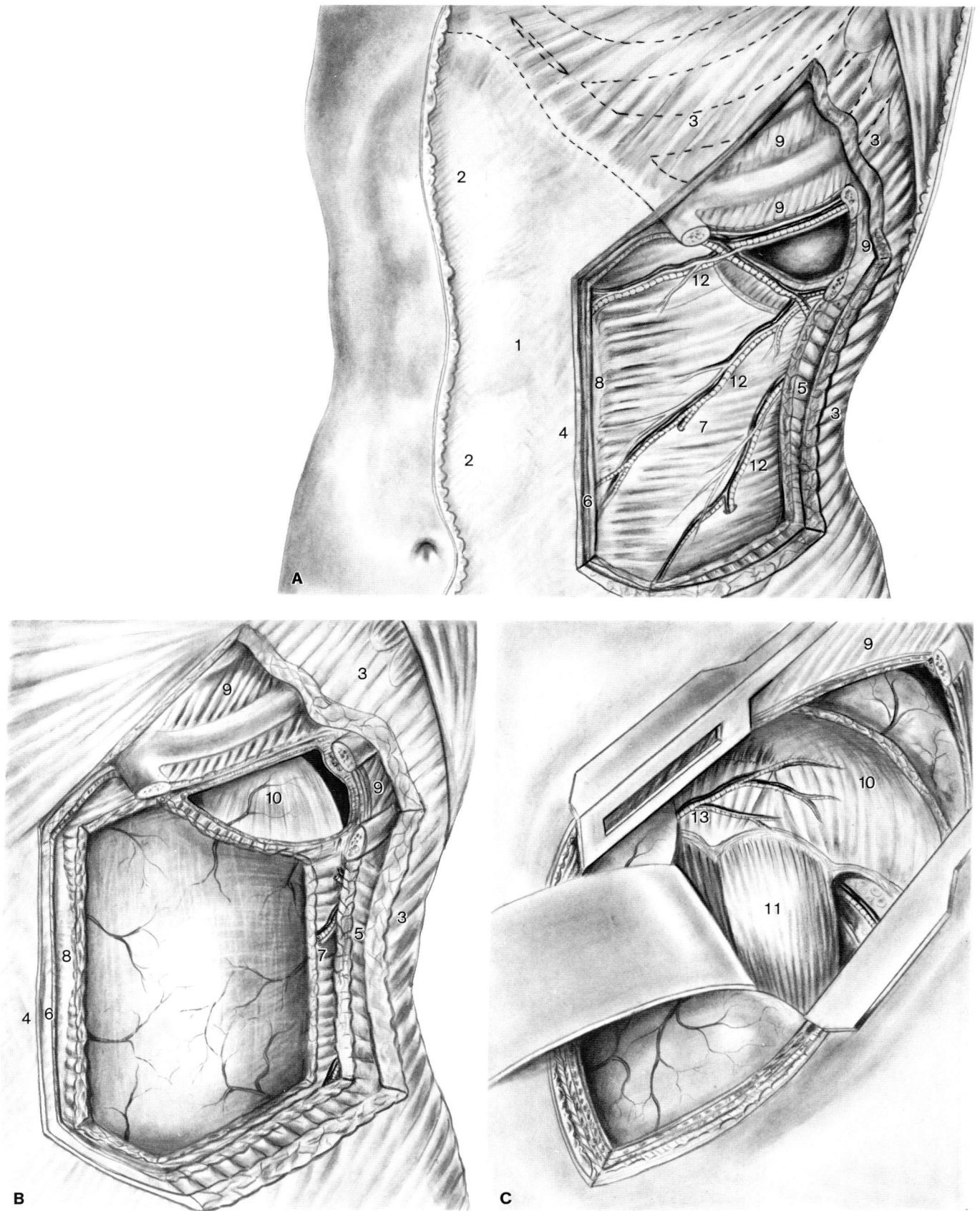

Figure 103 A–C

B

C

A The deepest layer of the anterolateral thoracoabdominal wall

B The serous layer of the anterior thoracoabdominal wall with the pleura opened and the peritoneal envelope exposed

C Displacement of the peritoneal envelope and exposure of the posterior abdominal wall and disphragmatic crura

1 m. rectus abdominis   *2* vagina m. recti abdominis (lamina ant.)
3 m. obliquus externus abdominis   *4* aponeurosis m. obliqui abdominis externi   *5* m. obliquus internus abdominis   *6* aponeurosis m. obliqui interni abdominis   *7* m. transversus abdominis   *8* aponeurosis m. transversi abdominis   *9* mm. intercostales interni   *10* diaphragma   *11* m. quadratus lumborum   *12* v., a., and n. intercostalis   *13* a. and v. phrenicae inf.

(7) Diaphragm (continued)

At the level of the lower intercostal spaces the fibers insert on the tip of the costal cartilage and on the arcuate fibrous bands lying between the cartilaginous segments. The lumbar (vertebral) portion of the diaphragm inserts on two pairs of fibrous arches and one pair of crura. The left and right crura originate on each side of the lumbar spinal midline. The much longer right crus originates from the first three or four lumbar vertebrae, whereas the shorter left crus originates from the first two or three lumbar vertebrae. The right and left crura fuse anterior to T12 to form an arch known as the median arcuate ligament delineating the aortic hiatus. Fibers extending from the arcuate ligament and from the left and (especially) right crura pass around the esophageal fibers of the crura to form an intermediate crus running towards the centrum tendineum. The medial lumbocostal arch (medial arcuate ligament or psoas arch), lying just lateral to the diaphragmatic crura, extends from the lateral part of the body of L1 or L2 to the tip of the transverse process of L1 or L2. It passes above the upper insertion of the psoas muscle, where it blends into the fascia iliaca. The fleshy fibers given off by this arch join the lateral leaves of the centrum tendineum. Further laterally lies the lateral lumbocostal arch, also known as the lateral arcuate ligament or arch of the quadratus lumborum, which inserts on the tip of the L1 transverse process and the tip of the twelfth rib, sometimes the eleventh rib when the twelfth is short. The lateral arch also gives off fleshy fibers to the lateral parts of the centrum tendineum. The muscle fibers of different arches delimit foramina allowing communication between the thoracic and abdominal cavities. The centrum tendineum is a shiny pearl-colored sheet resembling a three-leaf clover, the anterior leaf lying at some distance from the xiphoid process while the lateral leaves run more posteriorly and laterally, and is composed of tendinous bundles known as the semilunar bands. The upper band runs from the anterior toward the right lateral leaf of the centrum tendineum, whereas the lower band joins the right and left leaves. The foramen of the vena cava is a large quadrilateral orifice with rounded angles lying between the semilunar bands. Vessels and nerves run along the superior and inferior surfaces of the diaphragmatic cupulae, which are lined by serous membranes. The diaphragm is innervated by the right and left phrenic nerves arising from nerve roots C4 and C5 and to a lesser extent from C3. The right phrenic nerve approaches the right cupula on the right side of the inferior vena cava, where the nerve gives off three branches. The anterior branch supplies the anterior sternal and costal fibers of the diaphragm and gives off a retroxiphoid anastomosis to the left phrenic nerve. Lateral rami of the nerve supply the lateral costal part of the diaphragm. The posterior branch also passes through the foramen of the vena cava to appear on the lower surface of the diaphragm where it runs along the inferior phrenic (inferior diaphragmatic) artery. The posterior terminal branches of the right phrenic nerve join the diaphragmatic plexus and give off a few rami to the right semilunar ganglion of the solar plexus. The left phrenic nerve approaches the diaphragm slightly posterior to the tip of the heart and also gives off three branches passing through the centrum tendineum to reach the inferior surface of the diaphragm: an anterior branch anastomosing with the right phrenic nerve, a lateral branch, and a posterior branch. The posterior branch also innervates the diaphragmatic plexus and gives off rami to the solar plexus. Accordingly, transection of the muscle fibers radiating from the centrum tendineum towards the peripheral costal insertions of the diaphragm may cause injury to one of the branches of the phrenic nerve, thus depriving the muscle of part of its motor supply. Consequently, it is recommended that the diaphragm be incised in its peripheral zone in very close proximity to the costal insertions, since the terminal rami of the phrenic nerves do not pass in this region. The diaphragm receives arterial blood from vessels supplying its upper and lower surfaces. The upper surface receives the superior phrenic arteries, which branch off from the internal thoracic arteries and approach the muscle along with the rami of the phrenic nerve. On its lower surface the diaphragm is supplied by the two large inferior phrenic arteries, which arise as the first branches of the abdominal aorta and approach the diaphragm near the right and left crura to run upward on each side of the esophagus, giving off posterior and anterior branches to the lateral parts of the centrum tendineum. These arteries are paralleled by the inferior phrenic veins, which finally join the inferior vena cava, the gastric veins, or exceptionally the azygos vein. The upper surface of the diaphragm is covered by two types of serous membrane; the pericardial serosa on the anterior leaf of the centrum tendineum and the pleural serosa on the cupulae. These serous membranes, especially the pleural serosa, are rather firmly adherent to the diaphragm and thus contribute to diaphragmatic solidity when the transected muscle is sutured. The lower surface of the diaphragm is lined by the peritoneal serosa, which adheres intimately only to the centrum tendineum. Decollement of the peritoneal serosa is thus easy to achieve in the fleshy parts of the diaphragm.

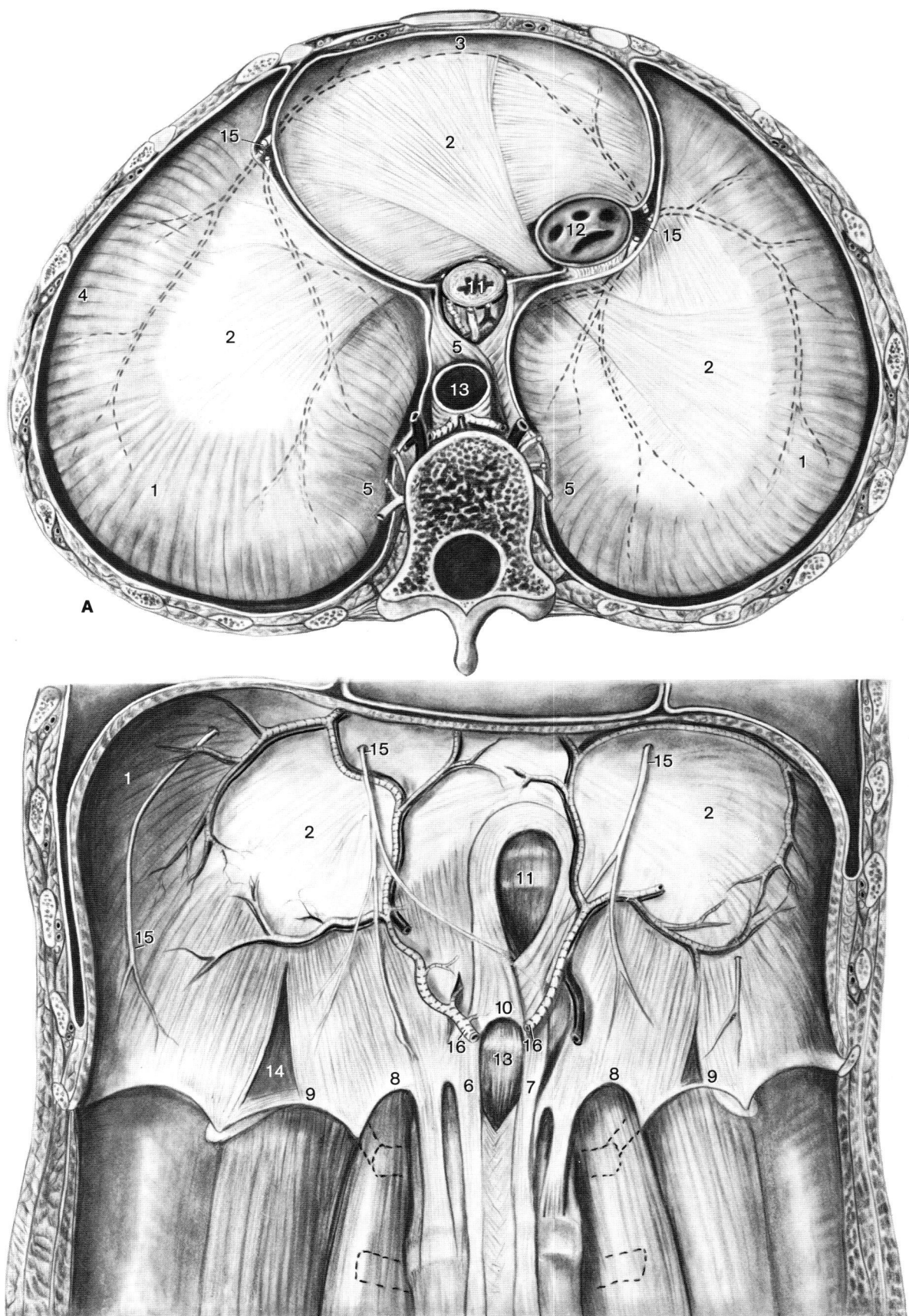

Figure 104 A, B

A The superior aspect of the diaphragm with the overlying pericardial and pleural serosae

B The inferior aspect of the diaphragm after removal of the intra-abdominal viscera

1 diaphragma   *2* centrum tendineum   *3* pars sternalis   *4* pars costalis
5 pars lumbalis   *6* crus dextrum   *7* crus sinistrum   *8* arcus lumbo-
costalis (lig. arcuatum mediale)   *9* arcus lumbocostalis (lig. arcuatum laterale)   *10* lig. arcuatum medianum   *11* hiatus oesophagus
12 foramen v. cavae   *13* hiatus aorticus   *14* trigonum lumbocostale
15 n. phrenicus   *16* aa. phrenicae inf.

f) Left Thoracolumbar Region

Prior to Transection of the Diaphragm

The left thoracolumbar region is composed of the following three sectors from bottom to top: the left subphrenic sector, exposed by displacing the abdominal viscera towards the midline; the left inframediastinal sector, lying anterior to and along the left flank of the spine, bounded by the lumbar and vertical part of the diaphragm, and extended laterally by the left costodiaphragmatic recess; and the left hemithoracic cavity, lying above the diaphragm. Owing to the presence of the diaphragm, the three sectors are independent. Furthermore, the thoracolumbar spine is surgically camouflaged by their contents.

After Transection of the Diaphragm

After transection of the diaphragm the region can be divided into lateral and medial parts.

The *lateral part* of the thoracolumbar region comprises three sectors from bottom to top.

In the lowest sector the posterior wall of the lateral region is essentially muscular. The lateral part of the posterior wall is formed by the quadratus lumborum, which is traversed above by the subcostal neurovascular (twelfth intercostal) bundle and below by the iliohypogastric and ilioinguinal nerves. The large psoas muscle lies medial to and extends in front of the quadratus lumborum, the two muscles forming a steplike mass.

The middle sector of the lateral thoracolumbar region contains the bandlike posterior insertions of the diaphragmatic crura represented by the lateral arcuate ligament (arch of the quadratus lumborum), the medial arcuate ligament (arch of the psoas), and the crus sinistrum. Opening of the aortic hiatus requires that the left crus be sectioned, thus removing the diaphragmatic boundary between the lumbar and thoracic regions.

The upper sector of the lateral thoracolumbar region contains the posterior segment of the lower left rib cage. The deep surface of the ribs and the internal costal spaces run very obliquely downward and laterally.

The *medial part* of the left thoracolumbar region contains the aorta and vertebrae, which lie anterior to the psoas muscle, thus forming a steplike region. The aorta runs along the left anterior surface of the thoracolumbar spine. Opening of the aortic hiatus exposes the continuity of the thoracic and abdominal segments of the aorta, which can be displaced toward the midline using a flexible retractor. Decollement of the abdominal structures from the lumbar region allows the aorta to be retracted to the right of the midline, permitting full exposure of the left thoracolumbar spine. Anterior to the aorta, the large vessels which arise from the anterior surface of the aorta and can be palpated through the pararenal fat pad are the inferior diaphragmatic arteries, the celiac trunk, the superior mesenteric artery, and the left renal artery. The heart and its surrounding pericardium lie anterior to the lower part of the thoracic aorta.

The *left anterolateral surface* of the lower thoracic and upper lumbar spine, with its protruding discs and depressed vertebral bodies, can be identified behind and to the left of the aorta. The rib heads are landmarks allowing identification of T11 and T12. During operation in this region the surgeon should first identify the vertical neural structures running between the aorta and spine, including the laterovertebral thoracic and lumbar ganglions and the emissary branches of the splanchnic nerve. The greater left splanchnic nerve passes through the medial diaphragmatic hiatus lateral to the left crus and then crosses over the left anterolateral flank of the aorta to join the left semilunar ganglion. The lesser splanchnic and inferior splanchnic nerves pass through the lateral diaphragmatic hiatus and then run along the left flank of the aorta to join the inferior ganglions of the solar plexus. The vessels of this region can be seen deep to the neural structures, and include the intercostal and lumbar bundles and the terminal part of the ascending lumbar vein near the origin of the hemiazygos vein. The internal tributary of the azygos vein joins the left renal vein and usually runs along the left flank of the aorta near the left splanchnic nerve. Finally, the thoracic duct can be identified as it runs upwards behind the aorta from the level of T12. The thoracic pleura lies over the left flank of the aorta superior to the left curs of the diaphragm.

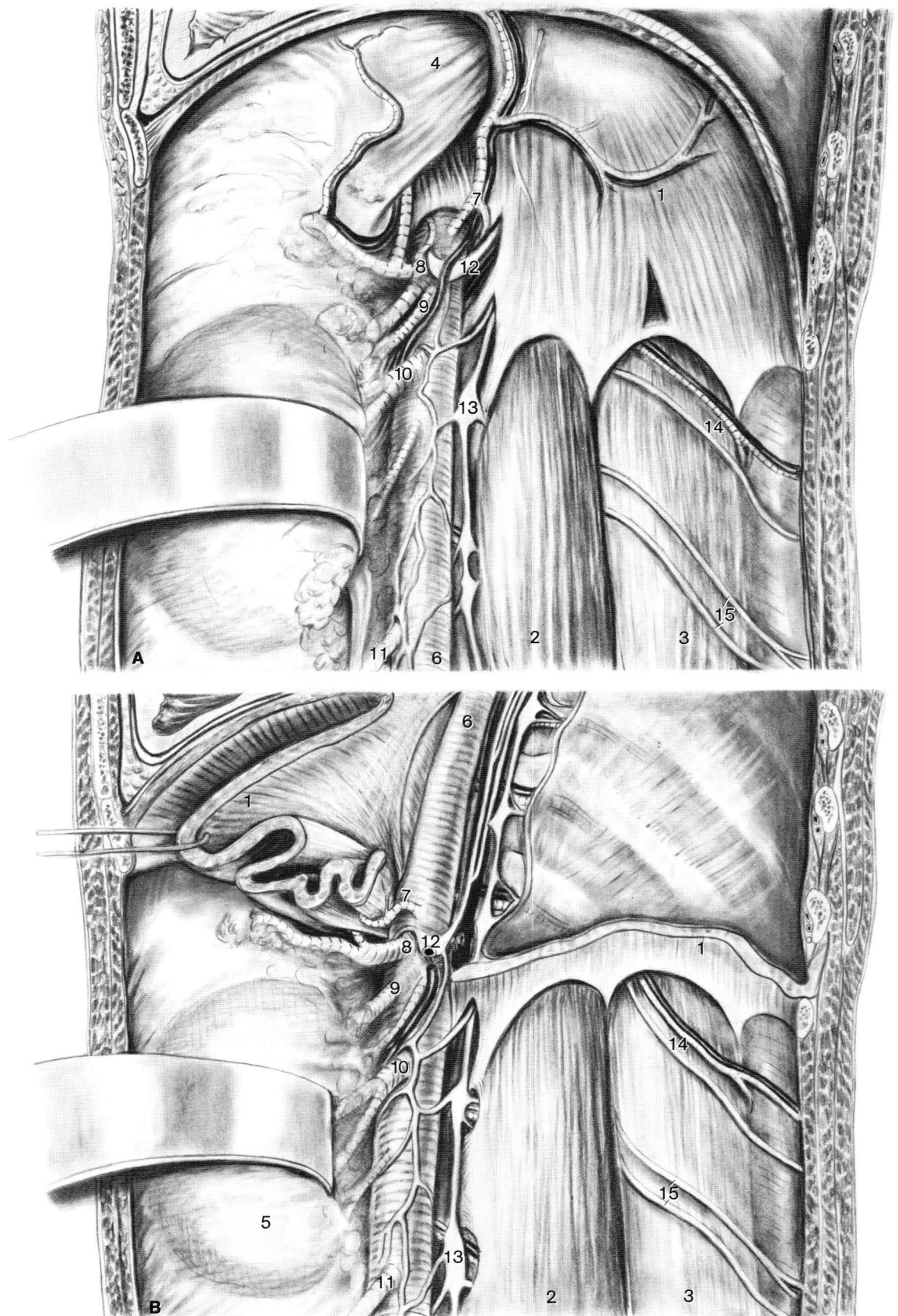

Figure 105 A, B

A The left subphrenic fossa
B The left thoracolumbar region after transection of the diaphragm

1 diaphragma *2* m. psoas *3* m. quadratus lumborum *4* gaster
5 peritoneum *6* aorta *7* a. phrenica inf. *8* truncus celiacus

9 a. mesenterica sup. *10* a. renalis *11* a. mesenterica inf. *12* ganglia celiaca and n. splanchnicus major *13* ganglia lumbalia *14* a. and v. subcostalis and n. intercostalis XII *15* n. iliohypogastricus and n. ilioinguinalis

g) Right Thoracolumbar Region

Prior to Transection of the Diaphragm

The right thoracolumbar region comprises three independent juxtaposed sectors:
The right subphrenic sector is exposed by displacing the liver and the right abdominal viscera towards the midline. Decollement of the liver from the abdominal surface of the diaphragm requires that the coronary ligament be sectioned.
The right part of the inframediastinal sector lies in the dihedral angle formed by the vertical lumbar part of the diaphragm and the anterior surface of the thoracolumbar spine. This narrow region is extended laterally by the right costo-diaphragmatic recess.
The right hemithoracic cavity, lined by the pleura, lies above the two preceding sectors. The three sectors together constitute an anterior obstacle to the spine. Exposure of the thoraolumbar vertebrae requires the transection of the diaphragm to achieve continuity between the three sectors.

After Transection of the Diaphragm

Transection of the diaphragm transforms the right thoracolumbar region into a vast posterior gutter of the trunk lying on the right flank of the spine. The region can be divided into a lateral and a medial part.

The *lateral part* of the right thoracolumbar region comprises inferior, middle and superior sectors:
The lateral zone of the essentially muscular lower sector is formed by the quadratus lumborum muscle, which is traversed by the subcostal (twelfth right intercostal) bundle and the iliohypogastric and ilioinguinal nerves. Medial to the quadratus lumborum lies the bulky psoas, the two muscles forming a steplike mass.
The middle sector is represented by the bandlike insertions of the diaphragmatic crura. These insertions are the lateral arcuate ligament (arch of the quadratus lumborum), the medial arcuate ligament (arch of the psoas), and finally the crus dextrum of the diaphragm. Suppression of the diaphragmatic barrier between the thoracic and lumbar regions requires that the aortic hiatus be opened by transection of the right crus.
The superior sector corresponds to the right posteroinferior part of the rib cage and the corresponding intercostal spaces lined by the mediastinal pleura.

The *medial part* of the right thoracolumbar region is centered on the inferior vena cava, lying on the right flank of the spine, which can be identified as a large, bluish, fragile, and depressible structure. The upper lumbar part of the vein is camouflaged by the overlying liver, which must be cautiously and progressively displaced toward the midline to expose the inferior vena cava and the spine. The heart, with its overlying pericardium, extends the inferior vena cava above the centrum tendineum. The bulky abdominal mass and the renal fossa lie anterior to the inferior vena cava, which is exposed by displacing them toward the midline. The diaphragm lies posterior to the liver. Neural and vascular structures lie in the dihedral angle formed by the posterior surface of the right flank of the spine and the right lateral margin of the inferior vena cava. The neural structures include the right laterovertebral plexus, running anterior to the rib heads and the psoas arches. The splanchnic nerves enter this region anterior to the laterovertebral plexus. The greater right splanchnic nerve is barely visible, since it passes behind the inferior vena cava. The inferior and lesser splanchnic nerves also pass posterior to the vena cava to join the ganglions of the solar plexus. The vascular structures of this part lie deep to the nerves, and include the intercostal and lumbar bundles and the vertical venous axis of the ascending lumbar vein and the azygos vein. The medial root of the azygos vein forms a transverse bar across the sectioned right crus of the diaphragm before joining the posterior surface of the inferior vena cava. Exposure of the lower thoracic vertebrae requires that the mediastinal pleura be opened.

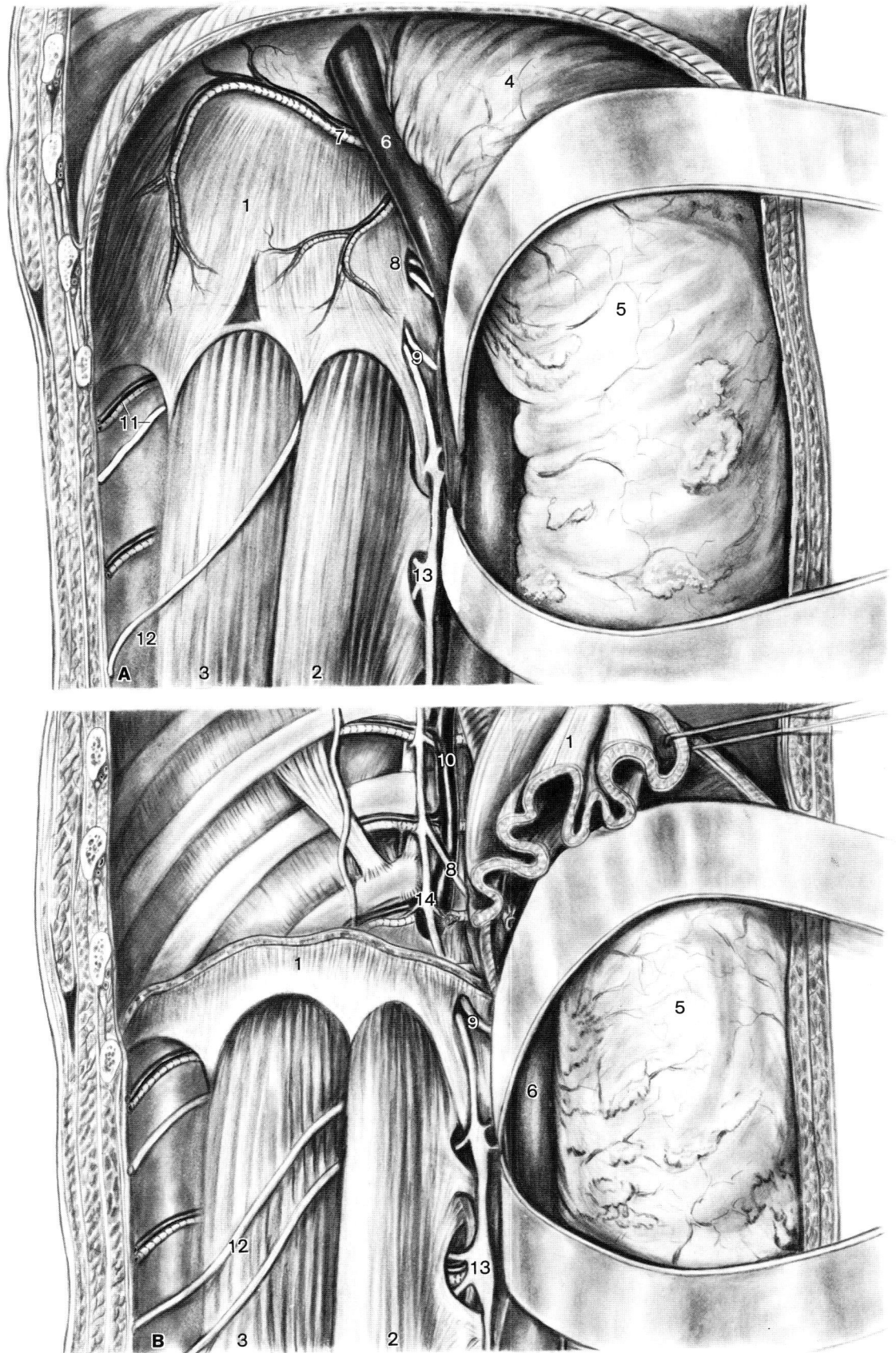

Figure 106 A, B

A   The right subphrenic fossa
B   The right thoracolumbar region
    after transection of the diaphragm

1 diaphragma 2 m. psoas 3 m. quadratus lumborum 4 hepar
5 peritoneum 6 v. cava inf. 7 a. phrenica inf. 8 n. splanchnicus
major 9 n. splanchnicus minor 10 v. azygos 11 a. and v. subcostalis
and n. intercostalis XII 12 n. iliohypogastricus 13 ganglia lumbalia

h) Immediate Relations of the Thoracolumbar Spine

When approaching the thoracolumbar spine subsequent to surgical displacement of the thoracic and abdominal viscera, three things are required: mobilization of the great vessels, ligation of the parietal vessels, and preservation of the nervous structures.

The *great vessels* requiring mobilization are the thoraco-abdominal aorta and the inferior vena cava, which lie precisely over the anterior surface of the spine. Owing to its obviously greater structural resistance, it is the aorta that should be mobilized to allow left-sided access, expecially as the more fragile inferior vena cava lies deep to the liver, which is more difficult to mobilize than the abdominal viscera on the left side.

Mobilization of the great vessels requires the hemostasis of the *parietal vessels* lying between the spine and the posterior surface of the aorta and inferior vena cava. The lumbar and intercostal arteries arise in pairs very close to the aortic midline to run horizontally or slightly downward towards their respective intervertebral foramina. The upper lumbar arteries frequently traverse the fibrous prevertebral insertions of the main crura of the diaphragm, and so must be identified and then ligated prior to the surgical separation of the posterior surface of the aorta from the aponeurotic tissue of the crura. The lumbar veins running along with these arteries join the inferior vena cava near its posterior midline. The right and left intercostal veins anastomose with the azygos and hemiazygos veins respectively. Ligation of the intercostal veins can thus be avoided by retracting the azygos veins laterally. The thoracic duct can be identified posterior to the aorta and can generally be mobilized along with it. Surgical injury to the thoracic duct must be avoided: if it occurs, the two free ends should be ligated immediately to avoid a serious postoperative fistula. After passing over the flanks of the thoracolumbar spine the parietal vessels run in front of the intervertebral foramina, where they give off dorsal or lateral spinal branches. The site of choice for the ligation of these vessels is halfway between their origin and their point of passage at the level of the intervertebral foramina.

The *neural structures* in the anterior thoracolumbar region, from anterior to posterior, include the solar plexus, lying in front of the visceral branches of the abdominal aorta, the greater and lesser splanchnic nerves, which arise from the thoracic and lumbar laterovertebral plexuses and run along the lateral margins of the aorta, and the thoracic and lumbar spinal nerves, emerging from the intervertebral foramina. Care must be taken not to injure the spinal nerves when surgical rasping of the lateral surfaces of the spine is performed, especially at the level of the upper insertions of the psoas muscle.

Anterior Relations of the Thoracolumbar Vertebral Canal. Subsequent to exposure of the anterior thoracolumbar spine, operation may include rachiotomy to gain access to the vertebral canal. The first step of this procedure involves the traversing of the vertebral bodies and the intervertebral discs, especially over the anterior middle third of these structures. During this step numerous venous channels are opened, and require hemostasis with bone wax. The anterior surface of the posterior longitudinal ligament appears at a depth of 20–25 mm. The ligament is wide and adherent to the posterior surface of the discs and narrow and free near the middle part of the vertebral bodies. Many veins draining the intraspinal plexus penetrate through or run anterior to this ligament. The large antero-lateral venous plexuses of the vertebral canal lie on each side of the posterior longitudinal ligament. Hemostasis of these plexuses is difficult to achieve, but bleeding can be interrupted with Surgicel or avoided by making a midline incision of the ligament to gain access to the anterior surface of the dural envelope without mobilizing the plexuses. Hemostasis of the posterior longitudinal ligament is easy to accomplish by electrocoagulation. The intervertebral foramina containing the spinal nerves, the venous structures, and the spinal artery lie between the sectioned vertebral pedicles.

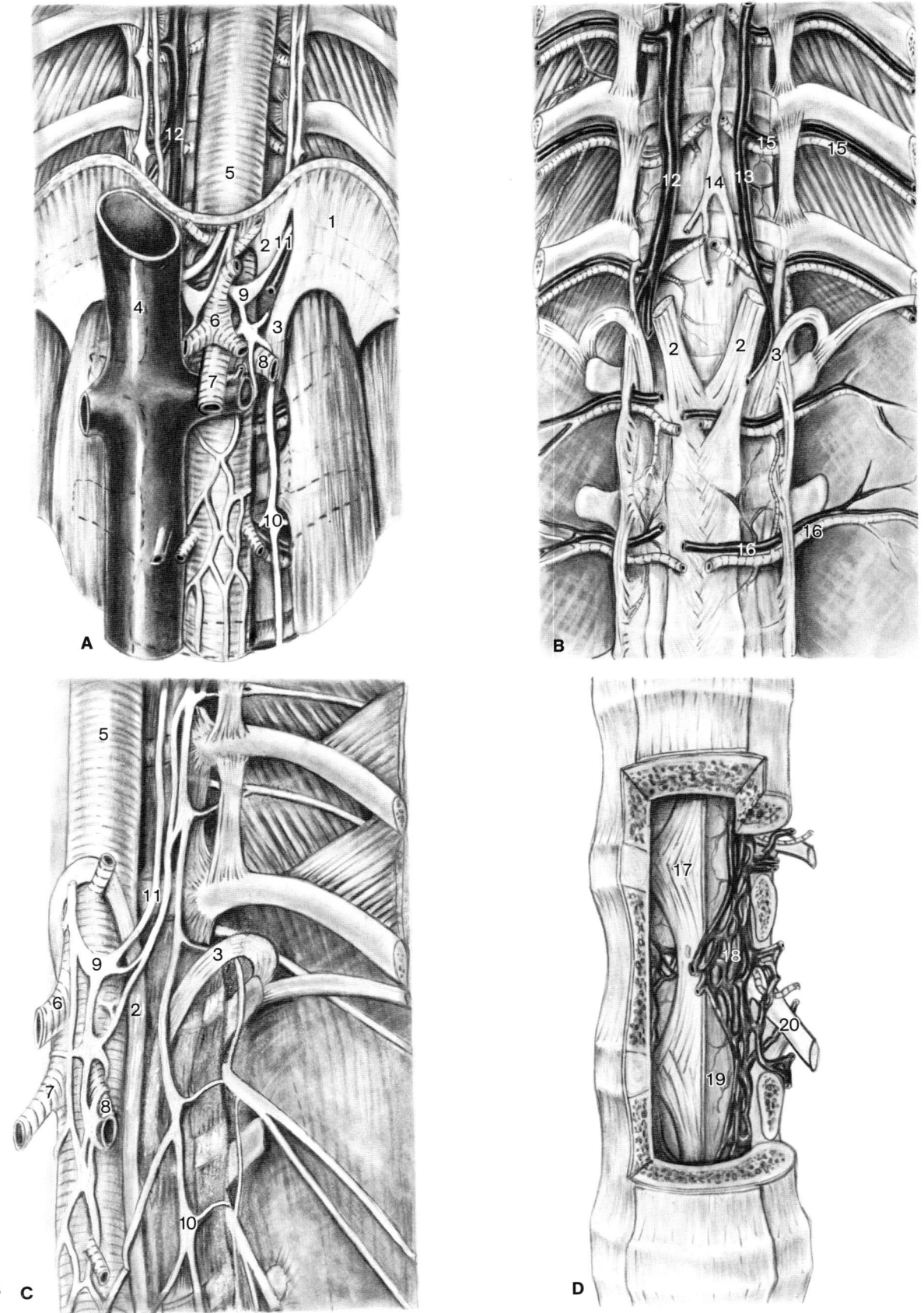

Figure 107 A–D

A   The great spinal vessels
B   Prevertebral collateral vessels
C   Pre- and laterovertebral nerves
D   Anterior rachiotomy

1 diaphragma 2 crus dextrum, crus sinistrum 3 lig. arcuatum mediale 4 v. cava inf. 5 aorta 6 truncus celiacus 7 a. mesenterica sup. 8 a. renalis 9 ganglia celiaca 10 ganglia lumbalia 11 n. splanchnicus major 12 v. azygos 13 v. hemiazygos 14 ductus thoracicus 15 a. and v. intercostales post. 16 a. and v. lumbales 17 lig. longitudinale post. 18 plexus venosi vertebrales interni ant. 19 dura mater 20 nn. spinales

i) Horizontal Section Through T12

This horizontal section clearly demonstrates that the thoracolumbar spine is the prominent structure of the posterior wall of the trunk at the junction of the thoracic and abdominal cavities. The presence of the vertebral canal containing the radiculomedullary structures and of the transverse processes extended by the ribs allows distinction of posterior dorsal and anterior ventral regions.

The *posterior dorsal region* is topographically more superficial and less complex, comprising the juxtaposed posterior arches of the ribs and the interlaminar spaces with their overlying spinal muscles, which are separated by interstices and traversed by neurovascular structures. From the anatomical standpoint, the median posterior approach allows the simplest route of access to the thoracolumbar spine.

The *anterior region,* comprising the vertebral bodies and intervertebral discs, presents far more complex anatomical relations. From posterior to anterior, five layers can be described.

The *first layer* is that of the *inframediastinal space* extended by the costodiaphragmatic sinus. The medial part of this layer contains the aorta, the vegetative nerves, the roots of the azygos veins, and the thoracic duct, and the lateral part corresponds to the pleural cul-de-sac. The *second layer* is formed by the *diaphragm,* especially the crura in the lumbar region. Transection of the diaphragm is required to gain anterior access to this spinal region. The *third layer* is that of the *retroperitoneal region,* containing the kidneys, the adrenal glands, the vascular pedicles of these organs, and the pararenal fat. The *peritoneal cavity* constitutes the *fourth layer,* with the duodenopancreatic fossa on the midline and the stomach and transverse mesocolon anteriorly. The liver lying anterior to the inferior vena cava occupies the entire right lateral part of the peritoneal cavity. Left lateral access to the thoracolumbar spine requir the displacement of the spleen and splenic flexure of the colon. The *fifth layer* corresponds to the *anterior wall of the abdomen,* comprising the rectus and large flat abdominal muscles. The abdominal wall is continued laterally and posteriorly by the intercostal spaces. Anterior access to the thoracolumbar junction is thus achieved by disinsertion or transection of the diaphragmatic crura. The parietal wall can be opened laterally in the region of the intercostal spaces, anteriorly in the upper part of the anterolateral abdominal wall, or straddling these two regions. The operative route then passes either posterior to the peritoneal and retroperitoneal viscera or through the peritoneal cavity with forward displacement of the structures in the renal fossa.

Anastomosis of the Parietal and Medullary Arteries

Anterior sugery of the thoracolumbar junction carries a theoretical risk of impairment of the spinal arterial supply owing to the frequent presence of the artery of the lumbar swelling (Adamckiewicz's artery) in this region. However, recent anatomical studies have shown that the spinalcord is protected by a rich system of arterial anastomosis, allowing adequate blood supply if the anastomotic crossroads are conserved during operation. The parietal arteries arising from the aorta run over the vertebral bodies and then anterior to the intervertebral foramina, where they branch off separately or as a common trunk to give rise to the spinal arteries supplying the spinal cord and the dorsal arteries supplying the posterior muscles, and then laterally toward the walls of the trunk.

The arteries arising near the intervertebral foramina participate in the formation of individual anastomotic systems. The spinal arteries (of variable caliber) run along the spinal nerves to enter the vertebral canal and finally reach the spinal cord. Contrary to classical theories, the spinal arteries exist at all metameric levels. Along with the anterior and posterior spinal arteries, they form a vertical perimedullary system of anastomosis. The different spinal arteries are thus not only supplied at each metameric level (especially by all the arterioles of the roots of the cauda equina), but also communicate with each other by the arcuate anastomoses located at the origin of the filum terminale. The dorsal arteries, metamerically distributed to the spinal muscles, form rich anastomoses within the muscle bodies. Finally, the parietal arteries anastomose with each other at the level of the intercostal spaces and the anterolateral abdominal wall. It is thus apparent that the arterial distribution to the spinal cord is formed by a network of horizontal metameric arteries interconnected by vertical systems running along the spinal cord and spinal muscles and in the wall of the trunk. Accordingly, the occurrence of medullary ischemia would require the alteration of a large number of the right and left metameric arteries to interrupt the anastomotic system or the alteration of the arterial crossroads in the region of the intervertebral foramina. It follows from these considerations that bilateral surgical procedures on the vertebral bodies and injury to the arteries in or near the intervertebral foramina must be avoided.

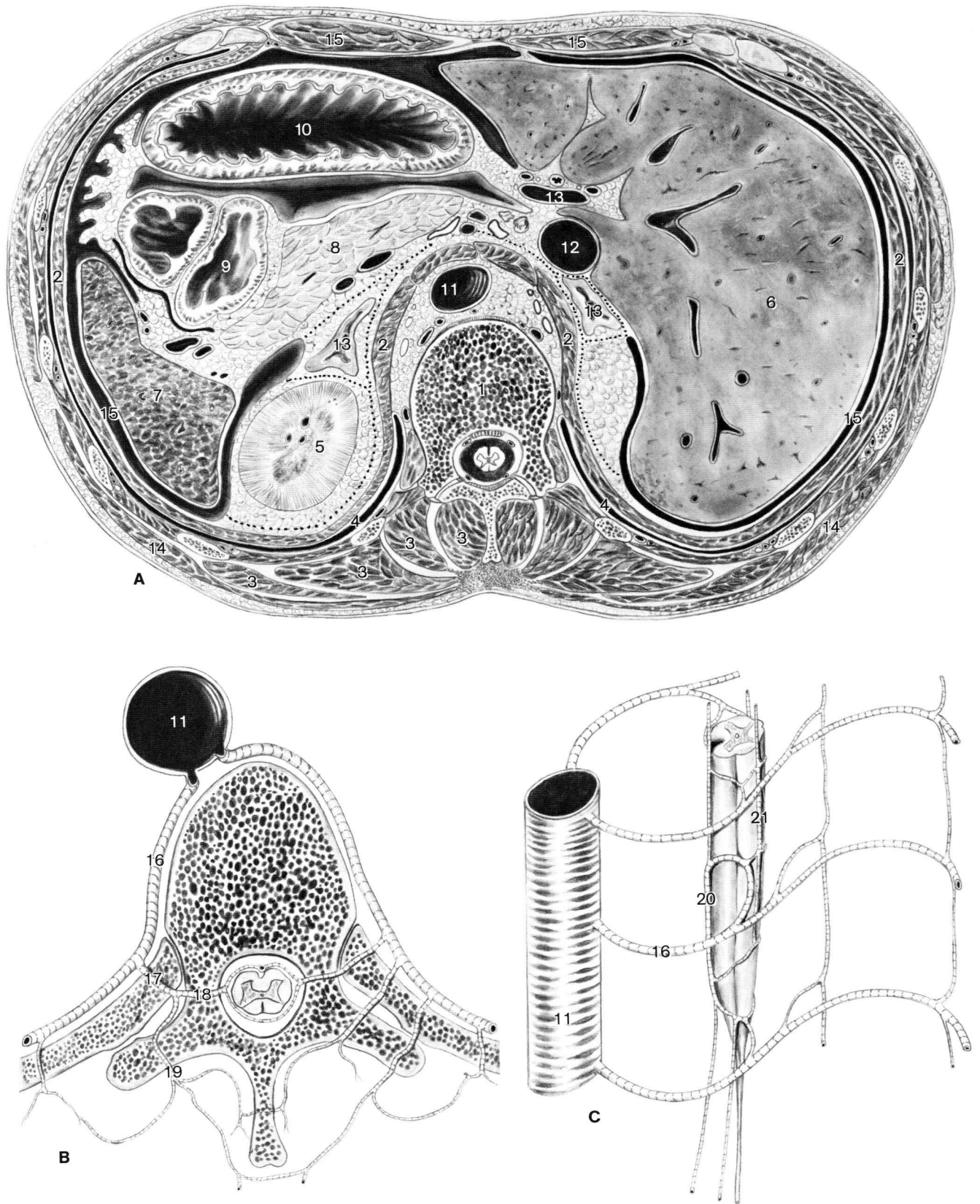

Figure 108 A–C

A   Horizontal section of the trunk through T12
B, C   The anastomotic system of the medullary arteries

10 gaster   *11* aorta   *12* v. cava inf.   *13* glandula suprarenalis
14 m. latissimus dorsi   *15* m. rectus abdominis   *16* a. lumbalis,
intercostalis   *17* truncus dorso-spinales   *18* ramus spinalis
19 ramus dorsalis   *20* a. spinalis ant.   *21* a. spinalis post.

1 vertebra thoracica XII   *2* diaphragma   *3* mm. dorsi   *4* cavum
pleurae   *5* ren. sinister   *6* hepar   *7* lien   *8* pancreas   *9* duodenum

2. Operative Approach

a) Left Thoracophrenolumbotomy

Our technique of thoracophrenolumbotomy presents two major modifications to that first described by Hodgson (1955). We have performed our procedure in over 100 cases with the patient in the supine rather than the lateral supine position, and with the incision made higher up on the ninth rib and contiguous abdominal wall rather than on the tenth and eleventh ribs. The aim is to gain access to the anterior surface of the thoracolumbar junction as close as possible to the midline. This procedure allows more reliable hemostasis, since dissection is carried out in closer proximity to the aorta and inferior vena cava. Furthermore, the median position of the surgical work greatly facilitates decompressive rachiotomy. Finally, arthrodesis with a median inlay bone graft and screw plate is easier to perform and more reliable than a lateral approach. The lateral position may induce curving of the spine with the risk of fixing the spine in this abnormal position on arthrodesis. Excluding scoliosis, most lesions of the thoracolumbar junction require reduction with the spine in lordosis, which is only possible with the patient in the supine position.

(1) Operative Position

The patient is placed supine on the operating table and anesthesia is delivered by endotracheal intubation. The table is then angled or a large pad placed under the thoracolumbar junction. With the patient's feet fixed to the table, spinal traction is applied by a headpiece wired to a tackle block and dynamometer. Even before incision, traction allows creation of lordosis, which helps to reduce the traumatic or static anomalies under monitoring with the image intensifier. The left upper limb is fixed to a metal arch support so that the forearm lies horizontally over the manubrium. The surgeon and first assistant work on the left of the patient and the second assistant on the right. Two operative fields are prepared, one for the left thoracophrenolumbotomy and one on the leg or iliac crest for the removal of bone-graft material. The patient is draped with three transverse double-thickness towels: one over the thorax and head, one lying between the two sites of incision, and one over the lower extremities. Two towels are then placed lengthwise to delimit the operative fields and isolate the anesthesiology zone. Transparent adhesive drapes are applied to the operative regions. The suction cannula is placed to the left of the surgeon and the electric cautery knife to the right.

(2) Skin Incisions

The most common incision to approach the thoracolumbar junction extends along the upper margin of the ninth rib, beginning on the midaxillary line, and continues in this direction onto the upper part of the anterolateral abdominal wall as far as the lateral margin of the rectus muscles a few cen-

timeters above the umbilicus. When the operation requires access to the spine below L2, the abdominal part of the incision should be curved to reach the lateral margin of the rectus muscles at the level of the umbilicus. The ninth rib is identified by first determining the position of the twelfth rib by radiography and palpation. A peg of fibular bone for grafting is taken through an incision of the left leg running on the line from the posterior margin of the head of the fibula to the posterior edge of the lateral malleolus. This incision should run along the depressed muscle region lying over the fibular bone, beginning near the middle of the fibular diaphysis and ending three fingers below the head of the fibula to avoid the zone where the common peroneal nerve crosses over the bone. Iliac bone-graft material is taken through an incision made along the anterior half of the iliac crest, beginning at a point lying two fingers lateral to the antero-superior iliac spine to avoid injury to the lateral cutaneous nerve of the thigh.

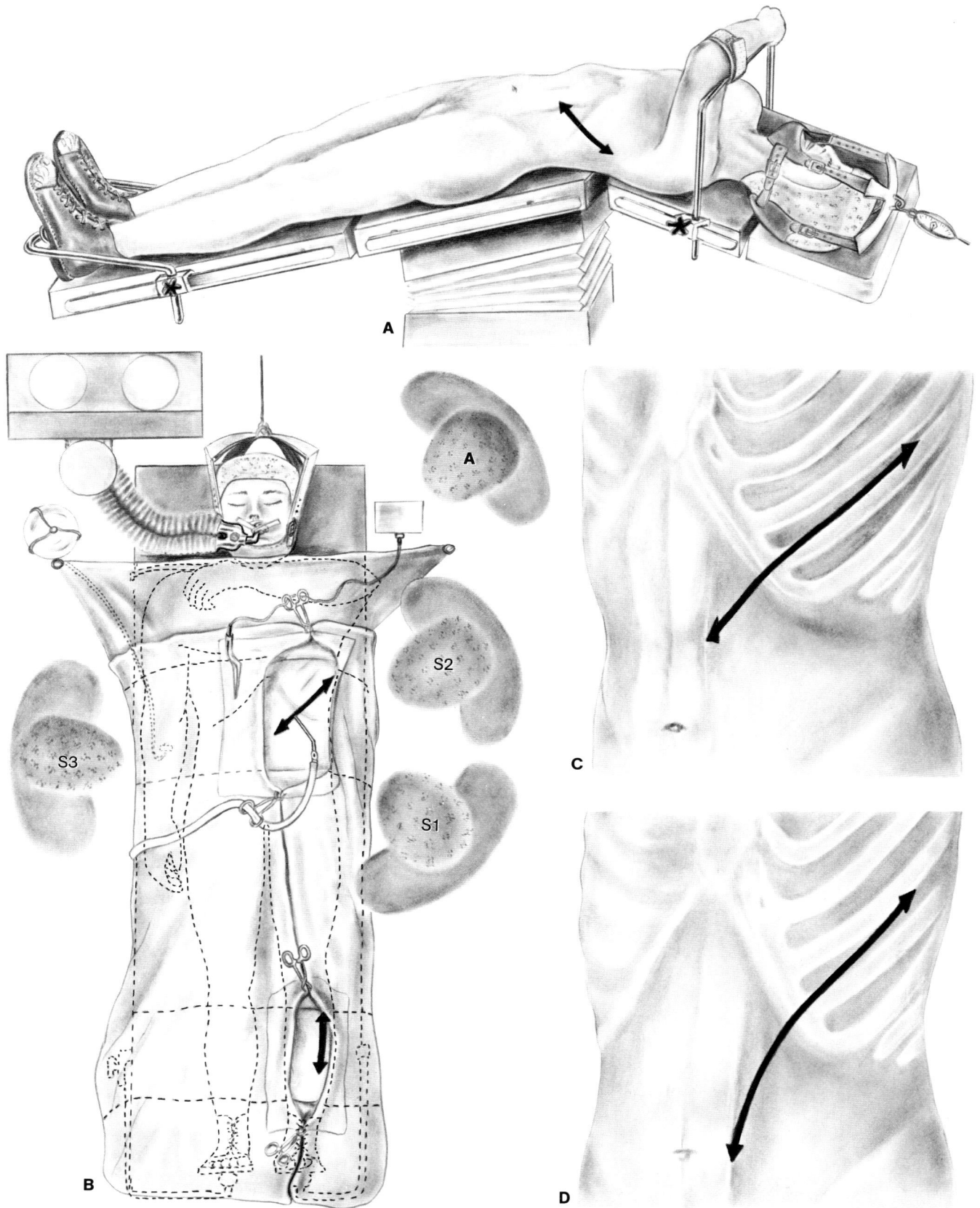

Figure 109 A–D

A   Operative position for left thoracophrenolumbotomy
B   Overhead view of the operative scene

C   Skin incision for left thoracophrenolumbotomy
D   Extension of the incision to the lumbar region

(3) Anterior Parietal Dissection

The full skin incision is made as a two-step procedure to allow progressive hemostasis. The electric cautery knife is then used to incise the subcutaneous tissue, followed by transection of the obliquus externus abdominis over the entire length of the operative field. As the muscle is transected its fibers retract to expose the underlying layer. Hemostasis of a few sites of bleeding is achieved by electrocoagulation. Work is then started in the abdominal segment of the operative field to expose the anterior part of the parietal peritoneum. The obliquus internus abdominis is carefully transected with the cautery knife to expose the fibers of the transversus muscle. Hemostasis of the cut muscle fibers is achieved by electrocoagulation. Flexible retractors are installed to retract the obliquus muscles and expose the transversus and its aponeurosis clearly. Alternate opening and closing of scissors is done in the horizontal plane to dissect the transversus muscle and expose the peritoneum, and clamp-held compresses are introduced under the transversus to separate it from the peritoneum without tearing the latter. Blunt dissection is continued down to the caudal end of the operative field. With the compresses under the transversus to protect the peritoneum, the muscle is then transected with the cautery knife. In cases where the peritoneum is opened inadvertently, immediate peritoneal closure should be carried out with a fine continuous suture, care being taken not to suture any underlying abdominal structures.

Work is now transferred to the thoracic part of the operative field. Incision is first made along the upper margin of the ninth rib using the cautery knife and a costal rasp is used to disinsert the intercostal muscles from the costal periosteum. Indeed, it is unnecessary to transect the intercostal muscles, since their disinsertion leads to immediate opening of the pleural cavity. At this stage the anesthesiologist is informed of the pleural opening so that appropriate measures are taken to ensure proper ventilation by the right lung. The section of the common cartilage between the ninth and eighth ribs is the next step. A large needle holder is first introduced under the common costal cartilage to separate it from the underlying layers, and then it is sectioned with the plain knife. This procedure often leads to minor bleeding resulting from the section of the phrenic branch of the internal mammary artery, but hemostasis can be achieved by electrocoagulation near the deep surface of the cartilage on each side of the sectioned tissue. An orthostatic retractor can now be installed to stretch the muscle fibers of the diaphragm between the opening in the cartilage, but should be opened only moderately to avoid dilaceration of the diaphragm. The operative field can now be divided into three sectors: lower peritoneal, middle diaphragmatic, and upper pulmonary. The left lung is protected by a warm moist compress. The operator now proceeds to decollement of the peritoneum from the abdominal surface of the diaphragm. This should be done in the lumbar region, where the peritoneum is only loosely adherent to the diaphragm, rather than in the region of the centrum tendineum, where it is strongly adherent. Clamp-held compresses are introduced between the peritoneum and diaphragm, and transection of the diaphragm is then begun at a point 10–15 mm from the peripheral costal insertion of the muscle, to leave a muscle stump suitable for reconstruction of the diaphragm at the end of the operation.

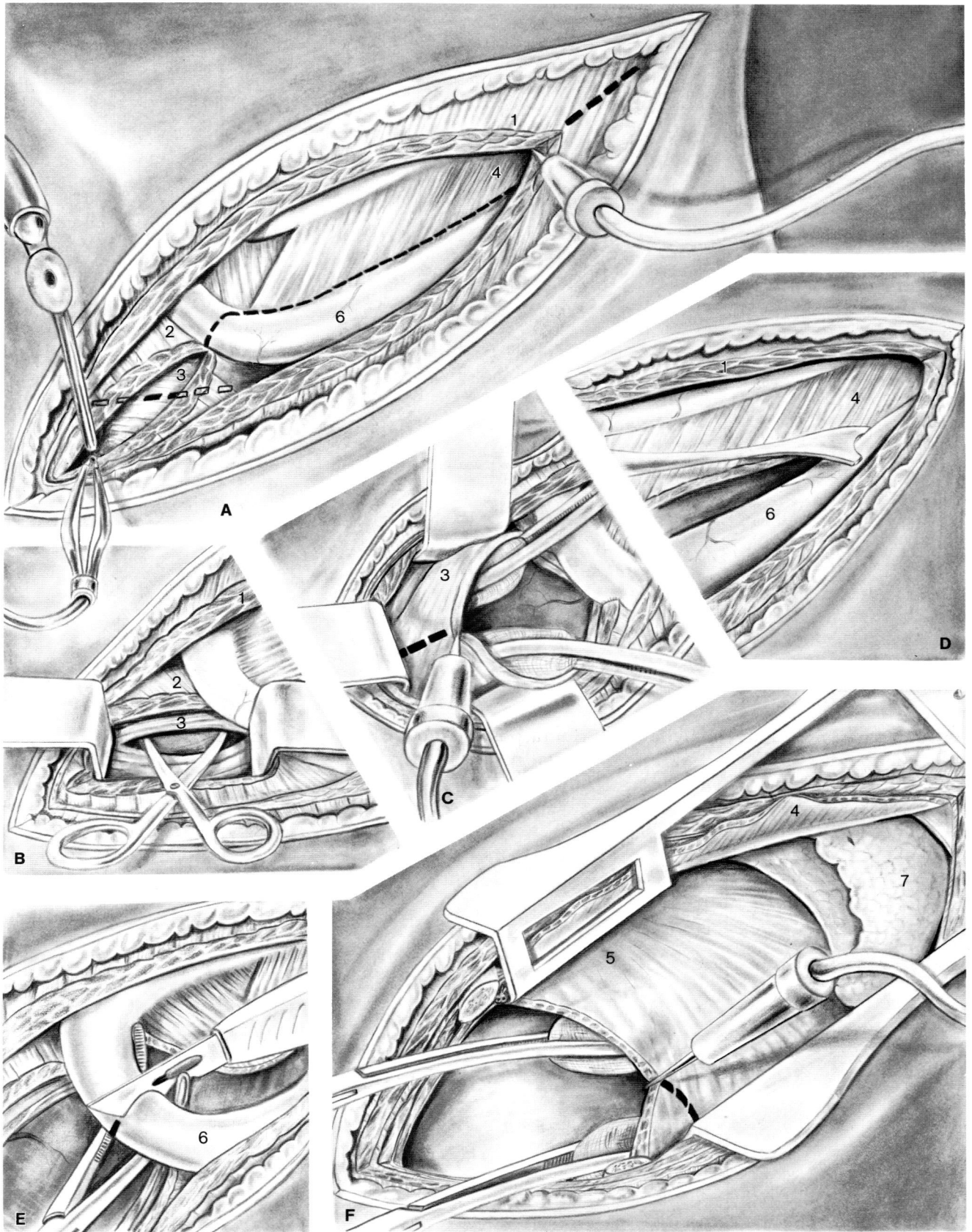

Figure 110 A–F

A Dissection of the superficial layers, comprising the obliquus externus and internus, and preparation of the intercostal section

B Dissection of the transversus muscle and exposure of the peritoneum

C Transection of the transversus muscle

D Disinsertion of the intercostal muscles along the upper margin of the ninth rib

E Section of the common costal cartilage

F Decollement of the peritoneum and progressive transection of the diaphragm

1 m. obliquus externus abdominis *2* m. obliquus internus abdominis
3 m. transversus abdominis *4* mm. intercostales *5* diaphragma
6 costa IX *7* pulmo

(4) Transection of the Diaphragm

Subsequent to anterior parietal dissection, operation is continued by the transection of the peripheral part of the diaphragm up to the aortic hiatus to eliminate the diaphragmatic barrier separating the thoracic and lumboabdominal cavities. As can be demonstrated by examination of the thoracic surface of the diaphragm on anatomical specimens, the preferred site of transection is 10–15 mm from the peripheral costal insertion, as transection in this region avoids the section of the superior and inferior diaphragmatic arteries and the motor branches of the phrenic nerves. Peripheral transection is obviously a more time-consuming procedure than a straight-line transection from the ninth rib through the centrum tendineum to the aortic hiatus, but the latter technique would lead to denervation of part of the posterior diaphragm and would require decollement of the peritoneum in its most adherent part, with the risk of injury to the peritoneum and subsequent protrusion of the intra-abdominal viscera into the operative field. Reconstruction of the peritoneum would also be difficult to achieve due to its thinness in the region of the centrum tendineum. The transection of the diaphragm from the ninth rib to the spine is accomplished by repetition of a series of three maneuvers: retraction of the abdominal viscera, section of the diaphragm, and opening of the orthostatic retractor. Decollement of the lumboabdominal mass is achieved using blunt dissection with clamp-held compresses, working along the deep surface of the peripheral insertions of the diaphragm and quadratus lumborum. As decollement progresses a large flexible retractor is used to displace the abdominal viscera towards the midline, thus clearly exposing the remaining adherent parts of the muscle. Once adequate exposure of the abdominal and thoracic surfaces of the peripheral diaphragmatic insertions has been achieved the diaphragm is transected with the electric cautery knife. Hemostasis of a few bleeding vessels of the cut muscle surface is required as transection is continued. Stay sutures to identify the transected muscle are not necessary and indeed, would complicate the operative field excessively. The operative field can be enlarged by opening the orthostatic retractor. The three maneuvers are then repeated until the transection has reached the region of the posterior crura of the diaphragm. The operator then proceeds to accomplish decollement of the anterior surface of the quadratus lumborum and lateral arcuate ligament. With the large flexible retractor bent over the psoas muscle, the abdominal viscera are dissected free of the muscle to expose the medial arcuate ligament. A second flexible retractor is then used to displace the remaining abdominal viscera upward to lie under the left cupula of the diaphragm. The first assistant has an important and laborious role during this stage of the operation, i.e., to stretch the fibers of the diaphragmatic crura by displacing the viscera toward the midline and upward under the left cupula. Decollement is continued with the clamp-held compresses until the abdominal aorta is felt or brought into view. The viscera lying over the aorta are retracted so that the aorta is constantly exposed, thus avoiding injury to it. The next important step for good transection is identification of the greater splanchnic nerve, which runs transversely anterior to the left crus to join the left semilunar ganglion anterior to the aorta. Transection can then be continued 1.5 cm above the lateral and medial arcuate ligaments to reach the left crus at a point just below the passage of the left greater splanchnic nerve. A needle holder is passed through the costodiaphragmatic sinus to emerge against the lateral surface of the abdominal aorta, allowing isolation of the left crus, which is then retracted and cut using scissors. This opens the aortic hiatus, after which the left cupula of the diaphragm can be completely displaced towards the abdominal mass. The barrier between the left hemithorax and the lumboabdominal region now no longer exists, and the continuity between the thoracic and abdominal parts of the aorta can be seen and palpated. In some cases a vein (hemiazygos root) must be interrupted in contact with the left crus. Hemostasis of this vessel is achieved by either ligation between two clips or electrocoagulation.

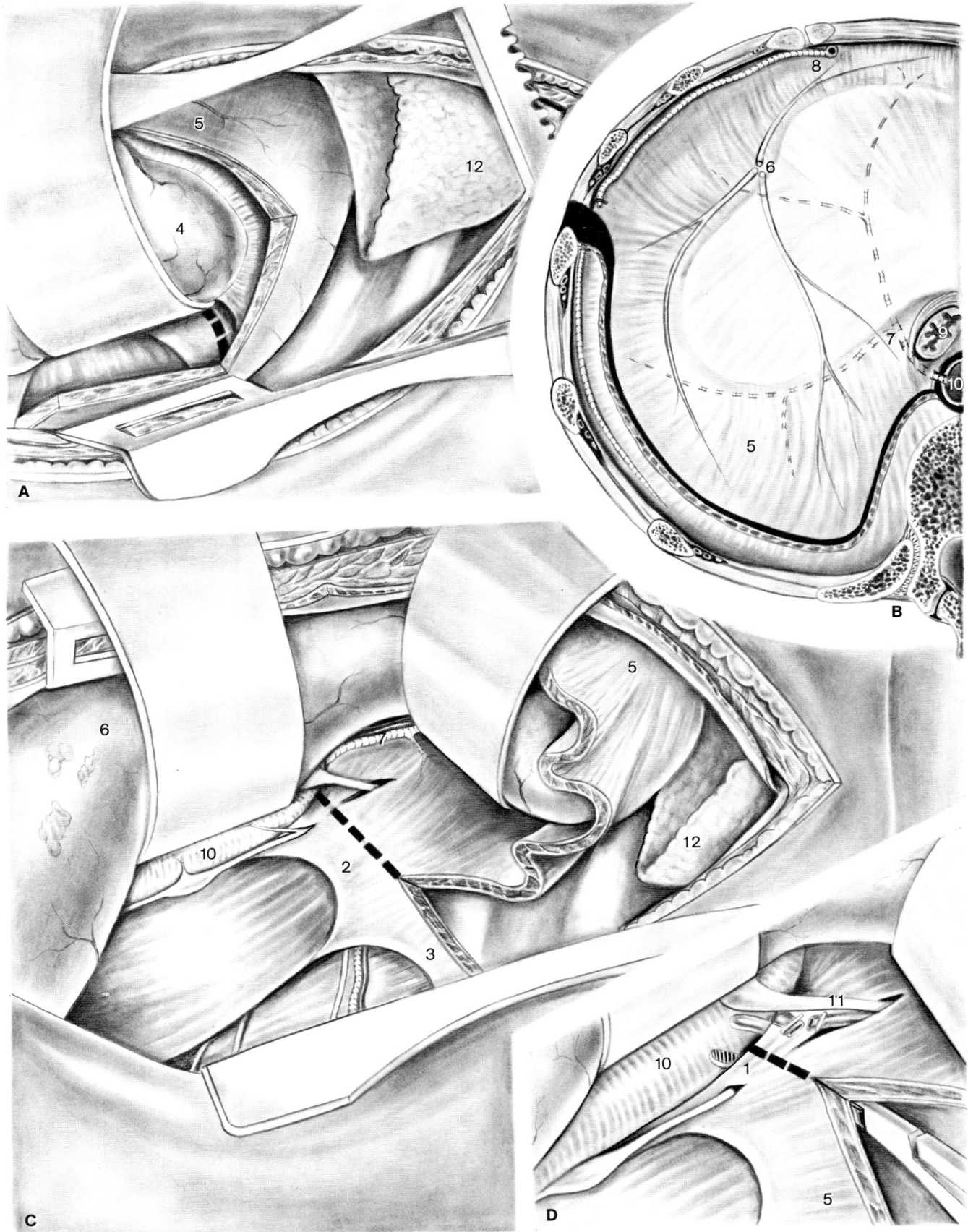

Figure 111 A–D

A   Transection of the lateral lumbar part of the diaphragm

B   Superior aspect of the diaphragm, showing the vascularization and centrifugal innervation from the centrum tendineum toward the periphery. The ideal transection is from a point 1 cm medial to the peripheral margin of the diaphragm to the aortic hiatus

C   Transection of the posterior part of the diaphragm in the region of the lateral crus (ligamenta arcuata mediale and laterale)

D   Transection of the crus sinistrum above the greater splanchnic nerve

1 crus sinistrum   2 lig. arcuatum mediale   3 lig. arcuatum laterale
4 organa abdominis   5 diaphragma   6 n. phrenicus   7 a. phrenica
inf.   8 a. thoracica interna, a. musculophrenica   9 oesophagus
10 aorta   11 n. splanchnicus major sinistrum   12 pulmo

(5) Vascular Sections

Transection of the diaphragm exposes the left anterolateral flank of the thoracolumbar spine, camouflaged by the aorta, the mediastinal pleura, and the collateral intercostal and lumbar vessels. Exposure of the spine requires that the aorta be mobilized by the section of one or several collateral vascular bundles. The procedure begins with sectioning the mediastinal pleura along the left lateral margin of the aorta to expose the lowest intercostal vessels. Blunt dissection is employed along the left anterolateral flank of the spine while the thoracoabdominal aorta is displaced slightly towards the midline with flexible retractors (manipulated by the assistant). This exposes the collateral vessels, lying mainly in the middle gutter of the vertebral bodies except the origin of the hemiazygos vein, which runs upward along the flank of the spine. At this stage a metal tag should be attached to allow precise identification of spinal level under the image intensifier. The vertebrae to be exposed and consequently the vessels to be interrupted are selected according to the site of the spinal lesion(s). The site of choice to interrupt the collateral vessels is the point where they change direction, i.e., between the anterior and left lateral surfaces of the vertebral bodies. When the vessels are ligated in this region, the remaining vascular stump arising from the aorta is of sufficient length to allow religation if the initial suture gives way. Furthermore, ligation at this point is sufficiently distant from the intervertebral foramina not to alter the spinal system of arterial anastomoses. Ligation can be achieved using metal clips or suture material, but in either case the vascular bundle or the artery and vein separately must be isolated by passing a long, slender, curved needle holder under the vessels. The suture material is then placed on each side of the arms of the needle holder or the clips placed on the vessels, and the section is made between two sufficiently spaced ligatures (5–10 mm apart). In the region of the left crus, which is frequently traversed by the lumbar vessels, ligation and section should be done on each side of the crus. Postoperative hemorrhage can be avoided by precisely placed ligatures and tight clips.

(6) Exposure of the Vertebral Bodies

Once the collateral vessels have been sectioned, displacement of the major prevertebral vascular structures (aorta and vena cava) is relatively easy to accomplish with a flexible retractor slightly bent to mold over the aorta. The assistant uses his retractor to lift the aorta slightly, thus creating a space between the aorta and the anterior surface of the vertebral bodies. A long, slightly curved large periosteal rasp is then used to displace all the soft tissue structures lying over the anterior longitudinal ligament towards the posterior wall of the aorta and vena cava until the instrument is brought in contact with the right surface of the spine. The raspatory should not be manipulated with force, since the connective tissue in this region is rather loose. Furthermore, forceful manipulation can lead to the instrument slipping and injuring the posterior surface of the inferior vena cava, so instrumental manipulation must be strictly controlled. Finally, clear exposure of the spine is accomplished be remodeling the flexible retractor to form an S shape, the distal part applied to the right lateral surface of the spine and the proximal part supporting the mass of abdominal viscera.

The above procedures apply to cases of noninflammatory lesions. The approach to a region of osteoarthritis accompanied by fibroconjunctive tissue covering the anterior surface of the spine requires a different technique. Indeed, in such cases visual identification of the intercostal and lumbar vascular bundles is practically impossible. The first step under these conditions is to incise the fibrous shell a few millimeters from the left margin of the aorta. The incision should be made in direct contact with the hard bony surface of the spine well in front of the intervertebral foramina. The electric cautery knife is used to cut through the full thickness of the fibrous shell, working along the full length of the lesion. Progressive occurrence of hemorrhage demonstrates the presence of a collateral vessel, and temporary hemostasis is achieved by placing a hemostat on each side of the cut fibrous lesion. Permanent hemostasis is then obtained by coagulation using the hemostat or by installing a suture around the tip of the clamp. Once the fibrous shell has been completely incised and full hemostasis achieved, a large periosteal rasp is used in contact with the bone to separate the soft tissue structures from the spinal bone and discs without attempting to identify the anterior longitudinal ligament.

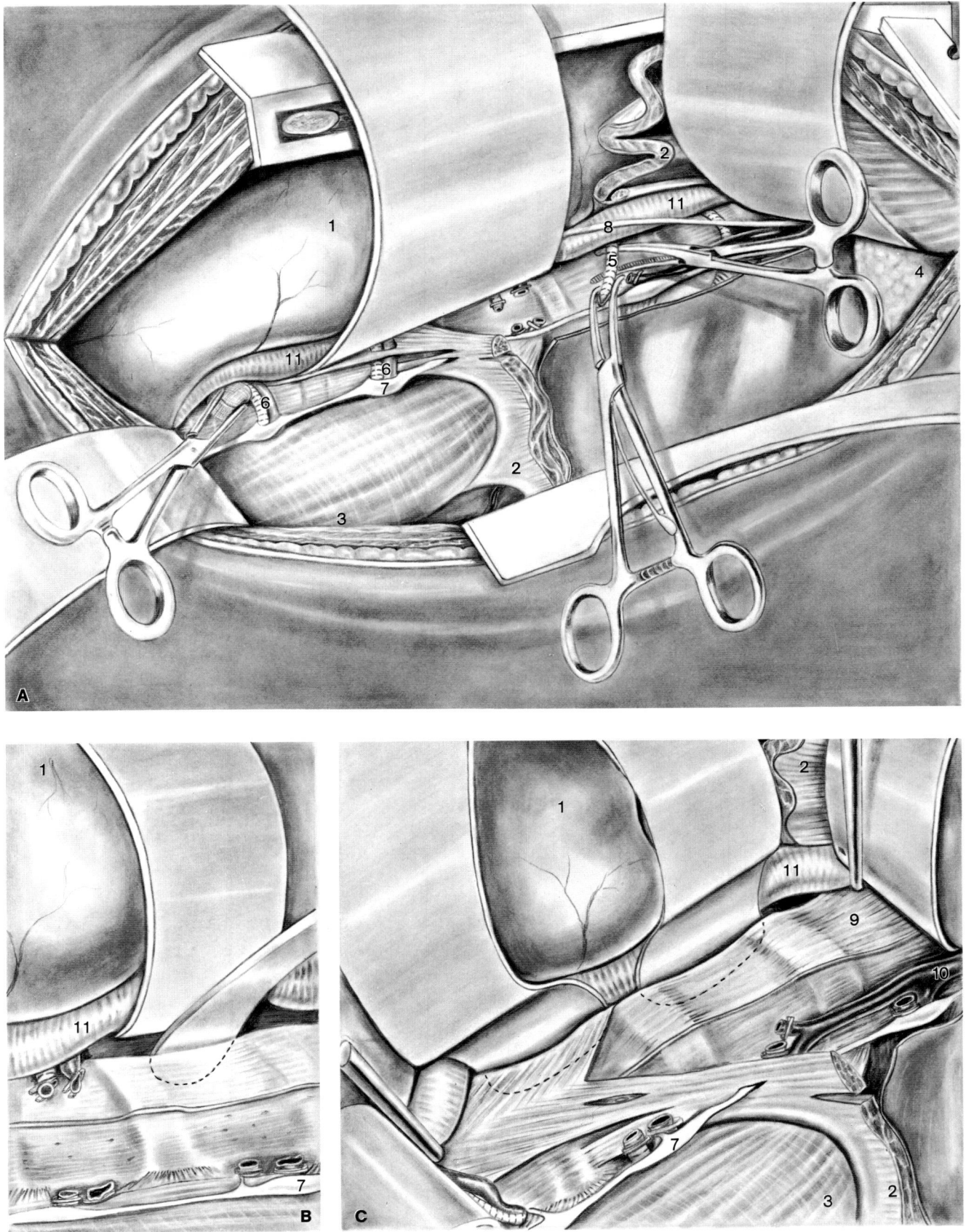

Figure 112 A–C

A Hemostasis of the parietal collateral vessels
B Exposure of the anterior and lateral surfaces of the spine
C Position of the flexible retractors to expose the spine

1 organa abdominis 2 diaphragma 3 psoas 4 pulmo 5 a. inter-costalis 6 a. and v. lumbales 7 truncus sympathicus 8 n. splanchni-cus major 9 lig. longitudinale ant. 10 v. hemiazygos 11 aorta

(7) Closure

Parietal closure begins with the reconstruction of the diaphragmatic insertion in the region of the left cupula. The two
ends of the left crus are identified and then approximated by
a figure-of-eight suture with nonresorbable monofilament using a curved needle with a round cross-section. The operator
should check that the reconstructed aortic hiatus is neither
stenotic nor too loose. The free lip of the diaphragm is then
presented anterior to the fixed lip (near the arcuate ligaments). Care should be taken to ensure that the assistant presents the two lips of the diaphragm correctly with the flexible
retractors. Nonresorbable monofilament is used to close the
diaphragm with interrupted sutures. It must be checked that
the needle also passes through the pleura lining the diaphragm, since the pleura affords solidity to the muscle. The
sutures are tied off on the abdominal side of the diaphragm.
Approximation of the diaphragm is pursued towards the lateral wall of the trunk. Next, release of the abdominal mass
leads to progressive "reinflation" of the diaphragmatic cupula, allowing proper alignment of the lips of the diaphragm in
the region of the anterior third of the cupula. The interrupted
sutures in this region are now knotted on the thoracic side of
the diaphragm. As closure progressively approaches the anterior end of the eighth and ninth ribs the orthostatic retractor is
relaxed to allow approximation of the final centimeter of diaphragm. Finally, the retractor is removed and the costal cartilage reconstructed by a transfixing figure-of-eight suture to
approach the cut edges exactly. Cartilaginous suture is highly
effective, as it leads to definitive consolidation in the proper
position. An everting suture should be avoided, since it can
lead to a rather unaesthetic ridge under the skin.

Two firm 8–10 mm diameter thoracic drains are then installed. One should exit through the tenth or eleventh intercostal space at the level of the posterior axillary line, to evacuate fluid, the other through the anterior part of the fourth or
fifth intercostal space, to allow evacuation of air from the
thoracic cavity. The intercostal space is then closed by two or
three full-thickness sutures running on each side of and perpendicular to the eighth and ninth ribs. Once the intercostal
sutures are tightened the intercostal muscles are practically in
contact with the ninth rib, thus obviating their fixation with
special sutures. The next step is to close the abdominal wall
with interrupted sutures of the transversus and obliquus internus muscles. The obliquus externus is closed as a separate
layer, using a continuous suture to obtain a tight seal. The
subcutaneous layer is approximated with a second hermetic
continuous suture, and finally skin closure is achieved with a
continuous suture. The anesthesiologist then applies positive
ventilatory pressure to reinflate the left lung and evacuate
most of the fluid and residual air in the thoracic cavity. The
drains are clamped and connected by a Y tube.

(8) Possible Complications

Dilaceration of the peritoneum with protrusion of the abdominal viscera in the operative field may occur when dissection is overforceful or poorly directed i.e., toward the diaphragmatic cupula rather than the lumbar region. The peritoneal wound can be closed by a continuous suture. Another
possible problem is difficulty in identifying the aortic hiatus
to allow transection of the left crus. The correct landmark to
allow identification is obviously the abdominal aorta, followed by the left splanchnic nerve lying above the left crus. In
case of difficulty the mediastinal pleura can be opened to allow identification of the hiatus from above. Hemostasis during surgery may be problematic. Untoward hemorrhage of a
vessel should be arrested immediately by finger pressure, followed by a warm moist compress. The vessel should then be
exposed slowly, and finally clamped with a hemostat. Injury
to a major blood vessel results from overaggressive maneuvers, which must be avoided. Nevertheless, hemostatic
clamps should be included among the instruments used in
thoracophrenolumbotomy. Injury to a large blood vessel
should be repaired by small interrupted sutures. Problems in
the identification of the spinal lesions can be avoided only by
systematic preoperative roentgenograms. Insufficient exposure of the vertebral bodies can be remedied by full dissection
anterior to the anterior longitudinal ligament in the absence
of inflammatory lesions of the spine, but when such lesions
are present dissection must be carried out in direct contact
with the vertebral bone. Proper use of the counterangled flexible retractors subsequent to freeing of the right flank of the
spine allows clear exposure. When difficulties are encountered in reconstructing the diaphragm, the operator should
painstakingly identify the lips of the transected diaphragm
and then check that they are properly aligned by manual testing. Postoperative pleuropulmonary complications can be
avoided by maintaning constant mild suction (50 cm H_2O) on
the thoracic drains for at least four days postoperatively. The
left lung should be properly inflated at the end of operation:
monitoring by auscultation and chest X-ray detects any residual or persistent collection of air or fluid. Roentgenographic
signs of partial or total atelectasis may indicate the presence
of bronchial obstruction, which should be remedied.

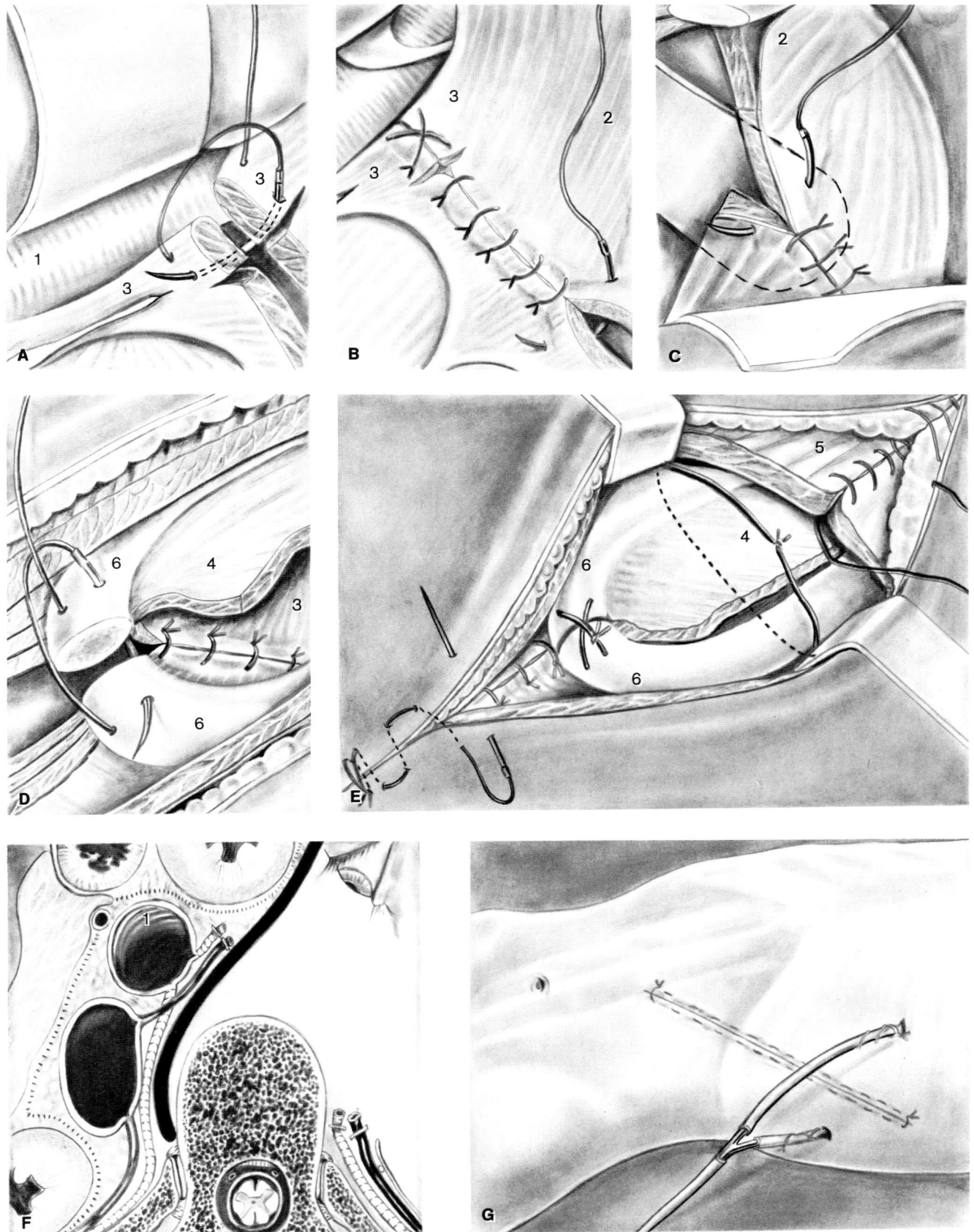

Figure 113 A–G

A   Suture of the crus sinistrum
B   Suture of the lateral arcuate ligament
C   Suture of the lateral and anterior part of the diaphragm
D   Reconstruction of the costal cartilage
E   Parietal closure

F   Horizontal section through T12 to show the operative field of vision
G   Skin closure and thoracic drainage

1 aorta   *2* diaphragma   *3* crus sinistrum   *4* mm. intercostales
5 m. obliquus externus abdominis   *6* costa, cartilago costalis

b) Left Lateral Thoracolumbotomy

In cases where the patient must be operated on in the lateral position (scoliosis) a more lateral approach can be used straddling the thoracic and anterolateral abdominal walls. This approach is similar to that described by Hodgson (1956).

(1) Operative Position

Access to the left flank of the spine is gained with the patient in the right lateral position. The pelvis is held in place by a pad supporting the sacrum and the pubis. The right lower limb is flexed to a 90° angle at the knee under the overlying extended left limb, and the lower limbs are held in place with a self-adhesive strap over the thighs. The right upper limb is elevated by a cushion placed under the axilla to allow proper flow of intravenous fluids. The left upper limb may be left to lie free over the thorax or attached to an upright support. The head should rest on a small cushion. Elevation of the right flank of the spine is not desirable if arthrodesis is to be performed.

(2) Skin Incision

The most commonly used incision runs along the tenth intercostal space and extends in the same direction onto the anterolateral wall of the abdomen. The tip of the eleventh rib should thus be identified and the incision made above this point. The incision can be extended at either end: upward along the lateral margin of the spinal muscles toward the lower thoracic wall, to approach the thoracic vertebrae; or downward obliquely toward the lateral margin of the rectus abdominis in the subumbilical region, to approach the lower lumbar vertebrae.

(3) Parietal Dissection

After incision of the skin and subcutaneous tissue the electric cautery knife is used to transect the obliquus externus abdominis and then the latissimus dorsi above the eleventh rib. The second muscle layer to be transected is that of the obliquus internus abdominis and the serratus posterior inferior. The third layer comprises the transversus abdominis and its aponeurosis, which must be transected cautiously so as not to open the peritoneal envelope lying immediately deep to the muscle. The more posterior intercostal muscles are disinserted from the upper margin of the eleventh rib using a raspatory, with hemostasis of the cut muscular surfaces. The direction of the incision normally obviates the section of an intercostal vascular bundle. The next step is to resect the eleventh rib by first sectioning its anterior end, leaving in place 1 cm of bone adherent to the abdominal muscles and diaphragm, then rasping along its deep surface and lower margin out to the level of the spinal muscles, where it is sectioned. This procedure largely opens the pleural cavity. The left lung is retracted and protected by a moist compress. The peritoneal envelope is dissected free of the lateral and posterior abdominal wall using clamp-held compresses, while the assistant retracts the abdominal mass forward and medially with a large flexible retractor. In cases where the operative field is enlarged towards the thoracic wall, one or two additional ribs are sectioned anterior to the costotransverse joints. With this approach the intercostal muscles and neurovascular structures are left intact, although their presence slightly hinders operation.

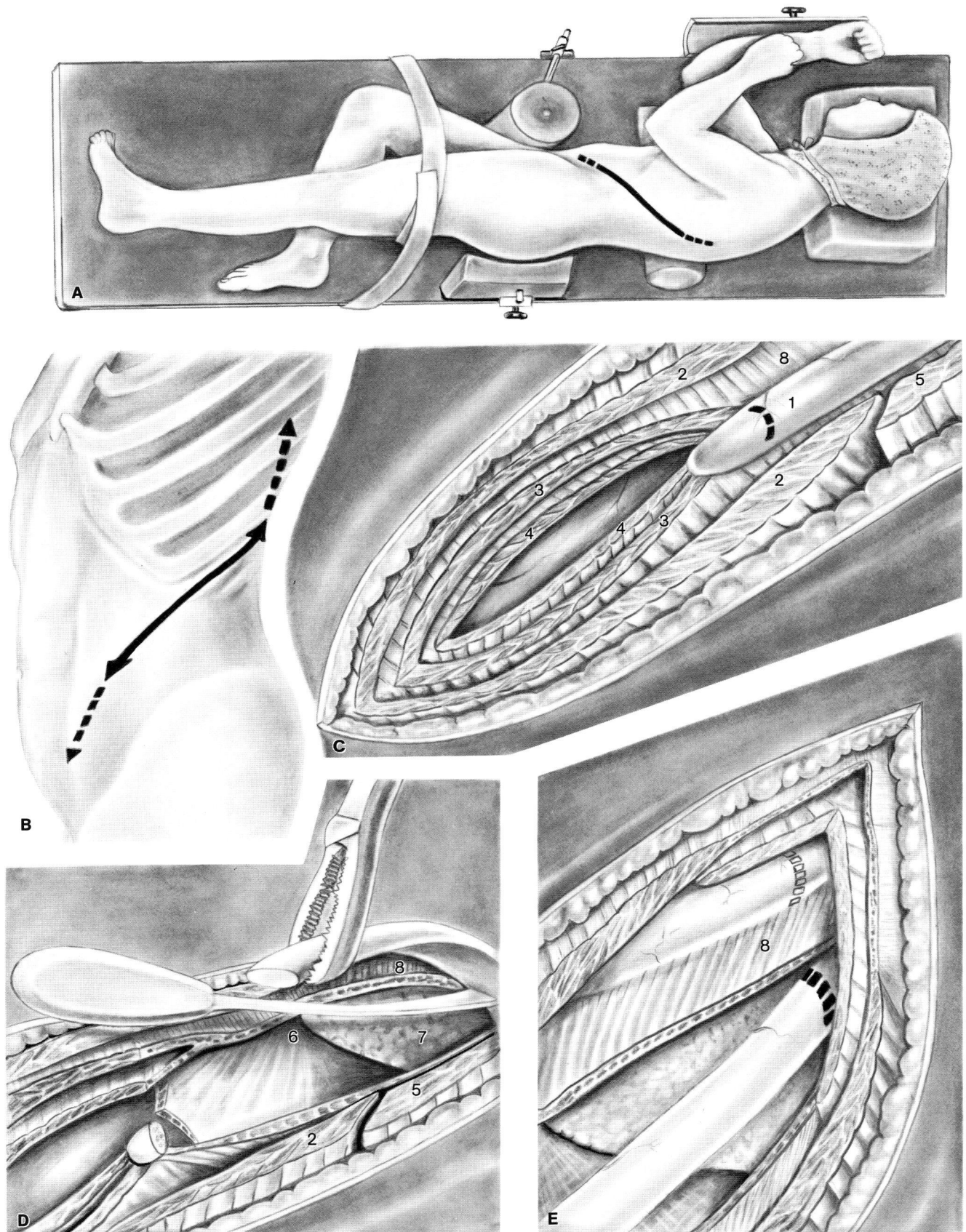

Figure 114 A–E

A   Overhead view of the operative position in left lateral thoraco-
lumbotomy

B   Skin incision and possible extension towards the thorax and abdomen

C   Parietal dissection

D   Exposure of the twelfth rib

E   Section of the posterior angle of the twelfth rib and occasionally the
eleventh rib

1 costa XII *2* m. obliquus externus abdominis *3* m. obliquus internus abdominis *4* m. transversus *5* m. latissimus dorsi *6* diaphragma *7* pulmo *8* mm. intercostales

(4) Disinsertion of the Diaphragm

With this approach the diaphragm is not regularly transected at some distance from its posterior insertions, but rather is disinserted from the remaining points of support, i.e., the tip of the twelfth rib, the ligamentous insertion on the transverse process of L1, and the crus sinistrum. The arcuate ligaments are thus detached from the posterior wall. To expose these points of disinsertion clearly the retroperitoneal fat must be completely freed by blunt dissection. This procedure is started at the quadratus lumborum and the subcostal (twelfth intercostal) bundle, proceeding to the bulky psoas and finally the left lateral wall of the spine, where the beating of the abdominal aorta can be felt. Manipulation of the clamp-held compresses between the abdominal aorta and the spine enables identification of the crus sinistrum and the neighboring lumbar sympathetic trunk and left splanchnic nerve. The crus is isolated by passing a needle holder under it from the psoas muscle to the left lateral margin of the aorta, and sectioned using scissors. After disinsertion the diaphragm can be retracted upward toward the thoracic cavity.

(5) Vascular Ligation

Exposure of the left flank of the spine requires the identification of the lesions to be treated and the vascular bundles to be sectioned. The lesions are identified radiologically, using a metal tag as a landmark. The intercostal and lumbar vascular bundles are found on the depressed middle part of the vertebral bodies halfway between the intervertebral discs, and are first clearly exposed by blunt dissection with the clamp-held compresses. Each bundle is then isolated on a needle holder and sectioned, between two ligatures or clips, at a point halfway between the aorta and intervertebral foramina. The first lumbar vascular bundle often runs through the crus sinistrum, and accordingly hemostasis must be effected on each side of the crus. It is not necessary to seek out the ascending lumbar vein lying in front of the intervertebral foramina. The left hemiazygos vein can usually be conserved by ligating the arteries lying anterior to it, but in some cases the medial root of the hemiazygos must be sectioned when it runs over the crus sinistrum and the lateral surface of the aorta.

(6) Exposure of the Spine

A large periosteal rasp is used to expose the left lateral and anterior surfaces of the spine. Rasping is started near the flank of the spine to disinsert the psoas arches without, however, fully reaching the intervertebral foramina, as rasping in this zone carries the risk of injury to the venous plexuses, the spinal nerve roots, and expecially the medullary arterial anastomotic system. Rasping then proceeds to the anterior surface of the spine while the assistant lifts the aorta very slightly with a flexible retractor. Work should be anterior to the anterior longitudinal ligament except in cases of inflammatory lesions. In cases where a shell of fibrous tissue is present, the correct plane of incision lies in direct contact with the bone,

i.e., deep to the anterior longitudinal ligament, which is practically free due to the inflammation. A counterangled flexible retractor (bent to form an S) is installed to hook onto the anterior surface of the spine and extend over to the beginning of the contralateral right surface of the spine. This lateral approach allows good visualization of only the left side of the spine, mediocre exposure of the anterior surface, and no access whatsoever to the right side of the spine. Opening of the vertebral canal can be achieved only by the lateral route in front of the intervertebral foramina, median access being impossible. It should be noted that when the initial incision is extended downward this approach allows access to L4 and even the left flank of L5. The operator should bear in mind that the ureter runs along the posterior surface of the peritoneum and should thus check that it is displaced along with the peritoneum when the latter is dissected free. In the lower operative field the arch of the inferior epigastric artery may cause obstruction between the obliquus internus and the transversus, in which case the artery should be solidly ligated and divided. Finally, the left common iliac artery and vein are in contact with L4, and should be mobilized subsequent to the ligation of a lumbar vascular bundle.

(7) Closure

Closure is begun by the reinsertion of the posterior diaphragmatic crura. The diaphragm is reinserted on the crus sinistrum, the transverse process of L1, and the tip of the twelfth and eleventh ribs with a nonresorbable figure-of-eight suture and a round needle. A few sutures are required to approximate the distended muscle fibers between the tenth rib and the tip of the eleventh. After installing one or two thoracic drains in the pleural cavity the different muscle layers are closed. Suction drainage can be installed in the lumbar region when perfect hemostasis has not been obtained. The bed of the resected eleventh rib can be closed by a continuous suture of the intercostal muscles initially lying on either side of the rib. The other muscle layers require closure by interupted sutures, since continuous sutures in the abdominal region may lead to muscle tearing when abdominal distension occurs postoperatively. The transversus, serratus posterior inferior, obliquus internus, obliquus externus, and latissimus dorsi are thus approximated in this way. The subcutaneous layer and skin should also be closed with interrupted sutures, giving greater elasticity than continuous closure.

Postoperative care and possible complications are identical to those described in the section on left thoracophrenolumbotomy.

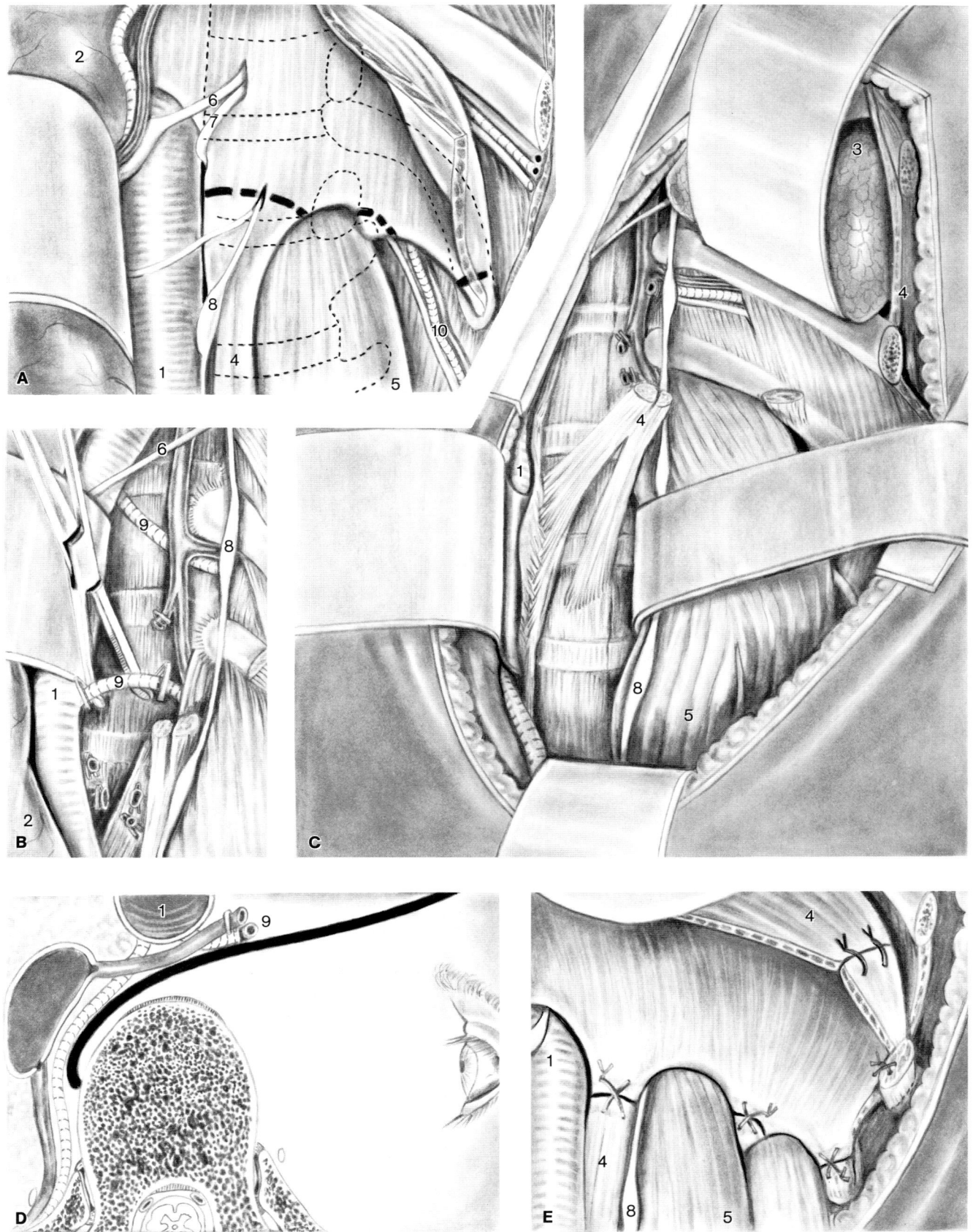

Figure 115 A–E

A Section of the ligamenta arcuata mediale and laterale and the crus sinistrum
B Hemostasis of the parietal collateral vessels
C Exposure of the left anterolateral surface of the spine
D The operative field of vision

E Reinsertion of the diaphragm and parietal closure

1 aorta *2* organa abdominis *3* pulmo *4* crus sinistrum *5* psoas *6* n. splanchnicus major *7* n. splanchnicus minor *8* truncus sympathicus *9* a., v., and n. intercostales *10* a., v., and n. subcostales

3 Lumbosacral Spine

I. Posterior Region

A. Topography

The lumbosacral region is bounded above by the spinous process of T12 and the twelfth rib, and below by the posterior iliac crest, the upper margin of the gluteal muscles, and the coccyx. Described below are the different layers penetrated to gain access to the posterior lumbosacral region.

1. Cutaneous and Subcutaneous Layers

The skin of the back is thick, mobile, and often bears hair. Various underlying structures are distinguishable, including on the midline the depressed region, corresponding to the spinous processes and the sacral crest, which continues into the intergluteal fold. In relatively muscular subjects the spinal muscles are easily palpable on each side of the midline. Lateral to the spinal muscles the flanks of the lumbar region extend down to the iliac crest and the neighboring large gluteal masses. The posterosuperior iliac spines can be deeply palpated as two fossettes and represent essential landmarks for the identification of the lumbar vertebrae. The horizontal line joining the fossettes transects the L5–S1 interspinous space.

2. Fascial Layer

The thoracolumbar fascia appears as a thick, shiny, white, resistant, and stretched sheet lying deep to the more or less thick fat pad in the lumbosacral region. The fascia adheres to the tip of the spinous processes and sacral crest on the midline and the iliac crests laterally. It blends above with the fleshy muscle bodies of the latissimus dorsi and below with the gluteal muscles and their fascia. It should be preserved and correctly reconstructed during surgery, as a surgical defect is practically impossible to repair owing to its lack of extensibility. Furthermore, proper reinsertion of the fascia on the spinous processes reestablishes normal lumbosacral morphology and ensures the resistance of the erector spinae muscles to effort. Finally, the correct repositioning of the fascia applies pressure to the muscles of the vertebral gutters, thus aiding the maintenance of postoperative hemostasis.

3. Erector Spinae Muscles

The erector spinae muscles completely fill the vertebral gutters on each side of the spinous processes and sacral crest down to the iliac tuberosities and out to the vertebral arches. One special feature of these muscles is that they are formed by overlapping bands, which thus create practically sagittal interstices. As opposed to the muscles of the appendicular skeleton, whose ends are attached to the bone but whose bodies can slide over the bone, the spinal muscles insert as a continuous sheet on the bony and fibrous structures of the vertebral gutters. Accordingly, there is no plane of incision against the bone to allow mobilization of these muscles without their disinsertion. Postoperatively, the spinal muscles must reconstitute their normal insertions, at the price of a temporary period of postoperative muscle fragility. Beginning on the midline and extending laterally, five muscle groups can be described. The interspinalis thoracis and lumborum lie between the spinous processes. The spinalis thoracis and lumborum originate at L2 and extend cranially to insert on the flanks of the spinous processes. The transversospinalis is formed of numerous bands originating on the transverse processes and inserting on the spinous processes. The lower origin of the transversospinalis group is the tubercle of the sacrum. The longissimus lumborum and thoracis muscles extend upwards from the mass of the spinal muscles to insert on the transverse processes and posterior angles of the ribs. Finally, the iliocostalis lumborum and thoracis originate from the mass of spinal muscles and the iliac crest and insert on the posterior angles of the ribs. Anterior to the erector muscles, the intertransversarii and quadratus lumborum form a boundary separating the posterior from the anterior lumbosacral region.

4. Vertebral Arches and Interlaminar Spaces

This osteoligamentous region comprises the sacral and lumbar vertebral arches with the interlaminar and intertransverse spaces intervening between the mobile segments. These spaces are absent in the sacral region, except in cases of lumbalization of the sacrum. The possible presence of spine bifida creating a fibrous space should also be kept in mind, since in such cases the surgical approach could lead to injury of the lumbosacral canal. The sacral groove, allowing identification of the sacrum, is a continuous structure lacking interlaminar spaces, slanting very obliquely forward in its cranial region and totally lacking mobility when traction is applied to the sacral crest. Conversely, the vertebral laminae are regularly interrupted by the interlaminar spaces and can be mobilized by manipulating the spinous processes. The presence or absence of mobility permits identification of the various bony structures in this region if the possible existence of a transitional anomaly is not overlooked. The bulky zygapophyseal (posterior) articulations lie lateral to the interlaminar spaces. The interface of these cartilage-lined joints, corresponding to that seen on X-ray, can be identified only by using a sharp instrument subsequent to mobilization of the spinous processes. The depressed areas between the zygapophyseal articulations correspond to the isthmic regions and the region of passage of the dorsal neurovascular bundles. This zone must be respected during disinsertion of the muscles by avoiding work extending beyond the lateral margin of the isthmic regions. As with the vertebral bodies, the depressed regions of the posterior arches contain the dorsal neurovascular bundles. This region of passage in the lumbar spine, sometimes referred to as the posterior intervertebral foramen, corresponds to the posterior sacral foramen at the level of the sacral spine. An intertransverse ligament separates the medial and lateral branches of the dorsal nerves. Some branches run along the posterior surface of the laminae and zygapophyseal joints. Injury to these nerve fibers can be avoided by working in very close contact with the bone during muscle disinsertion.

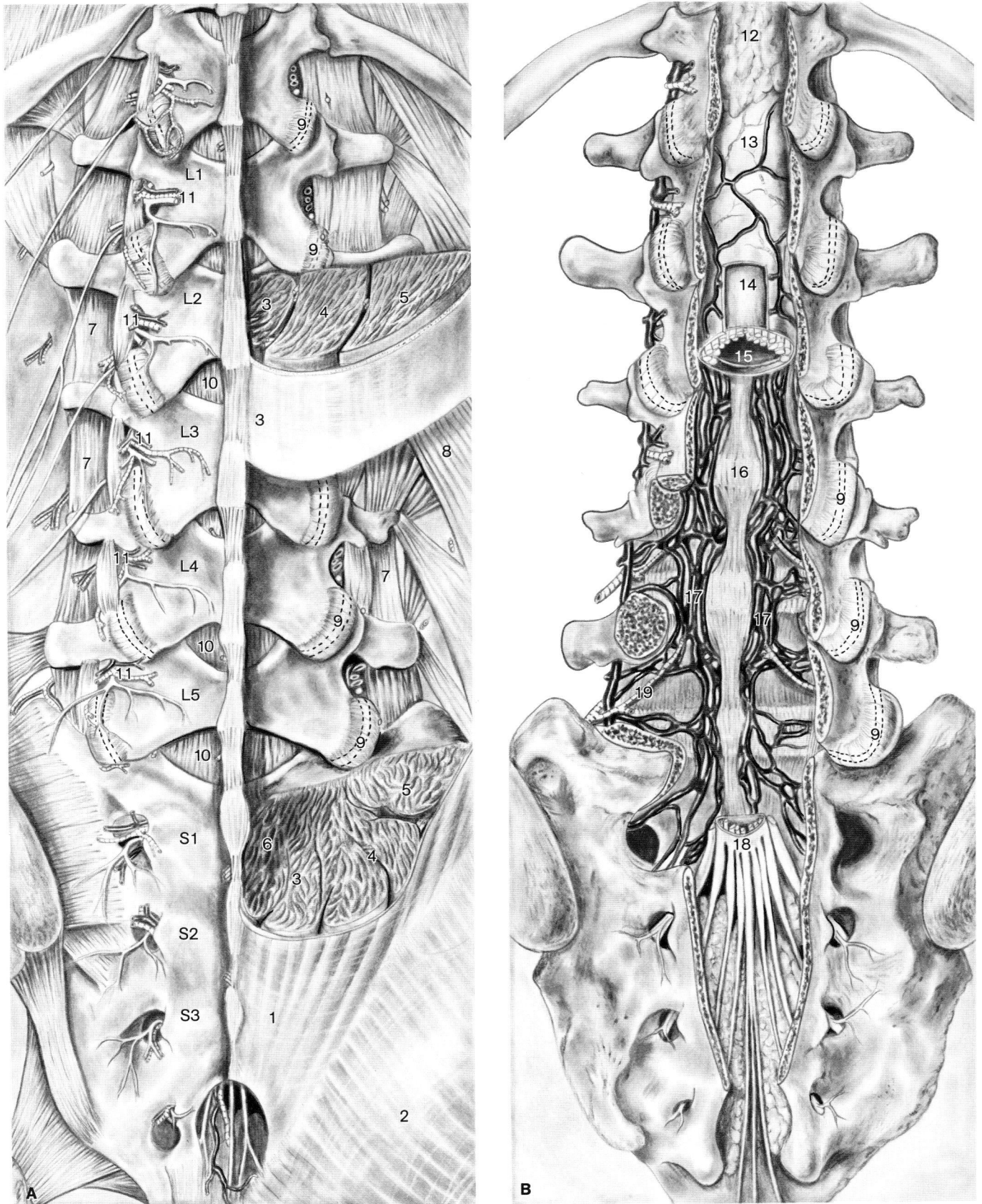

Figure 116 A, B

A   Posterior superficial aspect of the lumbosacral spine
B   Deep structures of the posterior lumbosacral spine after lower left
    laminectomy and foraminotomy

1 fascia thoracolumbalis   2 fascia glutea   3 m. spinalis thoracis
4 m. longissimus thoracis   5 m. iliocostalis thoracis and lumborum
6 mm. multifidi   7 mm. intertransversarii laterales lumborum

8 m. quadratus lumborum   9 juncturae zygapophyseales, capsula
articularis   10 lig. flavum   11 rami dorsales   12 corpus adiposum
cavi epiduralis   13 duramater spinalis   14 arachnoidea spinalis
15 cavum subarachnoideale, radices n. spinalium   16 lig. longitudinale
post.   17 plexus venosus vertebralis internus   18 fundus durae matris
spinalis, pes anterius   19 ramus anteriosus spinalis

5. Vertebral Canal and Intervertebral Foramina

The vertebral canal and the intervertebral foramina contain the spinal nerves with their sheaths and their associated vessels. Resection of the vertebral arches exposes the median region of the vertebral canal, which widens progessively in the caudal direction down to the level of the L5–S1 intervertebral disc, and then narrows again from the sacrum downward to open at the sacral hiatus near S4. The vertebral canal communicates laterally with the intervertebral foramina at the level of each intervertebral space and with the sacral foramina. The most superficial part of the lumbosacral canal contains the epidural fat, traversed by a few very small blood vessels. Displacement of the epidural fat exposes almost the full length of the dural envelope, which tapers down to its termination at the level of S1 or S2. The space containing the fat surrounding the dural envelope and spinal nerve roots is known as the epidural space, and can be used to allow surgical dissection or to administer anesthetic (epidural anesthesia) or contrast material (epidurography). Opening of the dura mater on the midline exposes the subdural space lying between the spinal dura mater and the transparent arachnoidea, which bulges outward due to the CSF pressure. Opening of the arachnoidea leads to leakage of CSF and allows direct visualization of the paired sensory and motor spinal nerve roots. These nerve roots, fanning out to form the cauda equina, can be followed visually to their point of dural penetration. It should be noted that the sensory roots are posterior to the motor ones; this allows easy identification when sensory radicotomy is to be performed. The roots of the cauda equina are not arranged in random fashion, but rather lie in a coronal plane with marked anterior concavity. At the conic termination of the dural envelope the emergence of the various sacral nerve roots resembles the foot of a goose. Anterior to the dural envelope, the posterior longitudinal ligament and the anterolateral intraspinal venous plexuses can be seen to run over the posterior and lateral surfaces of the vertebral bodies and intervertebral discs. In addition to the spinal nerves, the intervertebral foramina contain the veins, specially large where they lie in contact with the pedicles, and the spinal arteries, which accompany each spinal nerve to reach the cauda equina and finally the lumbosacral spinal cord. The intervertebral foramina are limited posteriorly by the zygapophyseal joints, so that liberation of the foramina leads to suppression of the articular facets of the corresponding joint (foraminotomy).

6. Vertebroradicular and Vertebromedullary Topography

In our experience the spinal cord terminates just above or below the L1–L2 intervertebral disc in 75% of cases. In certain exceptional cases spinal cord termination was observed at the level of L4, and in one case at S4. The termination of the dural envelope is also variable; from the S1–S2 disc to the S3–S4 disc. The association of spinal cord and dural envelope terminations permits description of two common types, the L1–S1 and L2–S2 terminations.

L1–S1 Termination. In this case the conus medullaris terminates posterior to the body of L1 above the level of the L1–L2 intervertebral disc. Nerve roots L1 and L2 traverse the dura mater at the level of the middle of the numerically corresponding vertebral bodies. The L3 root traverses the dura mater at the upper third of the body of L3, the L4 root at the upper quarter of L4, the L5 root at the upper fifth of L5, and the S1 root at the upper margin of or a few millimeters cranial to the L5–S1 disc.

L2–S2 Termination. In this type of termination the conus medullaris lies at the level of the L1–L2 intervertebral disc and the upper half of the body of L2. Nerve roots L1, L2, and L3 traverse the dura mater at the level of the middle of the numerically corresponding vertebral bodies. The L4 root emerges through the dura mater at the upper third of L4, the L5 root at the level of the upper quarter of L5, and the S1 root at the lower margin of the L5–S1 disc.

The spinal roots and nerves lie diagonally in the intervertebral foramina and run between the medial surface of the upper vertebral pedicle and the lateral surface of the lower pedicle. Neural and osseous topography, based on the identification of the vertebral arches, can be determined using the geometric projection of the intervertebral discs on the arches, i.e., the cranial half of the zygapophyseal joint lies at the level of the disc.

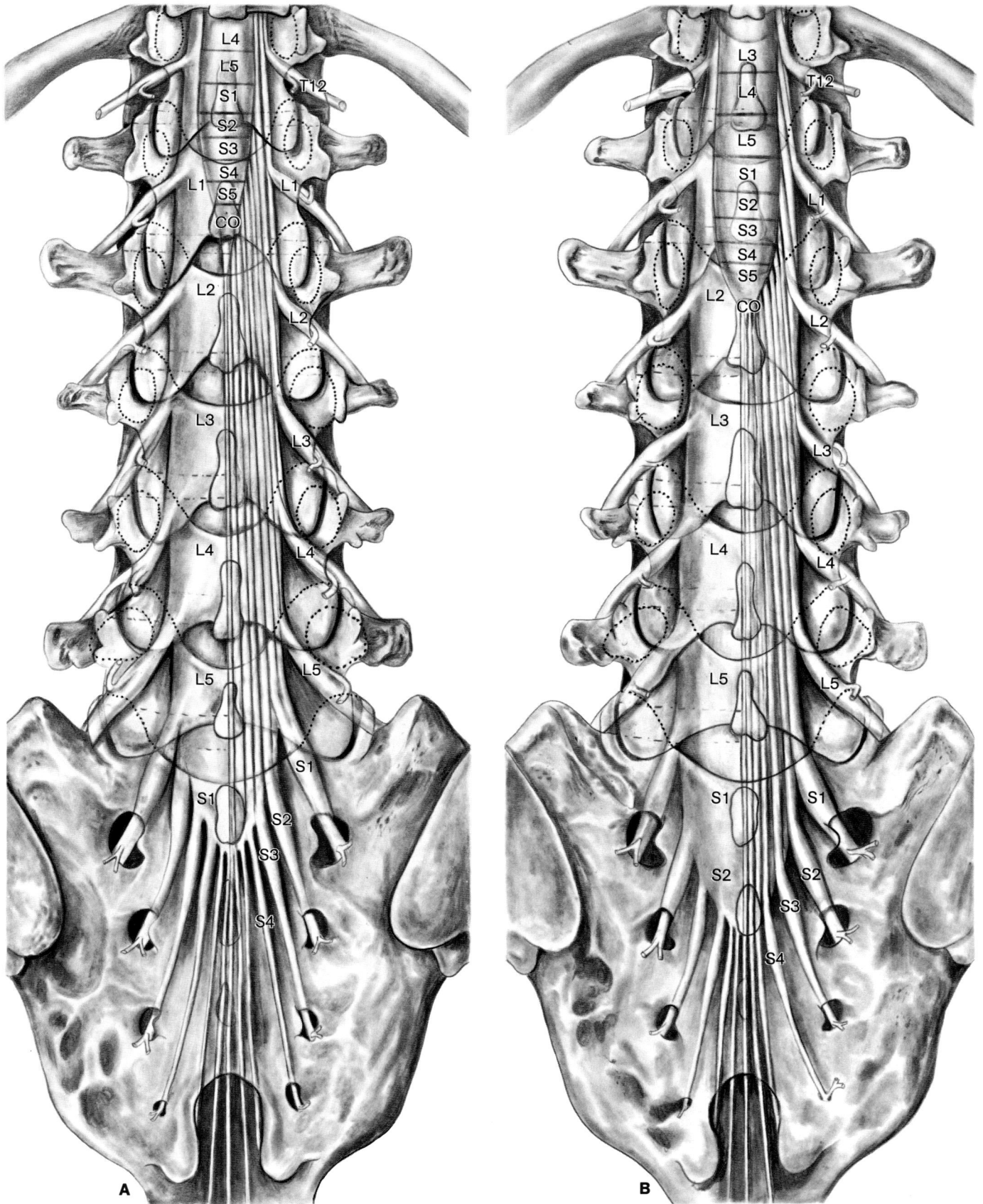

Figure 117 A, B

A Posterior view of the vertebromedullary and vertebroradicular relations as seen by transparency in the L1–S1 type of termination

B Posterior view of the spinal cord and nerve roots as seen by transparency in the L2–S2 type of termination

B. Posterior Operative Approach

1. Operative Positions

Access to the lumbosacral spine can be achieved with different positions according to the aim of operation; decompression or arthrodesis.

a) Standard Prone

The standard prone position is the basic position for the posterior approach to the lumbosacral spine, permitting the whole range of surgical techniques, and should be mandatory when the aim is to achieve stable spinal fusion, since the prone conditions best correspond to those of lumbosacral statics in the upright position. Anesthesia is induced conventionally with the patient lying supine on a wheeled stretcher next to the operating table. The patient is then turned cautiously over to lie prone on the operating table, previously prepared with different types of support. One technique of support is the orthopedic frame specially designed for spinal surgery and featuring four fully adjustable points of support, two for the thorax and two for the ilioinguinal region. This frame can be replaced by three rubber blocks allowing homogeneous support and adequate elevation (15–25 cm) of the sternum and the lateral part of the left and right ilioinguinal regions. The aim of such support is to eliminate any compression of the abdominal region, which in fact must be loosely suspended over the operating table to avoid interference with respiration and compression of the venous return of the inferior vena cava, the latter being the source of increased intraspinal venous pressure leading to peroperative hemorrhage. The operator should therefore check that the three points of support are correctly positioned. The sternal support should not extend to the cervical or epigastric region, and the ilioinguinal supports should not lie under the region of the femoral vessels. Furthermore, it should be verified that the head, slightly turned to one side, is not excessively compressed against the operating table. The upper limbs, flexed to 90° at the elbows, should be aligned with the shoulders. Soft pads are placed under the elbows to protect the cubital nerves against compression. A self-adhesive belt is used to hold the thighs in place, thus avoiding any inopportune movement by the patient if anesthesia should turn out to be insufficient. Finally, the dorsa of the feet should rest on cushions to avoid compression.

b) Flexed Prone

When the aim of operation is to gain access to the vertebral canal and to widen the interlaminar spaces, it is desirable to create lumbosacral flexion. This position can be achieved by angling the operating table to 90° at two different points, the ilioinguinal region and the knees. The three points of thoracic and ilioinguinal support are positioned as described in the standard prone position. The table should be tilted slightly downward at the head to stop the patient sliding caudally.

c) Genupectoral

The genupectoral position is the position of choice when operating on a prolapsed intervertebral disc, as lumbosacral hyperflexion induces maximum opening of the interlaminar spaces. However, the disadvantage is that the spinal roots and nerves are stretched, thus rendering their mobilization difficult and possibly inducing neurological microtrauma. Subsequent to induction of anesthesia the patient is transferred to the prone position on the operating table. The lower limbs are then folded under the abdomen while two assistants, one on each side of the table, link their hands together under the abdomen to maintain the patient in the elevated position. A rubber pad which can be adjusted in the vertical direction is then placed under the thighs so that the angle between the thighs and the legs is about 40°. Indeed, hyperflexion of the popliteal regions must be avoided at all costs in order to eliminate the risks of irreversible postoperative vascular disturbances of the feet subsequent to a prolonged operation. The knees are slightly displaced laterally to increase stability. A 20–30 cm rubber support pad is placed under the sternum. The upper limbs are flexed to 90° at the elbows aligned with the shoulders. The cubital regions should be protected against compression. The head is placed on a small soft sponge cushion with a concave upper surface. The operating table is then tilted to elevate the head slightly, stabilize the patient, and bring the lumbosacral region to the horizontal position. The risk of lateral displacement of the patient is avoided by fixing the trunk to the operating table with a self-adhesive belt. In this way, the patient can be tilted towards the surgeon to allow a better view of the field during operation.

d) Lateral

In exceptional cases operation can be performed with the patient lying in the lateral position, e.g., when the anterior and posterior approaches to the lumbosacral spine are used during the same operation. However, it must be underlined that this position is inconvenient, bleeding is always more pronounced, and it is difficult to maintain the orthostatic retractors in a symmetrical position.

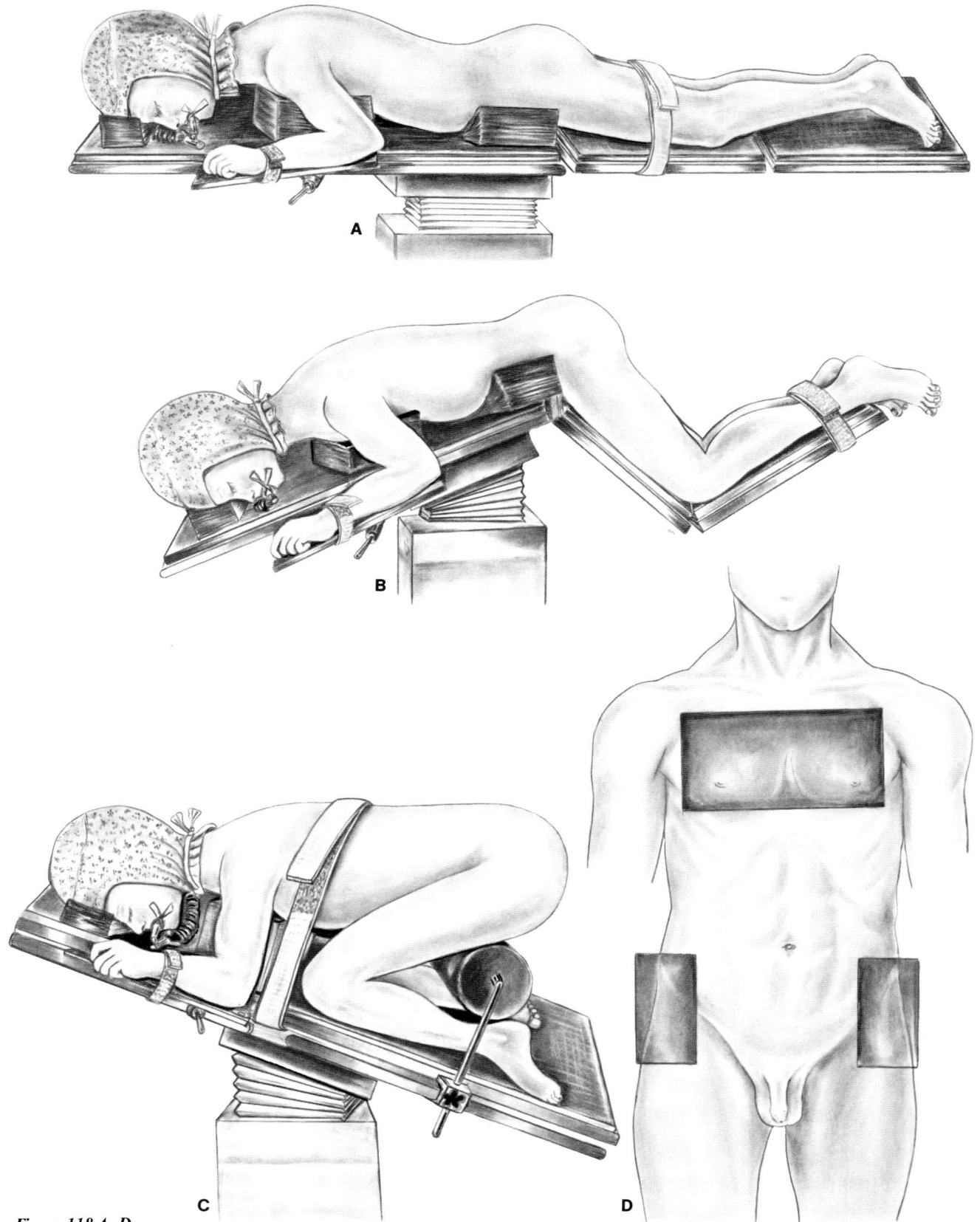

Figure 118 A–D

A   The standard prone position
B   The prone position with flexion

C   The genupectoral position
D   The points of thoracic and ilioinguinal support to free the abdomen in the prone position

2. Median Posterior Approach

a) Identification of Lesions

Prior to tracing the site of incision and draping of the operative field, it is necessary to identify the level of the lesions with the patient in the operative position. Indeed, mistaken identification of the lesional level often occurs, leading to operative failure or unduly prolonged intervention. The presence or absence of a transitional anomaly as evidenced by standard X-rays must be taken into account. The most reliable technique for identifying the level of the lesions is the image intensifier. Good precision for identification of the lesional level can also be obtained using the posterosuperior iliac spines as landmarks. Palpation of the two fossettes lying over these spines enables identification of the L5–S1 interspinous space. However, this landmark is truly reliable only when the patient is in the standard prone position. When the lumbosacral spine is in flexion or hyperflexion, the posterior bi-iliac line lies 2 cm cranial to the level of the L5–S1 intervertebral disc. A small file is useful to mark the skin landmarks permanently by tracing a median posterior line and the upper and lower limits of the site of incision.

b) Preparation of the Operative Field

After thorough wide disinfection of the lumbosacral region, the operative towels are draped on the cranial and caudal sides of the skin marks corresponding to the site of incision. A transparent adhesive plastic sheet is placed on the operative field. The electric cautery knife and the suction cannula are fixed to the right and left of the operator respectively.

c) Superficial Dissection

The skin is incised strictly on the midline with the blade of the scalpel in the vertical position. The incision is made down to but not including the superficial fat layer, to allow immediate disinfection of the cutaneous wound and hemostasis of the subdermal vessels. A warm compress is applied to the incision, which is then uncovered progressively as electrocoagulation hemostasis is performed. The coagulation apparatus should be adjusted to allow hemostasis without burning the skin. Use of the aspiration cannula over the sites of bleeding enables precise coagulation hemostasis. With this progressive procedure full hemostasis should be achieved when the entire incision is finally exposed. Indeed, it is of great importance to achieve full hemostasis of all operative layers – similar to that required in neurosurgery – to avoid operating without clear exposure, which may lead to inadvertent injury to the neural structures of the spine. The next step is to incise the fat with the cautery knife until the thoracolumbar fascia is exposed. Incision of the thoracolumbar fascia is prepared by first identifying the spinous processes and sacral crest using the finger or a dissector. According to whether or not laminectomy is to be done, there are two modes of incision. If the crest of spinous processes is to be conserved then the fascia should be incised along two parallel lines, one on each side of the processes, leaving a band of fascia on the processes onto which the detached fascia can be reinserted when spinal surgery is terminated. When laminectomy is to be performed the fascia must be incised strictly along the midline of the spinous processes to leave sufficient fascial tissue to allow closure at the end of operation.

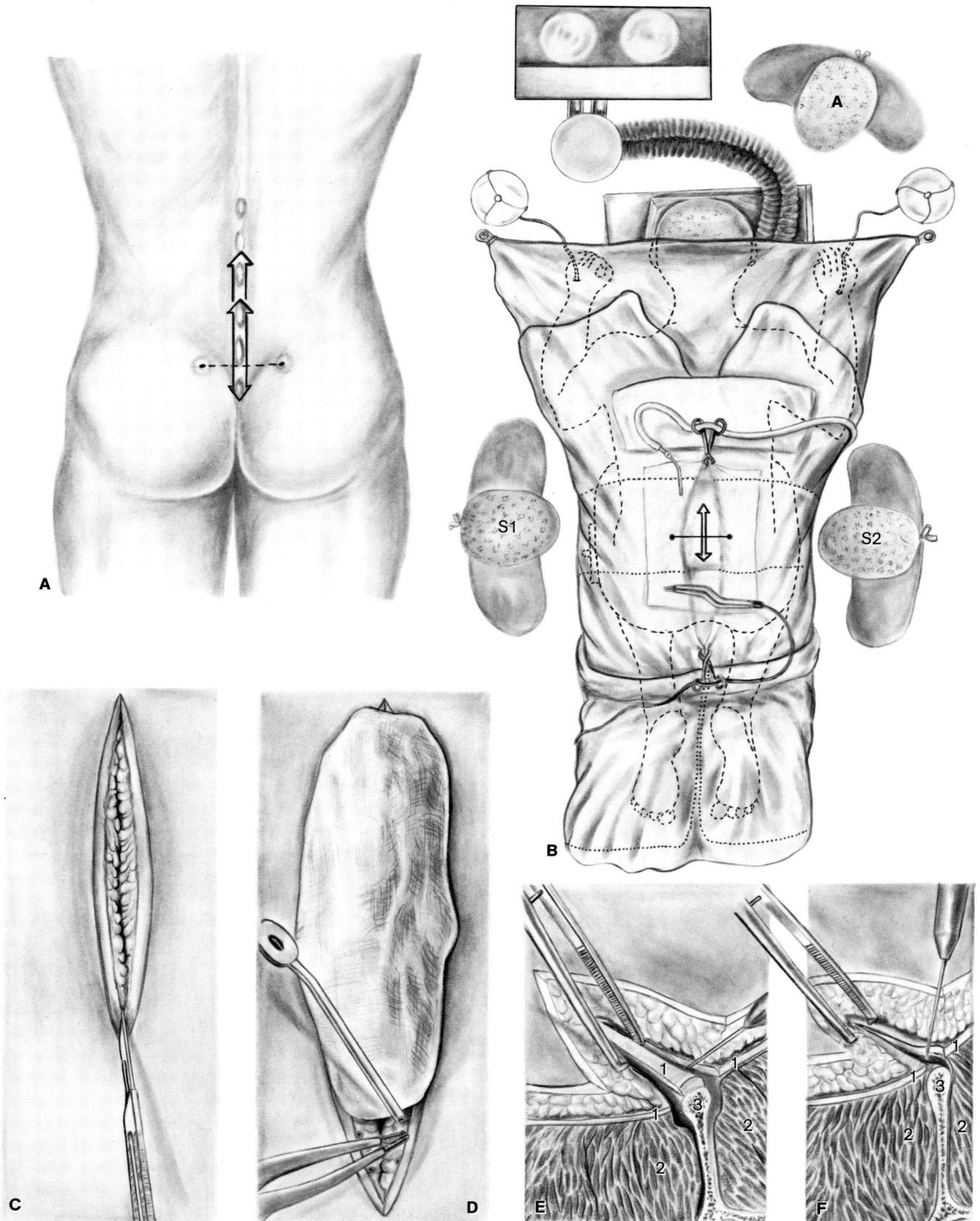

Figure 119 A–F

A Median posterior lumbosacral incisions. The posterior bi-iliac line is used as a landmark

B Overhead view of the genupectoral operative position after draping of the operative field

C Midline skin incision

D Hemostasis of the subdermal layer

E Incision of the thoracolumbar fascia with the electric cautery knife on each side of the spinous processes when laminectomy is not planned

F Incision of the thoracolumbar fascia on the spinous process midline when laminectomy is planned

1 fascia thoracolumbalis *2* m. erector spinae *3* processus spinalis

d) Muscle Disinsertion

Exposure of the vertebral arches requires that the spinal muscles attached to these structures be disinserted. In the absence of a plane of incision between the muscles and vertebral arches, uniform muscle disinsertion must be carried out over the entire operative field. Because these muscles receive their vascular and nervous supply from the interarticular regions, median disinsertion does not lead to neurovascular injury. Disinsertion should be performed with sharp instruments, e.g., a raspatory or a large periosteal rasp. The instrument should be sufficiently wide (15–20 mm) not to slip off track through an interlaminar space or a zone of spina bifida into the vertebral canal. Disinsertion is begun in the sagittal plane, working against the lateral surfaces of the spinous processes and sacral crest until contact is made with the laminae. At this stage disinsertion is carried out in the coronal plane to allow sufficient lateral exposure, the extent depending on the operative procedures to be performed. In cases where only decompression of the vertebral canal is to be performed, muscle disinsertion need not extend beyond the medial margin of the zygapophyseal joints. Conversely, when arthrodesis is to involve fusion of these joints, disinsertion must extend to their lateral margin. Care must be taken to avoid instrumental maneuvers capable of injuring the dorsal neurovascular bundles in the interarticular region, i.e., flush with the isthmic zones of the lumbar vertebrae. Temporary hemostasis is achieved by packing a warm moist compress into the exposed spinal gutters. When both gutters have been exposed, the compresses are removed and an orthostatic retractor installed. Sufficiently resistant retractors should be used, owing to the strength of the spinal muscles and their fascia; a lock-toothed mechanism is preferable to a hinge type. A retractor with interchangeable blades of different length should be used to adapt to the obliquity of the lumbosacral region and varying degrees of corpulence. Finally, the deep tip of the retractor blades should be slightly hooked to retain the powerful spinal muscles.

e) Exposure of the Vertebral Arches

A curette is used to remove any remaining muscle fibers on the vertebral arches. Hemostasis of the different sites of bleeding is then achieved in the interspinous, interlaminar, and interarticular spaces. At this stage of operation it is useful to rinse the operative field with saline-antibiotic solution to prevent infection. The spinal level of the exposed vertebral arches is then checked by referring to the sacrum, identified by its lack of mobility when force is applied to the sacral crest, its upward tilt, and the absence of interlaminar spaces.

f) The Interlaminar Approach

Access can be gained to the vertebral canal without laminectomy by the approach through the interlaminar spaces. The L5–S1 space is usually large enough to allow access without wide bone resection. Access through the L4–L5 and especial-ly the suprajacent interlaminar spaces, however, requires extensive bone resection in addition to removal of the ligamentum flavum. The approach is begun with the decollement of the ligamentum flavum from the lower margin of the lamina delimiting the upper part of the interlaminar space, using a sharp dissector, followed by resection of the inferior margin of the exposed lamina with long slender gouge forceps. Resection should extend horizontally to remove one third to one half of the laminar bone, and laterally until contact is made with the inferior articular process. Bone wax is applied to the cut bone with a clamp-held compress, and the operator proceeds to excise the ligamentum flavum in two steps. The first step begins with incising the medial inferior margin of the ligamentum flavum, using a long, fine scalpel along the spinous processes to expose the epidural fat. The lateral lip of the incised ligament is then grasped with toothed forceps while disinsertion is pursued along the upper margin of the subjacent lamina with the knife. The second step is to use a sharp, middle-sized curette introduced between the epidural fat and deep surface of the ligamentum flavum to disinsert the ligament. The curette must be manipulated in contact with the ligament to avoid injury to a spinal nerve root. Use of the curette is pursued laterally until the ligamentum flavum is disinserted anterior to the zygapophyseal articulation and finally from the upper lamina. It is also sometimes necessary to widen the lower part of the operative field by resecting the upper margin of the lower lamina with a rongeur. The resulting window in the interlaminar space should be rectangular, with vertical and not beveled cut surfaces in order to allow maximum exposure. The vertebral canal can now be explored using a blunt dissector and small-caliber suction cannula. The epidural fat is retracted toward the midline. The lateral convex margin of the dural envelope is identified, followed by the emergence of a nerve root, which is displaced towards the midline using a supple retractor. This procedure exposes the intraspinal venous plexuses, which should be coagulated preventively prior to approaching the posterior surface of the intervertebral discs or vertebral bodies. Access to the intervertebral foramina should be gained via this approach without resection of the zygapophyseal articulation, in order not to destabilize the spine. Foraminotomy by resection of a zygapophyseal joint should only be performed when the lesions are not accessible by the median route.

Figure 120 A–H

A   Disinsertion of the spinal muscles and hemostasis with a compress
B   Installation of the orthostatic retractor and exposure of the vertebral arches with hemostasis
C   Decollement of the ligamentum flavum
D   Widening of the interlaminar space by resection of the upper lamina with preservation of the zygapophyseal joint
E   Section of the medial inferior margin of the ligamentum flavum with the plain knife
F   Disinsertion of the lateral and upper margins of the ligamentum flavum using the curette

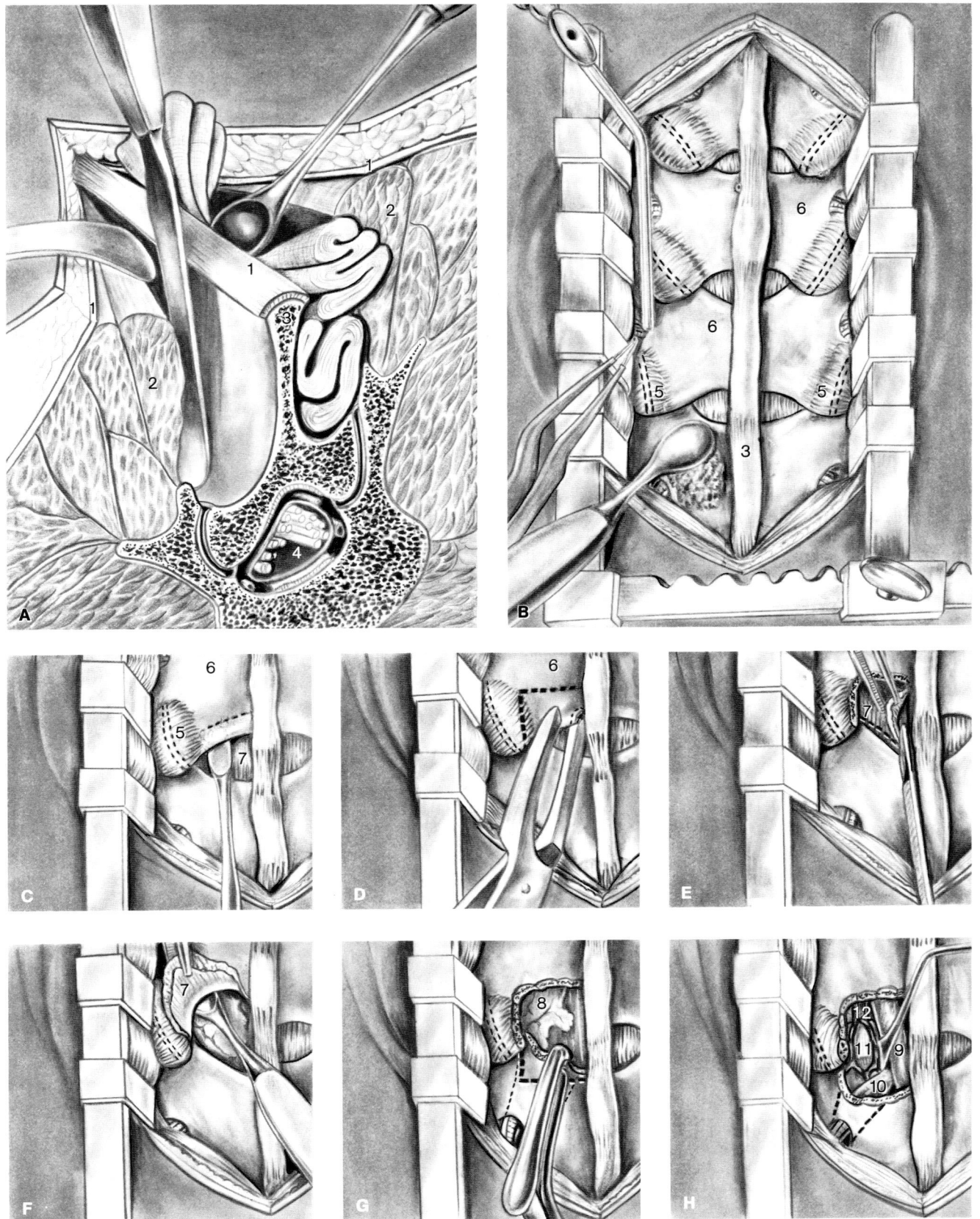

Figure 120 A–H

G   Widening of the interlaminar space by resection of the lower lamina with a rongeur

H   Exposure of the posterior surface of the intervertebral disc and internal intraspinal venous plexuses. The dural envelope and a spinal nerve root are displaced towards the midline with a retractor

1 fascia thoracolumbalis   2 m. erector spinalis   3 processus spinalis
4 duramater spinalis, cauda equina   5 articulatio zygapophysealis, capsula articularis   6 lamina arcus vertebrae   7 lig. flavum   8 corpus adiposum cavi epiduralis   9 duramater spinalis   10 n. spinalis
11 discus intervertebralis   12 plexus venosus vertebralis internus

g) Lumbosacral Laminectomy

Laminectomy is required when the aim of operation is to perform wide exploration of the lumbosacral canal at several intervertebral levels. The procedure is begun with the resection of the spinous processes and sacral crest using large strong gouge forceps. The entire spinous process should be removed, with care being taken not to bite so deeply into the bone as to lead to simultaneous resection of the laminae and midline opening of the vertebral canal, which would cause immediate injury to the dura mater. Hemostasis of the cut surfaces of bone is achieved by applying bone wax with a clamp-held compress. The operator proceeds with the décollement of the ligamenta flava from the lower margin of the laminae delimiting the upper part of the interlaminar spaces. The laminae are then resected by alternating bone removal on the right and left sides using middle-sized gouge forceps. Laminectomy should not extend laterally beyond the line tangential to the zygapophyseal joints. The walls of the cut bone should be vertical and not beveled in order to avoid reduction of the operative field. The opening in the bone is terminated using either long slender gouge forceps or a rongeur. The next step is to excise what remains of the ligamenta flava, accomplished by lifting and deeply disinserting the ligaments in front of the zygapophyseal joints with a large sharp curette, followed by their incision on the midline with the plain knife. The curette must constantly be manipulated in contact with the deep surface of the ligament to avoid injury to a spinal nerve root. Excision of the ligamenta flava exposes the posterior surface of the dural envelope with its overlying fat traversed by a few vessels, mainly veins. Hemostasis of the epidural vessels is then achieved. The operator can now explore the convex lateral margin of the dural envelope and the emergence of the spinal nerve roots at the junction of the anterior and lateral walls of the dura. A supple retractor can be used to displace the dural envelope or the spinal nerve roots to allow the exploration of the lateral recesses of the vertebral canal containing the intraspinal venous plexuses. Hemostasis of the latter is often required as a preventive measure. Moistened rectangular cotton compresses with an identification thread should be used when exploring the vertebral canal, in order to ensure good hemostasis and protect the meningeal and neural structures from accidental instrumental damage and dessication in contact with the ambient air. If recurrent hemorrhage is encountered, a small piece of Surgicel can be moderately packed in contact with the site of bleeding.

In some cases only hemilaminectomy is performed, to explore one side of the lumbosacral canal. The same technique as described above is used, except that laminectomy and resection of the ligamenta flava are done only on one side, not extending medially beyond the spinous processes or laterally beyond the articular facets. Indeed, the articular pillars must remain in continuity, especially in the isthmic regions where an area of bone at least 5 mm wide should be left intact to avoid spondylolysis. Resection may involve 2–3 mm of the articular facets without interfering with their functional capacity.

h) Transdural Exploration

When the lesions to be treated are located within the dural envelope at the level of the cauda equina, intrameningeal exploration is necessary. In such cases, a long fine scalpel is used to make an interrupted superficial opening of the inferior part of the dural envelope on the midline. Fine scissors are then used to open the dural envelope on the midline upward to the desired level. The arachnoidea is often left intact and must then also be opened with the scissors, leading to evacuation of CSF and allowing visualization of the spinal nerve roots in the meningeal cavity. The nerve roots must be protected by cotton wads soaked in pure isotonic saline. The emergence of the nerve roots can easily be identified at the junction of the anterior and lateral surfaces of the dural envelope, each pair emerging at a common depression in the dura mater but through two distinct orifices separated by a small meningeal falx. The more posterior of the two orifices, giving passage to the sensory nerve, is an excellent landmark for sensory radicotomy.

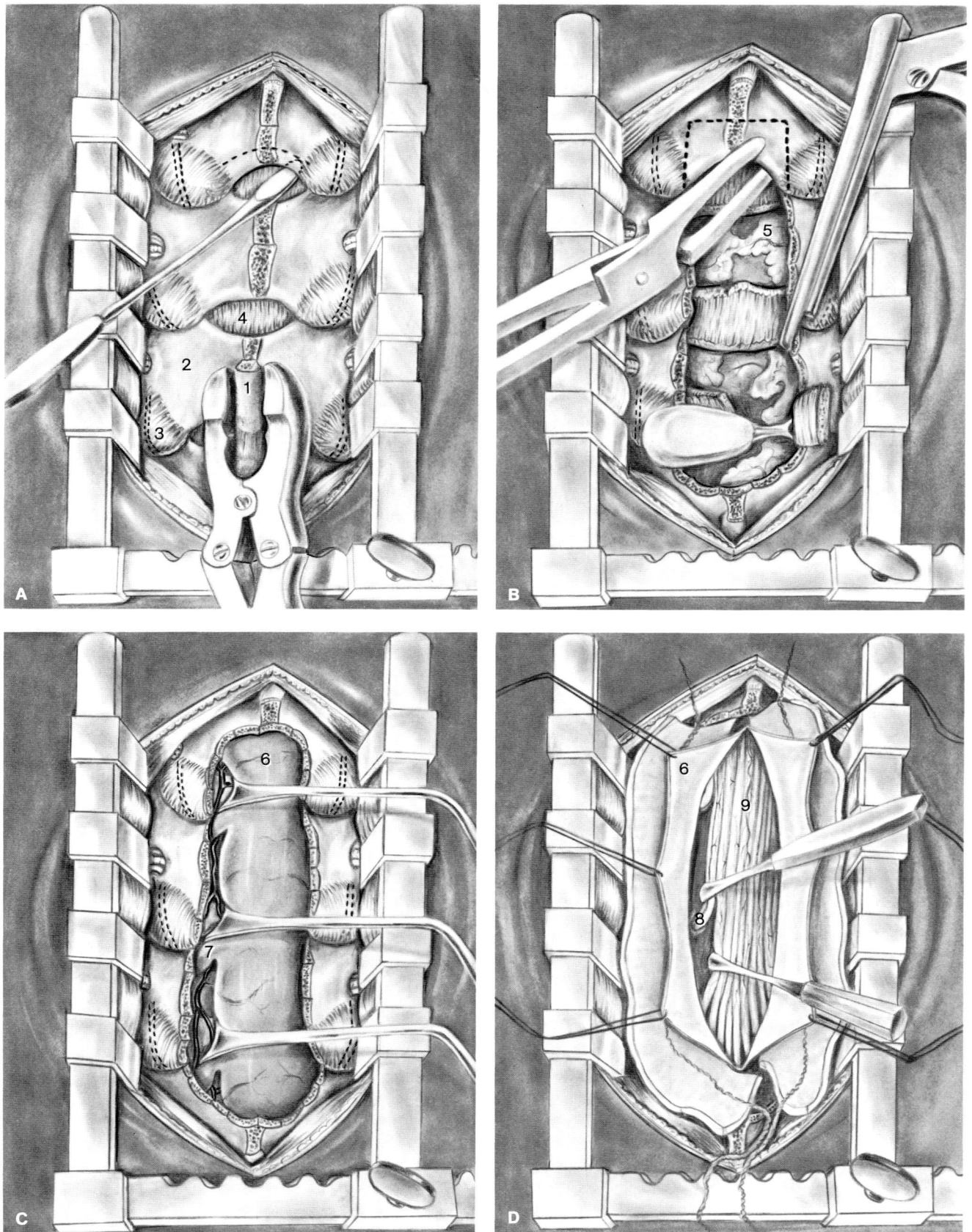

Figure 121 A–D

A The first stage of laminectomy, with the resection of the spinous processes and decollement of the lig. flava from the upper laminae

B The second stage of laminectomy, with rectangular resection of the laminae and excision of the ligamenta flava with the curette. Note that one of the posterior articular pillars is left intact

C Exploration of the vertebral canal by reflection of the dura mater and spinal nerve roots, with exposure of the lateral recesses, intraspinal veins, and intervertebral discs

D Opening of the dura mater, allowing both exploration of the subarachnoid space containing the nerves of the cauda equina and identification of the emergence of the nerve roots

1 processus spinalis *2* lamina arcus vertebrae *3* articulatio zygapophysealis, capsula articularis *4* lig. flavum, spatium interarcuale *5* corpus adiposus cavi epiduralis *6* duramater spinalis *7* canalis vertebralis *8* radices subarachnoideales *9* cauda equina

i) Dural Closure

Closure of the dura mater is achieved with a continuous suture, using fine nonresorbable monofilament mounted on a small curved needle with a circular cross section. When the suture is terminated a hermetic seal should be obtained. Isotonic saline is then injected into the subarachnoid space to replace the lost CSF. The injection is stopped when the dural envelope regains its normal cylindrical shape and manual palpation reveals normal pressure. This procedure is absolutely necessary to avoid postoperative vertigo or even cerebellar herniation through the foramen magnum. Furthermore, reestablishment of normal CSF pressure allows earlier postoperative ambulation, i.e., about two days after operation. It is also useful to place one or two pieces of Surgicel on the posterior surface of the dura mater to ensure hermetic closure of the suture and hemostasis.

j) Parietal, Subcutaneous, and Skin Closure

Subsequent to laminectomy the spinal muscles on the right and left sides are pulled towards the midline by a few full-thickness sutures with slow-resorbing material mounted on a large curved needle. The sutures should be tightened only moderately so as not to cut into the muscle fibers and cause postoperative pain. When good hemostasis has been obtained suction drainage is not necessary, and indeed leads to increased postoperative blood loss. In most cases parietal reconstruction with tension on the muscles deep to the thoracolumbar fascia suffices to avoid formation of a compressive hematoma. Drainage is required only when proper hemostasis has clearly not been obtained. Suction drainage is contraindicated when the dural envelope has been partially or fully opened, since in such cases it might lead to CSF depletion. The free lips of the thoracolumbar fascia are then sutured together using large-caliber slow-resorbing material. In cases where the spinous processes are intact, the muscles can be sutured by a few interspinous stitches or even left in place without suture. The fascia is then reinserted on the spinous processes, with the sutures passing twice through the fascia in order to reinsert each of the fascial commissures on the corresponding margins of the fascial band lying over the spinous processes. Parietal closure is followed by interrupted sutures of the subcutaneous tissue, care being taken not to leave dead space between the adipose tissue and the underlying fascia to avoid hematoma formation. Finally, skin closure is achieved with plain interrupted sutures or interrupted mattress sutures, the latter allowing better approximation without postoperative overlapping of the skin due to movement of the patient while bedridden. After closure the skin suture should be free of bleeding points, which might lead to superficial suppuration when the patient lies on the wound.

k) Postoperative Care and Possible Complications

In the absence of operative incision of the dural envelope the patient is allowed to get out of bed on the first postoperative day, and in other cases on the second to fifth day, when there is no headache. Except in special cases, postoperative administration of antibiotics or anticoagulants is not necessary. Patients having undergone arthrodesis should wear a corset brace to allow immobilization of the operative region.

A common peroperative complication is respiratory disturbance due to abdominal compression, especially in obese patients. A special operative support frame is very useful in avoiding this problem. Surgery may be complicated by erroneous identification of the level of the lesions, resulting from poor interpretation of the initial roentgenograms or the absence of peroperative identification under the image intensifier in difficult cases. Abundant bleeding from the intraspinal venous plexuses frequently creates an obstacle to good surgery, arising when the abdomen is compressed or overforceful surgical manipulations are performed in the lateral recesses of the vertebral canal. This complication can be avoided by gentler maneuvers with a blunt instrument and by preventive coagulation of all veins exposed in the operative field. Hemostasis should be achieved with a sheathed bayonet-shaped coagulation clamp, accompanied by suction with a small cannula. Clear operative exposure is also aided by packing moist cotton wads into the lateral recesses of the vertebral canal. Injury to the neural and meningeal structures is specially frequent when hemostasis is poor. Forceful and prolonged retraction of the spinal nerve roots should be avoided by intermittently relaxing the traction to reestablish the blood supply, momentarily interrupted by the pressure of retraction. Injury to the dura mater should be repaired by sutures whenever possible. In other cases, Surgicel or muscle fibers taken directly from the cut parietal muscles can be applied to the wound. Excluding factors inherent to the operating room, postoperative infection is related to poor hemostasis, the absence of frequent rinsing of the operative field, and the presence of debris due to microtrauma of the muscles and excessive coagulation. Poor parietal closure, leaving dead spaces with zones of skin burns, also leads to infection.

Late complications can be avoided with a few rehabilitation exercises. Radiculomeningeal adhesions in the vertebral canal can be avoided by having the patient elevate the extended lower limbs alternately several times a day while standing. The normal seated position should be forbidden during the first three postoperative weeks and no dynamic lumboabdominal exercises allowed for six weeks, the latter period being required to allow reinsertion of the spinal muscles and avoid very painful tearing.

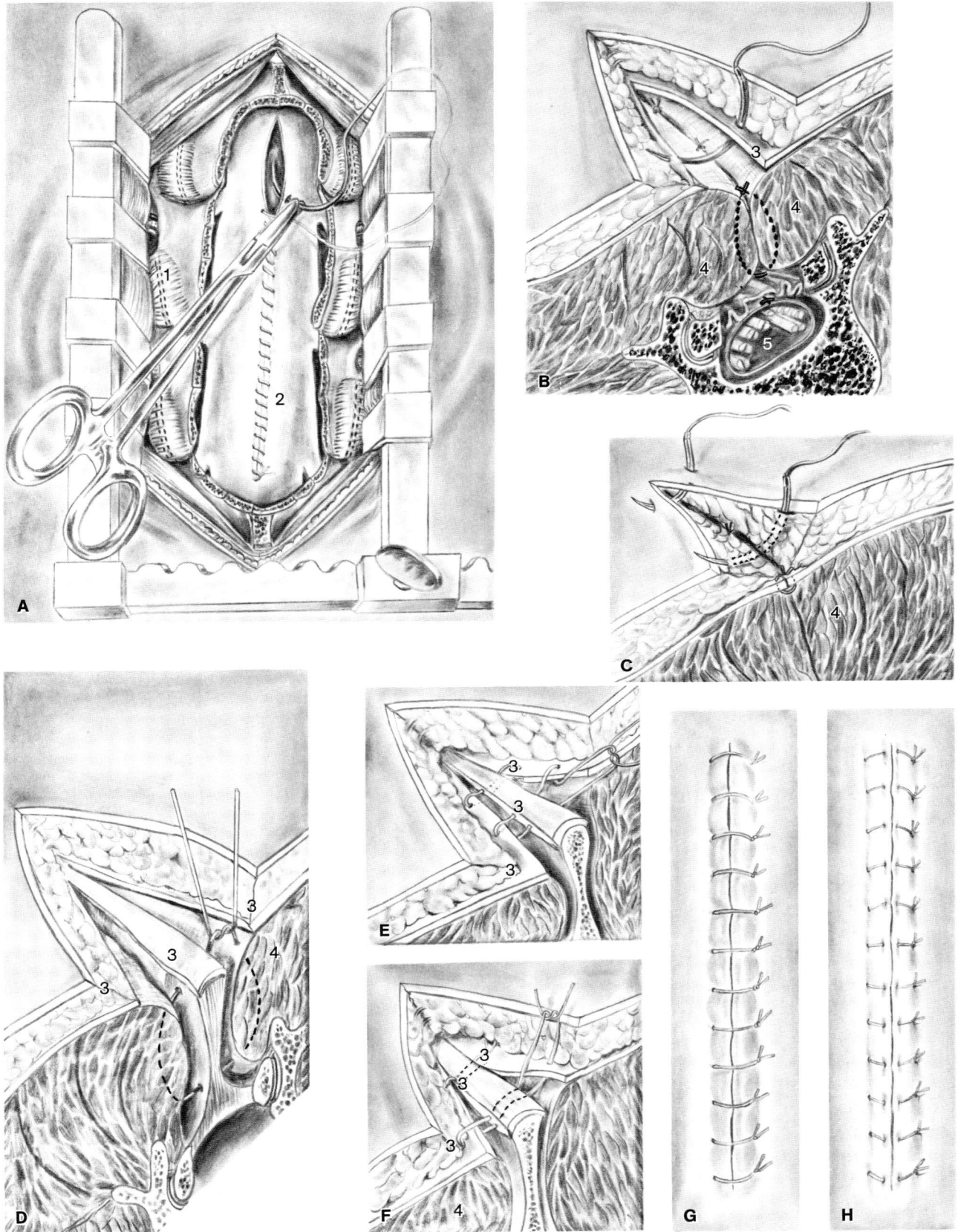

Figure 122 A–H

A   Closure of the dura mater with a continuous nonresorbable hermetic suture. Isotonic saline is then injected into the subarachnoid space

B   Closure of the musculofascial layers with interrupted sutures when laminectomy has been performed

C   Closure of the subcutaneous tissue and skin using interrupted sutures

D   Musculofascial closure in cases with preserved spinous processes

E   Reinsertion of the right and left fascial commissures on the supraspinous ligament. The suture is knotted deeply when rigid suture material is used

F   Reinsertion of the fascia on the supraspinous ligament using supple suture material

G   Skin closure with plain interrupted sutures

H   Skin closure with interrupted mattress sutures

1 articulatio zygapophysealis, capsula articularis   *2* duramater spinalis
3 fascia thoracolumbalis   *4* m. erector spinae   *5* cauda equina

II. Anterolateral Region

A. Topography

Access to the anterolateral surfaces of the lumbosacral spine is gained by the approach through the anterolateral abdominal wall. Incision through this part of the abdominal wall requires good acquaintance with its vascular and nervous supply, which should be preserved as far as possible.

1. Vessels of the Abdominal Wall

The *arterial supply* to the anterolateral abdominal wall comes from inferior, superior, and lateral sectors. The inferior sector is the iliofemoral region. Superficial to the fascia of the obliquus externus abdominis, the superficial epigastric artery runs toward the umbilicus and the superficial circumflex iliac artery along the inguinal fold. In the deep part of the abdominal muscles lying under the fascia transversalis, and 1 cm from the inguinal ligament, the external iliac artery gives rise to a medial branch, the inferior epigastric artery, and a lateral branch, the deep circumflex iliac artery. The inferior epigastric artery displays an arch with a superior and lateral concavity below the funiculus spermaticus, and then runs upward along the posterior surface of the rectus abdominis to penetrate between it and the posterior layer of the rectus sheath below the linea arcuata (Douglas' line). The artery penetrates progressively through the rectus muscle, finally anastomosing with the superior epigastric artery 5–6 cm above the umbilicus. The deep circumflex iliac artery runs upward along the posterior aspect of the inguinal ligament toward the iliac crest, where it gives off a branch running along the iliac crest to anastomose with its homologue branching off the iliolumbar artery. The deep circumflex iliac artery also gives rise to an ascending branch, which passes between the transversus and obliquus internus to anastomose with the lumbar arteries. The superior vascular sector comprises the terminal branches of the internal thoracic (mammary) artery: the abdominal branch (superior epigastric artery) and the musculophrenic branch. The superior epigastric artery penetrates the sheath of the rectus muscle posterior to the seventh costal cartilage and descends behind the rectus abdominis, finally entering the muscle and anastomosing directly with the inferior epigastric artery. In rare cases the two arteries are connected by a network of small anastomotic arteries. The musculophrenic artery, running along the posterior surface of the common costal cartilage, receives anastomoses along its lateral margin from the five or six lowest intercostal arteries. A network of anastomotic arteries lies in the triangular area between the two terminal branches of the internal thoracic artery. The lateral sector supplying the abdominal wall comprises three or four lumbar arteries arising directly from the aorta, running through the interstice separating the transversus and obliquus internus muscles, and diverging in radiate fashion toward the lateral margin of the rectus sheath. The three arterial sectors of the abdominal wall are anastomosed to each other.

The *venous circulation* of the abdominal wall is composed of paired veins accompanying the arteries described above. The superficial suprafascial veins run toward the umbilicus and the inguinal and axillary regions. The superficial veins of the epigastric region run toward the umbilicus to anastomose with the veins of the portal system via the round ligament of the liver (ligamentum teres hepatis). The veins of the lower part of the abdominal wall are drained by the great saphenous vein. Finally, the venous drainage of the lateral abdominal wall comprises a large anastomotic system, i.e., the thoracoepigastric veins anastomosing the iliofemoral and external thoracic (mammary) veins, the latter branching from the axillary vein.

2. Nerves of the Abdominal Wall

The sensory and motor nerves of the abdomen are arranged metamerically in parallel or slightly divergent bands, and comprise the thoracoabdominal nerves arising from the seventh through eleventh intercostal nerves and the subcostal or twelfth intercostal nerve. These nerves run through the abdominal wall in the interstice between the transversus and obliquus internus muscles to reach and penetrate the rectus sheath and terminate in the medial part of the rectus muscles. In their course they give off a lateral abdominal cutaneous branch and an anterior cutaneous branch. The tenth intercostal nerve reaches the midline near the umbilicus, the eighth halfway between the xiphoid process and umbilicus, and the twelfth above the symphysis pubis. The inferior part of the abdominal wall is innervated by the iliohypogastric and ilioinguinal nerves (small and large abdominogenital nerves), arising primarily from the first lumbar nerve and displaying an essentially cutaneous distribution in the inguinoscrotal region. The cutaneous femoral nerve leaves the abdominal wall just medial to the anterosuperior iliac spine.

Two types of incision can be recommended, based on the vascular and nervous topography of the anterolateral abdominal wall: median vertical incisions, and lateral incisions running obliquely downward and medially.

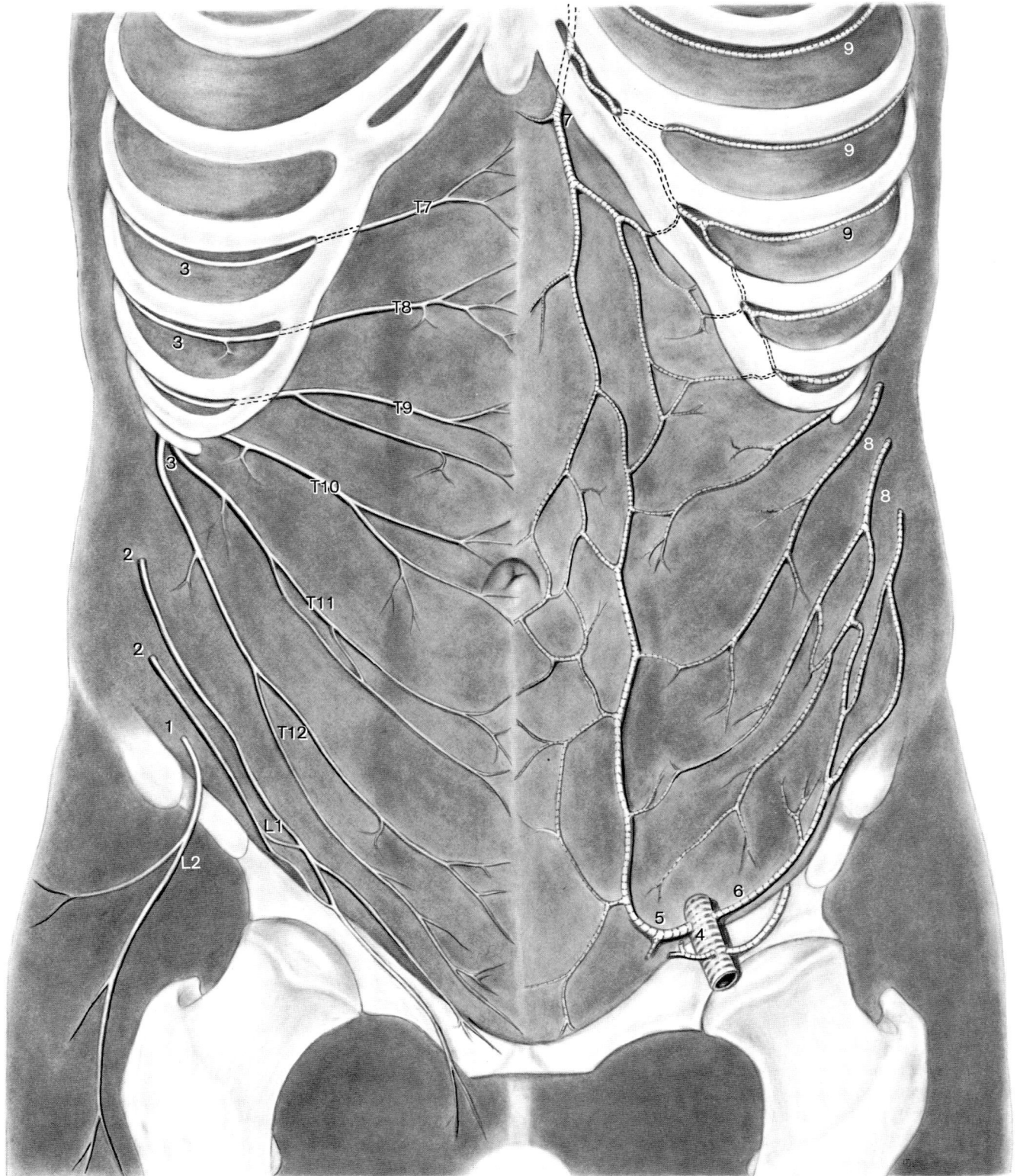

Figure 123. Arterial *(right)* and nervous *(left)* supply as seen by transparency through the abdominal wall

1 n. cutaneus femoris lateralis   *2* n. iliohypogastricus cranialis and caudalis   *3* nn. thoracici, nn. intercostales   *4* a. femoralis   *5* a. epigastrica inf.   *6* a. circumflexa ilium superficialis   *7* a. epigastrica sup.   *8* aa. lumbales   *9* aa. intercostales

3. Musculofascial Layers

The anterolateral abdominal wall is covered by skin and by a subcutaneous layer of greater or lesser thickness according to the individual. The musculofascial layers are three in number.

The *superficial layer* comprises the obliquus externus abdominis and the sheath of the rectus muscles. The obliquus externus inserts on the outer surface of the lower eight ribs, where its digitations blend with those of the serratus anterior and latissimus dorsi and often fuse with the external intercostal muscles. From their origin, the fibers of the obliquus externus converge obliquely downward and medially near the anterior part of the iliac crest. The lower end of the muscle gives rise to an aponeurosis which terminates as the reinforced inguinal ligament stretched between the anterosuperior iliac spina and tubercle of the pubis. The aponeurosis of the obliquus externus extends towards the midline of the abdomen by fusing with the superficial layer of the underlying obliquus internus abdominis. This anterior part of the rectus sheath forms the linea alba, which is narrow in the supraumbilical region and wide in the infraumbilical region. The umbilicus thus represents a cicatricial depressed zone near the middle of the linea alba, which can easily be identified without opening the rectus sheath in the region below the umbilicus. In the upper part of the abdomen the anterior layer of the rectus sheath receives the abdominal bundle of the pectoralis major. In the anterior part of the abdomen the aponeurosis of the obliquus externus is traversed at the level of the external inguinal ring by the funiculus spermaticus in men and the round ligament of the uterus (ligamentum teres uteri) in women.

The *middle layer* of the abdominal wall comprises the obliquus internus abdominis laterally and the rectus muscles medially. The obliquus internus originates from the fascia thoracolumbalis, the iliac crest, and the fascia iliaca. The fibers of the muscle run obliquely upward and medially towards the lowest three ribs to blend with the lowest three internal intercostal muscles. Slightly lateral to the rectus sheath the obliquus internus gives rise to its aponeurosis, which then divides to form two layers ensheathing the rectus muscles, the deep layer disappearing a few centimeters below the umbilicus. The lateral margin of the rectus sheath is thus formed by the bifurcation of the aponeurosis of the obliquus internus. The rectus muscle forms the medial part of the middle layer of the abdominal wall, and is long, thin, and relatively wide. The rectus muscle originates on the anterior surface of the xiphoid process and the fifth through seventh costal cartilages, and inserts on the crest and symphysis of the pubis. Three or more tendons traverse the muscle and fuse with the anterior layer of the rectus sheath.

The *deep layer* of the abdominal wall comprises the transversus abdominis and the posterior layer of the rectus sheath. The transversus originates from the fascia iliaca, the fascia thoracolumbalis, and the medial surface of the six lowest costal cartilages, where its fibers often blend with those of the diaphragm. The fibers of the transversus run horizontally towards the anterior abdominal region, save the lower fibers which run obliquely downward. The upper fibers run behind the rectus and then insert on the posterior layer of the rectus sheath. Conversely, the middle and lower fibers give rise to an aponeurosis whose upper two thirds fuses with the deep layer of the obliquus internus to form the posterior layer of the rectus sheath. The lower third of this aponeurosis passes completely anterior to the rectus muscles to constitute part of the anterior layer of the rectus sheath. Thus, a continuous aponeurosis runs posterior to the rectus muscles from the xiphoid process to its termination at the arcuate ligament (Douglas' line) a few centimeters below the umbilicus. Below this point the posterior surface of the rectus muscles is not lined by aponeurotic tissue. Finally, the deep surface of the transversus abdominis and its aponeurosis is lined by the cellular fascia transversalis. It should be borne in mind that the neurovascular bundles run mainly in the interstice between the transversus and obliquus internus, eventually penetrating the sheath and fleshy bodies of the rectus muscles.

4. Peritoneum

The posterior surface of the anterolateral abdominal wall is applied against the anterior surface of the peritoneal serosa. Decollement of the peritoneum is very easy to achieve in the region of the wide muscles of the abdomen, but less so in the region of the rectus muscles, where it is much thinner and more delicate.

The approach through the anterolateral abdominal wall can be made on the midline and through the linea alba, thus obviating transection of the muscles. Lateral oblique incisions can be made either by dissecting each muscle layer parallel to the muscle fibers or by transecting the fibers parallel to the neurovascular bundles. The midline approach obviously allows more solid reconstruction of the abdominal wall. Furthermore, with this approach adhesions between the planes of incision are avoided, thus maintaining the mobility of the different layers and normal function of the abdominal wall.

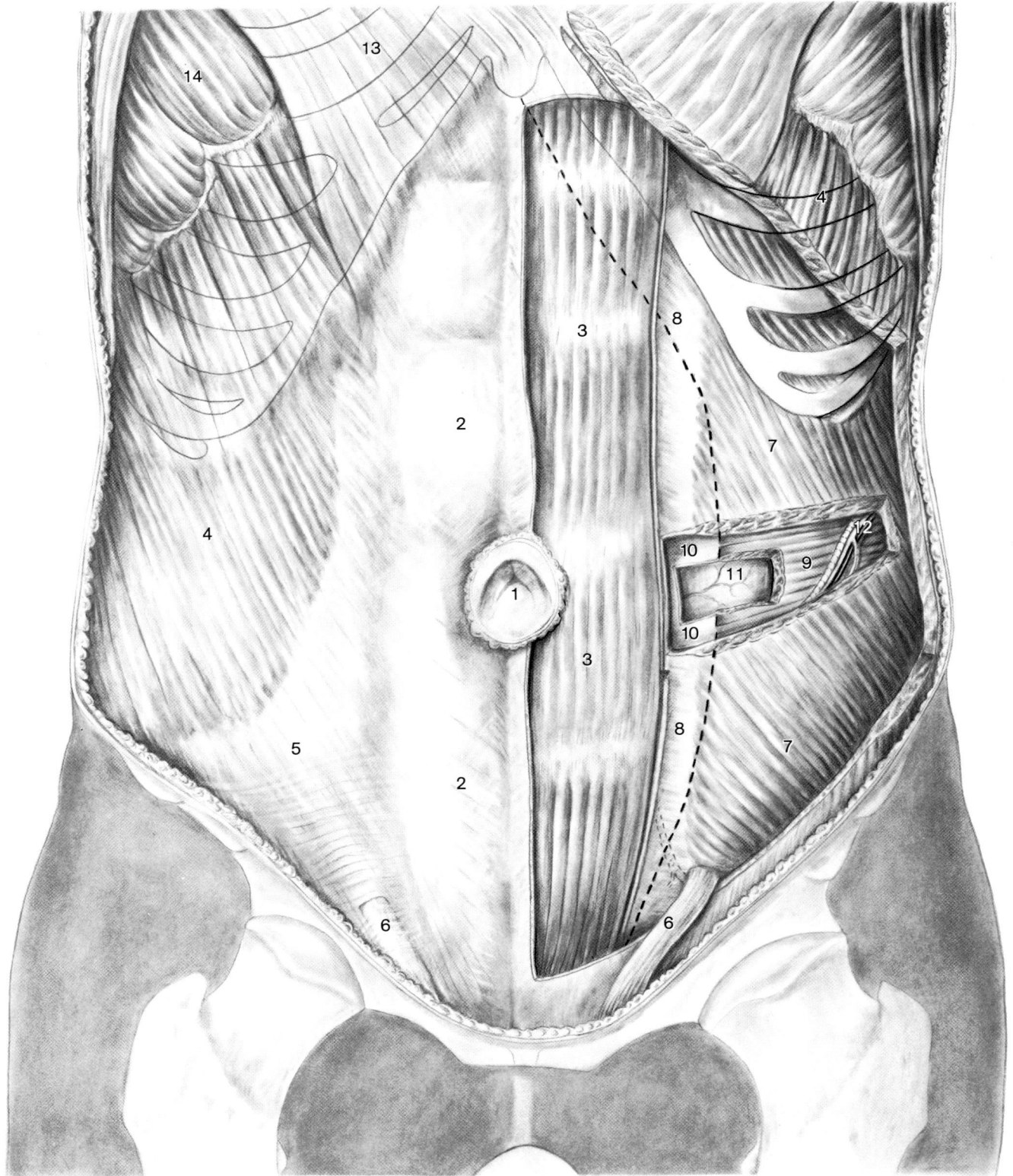

Figure 124. Musculofascial layers of the anterolateral abdominal wall: *right,* superficial layers; *left,* middle and deep layers

1 umbilicus *2* vagina m. recti abdominis *3* m. rectus abdominis *4* m. obliquus externus abdominis *5* aponeurosis m. obliqui externi

6 funiculus spermaticus *7* m. obliquus internus abdominis *8* aponeurosis m. obliqui interni abdominis *9* m. transversus abdominis *10* aponeurosis m. transversi abdominis *11* peritoneum *12* a., v., and n. lumbales *13* m. pectoralis major, pars abdominalis *14* m. serratus ant.

5. Anterolateral Relations of the Lumbar Spine

The ventral part of the lumbar spine lies deep on the midline of the posterior wall of the abdominal cavity and thus enters into relation with the neighboring visceral and peritoneal structures. The lumbar spine forms a prominent midline protrusion on the posterior abdominal wall, its flanks displaying relations to the muscles and nerves in this region. The central part of the lumbar spine is covered by the great prevertebral vessels and their collateral branches.

a) Serous and Visceral

Access to the flanks of the lumbosacral spine is gained by dissection in the retroperitoneal space between the peritoneal envelope, lying anteriorly and medially and lined deeply by the peri- and pararenal fat, and the deep surface of the transversus abdominis, lying posteriorly. Decollement of the peritoneal serosa is easily achieved from the region of the diaphragmatic crura to the iliac crest. The intraperitoneal viscera can be identified by transparency or palpation. The retroperitoneal viscera are camouflaged by the surrounding fat, save the ureter which can be mobilized with the posterior surface of the peritoneum in the region lying along the lateral margin of the psoas muscle. The ureter is easily identified owing to its cylindrical shape, its rich superficial vascular network, and its peristaltic movements at the slightest touched.

b) Muscular

Subsequent to exposure of the transversus abdominis, access is gained to a large muscular region resembling two steps, the first represented by the quadratus lumborum and the second, much higher, by the psoas muscle. The interstice between the two muscles is a poor route of access to the spine and should be avoided. Near the cranial part of this region, the psoas and quadratus lumborum are covered by the arcuate insertions of the diaphragm. Near the caudal part of the region, the quadratus lumborum inserts on the iliac crest and is extended by the iliacus muscle lying below the psoas. The anteromedial margin of the psoas muscle is attached to the flanks of the lumbar spine via arcuate insertions on the intervertebral discs.

c) Neural

Exposure of the retroperitoneal muscle layers enables identification of the neural structures in the lumbar region. The subcostal (twelfth intercostal) nerve lies lateral to the quadratus lumborum and under the diaphragmatic crura. The iliohypogastric nerve (abdominal branch of the abdominogenital nerve) and the ilioinguinal nerve (genital branch of the abdominogenital nerve) traverse the muscle layers at the level of the lateral margin of the psoas muscle and then descend diagonally toward the iliac crest. Similarly, the genitofemoral (genitocrural) and lateral cutaneous femoral nerves traverse the psoas to reach the iliac fossa. In the dihedral angle between the medial margin of the psoas and lumbosacral spine are found, in craniocaudal order, the splanchnic nerves, passing through the diaphragmatic crura and the lumbar sympathetic nervous tract, and the lumbar ganglions, linked together by connecting fibers and giving off rami to the intervertebral foramina and efferents to the mesenteric plexuses. Of these efferents, the most important from the functional standpoint are those arising at the level of L2, since they are almost always involved in the control of ejaculation. Exposure of the other nerves in the lumbosacral region requires the displacement of the psoas muscle up to the area around the intervertebral foramina. The nerves concerned are the spinal nerves constituting the lumbar plexus, which lies longitudinally parallel to the flanks of the spine anterior to the transverse processes.

d) Vascular

The anterior part of the lumbar spine is camouflaged by the great prevertebral vessels, the aorta on the left and the inferior vena cava on the right. The aorta is far more resistant to manipulation than the relatively fragile vena cava. These two vessels are practically in contact with the anteromedial margin of the psoas and thus must be raised and retracted toward the midline in order to visualize the anterolateral surfaces of the vertebral bodies and intervertebral discs. Separation of the aorta and inferior vena cava exposes the metameric lumbar vascular bundles, which usually lie over the middle depressed part of the vertebral bodies halfway between two discs. Each metameric artery and vein extends from the posterior surface of the aorta or vena cava to the intervertebral foramen, where it bifurcates. The large anastomotic ascending lumbar vein, which runs in front of the lumbar plexus at the level of the intervertebral foramina and is camouflaged by the arcuate psoas ligaments, drains the blood from the extraspinal venous plexuses.

e) Discocorporeal Layer

The retroperitoneal approach exposes the anterior and right and left lateral surfaces of the lumbar spine. According to the area of the operative field L1 to L5 and the intervening intervertebral discs can be exposed.

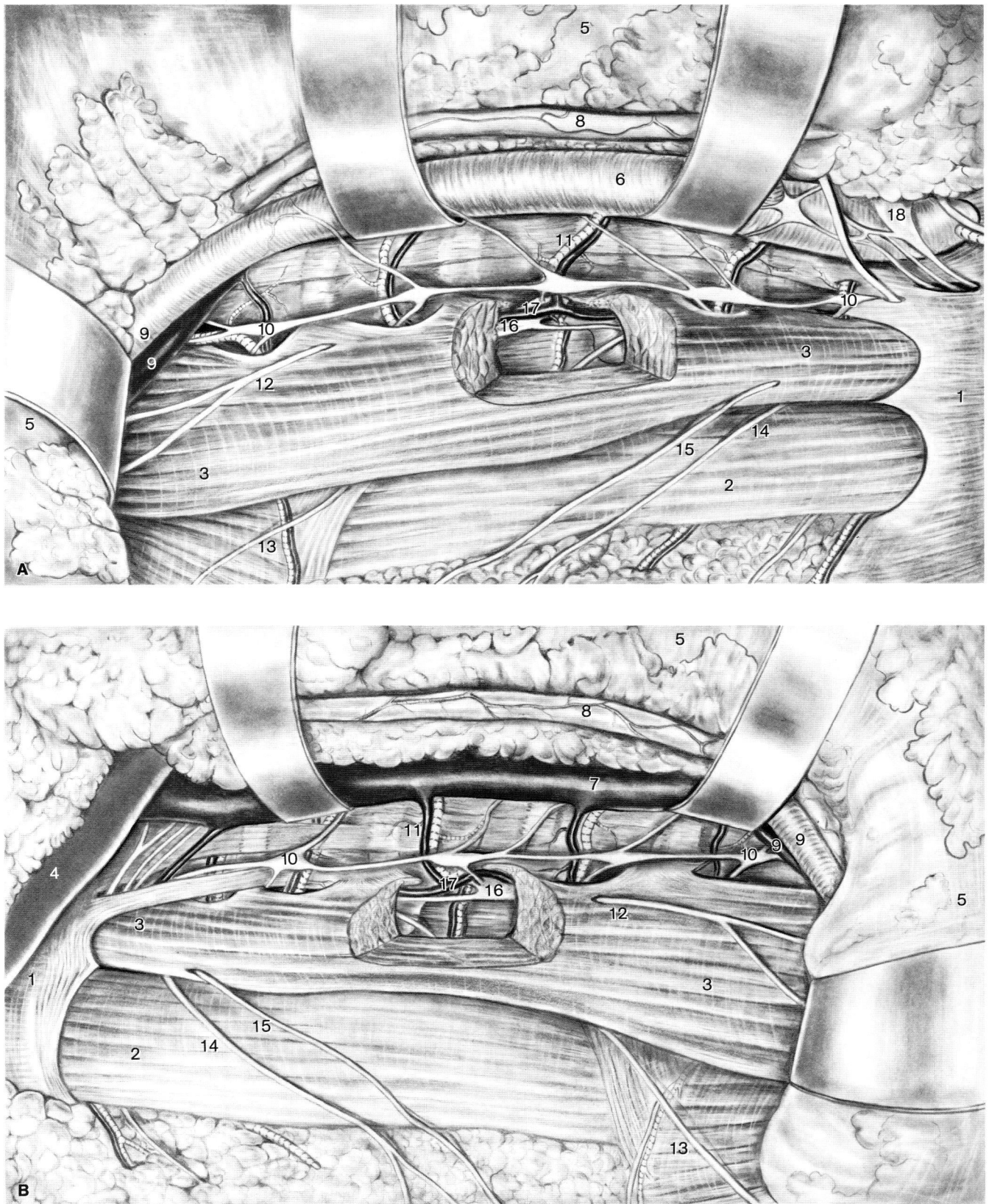

Figure 125 A, B

A   Anatomical relations of the left surface of the lumbar spine after retraction of the abdominal mass and the abdominal aorta. A window has been cut in the psoas to show the third lumbar spinal nerve

B   Anatomical relations of the right lateral lumbar spine after retraction of the abdominal mass and the inferior vena cava. A window has been cut in the psoas to show the third lumbar spinal nerve

1 diaphragma *2* m. quadratus lumborum *3* m. psoas *4* hepar
5 organa abdominis and capsula adiposa renis *6* aorta *7* v. cava inf.
8 ureter *9* a. iliaca communis *10* truncus sympathicus *11* a. and v. lumbales *12* n. genitofemoralis *13* n. cutaneus femoris lateralis
14 n. iliohypogastricus cranalis *15* n. iliohypogastricus caudalis
16 n. lumbalis *17* v. lumbalis ascendens *18* ganglia celiaca

6. Arterial Angiography

Precise investigation of the arterial system lying anterior to the lumbosacral spine is particularly helpful to the surgeon. Indeed, it is necessary to identify the great vessels to be protected and mobilized, the collateral vessels to be sectioned to expose the spine, and the spinal branches to be preserved to avoid neurological injury.

a) Great Vessels

The abdominal aorta and its branches, the right and left common iliac arteries, must be protected during surgery. The aorta lies on the left anterolateral part of the spine running progessively toward the midline, where it bifurcates at the level of the L4–L5 intervertebral disc. The common iliac arteries run diagonally over the flanks of L5, thus considerably hindering access to this vertebra by the lateral approach. The insterstice between the aorta and anterior longitudinal ligament is always sufficiently large to allow mobilization of the aorta without the risk of rupturing the lumbar arteries, since the latter can almost always be stretched at the posterior surface of the aorta.

b) Metameric Collaterals

The lumbar arteries usually arise near the posterior midline of the aorta above the level of the intervertebral foramina into which they penetrate, thus running downward. In a few cases, however, they run horizontally, or even in a recurrent upward direction like their homologues in the upper thoracic region. Regardless of these anatomical differences, the middle part of each lumbar artery lies over the central depressed region of the lateral surface of the vertebral body, like a river in its bed. They eventually enter the intervertebral foramina at the level of the lower half of the vertebral body, where they give off various branches. The spinal branches supply the structures lying within the vertebral canal, while the dorsal and lateral branches supply the posterior and lateral parietal regions respectively. The anatomical varieties of the collateral arteries are described in the section on the thoracic spine. It may be recalled from that description that a common trunk may give rise to the right and left arteries at a given level or to two contiguous metameres on one side, with division occurring anterior to the intervertebral foramen. In the lower part of the lumbar spine, at the level of L4 or L5, some of the lumbar arteries may arise not from the aorta but from the middle sacral or common iliac artery. Along their course the lumbar collaterals give off many branches to the anterior longitudinal ligament and the bodies of the vertebrae. Mobilization of these arteries thus sometimes leads to minor hemorrhage, which can easily be controlled by electrocoagulation or the application of bone wax. The site of choice for the section and hemostasis of a metameric artery allowing access to the lumbar spine is halfway between the retroaortic origin of the artery and its point of passage in front of the intervertebral foramen. In this way, the remaining arterial stump is sufficiently long to allow religation when a suture gives way, and hemostatic procedures are avoided near the intervertebral foramina where the risk of reducing blood supply to the spinal cord is greatest.

c) Spinal Arteries and Radiculomedullary Circulation

The spinal arteries arise from the lumbar arteries near the intervertebral foramina. The artery of the lumbar swelling (Adamciewicz's artery) may arise in this region, especially at the level of the first and second lumbar intervertebral foramina but exceptionally near the middle or lower lumbar foramina. As previously described in the thoracolumbar region, the spinal arteries form a rich network of anastomoses ensuring adequate protection of radiculomedullary vascular supply, comprising longitudinal and horizontal anastomoses over the full length of the spinal cord, including the arterioles of the roots of the cauda equina. The system is also furnished by the dorsal and parietal branches of the metameric arteries, via the arterial carrefour corresponding to the divisions of the spinal arteries in the region of the intervertebral foramina. Accordingly it is strongly recommended that the region of the intervertebral foramina be respected, as it is a veritable arterial crossroads supplying the different anastomotic networks protecting the radiculomedullary structures.

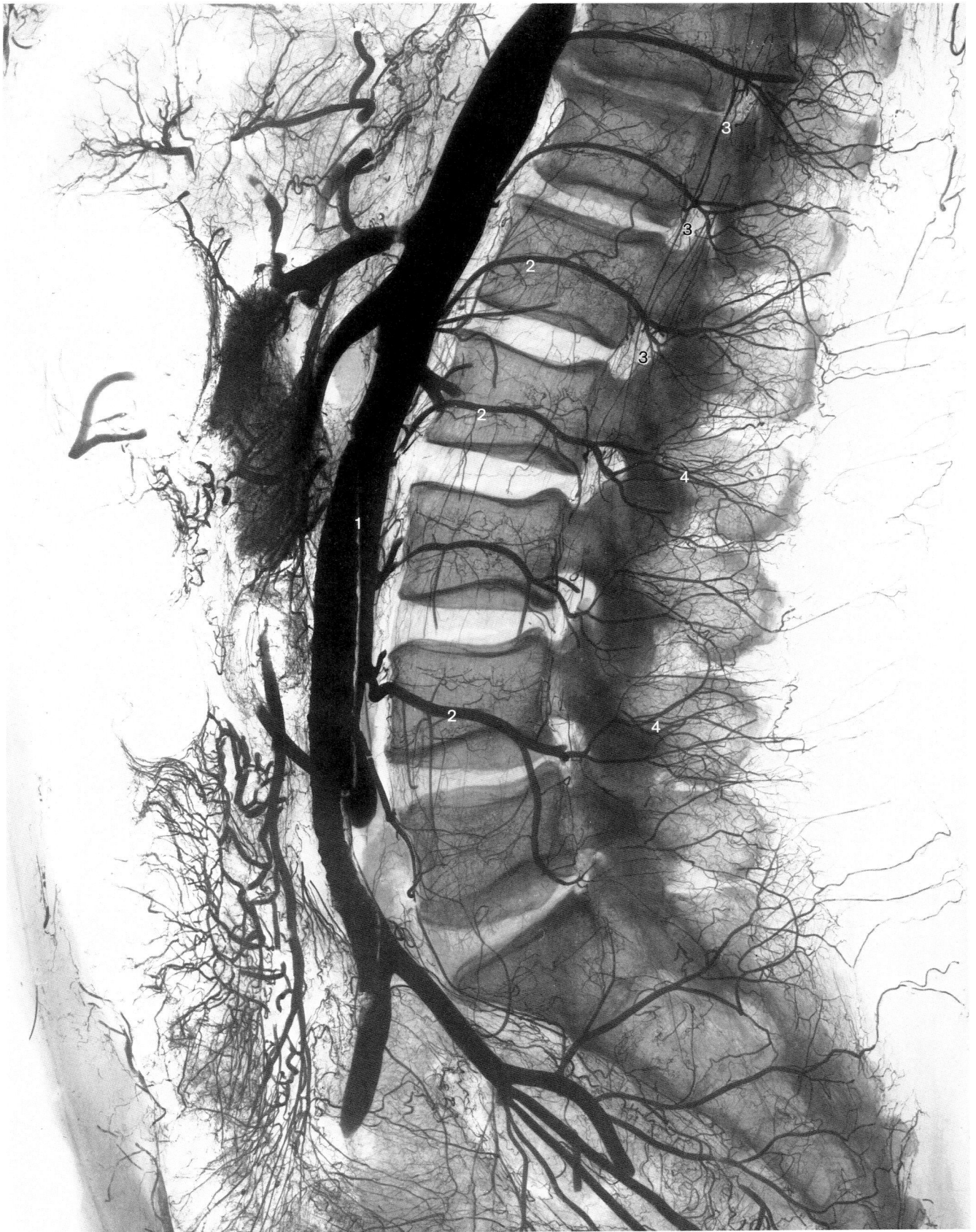

Figure 126. Roentgenogram of a sagittal section of the abdomen after injection of contrast material into the aortic system. Note the lumbosacral spine with the aortic system and its parietal intercostal, lumbar, and sacral arteries. The artery of the lumbar swelling is visible in the vertebral canal. The parietal arteries run over the middle of the vertebral bodies and in the region of the intervertebral foramina

1 aorta *2* a. lumbalis *3* a. spinalis ant. *4* rami dorsales arteriae lumborum

7. Venous Angiography

Knowledge of the venous structures around the lumbosacral spine enables one to understand the regional vascular drainage and to interpret venous angiograms on cavography or lumbar phlebography. The results of these investigations help to guide surgical procedures in this region. The lumbar venous system can be divided into three main parts: the large trunk of the inferior vena cava, the metameric tributaries, and the spinal venous plexuses.

a) Inferior Vena Cava

The inferior vena cava lies against the convex anterior surface of the lumbar spine. The vein originates at about the level of L5 with the confluence of the right and left common iliac veins and runs upward along the spine to the retrohepatic and prediaphragmatic region, finally traversing the diaphragm and joining the lower surface of the right atrium. According to Gillot the inferior vena cava can be divided into two parts: a frankly vertebral sector from L5 to L2, draining blood from the lower limbs, and a visceral sector from L1 to the termination of the vein, draining blood from the kidneys and liver. The inferior vena cava most often originates slightly to the right of the midline at the level of the body of L5, but in some cases the origin is at the L4–L5 intervertebral disc and in rare cases at the lower half of the body of L4. The vein then runs upward along the right half of the lumbar vertebral bodies to the level of the right diaphragmatic crus, which is covered by the vein. Its mean caliber is 26 mm. On exposure the inferior vena cava appears as a relatively fragile, easily depressible, bluish structure. It can nevertheless be mobilized during surgery, since its venous attachments are not fully stretched in the normal anatomical position.

b) Metameric Tributaries

The metameric arrangement of the lumbar veins is less typical than in the thoracic region. In 70% of cases a lumbar vein runs over the middle part of its corresponding vertebral body. The vein originates in the muscles of the anterolateral and posterior walls of the abdomen (quadratus lumborum, spinal muscles, psoas) and anastomoses with the spinal plexuses at the level of the intervertebral foramina and lumbar venous plexuses, finally joining the inferior vena cava or one of its major tributaries, the common iliac, the internal iliac, or the lateral or middle sacral vein. The left lumbar veins are longer than their homologues on the right, as they join the inferior vena cava on the right side of the spine. A lumbar vein often terminates at the level of the vertebral body over which it runs, although in some cases it joins the vena cava one vertebral body lower, and occasionally higher. This classical arrangement is disrupted by numerous variations due to the existence of vertical anastomoses, either within the psoas muscle or in front of its arcuate ligaments posterior to the inferior vena cava, which form common venous trunks uniting two or three metameric veins. Within the psoas, on each side of the trunks

giving rise to the lumbar venous plexus, a longitudinal venous system can be found forming either an anastomotic network or a fairly well individualized vein known as the ascending lumbar vein. According to Gillot the ascending lumbar vein is actually an anastomotic system between two venous groups, that of the descending iliolumbar vein and that of the ascending second lumbar vein and lateral root of the azygos vein. The iliolumbar vein joins the posterior surface of the common iliac vein and represents a sort of terminal for the fifth lumbar vein. The second lumbar vein drains blood toward the inferior vena cava or the azygos system depending on the degree of intra-abdominal and intrathoracic pressure. On the left the ascending system also anastomoses with the left renal vein, forming in some cases the renoazygolumbar venous trunk. Via the azygos system, the metameric veins constitute an anastomotic system between the drainage territories of the inferior and superior venae cavae.

c) Spinal Venous Plexuses

The ascending lumbar vein, the iliolumbar vein, and the lateral root of the azygos vein form a sort of extraspinal venous plexus in front of the intervertebral foramina, constituting an obstacle to surgery due to hemorrhage when operative maneuvers are performed in contact with the veins. It should also be noted that the metameric lumbar veins receive anastomoses from the alveolae of the cancellous vertebral bone. Sometimes voluminous, these anastomoses bleed on surgical exposure of the vertebral bodies, their hemostasis requiring the application of bone wax. Clearly visible on lumbar phlebograms, the intraspinal venous plexuses give a reliable picture of compression of the vertebral canal, sine they are in intimate contact with the posterior surface of the vertebral bodies and intervertebral discs. Access to the vertebral canal requires the identification and subsequent protection or preventive hemostasis of the intraspinal plexuses.

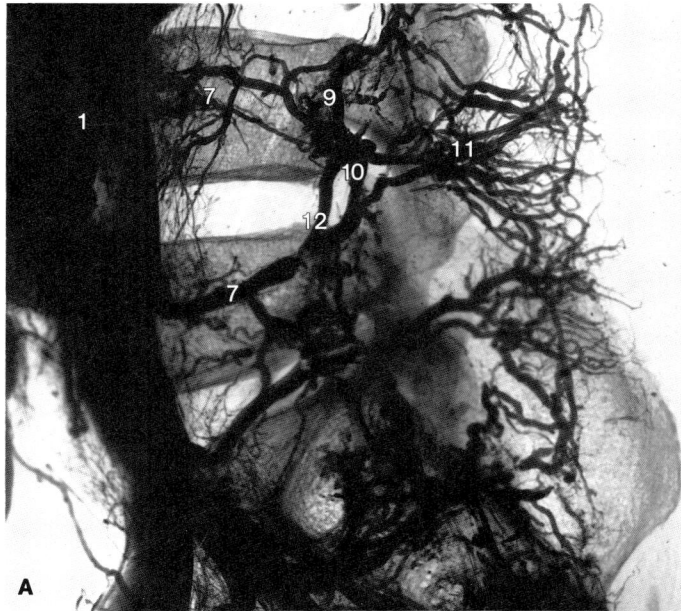

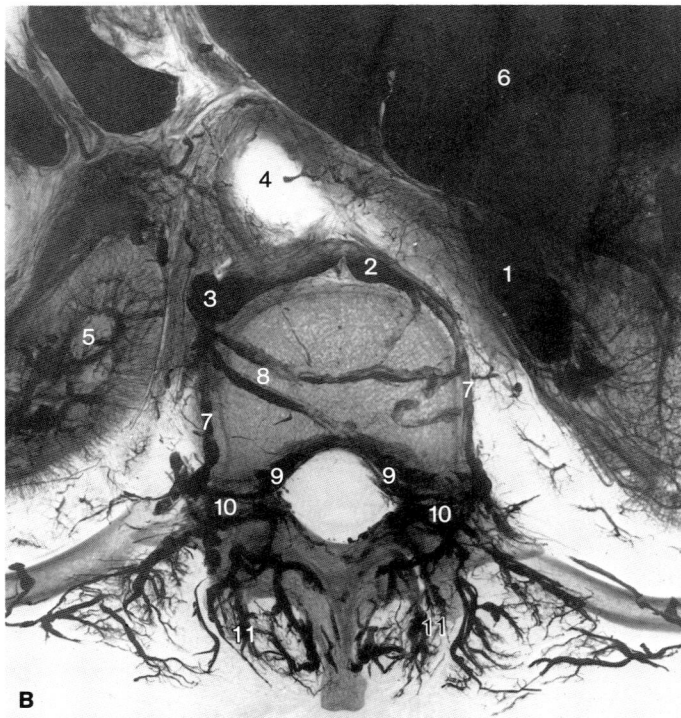

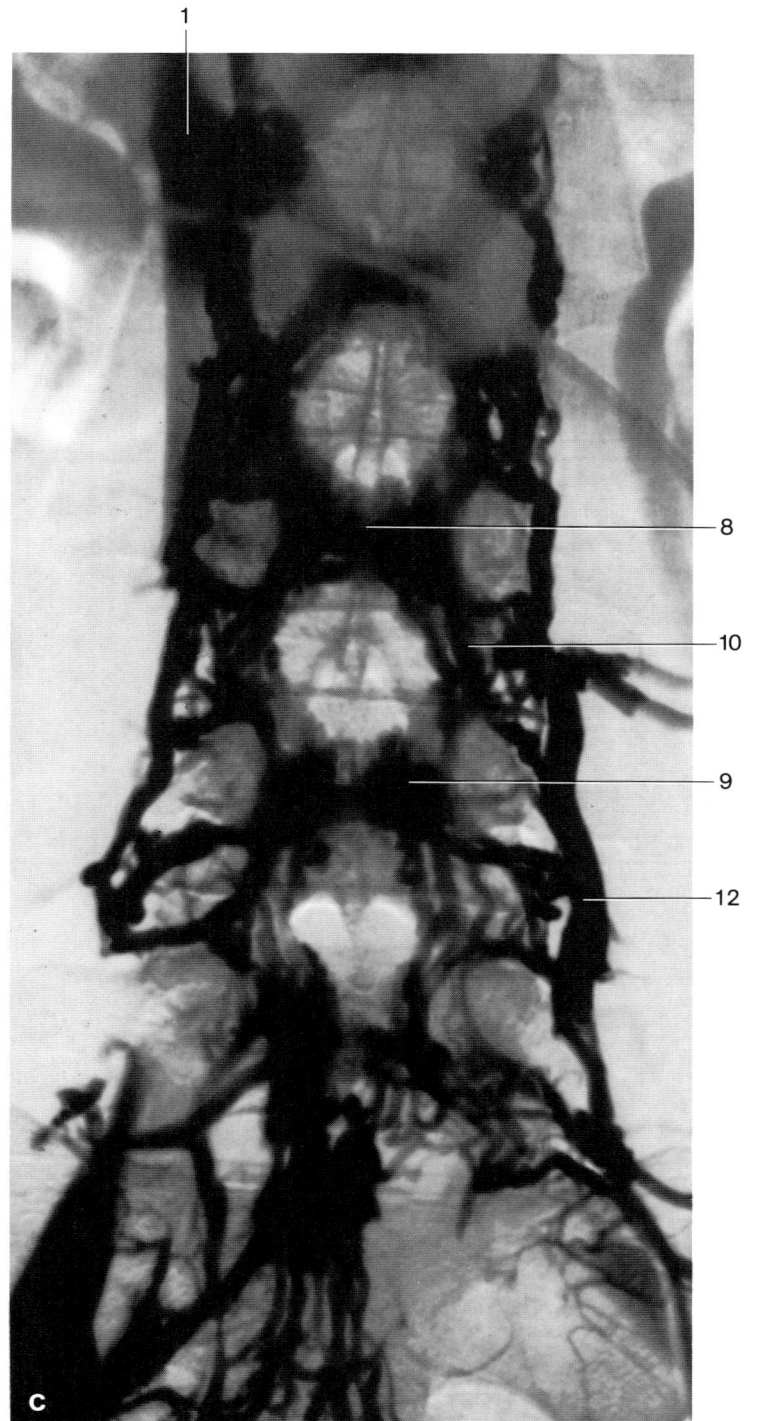

Figure 127 A–C

A Lateral aspect of the lumbosacral spine after intravenous injection of contrast material

B Horizontal section through T12 after intravenous injection of contrast material

C Lumbar phlebography
   (courtesy of Dr. Corbeau and Prof. J. P. Clément, Marseilles)

1 v. cava inf. *2* v. azygos *3* v. hemiazygos *4* aorta *5* ren *6* hepar *7* v. lumbalis *8* vas anastomicum *9* plexus venosus vertebralis internus *10* plexus venosus foraminis intervertebralis *11* rami venosi dorsales *12* v. lumbalis ascendens

The spine contains anterointernal and posterior longitudinal venous plexuses. The anterointernal plexuses are the more important, lying in the lateral third of the vertebral canal in contact with its anterior wall and displaying transverse anastomoses flush with the middle part of the vertebral bodies. Avascular spaces between the transverse anastomoses form windows in the venous system over the middle part of the intervertebral discs. The posterior intraspinal plexuses are formed of minuscule veins, practically invisible on phlebography, which lie in the epidural fat along the posterior surface of the dural envelope. Horizontal veins leave the longitudinal plexuses in three directions: The large centrovertebral diploic veins run horizontally forward to the body of the vertebrae, anastomosing the intraspinal and extraspinal venous plexuses via the metameric veins. The diploic veins run along the margins of, or penetrate the posterior longitudinal ligament. The anterointernal venous plexuses also give rise to lateral veins, which run horizontally toward the intervertebral foramina, and anterior to them anastomose with the extraspinal venous plexuses. Operative work in the intervertebral foramina is considerably hindered by the presence of these veins. Finally, dorsal veins run through the interlaminar spaces to anastomose with the veins of the spinal muscles.

8. Lumbar Arteriography: Horizontal Section Through L2

From posterior to anterior, six vascular regions can be described.

Posterior Spinal Region. Lying posterior to the vertebral arches, this region is subdivided by the spinous processes into two zones, and comprises essentially the erector spinae muscles traversed by the dorsal branches of the metameric lumbar arteries. These arteries enter the region as vascular bundles, mainly on the lateral concave margin of the interarticular (isthmic) regions, and their terminal branches run through the spinal muscles in the parasagittal plane.

Vertebral Canal and Intervertebral Foramina. This region is supplied by the spinal arteries, arising from the metameric lumbar arteries flush with the intervertebral foramina or from a common arterial trunk with the dorsal branches, which enter the vertebral canal along with the spinal nerve roots to supply the cauda equina and spinal cord or the osteoligamentous and meningeal structures of the canal. Care must be taken not to damage these arteries supplying the neural structures by avoiding bilateral electrocoagulation at the level of several intervertebral foramina.

Prevertebral Region. This region contains the two major vascular axes of the body: the aorta running over the left half of the vertebral bodies and the inferior vena cava over the right half. The aorta and inferior vena cava respectively give off and receive paired collaterals, which run on the right and left over the depressed central part of the vertebral bodies to enter the region of the intervertebral foramina below the vertebral pedicles. In their course the lumbar arteries give off a few direct branches to the vertebral bodies and finally, near the intervertebral foramina, give off spinal and dorsal branches prior to entering the lateral wall of the trunk. The anatomy of these metameric arteries thus accounts for the fixity of the aorta and inferior vena cava to the spine, and mobilization of the aorta and vena cava to expose the anterolateral aspects of the lumbar vertebrae requires that the arteries be sectioned near the posterior surface of the aorta or the anterior surface of the spine. The site of choice for vascular ligation and division is a point halfway between the medial margin of the psoas and the lateral margin of the aorta or inferior vena cava. The aorta and inferior vena cava are not in direct contact with the bodies of the vertebrae, as a band of adipocellular tissue separates the spine from the aorta by 1 cm and from the vena cava by 2 cm. Mobilization and dissection of these great vessels is thus relatively easy to achieve. The metameric lumbar arteries run under the arcuate ligaments of the psoas and their juxtavertebral parts are camouflaged by the body of the psoas. Exposure of these arteries requires the disinsertion of the arcuate ligaments.

Retroperitoneal Region. Branches of the aorta and inferior vena cava arise at the level of the L1–L2 intervertebral disc to form the renal (lateral visceral) vascular bundles, which are sufficiently long to allow the easy mobilization of the structures in the renal fossa towards the midline. This procedure is greatly facilitated by the division of one or several bundles of metameric lumbar vessels on the side of mobilization. The gonadal vessels join the aorta and inferior vena cava in the same lateral plane. The renal vascular bundles would constitute a major obstacle if the lateral approach to the lumbar spine were used, so the most reasonable approach is the anterolateral route posterior to the renal fossa: the structures within the fossa and the renal bundle can be displaced forward toward the midline to expose the bodies of the lumbar vertebrae.

Peritoneal Region. The abdominal viscera lying within the peritoneal envelope are supplied or drained by three main vascular structures anterior to the aorta and inferior vena cava: the celiac trunk, the portal vein, and the superior and inferior mesenteric vessels. These vessels and their branches, lying in the coronal plane anterior to the spine, constitute a major obstacle to the strictly anterior transperitoneal approach to the lumbar spine. The duodenopancreatic mass lies just over the anterior surface of the spine from L1 to L3. Accordingly, the best route of access to the lumbar spine is by the subperitoneal approach, with displacement of the intra- and retroperitoneal viscera toward the midline.

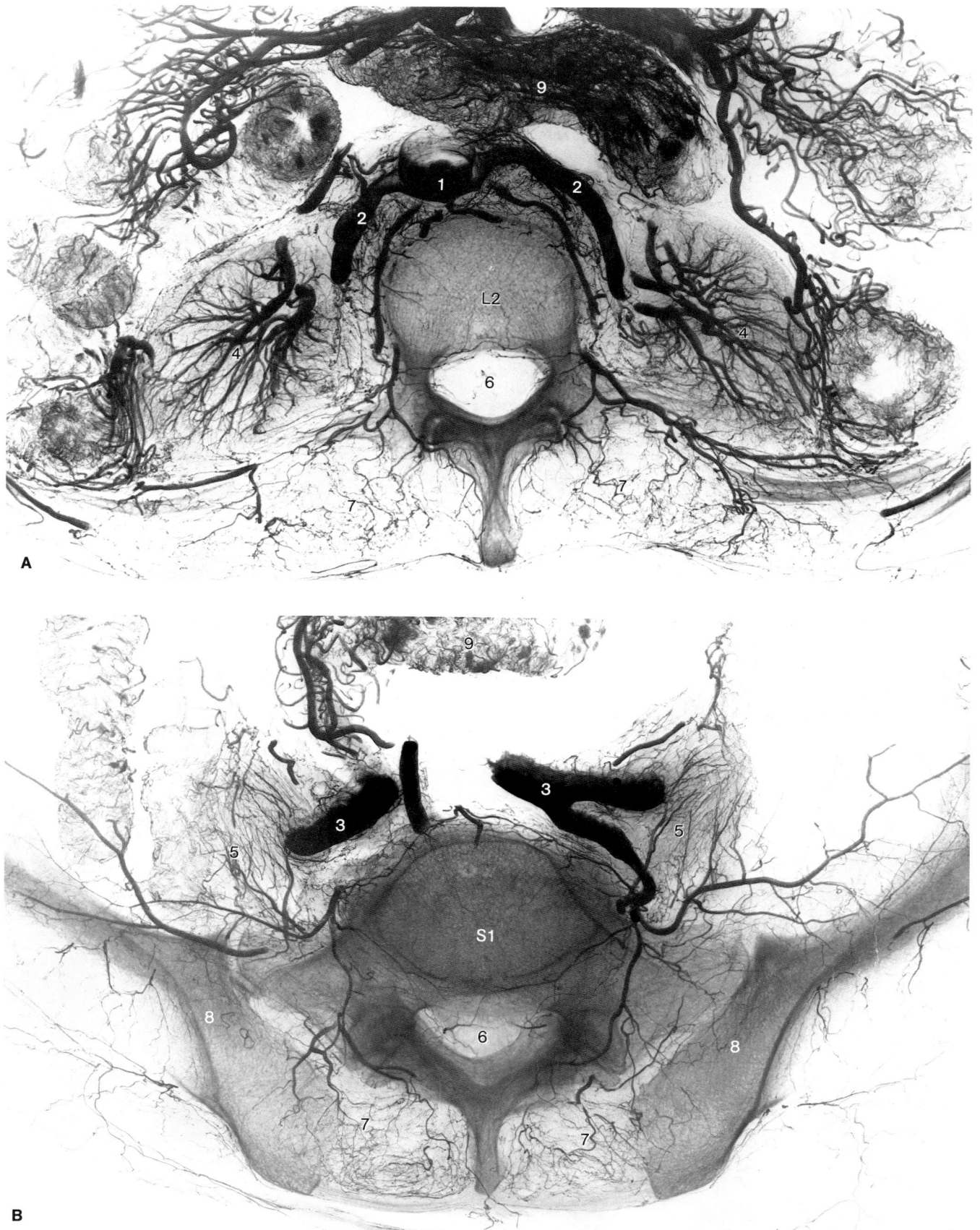

Figure 128 A, B

A   Horizontal section through L2 after intra-arterial injection of contrast material

B   Horizontal section through S1 after intra-arterial injection of contrast material

1 aorta abdominalis   2 a. renalis   3 iliaca communis   4 ren
5 psoas major   6 canalis vertebralis   7 m. erector spinae   8 tuberositas iliaca   9 jejunum, ileum (intestinum tenue mesenteriale)

Anterolateral Parietal Region. The most anterior vascular region on transverse section through L2 is represented by the vessels of the anterolateral wall of the abdomen. The epigastric arteries from a vertical network on the posterior surface of the rectus muscles. The terminal part of the metameric lumbar and intercostal vessels forms oblique axes running between the middle and deep layers of the lateral muscles of the abdomen. Two approaches through the parietal wall can be used to gain anterior access to the spine: the oblique route through the large abdominal muscles parallel to the metameric vessels, or a vertical incision within the sheath of the rectus muscles. However, the latter route leads to denervation of the muscle fibers lying between the abdominal midline and the incision.

9. Transverse Section of the Abdomen Through L2

The lumbar spine can be seen to occupy the posterior half of the sectional area. In thin subjects the bodies of the lumbar vertebrae can be palpated deep to the anterior wall of the abdomen. The anatomically simple posterior lumbar region lies behind the vertebral canal and transverse processes, and comprises the vertebral arches with their joints, the erector spinae muscles, and the dorsal skin. The abdominal cavity with its wall and contents lies anterior to this region. The walls of the abdomen are inserted on the lumbar spine, whose vertebral bodies and intervertebral discs protrude prominently into the abdominal region. The psoas muscles, displaying bundles of fibers inserting on the vertebral bodies and transverse processes, lie on each side of the spine. The lumbar nervous plexus and the ascending lumbar vein lie between the two psoas muscle bundles. These different structures form a considerable obstacle to the strictly lateral route of access to the lumbar vertebrae. Laterally, the abdominal wall is continued by the quadratus lumborum and latissimus dorsi followed by the three large muscles of the abdomen; the deep-lying transversus, the middle obliquus internus, and the superficial obliquus externus.

The anterior wall of the abdomen is formed by the rectus muscles and their sheath with the intervening linea alba on the midline. The fibrous sheet lining the deep surface of this layer comprises the fascia iliaca anterior to the psoas, and the fascia transversalis from the quadratus lumborum to the posterior wall of the rectus sheath.

The abdominal viscera can be divided into peritoneal and retroperitoneal sectors. The peritoneal sector lies in front of the coronal plane which passes anterior to the vertebral bodies. The parietal peritoneum lines the deep surface of the fascia transversalis, the anterior surface of the renal fossae, and the duodenopancreatic mass in front of the midline prevertebral vessels. The abdominal cavity contains the colon and loops of small bowel joined together by the mesentery. The renal fossae flanking the lumbar spine and psoas muscles contain the adrenal glands, kidneys, and ureters enveloped in the retroperitoneal fat. The great prevertebral vessels lie over the anterior surface of the lumbar spine, the aorta on the left and the inferior vena cava on the right. The periaortic ganglions lying along the left flank of the aorta are interposed between the

great vessels. The lumbar sympathetic trunk and metameric lumbar vessels lie between the great vessels and the anterior longitudinal ligament. The duodenopancreatic mass is located anterior to the pervertebral vessels.

Accordingly, access to the anterior part of the lumbar spine can in theory be gained by three routes:

1. The median transperitoneal route, requiring mobilization of the small bowel loops, the duodenopancreatic mass, and the prevertebral vessels. This approach is particularly deep and inconvenient, and is dangerous because of the number of major structures to be displaced.

2. The posterolateral route through the posterior part of the lateral abdominal muscles, displacing the renal fossae forward and finally passing between the quadratus lumborum and psoas muscles to reach the region of the intervertebral foramina. We strongly advise against this route, as dissection in this rich neurovascular region risks neural injury, hemorrhage through injury to the extraspinal venous plexuses, and medullary ischemia resulting from damage to the spinal arteries and their anastomotic system.

3. The lateral retroperitoneal approach, manifestly the route of choice. This approach allows decollement of the peritoneum and of the retroperitoneal fat from the walls of the abdomen to gain access to the anterior surface of the lumbar spine. Furthermore, access is in a zone where the metameric venous bundles can easily be dissected and ligated to mobilize the great vessels.

10. Prevertebral Vascular and Ureteral Anomalies

The surgeon must be familiar with these rare anomalies, which represent a serious operative risk.

Duplication of the inferior vena cava resultes from the persistence of the twin embryonic inferior venae cavae and features the presence of a large vein on the left lateral side of the aorta. The presence of such a structure would be a very unusual finding during the left lumbar approach. The supplementary vein can usually be mobilized by the division of the metameric vessels. Although not particularly dangerous, the ligation of the vein is generally not necessary.

A periaortic venous ring is due to the persistence of a large retroaortic anastomotic vein between the left renal vein and the inferior vena cava. This vein need not be ligated and divided during the mobilization of the great vessels.

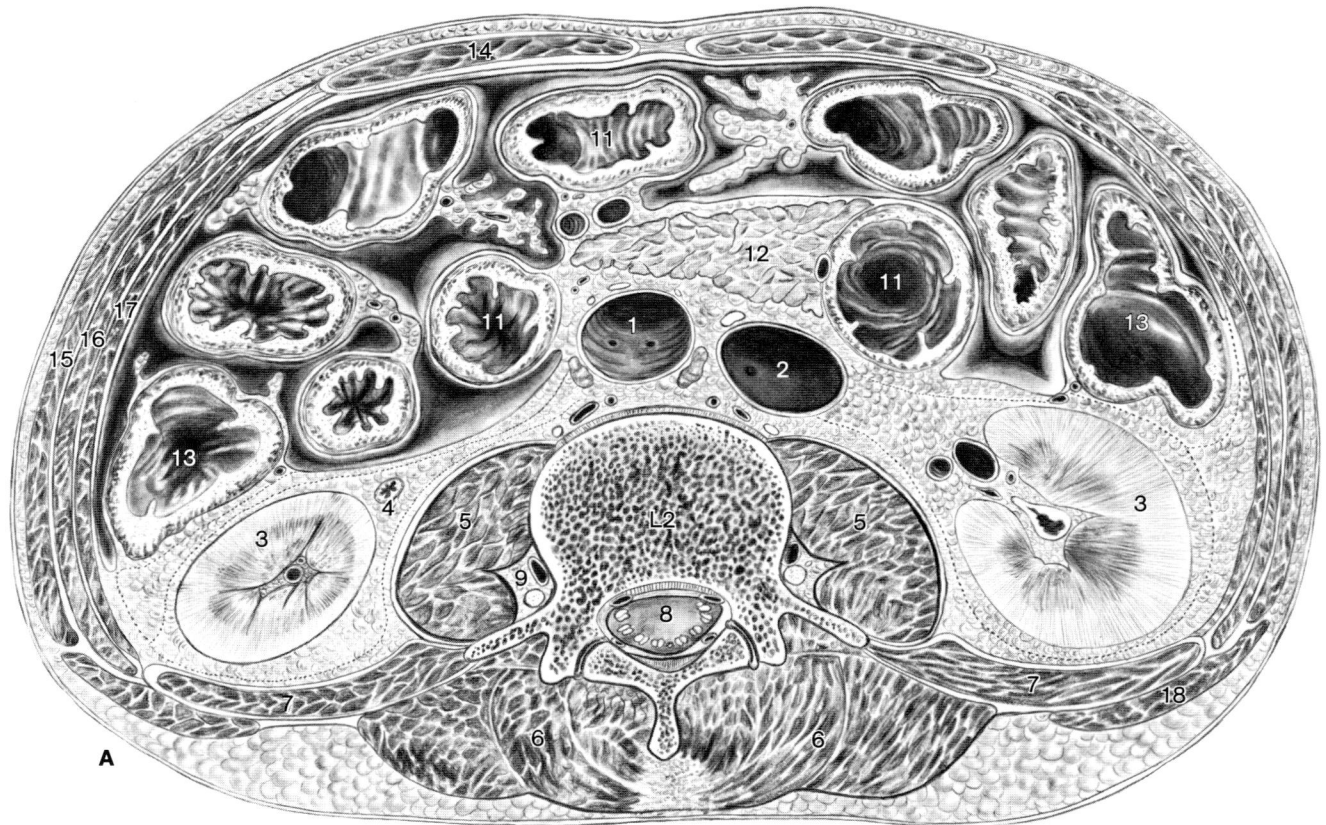

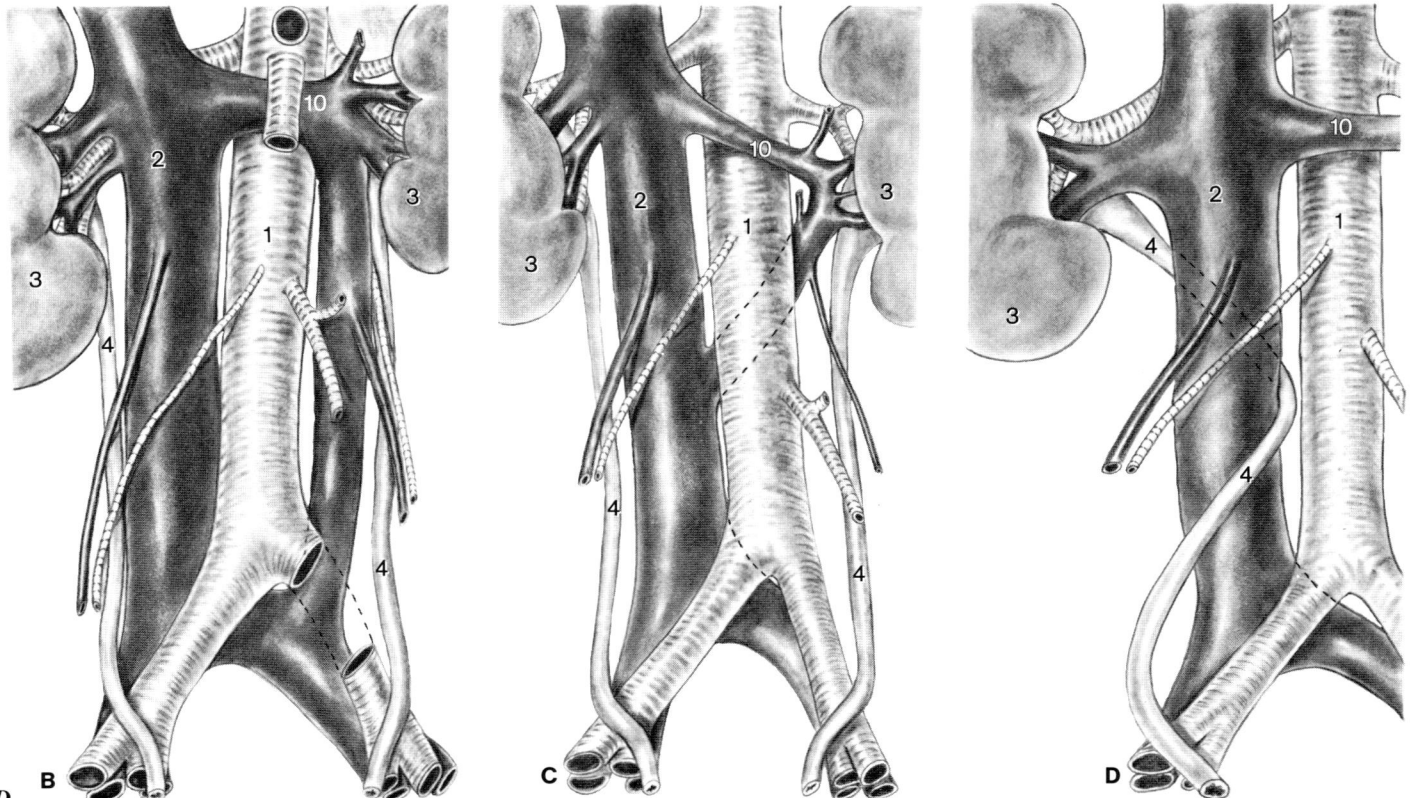

Figure 129 A–D

A   Horizontal section of the abdomen through L2
B   Duplication of the inferior vena cava
C   Periaortic venous ring
D   Retrocaval ureter

1 aorta *2* v. cava inf. *3* ren *4* ureter *5* psoas major *6* m. erector spinae *7* m. quadratus lumborum *8* cavum subarachnoidale, cauda equina *9* nn. spinales, v. lumbalis ascendens *10* v. renalis
11 jejunum, ileum (intestinum tenue mesenteriale) *12* pancreas
13 intestinum crassum *14* m. rectus abdominis *15* m. obliquus externus abdominis *16* m. obliquus internus abdominis *17* m. transversus abdominis *18* m. latissimus dorsi

A right retrocaval ureter is due to the anomalous fusion of the embryonic segments of the inferior vena cava; the right ureter passes behind the inferior vena cava and then between it and the aorta. Consequently, right lumbotomy with mobilization of the inferior vena cava would expose this large cylindrical retrocaval structure. Extreme care must be taken to identify the ureter and not confuse it with an anastomotic vessel.

B. Operative Approach: Left Lumbotomy

Left lumbotomy is preferred to approach from the right, since the aorta can be mobilized more easily and with less risk than the relatively fragile inferior vena cava.

1. Operative Position

The lateral position with the patient resting on a cushion, as used in lumbotomy to approach the kidney, is not recommended in spinal surgery except in cases of scoliosis with convexity on the side of approach. In all other cases we recommend the strictly supine position with elevation of the lumbar spine by angling of the table or use of a pad under the spine to render the vertebrae more superficial. Vertebral traction should be used when reduction is to be obtained. This position enables reestablishment of physiological lumbar lordosis and frontal rectitude of the spine after vertebral excision or reduction. The left upper limb is suspended at a 90° angle above the scapular girdle.

2. Skin Incision

The classical incision of lumbotomy runs from the costolumbar angle below the twelfth rib toward the lateral margin of the rectus at the level of the umbilicus. We prefer to use a more oblique incision, in view of the direction of the neural bundles of the anterolateral abdominal wall. Our incision is begun between the ends of the eleventh and twelfth ribs and is directed downward and medially toward the lateral margin of the rectus muscle to a point halfway between the umbilicus and symphysis pubis. This incision allows dissection between the eleventh and twelfth intercostal nerves without sectioning them. The incision can be extended cranially in the eleventh intercostal space and caudally along the lateral margin of the rectus towards the symphysis pubis. The subcutaneous tissue is then incised.

3. Parietal Dissection

The three large muscles of the abdomen can either be transected parallel to the skin incision or dissected parallel to their muscle fibers. Hemostasis of the cut muscle surfaces should be accomplished progressively by electrocoagulation to avoid retraction of the sectioned blood vessels. The neurovascular bundles run between the obliquus internus and transversus abdominis. Transection of the transversus must be done carefully after a buttonhole incision has been made in the muscle by alternately opening and closing the scissors to expose but not open the peritoneum. Decollement of the peritoneum is begun to allow clamp-held compresses to be passed deep to the transversus abdominis, which can then be transected with the electric cautery knife without injury to the peritoneum. Care must be taken at both ends of the operative field. At the cranial end, incision of the eleventh intercostal space should not extend within the zone lying 8 cm or less from the line of spinous processes, to avoid entry of the pleural cul-de-sac. If inadvertently opened, the cul-de-sac should be closed by suture while the anesthesiologist applies positive pulmonary pressure. Thoracic suction drainage would be required postoperatively only in cases where the lung cannot be fully inflated. In the caudal part of the operative field, the large inferior epigastric artery should be ligated under the transversus abdominis in cases where the incision is extended towards the symphysis pubis.

4. Retroperitoneal Decollement

Decollement of the anterior parietal peritoneum from the transversus abdominis is begun to allow installation of an orthostatic retractor. A large flexible retractor is used to displace the intraperitoneal structures towards the midline and to stretch the parietal adhesions of the peritoneum. The adhesions are then progressively suppressed by blunt dissection using clamp-held compresses. During decollement the deep surface of the transversus abdominis is brought into view first, followed by the anterior surface of the quadratus lumborum. Along the latter can be seen, in craniocaudal order, the twelfth intercostal nerve, the iliohypogastric nerve, the ilioinguinal nerve, and much farther down, the lateral cutaneous femoral nerve. Blunt dissection is pursued until contact is made with a pronounced muscle ridge corresponding to the lateral margin of the psoas muscle. Dissection should then extend over this ridge but not into the fissure separating the psoas and quadratus lumborum. Accordingly, the flexible retractor should be repositioned anteriorly and medially at this stage. During dissection along the anterior surface of the psoas the operator should seek to identify the ureter, which normally remains adherent to the posterior surface of the peritoneum. The ureter must not be mistaken for some other structure that would be ligated and divided. Features that help to identify it are its cylindrical shape, its peristaltic movements at the slightest touch, and its superficial network of anastomoses. Displacement of the abdominal contents toward the midline with one or two flexible retractors enables visualization of the medial margin of the psoas muscle with its arcuate ligaments inserting on the intervertebral discs. The aorta is now palpable and exposed in the vertebromuscular groove which also contains the lumbar sympathetic trunk posterior to the aorta.

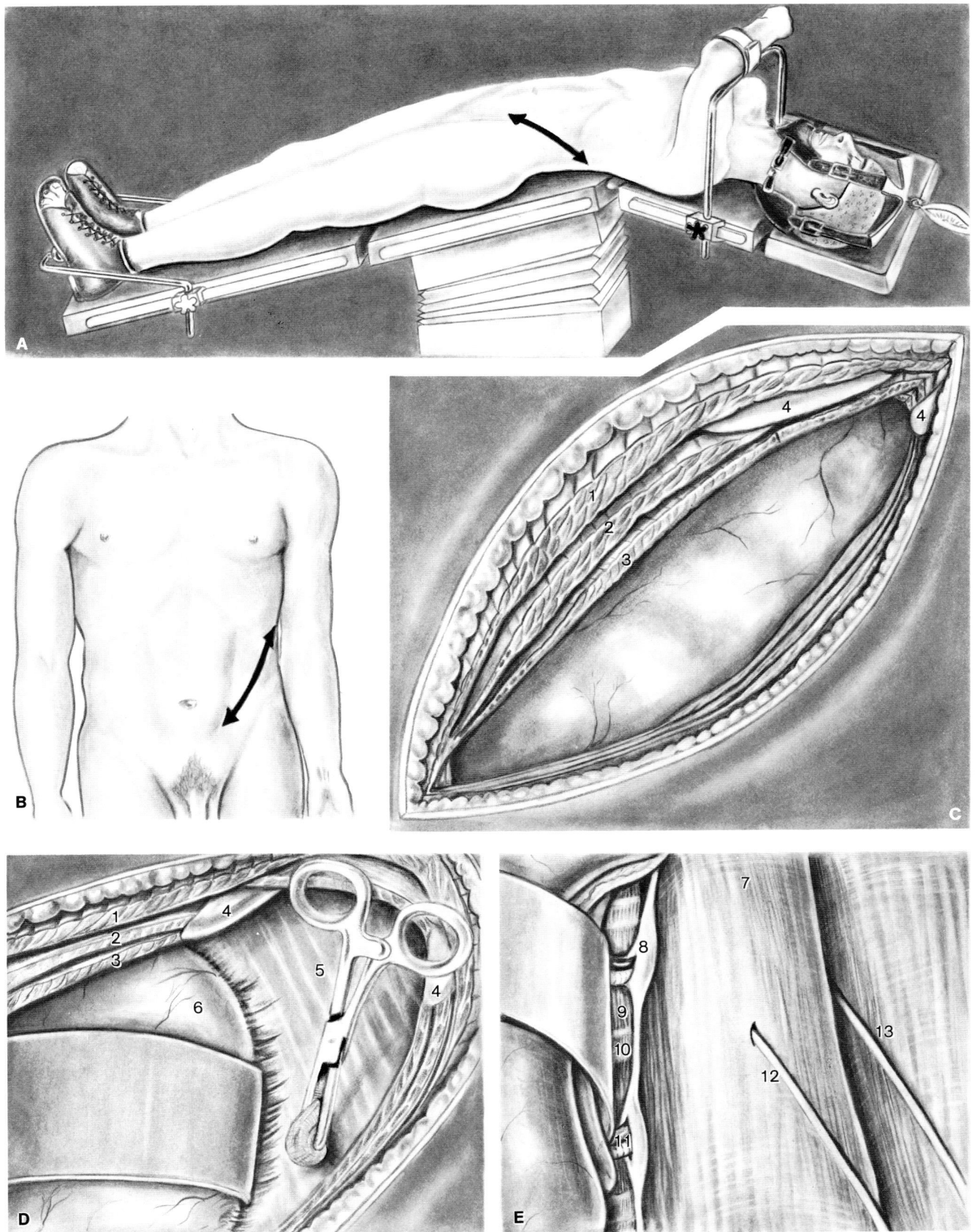

Figure 130 A–E

A Operative position in left lumbotomy
B Skin incision in left lumbotomy
C Parietal dissection
D Decollement of the peritoneal envelope and intraperitoneal viscera
E Exposure of the lumbar spine

1 m. obliquus externus abdominis *2* m. obliquus internus abdominis
3 m. transversus abdominis *4* costa *5* m. quadratus lumborum
6 cavum peritonei *7* m. psoas major *8* truncus sympathicus
9 vertebra lumbalis *10* discus intervertebralis *11* a. and v. lumbales
12 n. genitofemoralis *13* n. cutaneus femoris lateralis

5. Hemostasis of the Lumbar Vessels

Exposure of the intervertebral discs and vertebral bodies is begun by identifying the metameric vascular bundles and the prominent discs and pursued with blunt dissection between the aorta and psoas, using clamp-held compresses. The lateral part of the discs can usually be seen to be free of vessels, so the approach to a single disc can be achieved without the section of a lumbar vascular bundle. Conversely, exposure of the lateral surfaces of one or more vertebral bodies requires the identification, ligation, and division of a certain number of left lumbar arteries and veins. It should be remembered that the lumbar vessels run over the middle depressed part of the vertebral bodies. Each blood vessel is isolated on a long, curved, slender needle holder, clips are installed on each side of the instrument, and the vessel is divided between the clips. The vascular stumps should be sufficiently long to allow a second ligation if the clip gives way. Hemostasis can also be achieved by suturing the vessels with nonresorbable suture material, but coagulation should be avoided since these vessels are too large to allow adequate hemostasis with this technique. One exception to this rule is the case of sclerotic post-infectious lesions enveloping the vascular bundles, when electrocoagulation can be used.

6. Exposure of the Lumbar Spine

A large flexible retractor is bent to raise the aorta slightly and displace it toward the midline to expose the anterior surface of the lumbar spine. Exposure is completed using a large raspatory with a semicircular cutting edge, so as not to present a sharp acute-angled cutting surface in contact with the great vessels. The instrument is manipulated with its concave part over the convexity of the lumbar spine and in constant contact with the anterior longitudinal ligament. As the aorta is progressively displaced with the flexible retractor, the raspatory is gradually directed toward the left flank of the vertebral bodies. Once the desired region of the spine is exposed, the flexible retractor is molded into an S shape. One curve of the retractor is placed around the left flank of the lumbar spine while the second retains both the great vessels and the intraperitoneal viscera near the midline. Steinmann pins, planted in the bodies of the vertebrae at the upper and lower ends of the operative field, can be used to help obtain good exposure. An orthostatic retractor is then installed to relieve the assistants. This approach also allows correct exposure of the anterior and right lateral surfaces of the spine from the L1–L2 disc to the L4–L5 disc.

7. Closure

At the end of the operation it should be checked that good hemostasis has been achieved. Surgicel can be used to complete hemostasis in regions where coagulation and clipping are not appropriate. In cases where blood leakage persists, suction drainage should be installed in the retroperitoneal space, but in the presence of proper hemostasis drainage is not required.

Removal of the flexible retractors and orthostatic retractor results in full immediate occlusion of the lumbar fossa by the peritoneum and the viscera contained within. The next step is to reconstruct the different layers of the anterolateral abdominal wall using interrupted nonresorbable sutures for each muscle layer. Finally, the subcutaneous layer and the skin are closed with interrupted sutures. Continuous sutures should not be used, since this region is specially mobile and abdominal distension could lead to rupture of a continuous suture.

8. Possible Complications

Poor initial technique may lead to the section of the nerve bundles of the anterolateral abdominal wall when the skin incision is not sufficiently oblique. Over-forceful dissection can lead to opening of the peritoneum. If this happens the peritoneum should be closed with one or more continuous sutures and a moist towel should be placed against the peritoneum to avoid further injury. During decollement of the peritoneum, ligation of the ureter if mistake for a blood vessel is a serious complication which can be avoided simply by bearing in mind the anatomical features of the ureter. The most severe complications arise from injury to major vascular structures. Mobilization of the great vessels must be performed using flexible retractors with rounded edges and by manipulating the instruments firmly but not with so much force as to overwhelm the elasticity of the vascular tissue. Finally, proper hemostasis of the metameric vessels is prepared by good exposure.

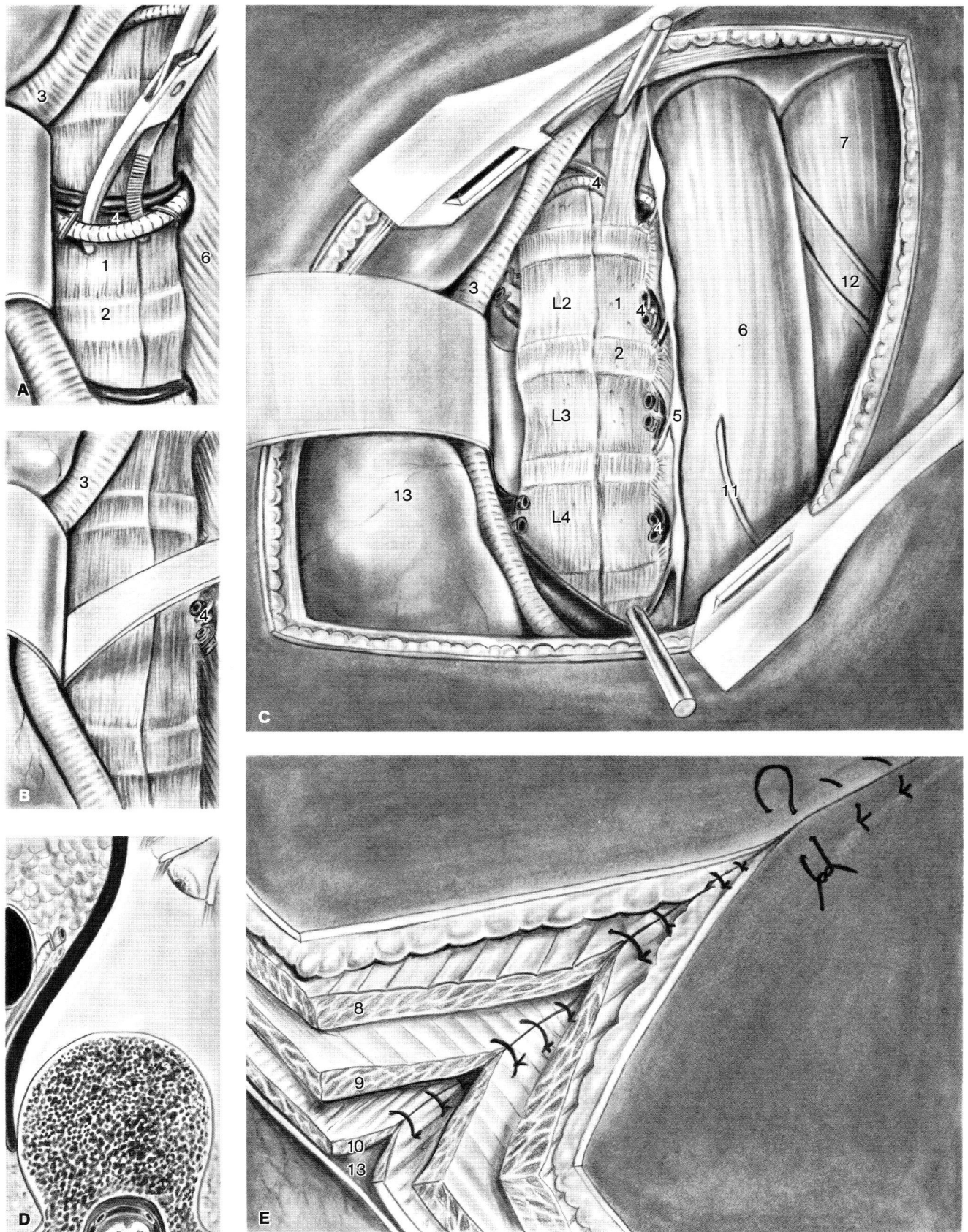

Figure 131 A–E

A   Ligation of a lumbar vascular bundle
B   Exposure of the vertebral bodies with the raspatory
C   Exposure of the anterior and lateral surfaces of the lumbar spine
D   The operative field of vision
E   Parietal closure

1 corpus vertebrae lumbalis   2 discus intervertebralis lumbalis
3 aorta abdominalis   4 a. and v. lumbales   5 truncus sympathicus
6 m. psoas   7 m. quadratus lumborum   8 m. obliquus externus
abdominis   9 m. obliquus internus abdominis   10 m. transversus
abdominis   11 n. genitofemoralis   12 n. iliohypogastricus, n. ilioinguinalis   13 peritoneum

III. Anterior Region

A. Topography

1. Anterior Parietal Structures

It can be recalled that the anterolateral wall of the abdomen is formed on each side of the midline by the rectus muscles and laterally by the obliquus muscles of the abdomen. The rectus muscles, forming a band three to four fingers in width above and below the umbilicus, are transversely intersected by tendons. They are enveloped by the rectus sheath, whose anterior layer is continuous, whereas the posterior layer lines only the upper two thirds of the muscles. On the midline, the anterior and posterior layers of the sheath fuse to form the linea alba, with the umbilicus lying in its center. The linea alba is widest below the umbilicus and thus should be opened initially in this region when a median anterior incision is made. On each side of the rectus muscles (from superficial to deep) lie the obliquus externus, the obliquus internus, the transversus abdominis. The deep part of the transversus and the posterior surface of the rectus sheath are lined by the fascia transversalis. The anterolateral part of the abdominal wall is traversed by neurovascular bundles running obliquely (parallel to the intercostal spaces) toward the linea alba. It may be recalled that the tenth intercostal bundle runs toward the umbilical region and the twelfth toward the symphysis pubis.

2. Peritoneal Structures

The lumbosacral region lies deep to the peritoneal cavity. The anterior layer of the peritoneum is located posterior to the rectus sheath and the posterior layer anterior to the great prevertebral vessels. The contents of the peritoneal cavity are the colon and mesocolon. The ascending mesocolon continues the posterior parietal peritoneum to the right, the descending mesocolon continues it to the left, and the mesosigmoid continues it toward the pelvic cavity. The intersigmoid recess is interposed between the mesosigmoid and the posterior parietal peritoneum. The insertions of the mesosigmoid limiting the intersigmoid recess lie on the presacral midline and extend along the common and left external iliac vascular bundle. The mesentery, lying anterior to the right mesocolon, inserts in bayonet fashion on the duodenojejunal flexure, the region of the anterior surface of the inferior vena cava, and along the common and right external iliac vascular bundle. Access to the lumbar spine thus requires the displacement of the small bowel loops and colon towards their respective mesocolons in order to expose the lumbosacral region with only the posterior parietal peritoneum remaining on the midline. Dissection of the posterior peritoneum exposes the prevertebral neurovascular structures.

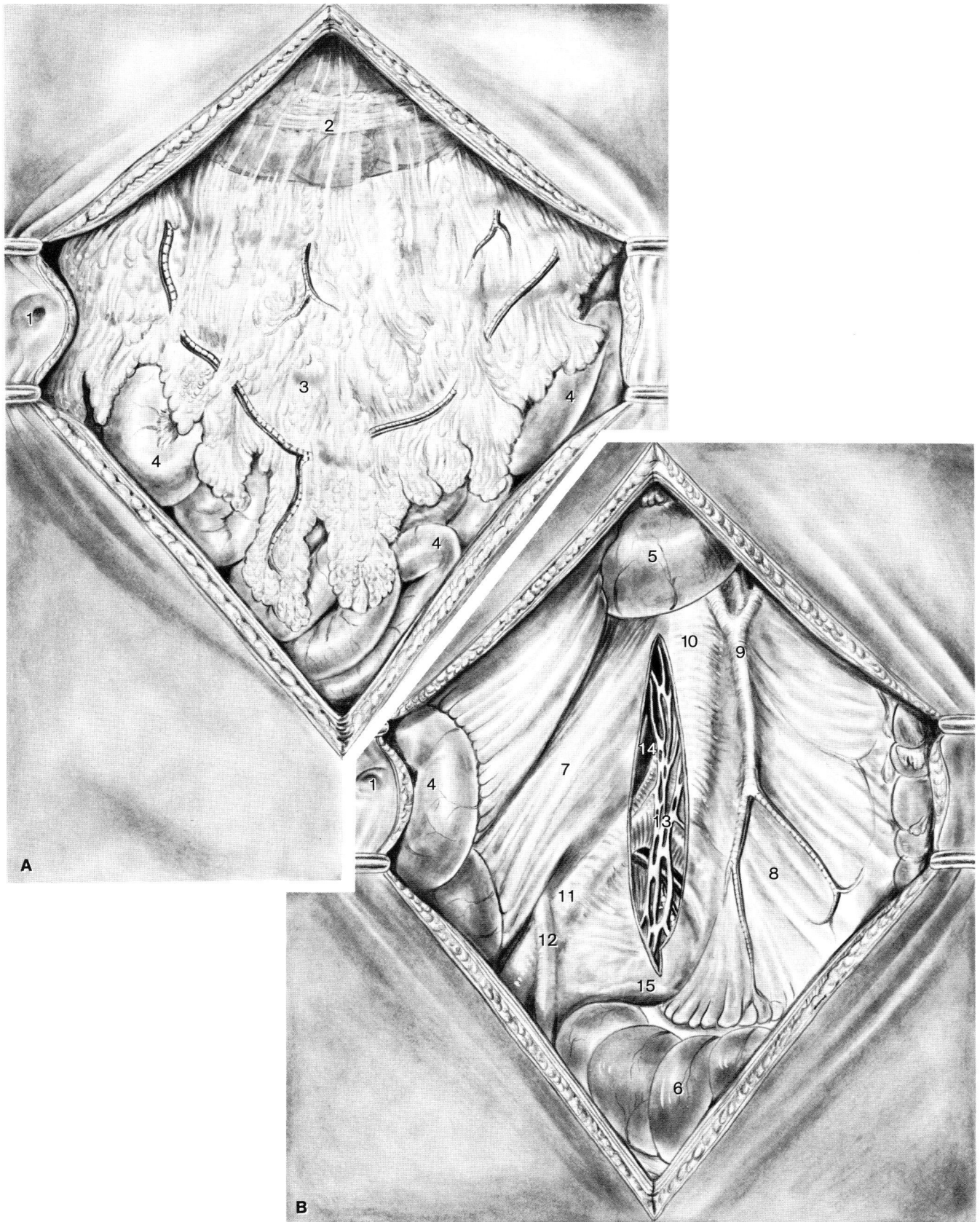

Figure 132 A, B

A Transperitoneal opening of the abdominal cavity
B Opening of the posterior parietal peritoneum lying over the
   lumbosacral junction

1 umbilicus *2* colon transversum *3* omentum majus *4* intestinum
tenue *5* duodenum, pars horizontalis *6* colon sigmoideum
7 mesenterium *8* mesocolon sigmoideum *9* a. mesenterica inf.
10 aorta abdominalis *11* a. iliaca communis *12* ureter *13* plexus
hypogastricus sup. *14* v. cava inf. *15* promontorium ossis sacri

3. Prevertebral Vascular Structures

The anterior surface of the lumbosacral region lies deep to the aortocaval axis and its collateral vessels. The topographical arrangement of these vessels is variable.

Aortocaval Axis. The termination of the aorta and the origin of the inferior vena cava each form a Y-shaped bifurcation, that of the aorta lying anteriorly and to the left side, that of the vena cava posteriorly and to the right side. The topography of the aortic terminal and origin of the inferior vena cava is summarized in the table below, based on our experience (1971):

Spinal level	Termination of aorta (%)	Origin of inferior vena cava (%)
L3	6	–
L3–L4	22	–
L4	43	21
L4–L5	24	30
L5	5	46
L5–S1	–	3

In Europeans the angle of aortoiliac bifurcation is 70°, whereas in our experience it is 45° in black Africans. Conversely, the iliocaval angle is 65° in the former population and 72° in the latter. The iliac bifurcations lie at the level of or slightly above the sacral promontory.

Collateral Vessels. The collateral branches of the aortocaval axis lying anterior to the lumbosacral spine comprise the inferior mesenteric artery, the middle sacral bundle, and the fourth and fifth lumbar bundles. The inferior mesenteric artery arises from the anterior surface of the aorta between the L2–L3 and L3–L4 intervertebral discs, usually in the region posterior to the third segment of the duodenum, and enters the left mesocolon. The middle sacral vascular bundle lies anterior to the sacrum near the midline (36% of cases), on the right (24%), or on the left (40%) of the sacrum. The middle sacral artery arises from the posterior surface of the aortic bifurcation, while the middle sacral vein joins one of the structures comprising the iliocaval confluent. The fourth lumbar vascular bundle runs metamerically towards the body of L4, whereas the fifth lumbar vessels display a more variable, dispersed course. In decreasing order of frequency the fifth lumbar artery may arise from the iliolumbar, fourth lumbar, or middle sacral arteries, or from the aorta. The fifth lumbar vein anastomoses with any one of the other veins in this region.

Topographical Varieties. Five types of aortocaval axes can be described according to the level of the bifurcation of the aorta and origin of the inferior vena cava. In the first so-called *classical* type (63.5% of cases) the aorta bifurcates at the level of the L4–L5 intervertebral disc while the common iliac veins join together just below this point. In the second *paradoxical* type (6.4%) the aortic bifurcation lies caudal to the origin of the inferior vena cava. The third type (15.4%) is an unusually *high* position of the aortic bifurcation, cranial to the L3–L4

disc, and of the origin of the inferior vena cava, above the L4–L5 disc. In the fourth type (5.1%) the bifurcation of the aorta and the origin of the inferior vena cava are unusually *low,* near the center of L5 and at the L5–S1 disc respectively. The fifth type (9.7%) is termed *dissociated:* the aortic bifurcation lies more than one vertebra cranial to the origin of the inferior vena cava. Knowledge of these topographical varieties enables determination of both the surgical maneuvers required to mobilize the great vessels and the sites of hemostasis of the collateral vessels for proper access to the anterior lumbosacral region.

4. Prevertebral Neural Structures

The bodies of the lumbosacral vertebrae display anatomical relations to the vegetative neural structures anteriorly and the lumbar plexus laterally. The lumbar *vegetative neural structures* comprise the right and left lumbar sympathetic trunks with their connecting rami and ganglions, and lie in the dihedral angle formed by the anterolateral surface of the vertebral bodies and the arcuate ligamentous insertions of the psoas muscle. The presacral nerve (superior hypogastric plexus) lies on the midline. Knowledge of the anatomy of this nerve is essential to the surgeon to avoid inducing sexual disturbances subsequent to the anterior approach to the lumbosacral junction. The following description is based on the studies by Delmas and Laux (1952), Winckler (1966), Taghavi (1970), and Maresca and Ghafar (1979). The presacral nerve lies on the anterior surface of the aortic termination below the origin of the inferior mesenteric artery, and is formed by the confluence of three groups of rami: lateral rami from the lumbar sympathetic trunk and median rami from the celiac plexus and from the superior and inferior mesenteric plexuses. The presacral plexus then spreads out downward between the common iliac arteries to divide slightly caudal to the sacral promontory to form two terminal branches, the hypograstic nerves.

Figure 133 A–F

A The common position of the aortic termination and origin of the inferior vena cava

B Anatomical arrangement of the aortocaval collateral vessels

C Paradoxical aortocaval axis with the origin of the inferior vena cava cranial to the aortic bifurcation

D Unusually low aortic bifurcation and origin of the inferior vena cava

E Unusually high aortic bifurcation and origin of the inferior vena cava

F The dissociated anatomical position, with the aortic bifurcation markedly cranial to the origin of the inferior vena cava

1 aorta abdominalis *2* v. cava inf. *3* a. iliaca communis *4* v. iliaca communis *5* promontorium ossis sacri *6* a. and v. lumbales IV *7* a. and v. sacralis mediana *8* a. and v. lumbales V

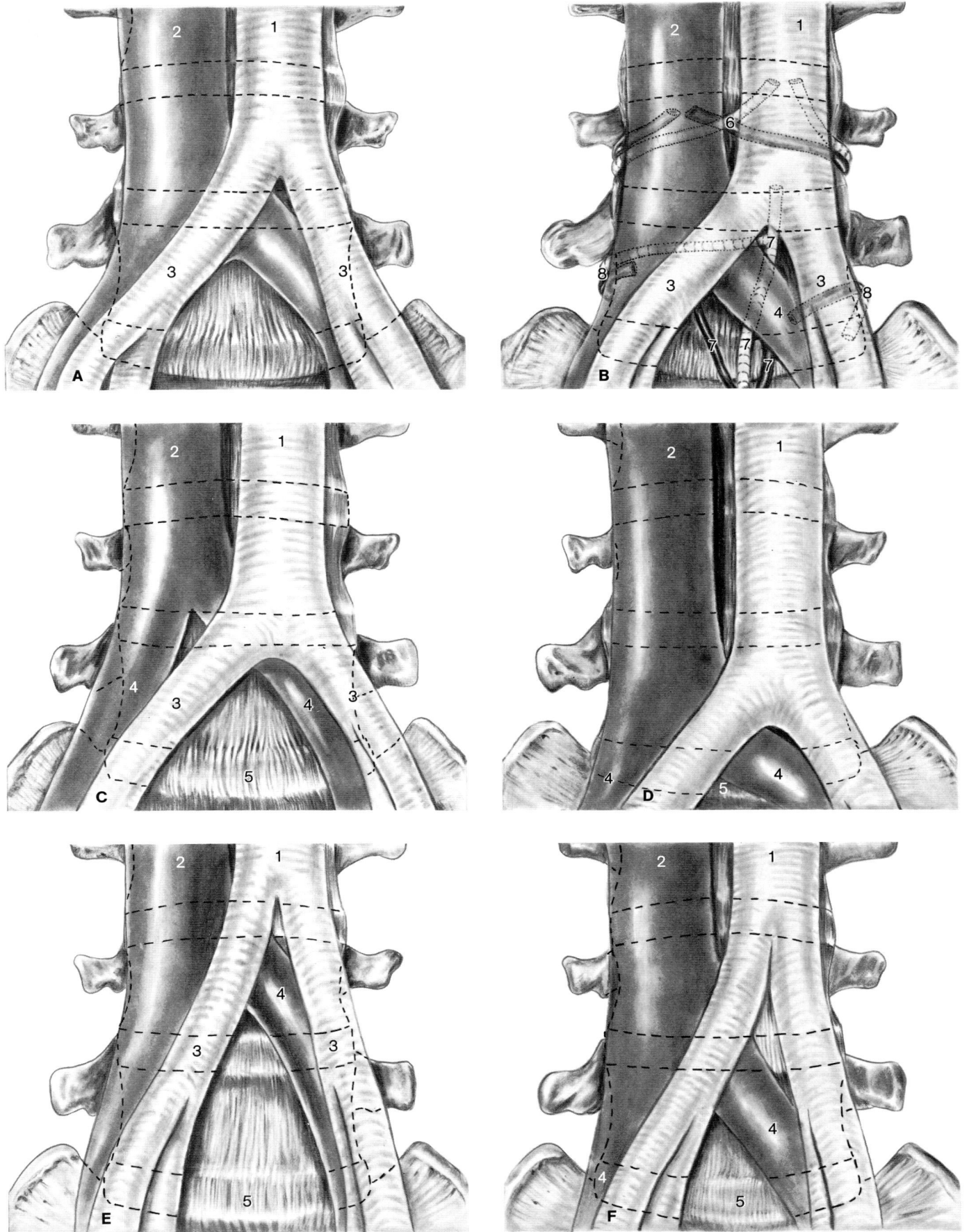

Figure 133 A–F

The four lumbar sympathetic ganglions give off lateral efferents to the right and left. The nerve fibers of the efferents on the right pass behind the inferior vena cava and then between the aorta and vena cava, finally reaching the anterior surface of the aorta. The two lowest fibers, originating at the level of L3 and L4, display a more variable course, i.e., pre- or retrovenous and retroarterial. The much shorter efferents on the left side run along the left lateral surface of the aorta. The efferents in the lumbosacral region are present with variable frequency, as shown in the following table:

Level	Right efferents (%)	Left efferents (%)
T12	2.6	0
L1	78.6	68
L2	98.6	84
L3	33.3	16
L4	45.3	32

The most commonly encountered efferents arise from the first and second lumbar ganglions. These efferents are specially involved in the ejaculatory function in men, and must therefore be protected during anterior surgery of the spine. The medial efferents comprise both sympathetic and parasympathetic (pneumogastric) fibers emanating from the celiac and mesenteric plexuses. The trunk of the presacral nerve extends anterior to the aorta from the inferior mesenteric artery to the termination of the left common iliac vein, the body of L5, and the L5–S1 intervertebral disc. The presacral nerve resembles one of three morphological types: the *truncal* type, in which the nerve comprises two or three longitudinal trunks linked together by a few fine fibers (38.6% of cases); the *plexiform* type, comprising three to five nerve trunks joined together by numerous anastomotic fibers (44%) and the *lamellar* type, in which the numerous anastomotic fibers constitute a veritable flattened network resembling a stretched-out nerve ganglion (17.3%). The presacral plexus (also referred to as the superior hypogastric plexus) is formed by longitudinal nerves, with numerous vegetative ganglions among its constituent fibers. It terminates to form a bifurcation at the level of the sacral promotory, giving rise to the right and left hypogastric nerves, which enter the pelvis to join the inferior hypogastric plexuses. The termination of the presacral plexus varies as follows:

Level of termination:

–Body of L5   4.0%
–L5–S1 disc   16.0%
–Body of S1   74.7%
–Body of S2   5.3%

In 80% of cases the bifurcation lies caudal to the promontory, thus requiring the lateral displacement of the presacral nerve to allow access to the two lowest lumbar discs.
The neural trunks of the lumbar plexus lie in a very lateral position in the angle formed by the transverse processes and bodies of the lumbar vertebrae, i.e., between the insertions of the psoas muscle on the transverse processes and vertebral

bodies. Access to these nerves requires the surgical detachment of the psoas insertions. The lumbosacral nerve trunk can be exposed along the posterolateral margins of the lumbosacral intervertebral disc.

5. Maneuvers to Mobilize the Prevertebral Neurovascular Structures

The aim of the anterior approach to the lumbosacral spine is to expose the bodies of the three lowest lumbar vertebrae, the body of the sacrum, and the intervening intervertebral discs. Anterior surgery thus requires the mobilization of the aortocaval axis and presacral nerve without causing injury to them, regardless of the topographical type encountered. The following five maneuvers enable the surgeon to achieve this goal.

Interiliac Route. The most frequently used, this route passes between the two common iliac vascular bundles below the origin of the inferior vena cava and aortic bifurcation. This approach allows easy access to the L5–S1 intervertebral disc and, in cases where the origin of the vena cava lies unusually high, the L4–L5 disc.

Inter- and Transiliac Route. This route also passes between the right and left common iliac vessels, followed by isolation and separation of the left common iliac vein from the left common iliac artery. This approach, particularly useful when the large left common iliac vein hinders access to the body of L5, allows access to the two lowest lumbar intervertebral discs. When this approach or the interiliac approach is used, the presacral nerve is usually displaced towards the left side. Hemostasis of the middle sacral vessels is required to expose the anterior surface of the disc.

Left Lateroaortic Route. This is the route of choice to gain access to the L4–L5 intervertebral disc, subsequent to ligation of the fourth and sometimes the fifth lumbar vessels on the left side. The presacral nerve is left in contact with the aorta, which is mobilized towards the right half of the anterior surface of the lumbar vertebral bodies.

Interaortocaval Route. The route of choice to the L3–L4 intervertebral disc, this approach requires the ligation of the third and fourth lumbar vessels and the displacement of the inferior vena cava to the right and aorta to the left. The sympathetic lumbar nerve fibers lying in the upper part of the interaortocaval space and arising from the first and second lumbar ganglions must be preserved.

Right Laterocaval Route. This inconvenient approach is rarely used. Access can be gained to the right lateral surface of L5 and L4 by the displacement of the inferior vena cava and right common iliac vein towards the midline, after ligation of one or two lumbar vascular bundles.

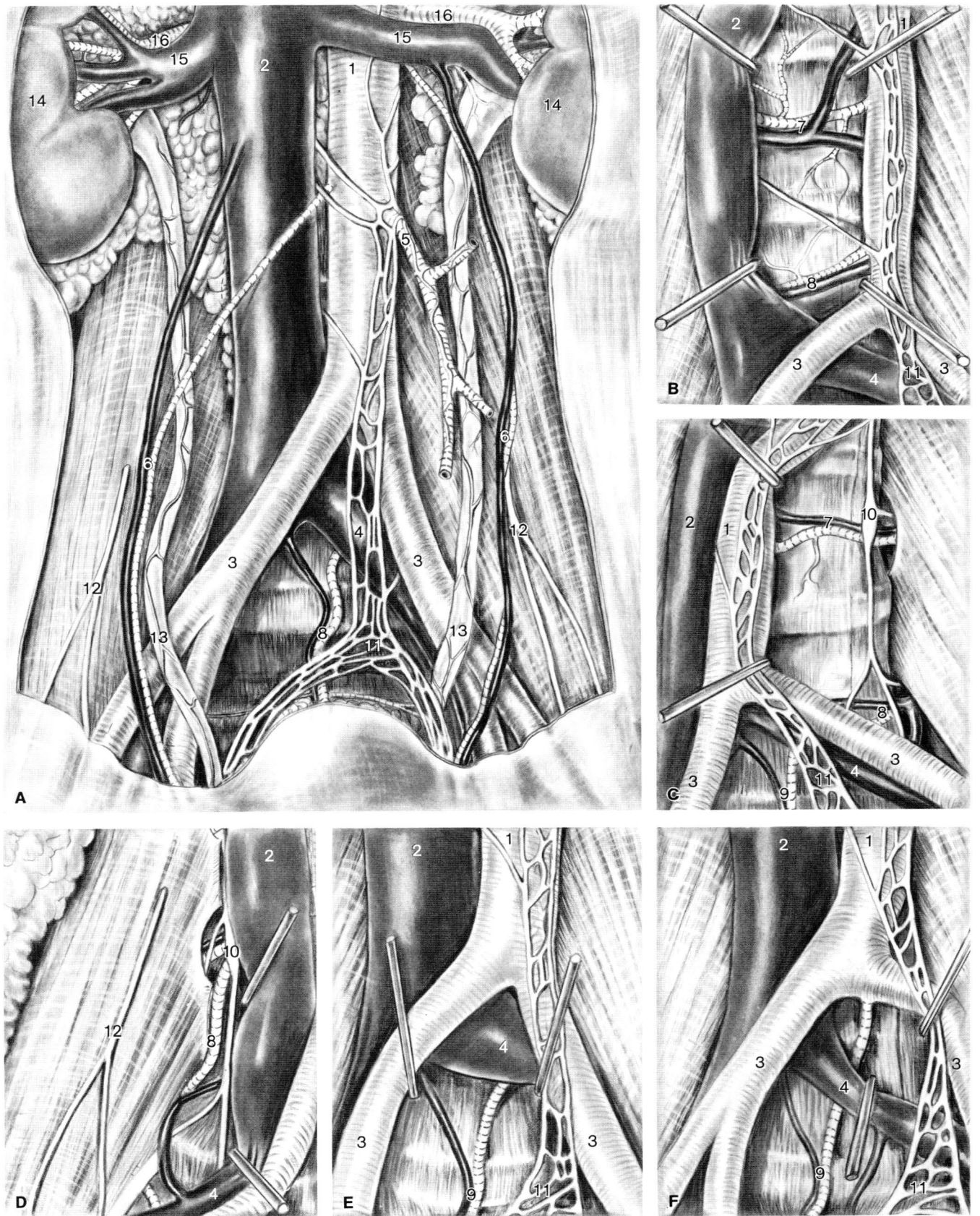

Figure 134 A–F

A   The arteries and veins in the anterior lumbosacral region
B   The interaortocaval approach to L3–L4
C   The left lateroaortic approach to L4–L5
D   The right laterocaval approach to L5
E   The interiliac approach to L5–S1 and occasionally L4–L5
F   The inter- and transiliac approach to L4–L5

1 aorta abdominalis 2 v. cava inf. 3 a. iliaca communis 4 v. iliaca
communis 5 a. mesenterica inf. 6 a. and v. testiculares or a. and
v. ovaricae 7 a. and v. lumbales III 8 a. and v. lumbales IV 9 a. and
v. sacralis mediana 10 truncus sympathicus 11 n. hypogastricus sup.
12 n. genitofemoralis 13 ureter 14 ren 15 v. renalis 16 a. renalis

6. Horizontal Section of the Trunk Through L5

The region shown by this horizontal section is a zone of transition between the lumbosacral spine and the abdominal and pelvic cavities. The transverse processes and wings of the iliac bones form a coronal barrier topographically separating the anterior and posterior parts of the region. The posterior sector contains the lumbar and gluteal regions, and the two visceral regions, the peritoneal cavity and the retroperitoneal fossa, lie anteriorly.

The *right and left lumbar regions* lie posterior to the region of the transverse processes containing the erector spinae muscles and their corresponding neurovascular bundles.

The *gluteal regions* contain the gluteal muscles and their corresponding neurovascular bundles occupying the full area of the external iliac fossae, and constitute a barrier to the direct access to the abdominal cavity.

The *retroperitoneal fossa (or space)* extends on each side of the midline in front of the vertebral bodies to the internal iliac fossae, being limited by the posterior parietal peritoneum anteriorly and by the psoas and internal iliac muscles laterally. The aortocaval axis, the common iliac vessels, and the middle sacral artery lie on the anterior surface of the vertebral bodies. The presacral nerve lies in the interiliac position. The lumbar sympathetic trunk runs along the dihedral angle formed by the convex part of the vertebral bodies and the psoas muscle. The constituent structures of the lumbar plexus lie in the interstice separating the posterior surface of the psoas muscles and the angle formed by the bodies and transverse processes of the vertebrae. At the level of L5 these constituent structures comprise the crural (or femoral) nerve and the anastomotic fibers between the fourth and fifth lumbar nerves. The ureters, the genitofemoral nerves, and the gonadal (testicular or ovarian) vessels lie behind the posterior parietal peritoneum. The lateral cutaneous femoral nerves run along the anterior surface of the iliac muscles. The iliolumbar vessels run vertically between the branches of the lumbar plexus.

The Peritoneal Cavity. The anterolateral wall of the abdomen is formed by the rectus muscles and their sheath and the large abdominal muscles laterally. The posterior parietal peritoneum forms the anterior and posterior boundaries of the retroperitoneal space and peritoneal cavity respectively. The right mesocolon and cecum are attached to the right part of the posterior parietal peritoneum, while at the level of the right iliac vessels the root of the mesentery with its appended loops of small bowel is adherent to the peritoneum. On the left side, the left mesocolon and mesosigmoid (separated from the psoas muscle and left iliac vessels by the intersigmoid recess) are attached to the posterior peritoneum. The transperitoneal approach thus requires the mobilization of these different visceral structures adherent to the posterior parietal peritoneum.
This transverse section through L5 clearly illustrates the different possible approaches to the lumbosacral spine, underlining their advantages and disadvantages:

The *lumbar approaches* allow direct access to the vertebral canal by laminectomy or the interlaminal route. However, use of a lumbar approach to gain access to the anterior part of the spine requires the prior resection of the transverse processes and the mobilization of the components of the lumbar plexus, and the approach is thus a narrow one between the articular pillars and iliac tuberosity.

The *transgluteal approach* requires the resection of part of the iliac bone to gain lateral access through the retroperitoneal space to the vertebral bodies lying immediately posterior to the aortocaval axis, and is thus a narrow, complex, and deep approach to the lumbosacral spine.

The *anterolateral retroperitoneal approach* passes through the large muscles of the abdomen with displacement of the peritoneal envelope to gain access to the anterior surface of the psoas and bodies of the vertebrae, and requires the mobilization of the great vessels and the ligation of a few collateral vessels. It should be noted that with this approach the vertebral bodies and intervertebral discs can be viewed from one side only.

The *anterior transperitoneal approach* is in our opinion the route of choice to visualize the full surface of the vertebral bodies and intervertebral discs. It requires midline dissection with displacement and protection of the intestinal loops, and the posterior parietal peritoneum must be opened in the interiliac angle and the great vessels mobilized after ligation of one or several lumbar vascular bundles.

7. Ectopic Iliac Kidney

The abnormal position of one of the kidneys in the lumbosacral region is obviously a dangerous obstacle to the anterior approach of the lumbosacral junction. An ectopic kidney may display several primary vessels, i.e., main renal artery arising a few centimeters cranial to the termination of the aorta with accessory arteries arising from the aortic bifurcation, the middle sacral artery, or the common iliac artery. The veins draining the ectopic kidney merge with the inferior vena cava or the common iliac vein. Furthermore, some of these different vessels may penetrate the renal parenchyma at one of the poles of the kidney instead of the region of the hilus. Preservation of the main vascular bundle is sufficient to ensure adequate function of the kidney. A more severe form of ectopy is the horseshoe kidney implanted directly on the termination of the aorta. In some cases the horseshoe kidney can be mobilized subsequent to the midline division of the organ, but in others this anomaly represents a formidable obstacle to anterior surgery of the lumbosacral spine.

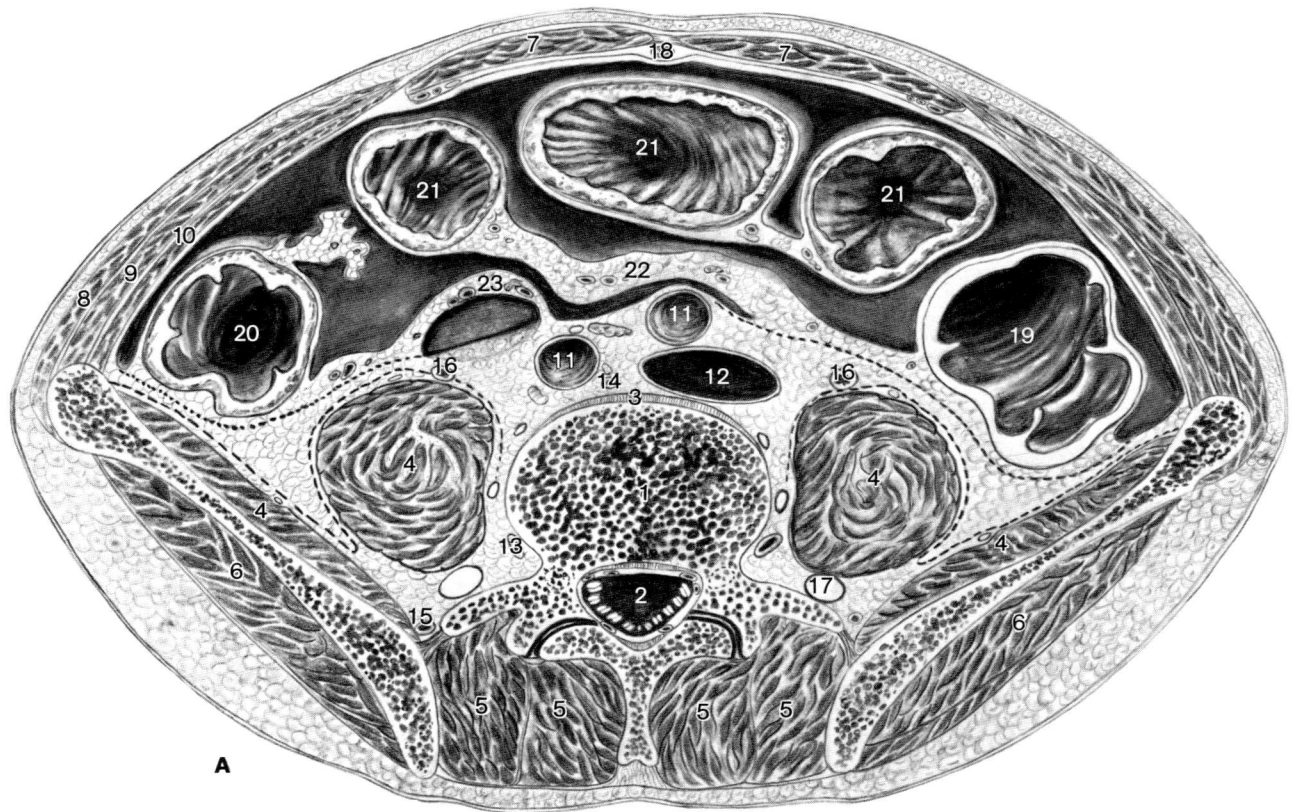

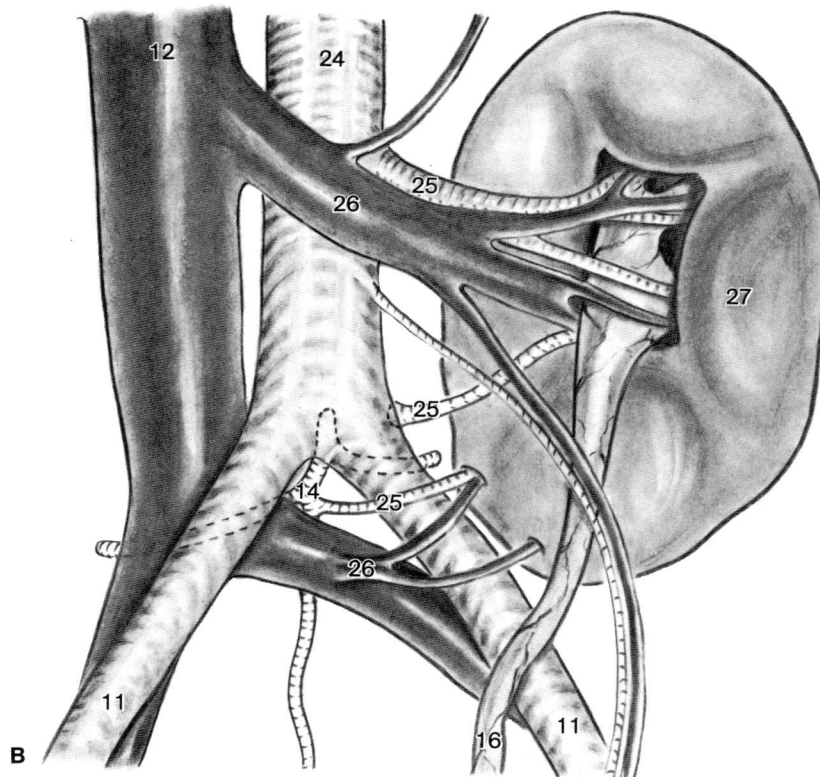

Figure 135 A, B

A   Horizontal section of the trunk through L5
B   Ectopic left iliac kidney

1 vertebra lumbalis V *2* cavum subarachnoidale, cauda equina
3 lig. longitudinale ant. *4* m. iliopsoas *5* m. erector spinae
6 m. glutaei *7* m. rectus abdominis *8* m. obliquus externus
abdominis *9* m. obliquus internus abdominis *10* m. transversus
abdominis *11* a. iliaca communis *12* v. cava inf. *13* v. lumbalis
ascendens *14* a. sacralis mediana *15* a. circumflexa ilium profunda
16 ureter *17* n. femoralis *18* plica umbilicalis mediana *19* cecum
20 colon descendens *21* intestinum tenue *22* mesenterium
23 mesocolon sigmoideum *24* aorta *25* a. renalis *26* v. renalis
27 ectopic left iliac kidney

B. Anterior Transperitoneal Approach

1. Preparation and Anesthesia

As in all types of abdominal surgery, preparation includes an enema on the eve of operation and evacuation of the bladder just prior to surgery, and an indwelling urinary catheter may be used during operation. The abdomen and pubis are thoroughly shaved. Endotracheal intubation is installed with the patient supine prior to the induction of anesthesia. In obese patients or where there is a risk of intestinal hypomotility a gastric tube can be installed. When cephalic traction is to be used the intubation tube should be protected from the teeth by a rigid tube slipped over it.

2. Operative Position

With the patient supine, the sacral region is elevated by a cushion, or preferably by angling the operating table under the sacral region. According to the type of spinal lesion, the table angle should be 30°–50°. As a general rule bipolar spinal traction is very helpful, and this is achieved by fixing the feet to the operating table and installing cephalic traction with a headpiece wired to a dynamometer. Traction should be applied parallel to the long axis of the trunk, i.e., obliquely downward in most cases. The right upper limb, bearing the intravenous infusion line, is laid along the trunk while the left upper limb is placed on a support to lie over the sternum. It is often necessary to prepare an iliac or fibular region for the removal of bone-graft material. The patient is then draped to isolate the anesthesiologists and to expose the abdominal operative field and site of bone removal. The surgeon usually works on the right and the two assistants on the left of the patient.

3. Incisions

The transperitoneal approach requires a midline abdominal incision, whose position varies according to the lumbosacral segment to be exposed. The approach to the L5–S1 intervertebral disc is achieved by making a subumbilical incision down to a point three fingers above the pubis. Access to the L4–L5 disc is achieved by a 15–20 cm incision straddling the umbilicus, one third of the incision being made above and two thirds below the umbilicus. Exposure of the L3–L4 disc also requires a 15–20 cm incision straddling the umbilicus, but with two thirds of the incision above and one third below. Access to the L5–S1 disc is also possible using a cosmetic transverse incision (Pfannenstiel's incision) lying two fingers above the pubis. After the incision of the skin and subcutaneous tissue the decollement of the commissures of the incision enables commencement of parietal dissection through the linea alba. Owing to the wide decollement, closure of the incision will require suction drainage of the subcutaneous layers. Prior to tracing the incision, it is often useful to identify the level of the spinal lesions using the image intensifier. Fibular bone for grafting is removed through an incision made along the line tangential to the posterior margin of the fibular epiphyses. The incision begins proximally at a point three fingers below the head of the fibula, and is continued downward for 10–15 cm according to the amount of fibular diaphysis to be removed. The incision should be made along the depressed muscular region which can be palpated between the peroneal and soleus muscles. When iliac bone material is to be taken for grafting, the incision is made along the anterior half of the iliac crest to a point two fingers from the anterosuperior iliac spine. The length of the incision depends on the amount of bone required for grafting. Prior to making the incision the abdominal wall should be compressed above the iliac crest to remove the prolapse of the abdominal muscles under the crest.

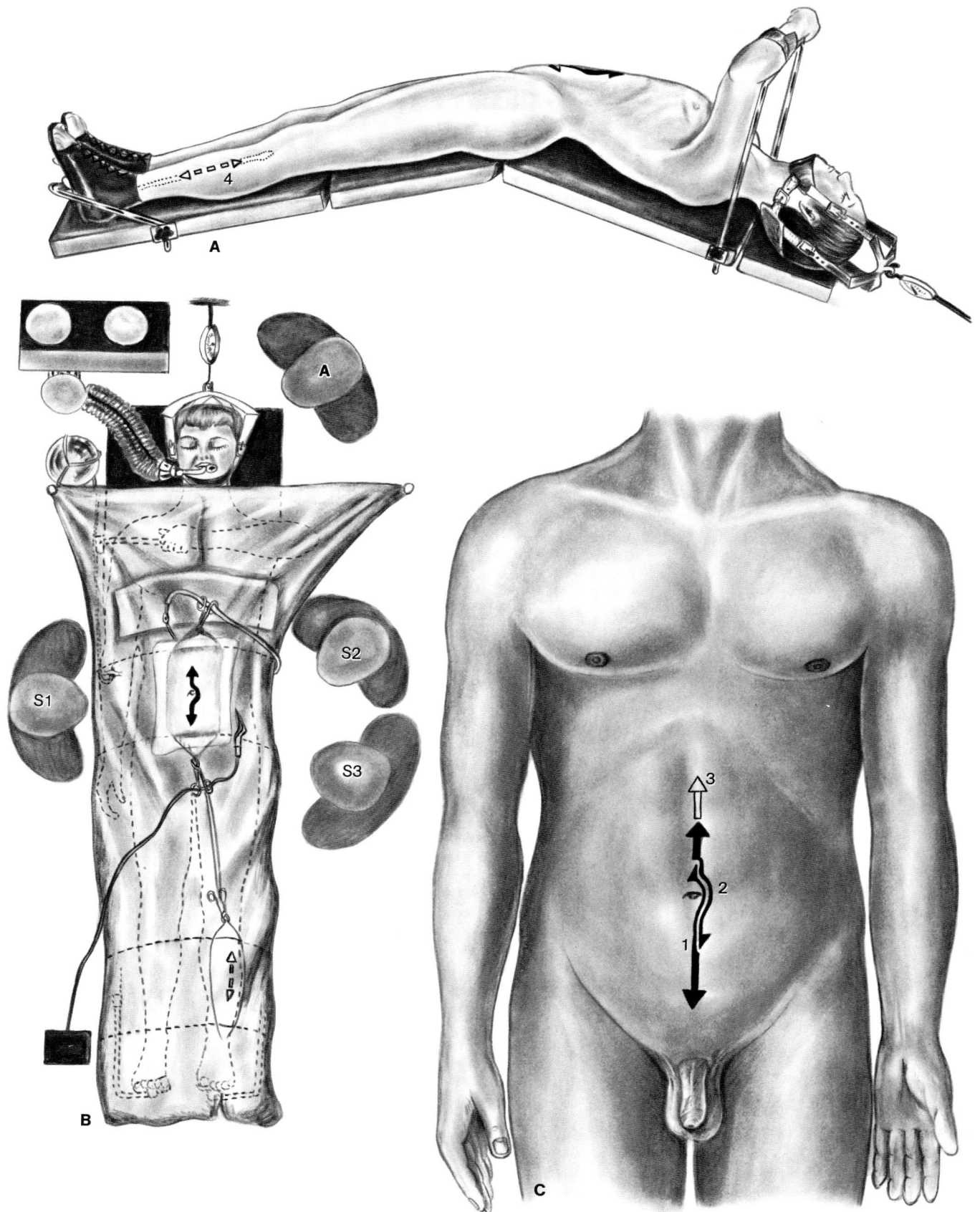

Figure 136 A–C

A   Operative position
B   Overhead view of the operative setting
C   Different types of incision used in the anterior transperitoneal approach

1 incision to approach the L5–S1 disc   *2* incision to approach the L4–L5 disc   *3* extension of the incision to approach the L3–L4 disc
4 incision for the removal of fibular graft material

4. Transection of the Abdominal Wall

When making the incision, the umbilicus should be pulled to the right of the line of incision using a towel clamp. In this way the knife can be used to trace a straight line of incision, avoiding penetration of the umbilicus without having to work around it. The incision should be made strictly on the midline down to the subcutaneous fat pad. After disinfection of the commissures of the incision, the opening is covered by a moist compress, which is then gradually removed to uncover the wound and allow progressive hemostasis of the subdermal vessels with electrocoagulation. The subcutaneous tissue is incised down to the fascial layer with the electric cautery knife, which is then used to nick the tissue of the linea alba just below the umbilicus (where the linea alba is widest). Next, scissors are introduced through the fascial buttonhole incision to free the fascia, which is then cut strictly on the midline to avoid opening the rectus sheath. The peritoneum is freed from the fat tissue near the umbilicus to allow a plicature of peritoneum to be grasped with large blunt forceps (Péan's forceps), care being taken not to trap an intraperitoneal visceral structure. The plain knife is then used to open the peritoneum cautiously through the transverse plicature until the lumen of the abdominal cavity is brought into view. The peritoneal opening is continued with scissors while the commissures of the parietal peritoneum are pulled to separate the peritoneum clearly from the underlying viscera. An orthostatic retractor can now be installed. The retractor is opened only moderately to avoid reduction of the operative field. It is not necessary to protect the commissures of the operative field with moist compresses as in general surgical procedures of the abdomen, since septic opening of the intestines is not performed during spinal surgery.

5. Exposure of the Posterior Parietal Peritoneum

The patient is tilted slightly toward Trendelenburg's position to free the loops of small bowel from the pelvic region, and the bowel loops are manipulated gently, manually or with compresses mounted on forceps. The greater omentum is then reflected towards the upper part of the operative field, and the loops of small bowel are displaced towards the right parietocolic gutter while an assistant elevates the right commissure of the operative field with a flexible retractor. The bowel loops are held in place by a moist rolled operative towel wedged between the right end of the retractor and the posterior wall of the abdomen. Similarly, the left commissure of the operative field is retracted and the sigmoid bowel and a few jejunal loops are displaced into the left parietocolic gutter, the bowel segments being held in place by another rolled moist operative towel sandwiched between the retractor and the posterior wall of the abdomen. Finally, the remaining loops of small bowel and the transverse colon are displaced toward the upper part of the operative field and held by a third rolled towel placed transversely between the right and left parietocolic gutters and anterior to the great prevertebral vessels. These procedures should expose the posterior parietal peritoneum fully, with the mesosigmoid displaced to the left and the mesentery to the right, and the operative field free of any bowel loops. To retract the rectum from the anterior surface of the sacrum a flexible retractor is introduced deeply anterior to the sacrum and bent over the pubic region.

6. Presentation of the Prevertebral Neurovascular Structures

The sacral promontory, the pulsatile aorta, and the iliac arteries are identified mainly by palpation. The posterior parietal peritoneum is grasped with toothless dissecting forceps and then incised with scissors, strictly on the midline, from the promontory up to the terminal centimeter of the abdominal aorta. The electric cautery knife is used to obtain hemostasis of the small points of bleeding on the lips of the peritoneal opening. Clamp-held compresses are then used to pursue dissection to expose the aorta and its terminal branches, the inferior vena cava, the left common iliac vein, and finally the presacral plexus. It is of utmost importance to identify within the fat tissue the fine white anastomotic branches of the presacral nerve. Of indurated texture on palpation, these vegetative nerve fibers run between the iliac vessels from the anterior surface of the aorta to the anterior surface of the promontory: they must not be ligated and divided to expose the vertebral region. Indeed, all vegetative nervous structures must be painstakingly identified and then protected by mobilization to the side allowing the best exposure of the spine. During dissection some of the vasa vasorum of the aorta or iliac vessels may be damaged, in which case hemostasis is achieved with a fine coagulation clamp, which is used to pick up the bleeder before coagulation to avoid a burn-induced eschar of the great vessels. Warm moist compresses packed into the operative field and left in place for a few seconds are necessary to complete hemostasis. Ligation or clips should be used only on the collateral vessels of the aorta and inferior vena cava.

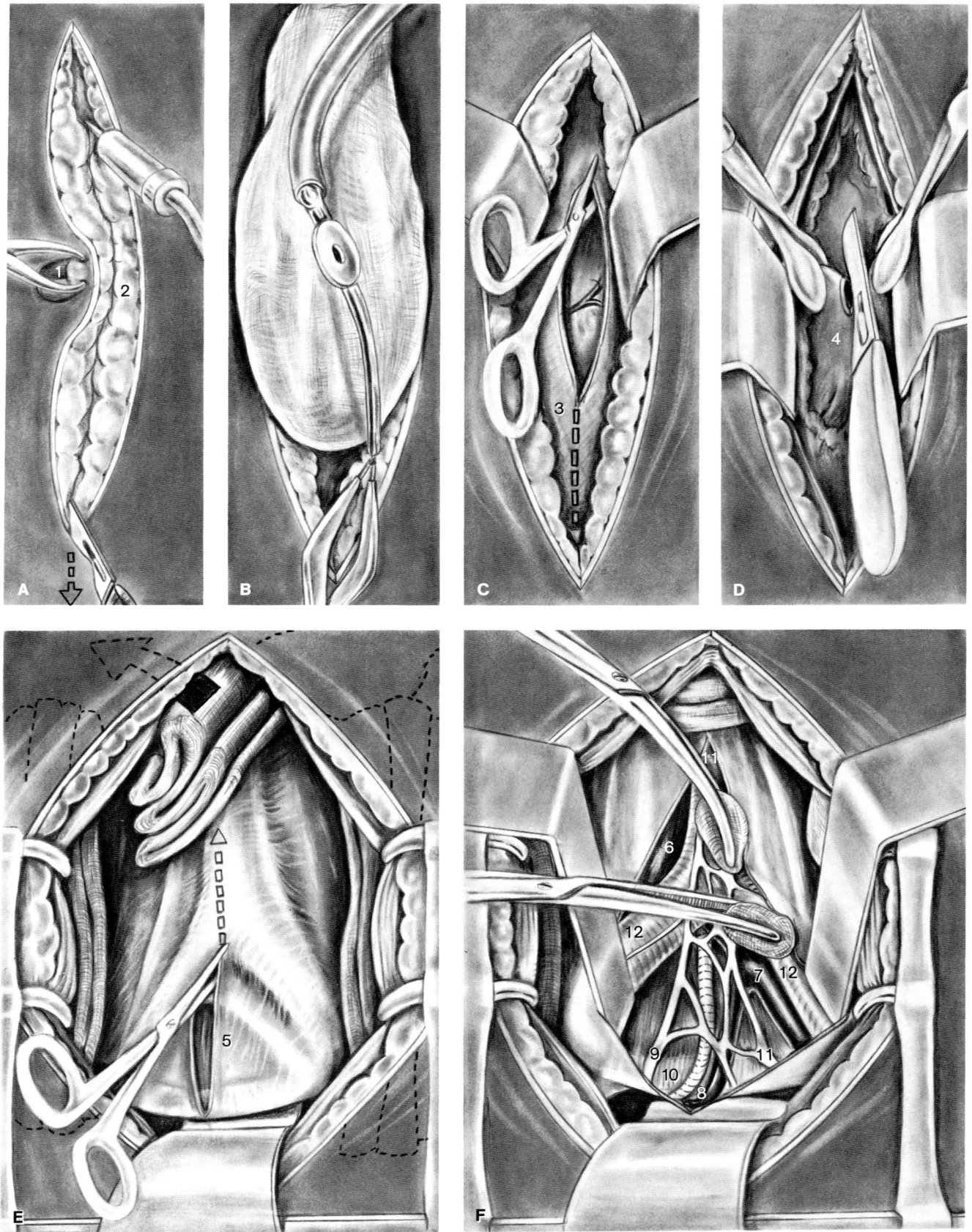

Figure 137 A–F

A   Skin incision
B   Subdermal hemostasis
C   Incision of the linea alba
D   Opening of the peritoneal cavity
E   Opening of the posterior parietal peritoneum
F   Blunt dissection of the lumbosacral prevertebral structures

1 umbilicus   *2* subcutis   *3* vagina m. recti abdominis, linea alba
4 peritoneum parietale ant.   *5* peritoneum parietale post.   *6* v. cava
inf.   *7* v. iliaca communis   *8* a. and v. sacralis mediana   *9* n. hypogastricus sup.   *10* a. and v. sacralis mediana   *11* n. hypogastricus sup.
12 promontorium

7. Mobilization of the Prevertebral Neurovascular Structures

According to both the topographic arrangement of the great vessels and the spinal region to be exposed, one or more of the following procedures can be used to mobilize the prevertebral vessels.

Interiliac Mobilization. This procedure exposes the triangular area between the common iliac arteries, thus allowing visualization of the middle sacral vessels. Once identified, the presacral nerve must be either left in place and lifted with an identification band or retracted toward the left iliac vascular bundle. The middle sacral vessels are then isolated on a clamp, clips installed, and the vessels divided. Each of the iliac vascular bundles is retracted as far as possible laterally, using clamp-held compresses to dissect the vessels free of the underlying bone. Next, Steinmann pins are positioned in the body of L5 to maintain the iliac vessels fully retracted. This procedure allows easy access to the L5–S1 and sometimes the L4–L5 intervertebral disc.

Inter- and Transiliac Mobilization. When a large left common iliac vein hinders access to the body of L5, and in some cases the sacral promontory, clamp-held compresses are used to separate the vein from the left common iliac artery. Curved forceps are introduced under each end of the vein, which can then be compressed by feeding suture material through a drain to "lasso" the vessel. In this way the vein collapses and no longer hinders access to the spine.

Left Lateroaortic Mobilization. To approach the L4–L5 intervertebral disc often requires the dissection of the left flank of the terminal aorta and the left common iliac artery until the fourth and in some cases the fifth lumbar vascular bundle is visible. The exposed lumbar vessels are then clipped and divided. Clamp-held compresses and flexible retractors and used to displace the aorta to the midline and finally to the right half of the vertebral bodies. Steinmann pins are planted in the vertebral bone to maintain the aorta in this displaced position. Excess tension on the iliac vessels must be avoided by decreasing the hyperlordosis of the lumbosacral spine.

Interaortocaval Mobilization. For access to the L3–L4 or L2–L3 intervertebral disc, clamp-held compresses are used to dissect the aorta free of the inferior vena cava, care being taken not to damage the scarce sympathetic nerve fibers running along the right lateral aspect of the aorta. The second or third lumbar vascular bundle is then ligated and divided. Steinmann pins are used to keep the great vessels retracted and afford clear exposure of the anterior surface of the lumbar spine.

8. Closure

Hemostasis is achieved by electrocoagulation, application of bone wax, and packing of Surgicel into the orifices made by the Steinmann pins. Once full hemostasis has been verified the posterior parietal peritoneum is closed by a fine continuous suture using slow-resorbing material mounted on a curved round needle. Drainage of this region is not required when good hemostasis has been obtained. The intestinal compresses are removed and the bowel loops anatomically repositioned, care being taken not to induce traction on the mesocolon in order to avoid torsion. The greater omentum is then placed over the intestinal structures. The orthostatic retractor is removed, followed by the closure of the abdominal wall using a flexible retractor to protect the intestines. The classic continuous suture of the anterior parietal peritoneum has been abandoned by most surgeons: the peritoneum can be left unsutured or taken up by the sutures of the fascia, which is closed with solid closely spaced (8 mm) interrupted sutures. The subcutaneous tissue and skin are finally closed as separate layers using interrupted sutures.

9. Postoperative Care

Nutrition is given by the parenteral route until gas is clearly passed, to avoid paralytic ileus. Antibiotics may also be given postoperatively. Anticoagulant therapy is indicated only in cases where there is a high risk of venous thrombosis. In certain obese patients a gastric tube can be left in place to siphon the gastric contents until gas is passed. An indwelling urinary catheter is not necessary.

10. Possible Complications

The presence of numerous peritoneal adhesions may hinder the operative approach or even render it impossible. However, weak adhesions can be dissected with clamp-held compresses or ligated and divided. Mistaken identification of the level of the spinal lesions can be avoided by peroperative radiography or radioscopy. One of the most feared complications is injury to one of the great vessels. When this occurs, the hemorrhage must immediately be arrested by direct compression with the finger or a moist compress while the hemostatic material, which should always be included among the instruments used in the transperitoneal approach, is prepared. The hemostatic instruments comprise vascular bulldog clamps or larger-angled clamps. Manual compression above and below the wound usually suffices to expose the vascular defect, which is then closed with a few very fine sutures using nonresorbable material mounted on a curved needle. In the most severe cases the inferior vena cava or aorta and the corresponding iliac vessels must be temporarily clamped or banded to reduce the hemorrhage, after which the defect can be closed. Immediate postoperative complications include mechanical ileus resulting from torsion of a bowel loop when the position of the mesentery has not been properly verified during closure. Paralytic ileus may occur when the patient is allowed to eat and drink prior to passage of intestinal gas. The presence of intestinal occlusion can be checked for on standard abdominal X-rays.

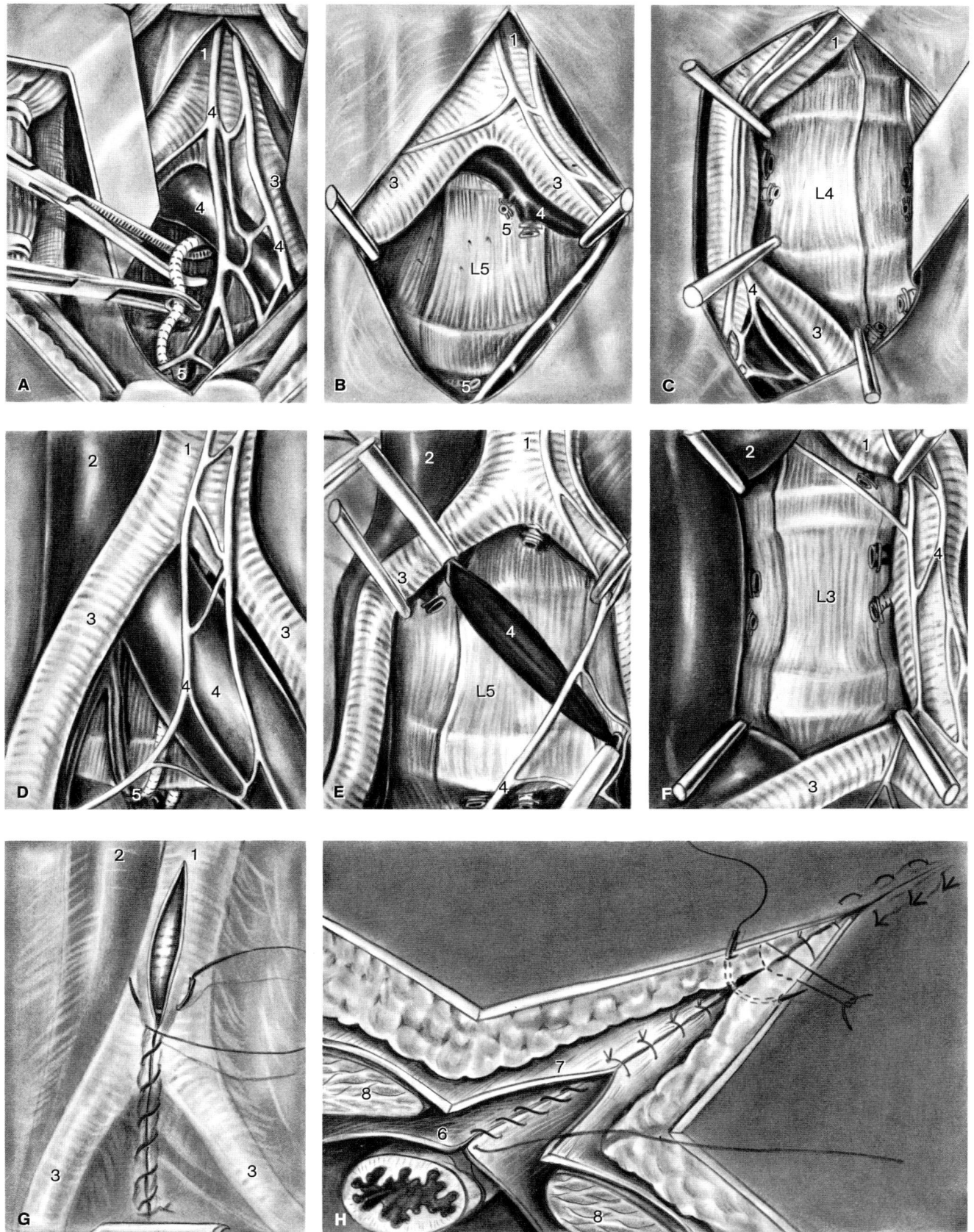

Figure 138 A–H

A Ligation and section of the middle sacral vessels
B Interiliac exposure of L5 and the sacral promontory
C Left lateroaortic exposure of L4 and the adjacent intervertebral discs
D Large left common iliac vein over the promontory
E Clamping of the left common iliac vein
F Interaortocaval approach to L3 and L4

G Closure of the posterior parietal peritoneum
H Parietal closure

1 aorta abdominalis *2* v. cava inf. *3* a. iliaca communis *4* v. iliaca communis *5* a. and v. sacralis mediana *6* peritoneum parietal ant. *7* vagina m. recti abdominis *8* m. rectus abdominis

Intestinal occlusion of mechanical origin requires surgical reintervention, whereas that of functional origin can be treated by gastric suction, balanced intravenous infusion of nutrients, and clinical and radiological monitoring of abdominal status. Reestablishment of intestinal transit may require two to five days. Sexual impotence is a very severe complication, due to widespread injury of the presacral nerve, but can be avoided by the correct identification and protection of the nerve.

IV. Lumbosacral Region: Special Operative Approaches

A. Subperitoneal Iliolumbar Approach

Incision. The patient is placed supine, or in rare cases in the lateral supine position. The incision is made along an oblique line beginning three fingers above the anterosuperior iliac spine and extending towards the tendinous pubic insertion of the rectus abdominis.

Parietal Dissection. In male patients care must be taken not to injure the funiculus spermaticus near the lower part of the incision. The inferior epigastric artery is ligated after dissection of the musculofascial layers of the large abdominal muscles. In the course of dissection the nerve bundles running practically parallel to the skin incision should be preserved. Subsequent to its exposure, the peritoneum is dissected free of the deep surface of the abdominal muscles using clamp-held compresses, and is then displaced toward the midline with a flexible retractor to visualize the ureter, the iliac vessels, and the left flank of the aorta. The ureter must be left adherent to the peritoneum.

Exposure of the Lumbosacral Spine. Mobilization of the great vessels requires the ligation of their left collaterals, i.e., the fourth lumbar vascular bundle and the iliolumbar vessels lying just lateral to the left iliac bundle. The great vessels are then displaced towards the midline with flexible retractors. This relatively narrow approach allows access to the left lateral surface and left half of the anterior surface of the bodies of L4 and L5 and the left aspect of the adjacent intervertebral discs.

Closure. Closure is achieved by relaxing the traction on the great vessels, performing very careful hemostasis, and allowing the peritoneum to regain its normal position in the right iliac fossa. Suction drainage is recommended. The anterolateral wall of the abdomen is closed layer by layer using interrupted sutures. The subcutaneous tissue and skin are closed as separate layers, also with interrupted sutures. Postoperative care requires routine procedures only. Oral feeding is allowed on the first evening after operation.

B. Posterolateral Transiliotransverse Approach

Operative Position and Incision. The patient is placed in the lateral supine position. The incision is made as a slightly curved line beginning at the level of the L3–L4 interspinous space at a point three fingers lateral to the midline and terminating in the gluteal region two fingers below the posterosuperior iliac spine.

Parietal Dissection. After incision of the skin and subcutaneous tissue the fascia thoracolumbalis is opened with the electric cautery knife. The fibers of the spinal muscles are dissected longitudinally parallel to the skin incision. A rectangular opening (3 cm × 3 cm) is made in the iliac tuberosity with removal of the posterosuperior iliac spine, and then the posterior surface of the ala sacralis is exposed. The transverse processes are resected close to their root of origin using narrow gouge forceps, taking care not to injure the structures lying in front of the transverse processes, i.e., the branches of the lumbar nervous plexus and the posterior surface of the common iliac vein. The dihedral angle formed by the transverse processes and vertebral bodies is thus exposed, although relatively hidden by the branches of the lumbar plexus and the iliolumbar blood vessels. Subsequent to the hemostasis of these vessels, clamp-held compresses are used to dissect the region to expose the posterolateral surfaces of the vertebral bodies and adjacent intervertebral discs lying under the network of fibers of the lumbar plexus. It must be underlined that this approach allows narrow access and should thus only be used in cases of small lesions.

Closure. A suction drain is installed, and the resected flap of the iliac tuberosity is then repositioned and held in place by one or two bone screws. The muscles and fascia thoracolumbalis are approximated, followed by interrupted closure of the subcutaneous layer and skin.

Figure 139 A–F

A   The iliolumbar incision
B   Operative vision of the subperitoneal field
C   Exposure of the lumbosacral spine
D   Incision of the transiliotransverse approach
E   Horizontal section through L4 showing the operative field of vision
F   Exposure of the operative field

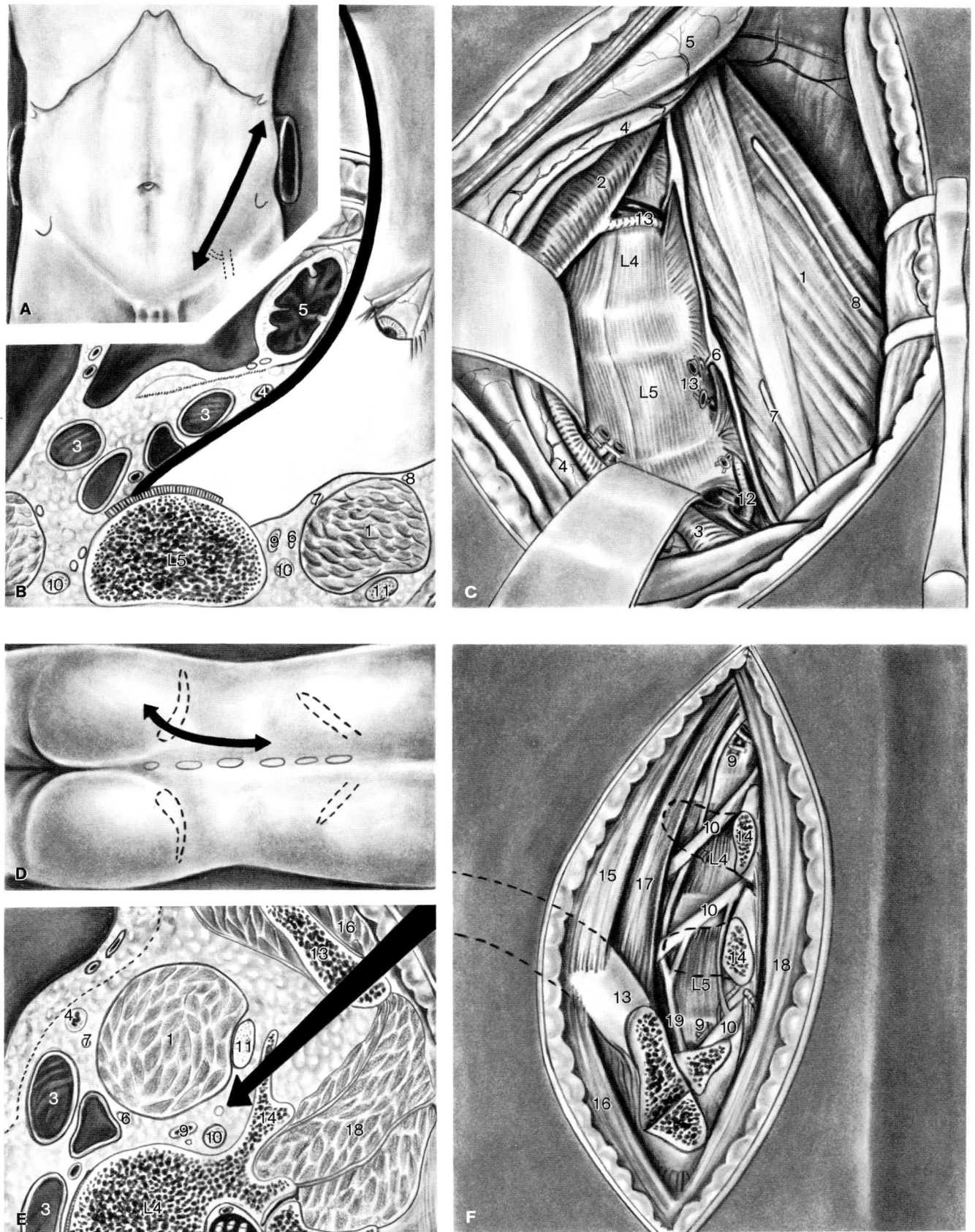

Figure 139 A–F

1 m. psoas   2 aorta abdominalis   3 a. iliaca communis   4 ureter
5 cavum peritonei   6 truncus sympathicus   7 n. genitofemoralis
8 n. cutaneus femoris laterale   9 v. lumbalis ascendens   10 n. spinalis
11 n. femoralis   12 a. iliolumbalis   13 crista iliaca   14 processus
transversus   15 m. obliquus externus abdominis   16 m. gluteus
maximus   17 m. quadratus lumborum   18 m. erector spinae
19 n. obturatorius

C. Paraspinal Approach

First described by Watkins (1953), this approach was developed by Wiltse (1964) to perform posterolateral spinal grafts.

Operative Position and Incision. There are usually two incisions, one on each side of the spinous processes two fingers from the midline, vertical and slightly curved toward the midline near the sacrum. The incisions begin at the level of the L3–L4 interspinous space and terminate one thumb's breadth below the posterosuperior iliac spines. In some cases a single, long, midline incision can be used with decollement of the skin and subcutaneous tissue to expose the lateral parts of the spinal muscles. Finally, a cosmetic horizontal incision through the L4–L5 interspinous space may be used in certain cases.

Parietal Dissection. The fascia thoracolumbalis is incised longitudinally at the junction of the lateral quarter and medial three quarters of the spinal muscles. The muscle fibers are then divided lengthwise until contact is felt with the transverse processes and ala sacralis. In addition to the transverse processes and ala sacralis, the operator should expose the zygapophyseal joints of L4–L5 and L5–S1. In the course of dissection, the dorsal bundles of the metameric vessels are prone to injury where they run along the lateral margin of the isthmic zones in the region between the posterior articulations. Hemostasis of the vessels can be achieved by electrocoagulation or by compression with Surgicel. This approach allows posterolateral arthrodesis extending to the interfaces of the zygapophyseal joints. Furthermore, foraminotomy can be achieved by excision of an articular pillar with decompression of the intervertebral foramen. Removal of a laterally prolapsed intervertebral disc can then be accomplished through the orifice of the foraminatomy, but this approach is not recommended for disc excision as spinal stability is reduced by the suppression of the articular pillar.

Closure. Suction drainage is optional. The spinal muscles, subcutaneous tissue, and skin are closed as separate layers by interrupted sutures.

Postoperative Care. As for the posterior approach to the lumbosacral spine, only routine postoperative care is required. Early ambulation is allowed, but the seated position should be avoided for several weeks after operation.

D. Transiliac Approach (According to Judet)

Operative Position and Incision. Operation is performed with the patient in the lateral prone position. A vertical incision is made along the lateral margin of the spinal muscles extending 10–12 cm above and below the iliac crest.

Parietal Dissection. Subsequent to incision of the subcutaneous tissue, the gluteal muscle is dissected free of the external iliac fossa to expose the great sciatic notch, taking care not to injure the gluteal artery where it passes around the upper margin of the great sciatic notch. If injury does occur it leads to pronounced hemorrhage, which should be treated by application of compression or repair of the defect using atraumatic sutures with a curved needle. Using a hammer and chisel, the external wing of the iliac bone is sectioned 5–6 cm anterior to the posterosuperior iliac spine. A retractor is then introduced into the osteotomy to displace the iliac tuberosity posteriorly, allowing the operator to section the anterior ligaments of the sacroiliac joint in the region of the medial surface of the iliac tuberosity. In this way, the cut iliac bone with its accompanying posterior spinal insertions can be reflected backward.

Exposure of the Spinal Region. Access is gained to the flank of L5, the ala sacralis, and the depressed region which contains the lumbosacral trunk, the obturator nerve, the iliolumbar artery, the common iliac vessels, and the S1 nerve roots. Nevertheless, this relatively narrow approach only enables treatment of localized lateral lesions of the lumbosacral junction.

Closure. Once good hemostasis has been achieved, the iliac bone is repositioned and held in place by two screw plates, and a suction drain is installed under the external iliac fossa. The muscles, subcutaneous tissue, and skin are closed layer by layer with interrupted sutures. Postoperative management is usually uneventful.

Figure 140 A–G

A Skin incision in the paraspinal approach
B Exposure of the transversoarticular region
C Horizontal section showing the regional anatomical relations
D Skin incision in the transiliac approach
E Iliac osteotomy
F Reflection of iliac bone showing the regional anatomy
G Closure with iliac reconstruction

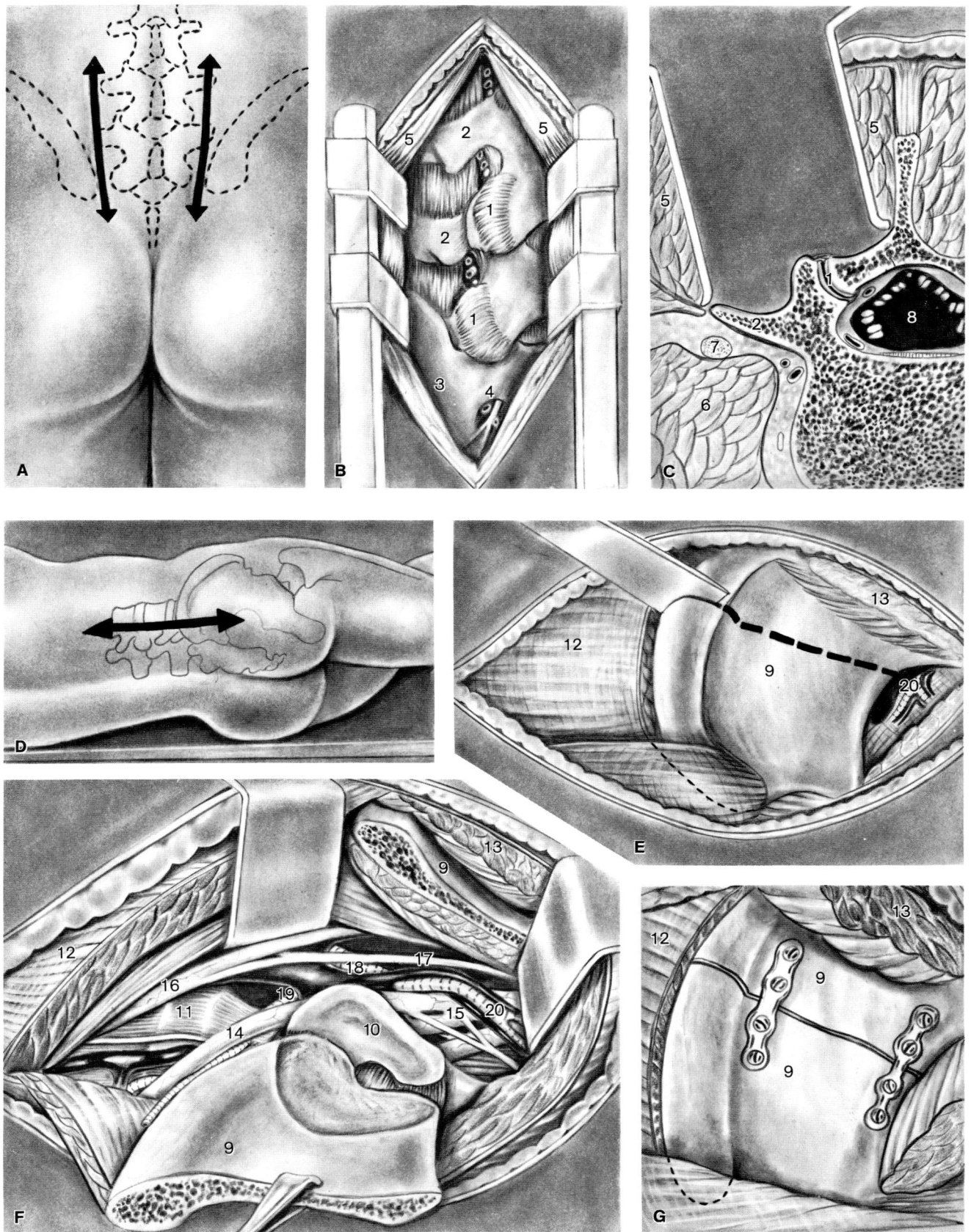

Figure 140 A–G

1 juncturae zygapophyseales, capsula articularis *2* processus transversus *3* ala sacralis *4* foramina sacralia, pediculus *5* m. erector
spinae *6* m. psoas *7* n. femoralis *8* duramater spinalis, cauda
equina *9* fossa iliaca *10* facies auricularis *11* discus intervertebrale,
L4–L5 *12* m. obliquus externus abdominis *13* m. glutaeus maximus
14 truncus lumbosacralis *15* plexus sacralis *16* n. spinalis L4
17 n. obturatorius *18* a. and v. iliacae communes *19* a. and v. ilio-
lumbales *20* a. and v. iliacae externae

References

Aasar YH (1938) Three cases of fusion of axis with third cervical vertebrae. J Anat 72:634

Abrams HL, McNeil BJ (1978) Medical implications of computed tomography (CT scanning). N Engl J Med 298:255

Abrams HM (1957) The cerebral and azygos venous systems and some variations in systemic venous return. Radiology 69:508

Adachi B (1928) Das Arteriensystem der Japaner. Ken Kuyusha, Tokyo Adamkiewicz A (1882) Die Blutgefäße der menschlichen Rückenmarkoberfläche. Verh Akad Wiss Math Nat Lk 85:101

Adams MA, Hutton WC, Stott JRR (1980) The resistance to flexion of the lumbar intervertebral joint. Spine 5/3:245

Aeby C (1879) Die Altersverschiedenheiten der menschlichen Wirbelsäule. Arch Anat Physiol 10:77

Aggraval ND (1979) A study of changes in the spine in weight lifters and other athletes. Br J Sports Med 13/2:58

Akeson WH, Woo SL, Taylor TK, Ghosh P, Bushell GR (1977) Biomechanics and biochemistry of the intervertebral disks: The need for correlation studies. Clin Orthop 129:133

Albers D (1954) Eine Studie über die Funktion der Halswirbelsäule bei dorsaler und vertebraler Flexion. ROEFO 81:606

Allbrook D (1957) Movements of the lumbar spinal column. J Bone Joint Surg [Br] 39:339

Anderson R (1951) Diodrast studies of the vertebral and cranial venous systems. J Neurosurg 8:411

Andersson GBJ, Örtengren R, Nachemson A (1976) Quantitative studies of back loads in lifting. Spine 1:178

Andersson GB, Ortengren R, Nachemson A (1977 a) Intradiscal pressure intra-abdominal pressure and myoelectric back muscle activity related to posture and loading. Clin Orthop 129:156

Andersson GBJ, Ortengren R, Herberts P (1977) Quantitative electromyographic studies of back muscle activity related to posture and loading. Orthop Clin North Am 8:85

Andersson GBJ, Schultz A, Nathan A, Irstam L (1981) Roentgenographic measurement of lumbar intervertebral disc height, Spine 6/2:154–158

Andreassi G (1961) L'origine des veines azygos et hémiazygos et sa valeur embryologique. CR Assoc Anat 47:69

Andriacchi TP, Schultz AB, Belytschko TB, Galante JO (1974) A model for studies of mechanical interaction between the human spine and ribcage. J Biomech 7:497

Anthonis PC (1970) A method for analysis of the articular movements of low amplitude applica to cervical intervertebral joints. Acta Anat 77/2:259

Apuzzo ML, Weiss MH, Herden JS (1978) Transoral exposure of the atlantoaxial region. Neurosurgery 3/2:201

Aquino CF (1970) A dynamic model of the lumbar spine. J Biomech 3/5:473

Argenson C, Francke TP, Sylla S, Dintimille H, Papasian S, Di Marino V (1979) Les artères vértébrales (segments V_1 et V_2). Anat clin 2/1:29–42

Arkin AM (1950) The mechanism of rotation in combination with lateral deviation in the normal spine. J Bone Joint Surg [Am] 32:180

Arnoldi CC (1972) Intravertebral pressure in patients with lumbar pain. A preliminary communication. Acta Orthop Scand 43:109

Arnoldi Linderholm M, Musselbichler M (1972) Venous engorgement and interosseous hypertension in osteoarthritis – J Bone Joint Surg [Br] 543:409

Asmussen E, Klausen K (1962) Form and function of the erect human spine. Clin Orthop 25:55

Atkinson PJ (1967) Variation in trabecular structure of vertebrae with age. Calcif Tissue Res 1:24

Austin G (1972) The spinal cord. Thomas Springfield

Badgley CE (1941) The articular facets in relation to lowback pain and sciatic radiation. J Bone Joint Surg 23:481

Baeyer EV (1960) Zennker's diverticulum and cervical block vertebra. AJR 84:1037

Bagnall KM (1977) A radiographic study of the human fetal spine. The sequence of development of ossifications centers in the vertebral column. J Anat 124/3:791

Bagnall KM, Harris PF, Jones PR (1979) A radiographic study of the human fetal spine. 3. Longitudinal growth. J Anat 128/4:777

Ball J, Meijers KAE (1964) On cervical mobility. Ann Rheum Dis 23:429

Banerjee T, Pittman HH (1976) Facet rhizotomy. Another armamentarium for treatment of low backache. NC Med J 37:354

Barbieri L, de Franceschi L (1974) Considération sur la biomécanique du disque intersomatique considéré comme un système visco-élastique. Chir Organi Mov 611:705

Barson AT (1970) The vertebral level of termination of the spinal cord during normal and anormal development. J Anat 106/3:489

Bartelink DC (1957) The role of abdominal pressure in relieving the pressure on the lumbar intervertebral discs. J Bone Joint Surg [Br] 39:718

Bartolozzi P (1977) Surgical treatment of the vertebral column using the anterior approach in Boston, Los Angeles, Hong Kong Centers. Arch Putti Chir Organi Mov 28:413

Batson OV (1940) The function of the vertebral veins and their role in the spread of metastases. Ann Surg 12:138

Batson OH (1957) The vertebral veins system AJR 78:195

Bauer R (1969) The problem of the rearrangement of the vertebral column. Acta Anat 72/3:321

Bauer R (1977) Postoperative surveillance and intensive care after orthopedic procedures of the vertebral column. Arch Orthop Unfallchir 90/2:157

Beadle OA (1931) The intervertebral discs. Med Res Coun (GB) Spec Rep Ser 161:6–9

Bearn JG (1961) The significance of the activity of the abdominal muscles in weight lifting. Acta Anat 45:83

Beaton GR (1966) The vertebral venous plexus. Leech. (Johannesb.) 363:84

Bell GH, Dunbar O, Beck JS (1967) Variations in the strength of vertebrae with age and their relation to osteoporosis. Calcif Tissue Res 1:75

Belytschko TB, Andriacchi TP, Schultz AB, Galante JO (1973) Analog studies of forces in the human spine. J Biomech 6:361

Belytschko T, Schwer L, Privitzer E (1978) Theory and application of a three – dimensional model of the human spine. Aviat Space Environ Med 49:158

Benjamin CP, Lee MD (1978) Computed tomography of the spine and spinal cord. Radiology 128:95

Bennett JG, Bergmanis LE, Carpenter JK, Skowlund HV (1963) Range of motion of the neck. J Am Phys Ther Assoc 43/45

Benson D, Schultz A, de Wald R (1976) Roentgengenographic evaluation of vertebral rotation. J Bone Joint Surg [Am] 58:1125

Berkson M, Schultz A, Nachemson A, Andersson G (1977) Voluntary strengths of male adults with acute low back syndromes. Clin Orthop 129:84

Bick EM (1952) The osteohistology of the normal human vertebra. J Mt Sinai Hosp NY 19:490

Bick EM, Copel JW (1950) Longitudinal growth of the human vertebra. J Bone Joint Surg [Am] 32:803

Billings EL (1955) Congenital scoliosis: An analytical study of its natural history. Proceedings of WOA. J Bone Joint Surg [Am] 37:404

Bloch-Michel H, Benoist M, Gallouin A (1973) Mesure du diamètre sagittal du canal rachidien à l'étage cervical. Technique radiologique. Etude statistique effectuée chez le sujet normal. Rev Rhum Mal Osteoartic 40/10:553

Blumel J, Evans EB, Hadnott JL, Eggers GWN (1962) Congenital skeletal anomalies of the spine: An analysis of the charts and roentgenograms of 264 patients. Ann Surg 28:501

Bogduk N (1975) The comparative anatomy of the dorsal lumbosacral region Masters thesis, University of Sydney

Bogduk N (1976) The anatomy of the lumbar intervertebral disc syndrome. Med J Aust 1:878

Bogduk N (1981) The lumbar mamillo-accessory ligament: Its anatomical and neurosurgical significance. Spine 6/2:162–168

Bogduk N, Long DM (1979) The anatomy of the so-called articular nerves and their relationship to facet denervation in the treatment of low back pain. J Neurosurg 51:172

Bogduk N, Long DM (1980 a) Lumbar medial branch neurotomy: A modification of facet denervation. Spine 5:193

Bogduk N, Long DM (1980 b) Percutaneous lumbar medical branch neurotomy: A modification of facet denervation. Spine 5/2: 162–168

Bolton B (1939) The blood supply of the human spinal cord. J Neurol Neurosurg Psychiatry 2:137

Borchwardt VG (1969) A relationship between the osseous and cartilageous stages in evolution of corpus vertebral. Arkh Anat Gistol Embriol 57/9:111

Bourret P, Louis R (1971) Anatomie du système nerveux central, 2e ed. L'Expansion Scientifique Française, Paris

Bowden REM, Abdullah S, Goodring MR (1967) Anatomy of the cervical spine, membranes, spinal cord, nerve roots and brachial plexus. In: Brain WR, Wilkinson M (eds) Cervical spondylosis. Saunders, Philadelphia

Bradford DL, Spurling RG (1945) The intervertebral disc. Thomas, Springfield

Bradford DL (1977) Techniques of anterior spinal surgery for the management of Kyphosis. Clin Orthop 128:129

Bradley KC (1974) The anatomy of backache. Aust NZ J Surg 44:227

Brailsford JF (1928/1929) Deformities of the lumbosacral region of the spine. Br J Surg 16:562

Brandner ME (1972) Normal values of the vertebral body and intervertebral disk index in adults. AJR 114/2:411–444

Braus H (1954) Anatomie des Menschen, Bd 1. Springer, Berlin

Breig A (1960) Biomechanics of the central nervous system. Almquist and Witsell, Stockholm

Breschet G (1828–1832) – Recherches anatomiques physiologiques et pathologiques sur le système veineux et spécialement sur les canaux veineux des os. Villaret, Paris

Broberg KG, Essen HO von (1980) Modeling of intervertebral discs. Spine 5/2:155–167

Brodelius A, Johansson BW, Sievers J (1962) Anomalous inferior vena cava with azygos and hemiazygos continuation. Acta Paediatr Scand 51:331

Brodetti A (1978) Vascularization of the spinal column in children in relation to the intervertebral disks. Arch Putti Chir Organi Mov 29:381

Brooke R (1924) The sacroilliac joint. J Anat 58:299

Brown MD (1969) The pathophysiology of the intervertebral disc. Anatomical, physiological and biomedical considerations. Master's thesis, Jefferson Medical College, Philadelphia

Brown MW, Templeton AW, Hodges FJ (1964) The incidence of acquired and congenital fusions in the cervical spine. AJR 92:1255

Brown T, Hansen RJ, Yorra AJ (1957) Some mechanical tests on the lumbosacral spine with particular reference to the intervertebral discs. J Bone Joint Surg [Am] 5:1135

Buck CA, Dameron FB, Dow MJ, Skowlund HV (1959) Study of normal range of motion in the neck utilizing a bubble goniometer. Arch Phys Med 40/390

Buckwalter JA, Cooper RR, Maynard JA (1976) Elastic fibers in human intervertebral discs. J Bone Joint Surg 58A1:73

Burton CV, Heithoff K, Kirkaldy-Willis W, Ray CD (1979) Computed tomographic scanning and the lumbar spine. Spine 4:356

Castaing J, Santini JJ (1975) Anatomie fonctionnelle de l'appareil locomoteur. Le rachis. Medicorama. Edit. EPRI, Paris

Cauchoix J, Binet JP, Evrard J (1957) Les voies d'abord inhabituelles dans l'abord des corps vértébraux, cervicaux et dorsaux. Ann Chir 74:1463

Cauchoix J, Binet JP (1957) Anterior surgical approaches to the spine. Ann R Coll Surg Engl 21:237

Cave AJE (1929/1930) On fusion of atlas and axis vertebra. J Anat 64:337

Charpy A (1921) Les vaisseaux de la moelle. Traité d'anatomie humaine. Masson, Paris

Chiro G, Schellinger D (1976) Computed tomography of spinal cord after lumbar intrathecal introduction of metrizamide (computer assisted myelography). Radiology 120:101

Clark AG, Taddonio RF (1979) Congenital atlantoaxial fusion: A case report Spine 4/1:9–11

Clemens JJ (1961) Die Venensysteme der menschlichen Wirbelsäule. De Gruyter, Berlin

Clemmesen V (1936) Congenital cervical synostosis (Klippel-Feil syndrome). Four cases. Acta Radiol 17:480

Cloward RB (1958) The anterior approach for removal of ruptured cervical disks. J Neurosurg 15:602

Cloward RB (1960) The clinical significance of the sinu-vertebral nerve of the cervical spine in relation to the cervical disc syndrome. J Neurol Neurosurg Psychiatry 23:321

Colachis SC, Strohm BM (1965) Radiographic studies of cervical spine in normal subjects, flexion and hyperextension. Arch Phys Med Rehabil 46:753

Colachis SC, Warden RE, Bechtol CO, Strohm BR (1963) Movement of the sacroiliac joint in the adult male: A preliminary report. Arch Phys Med Rehabil 44:490

Compere EL (1937) The operative treatment for low back pain. J Bone Joint Surg 19:749

Compere EL, Tachdjian MO, Kernakan WT (1958/1959) The Luschka joints – their anatomy physiology and pathology. Orthopedics 1:159

Cooper ERA (1960) The vertebral venous plexus. Acta Anat (Basel) 42:333

Corbin JL (1966) Recherches anatomiques sur la vascularisation artérielle de la moelle. Leur contribution à l'étude de l'ischémie médullaire d'origine artérielle. Thèse médecine, Université de Paris

Cordier P, Devols L, Delcroix A (1938) Essai de classification des variations du système azygos intrathoracique. CR Assoc Anat

Cossette J, Farfan H, Robertson G, Wells R (1971) The instantaneous center of rotation of the third lumbar intervertebral joint. J Biomech 4:149

Couinaud C (1973) Le système veineux vertébral. J Chir (Paris) 105/2:125

Coventry MB (1969) Anatomy of the intervertebral disc. Clin Orthop 67:9–15

Coventry MB, Ghormley RK, Kernohan JW (1945) The intervertebral disc: Its microscopic anatomy and pathology. Part I. Anatomy, development, and physiology. J Bone Joint Surg 27:105

Crock HV, Yoshizawa H, Kames SK (1973) Observations on the veinous drainage of the human vertebral body. J Bone Joint Surg [Br] 55:528

Crock HW, Yoshizawa H (1977) The blood supply of the vertebral column and spinal cord in man. Springer, Wien, New York

Crosby EC, Humphrey T, Lauer EW (1962) Correlative anatomy of the nervous system. Macmillan, New York

Cyron BM, Hutton WC (1978) The fatigue strength of the lumbar neural arch in spondylolysis. J Bone Joint Surg [Br] 60:234

Cyron BM, Hutton WC (1980) Articular tropism and stability of the lumbar spine Spine 5/2:168–172

Davis PR (1955) The thoracolumbar mortice joint. J Anat 3/153:370

Davis PR (1956) Variations of the human intra-abdominal pressure during weight lifting in different postures. J Anat 90:601

Davis PR (1959) The medial inclination of the human thoracic intervertebral articular facets. J Anat 68

Davis PR (1961) Human lower lumbar vertebrae: Some mechanical and osteological considerations. J Anat 3/159:337

Davis PR (1963) Some effects of lifting, pulling and pushing on the human trunk. Ergonomics. 4/64:303

Davis PR, Troup JDG (1964) Pressures in the trunk cavities when pulling, pushing and lifting. Ergonomics 7:465–474

Davis PR, Troup JDG, Burnard JH (1965) Movements of the thorax and lumbar spine when lifting: A chronocyclophotographic study. J Anat 4/65:13–26

Dechaume J, Antonietti V, Bouvier A, Duroux P (1961) Sympathique et arthroses cervicales. Documents anatomiques. J Med Lyon 42:493

Delmas A (1960) Valeur fonctionnelle de certaines vertèbres dans la posture. Bull Acad Natl Méd (Paris) 17–18:373

Delmas A, Depreux R (1951) Aspects graphiques des diamètres principaux de divers types de trous de conjugaison. CR Assoc Anat 67/IV:368

Delmas A, Pineau H (1959) Le poids des vertèbres comme élément significatif de leur interdépendance fonctionnelle. CR Assoc Anat 106:214

Delmas A, Pineau H (1967) Sur le canal vertébral de la colonne cervicale. CR Assoc Anat 134:282–289

Delmas A, Pineau H (1969) Signification de la quantité de matériau composant les vertèbres. Acta Anat (Basel) [Suppl] 56/73:139

Delmas A, Pineau H (1970) Sur le canal vertébral de la colonne lombaire. CR Assoc Anat 145:135–138

Delmas A, Pineau H (1970) Surface des apophyses articulaires lombo-sacrées. CR Assoc Anat 148:353

Delmas A, Pineau H (1975) Sur l'inclinaison des apophyses épineuses du rachis cervical. Bull Assoc Anat (Nancy) 59/166:601

Delmas A, Piwnica A (1957) Détermination des axes fonctionnels des vertèbres lombaires. Semaine des Hôpitaux. Arch Anat – Cytol Pathol 1, Paris

Delmas A, Piwnica A (1957) Le couple disco-vertébral lombo-sacré. CR Assoc Anat 43/94:272

Delmas A, Raou R, Piwnica A (1957) Forme du disque lombo-sacré et forme de L5. Importances relatives dans la constatation de la courbure lombaire. CR Assoc Anat 43/94:278

Delmas E, Ndjaga-Mba M, Vannareth T (1970) Le cartilage articulaire L4–L5 et L5–S1. CR Assoc Anat 55/147:230

De Palma AF, Rothman RH (1970) The intervertebral disc. Saunders WB, Philadelphia, p 262

De Seze S, Djian A, Abdelmoula M (1951) Etude radiologique de la dynamique cervicale dans le plan sagittal. Rev Rhum Mal Osteoartic 18:111 (Paris)

Dimmet J, Fischer LP, Gonon GP, Carret JP (1978) Radiographic studies of lateral flexion in the lumbar spine. J Biomech 11/3:143–150

Dinmore P (1977) A new operating position for posterior spinal surgery. Anesthesia Analgesia 82/4:377

Dolan KD (1977) Developmental abnormalities of the cervical spine below the axis. Radiol Clin North Am 15:167

Dommisse GF (1975) Morphological aspects of the lumbar spine and lumbosacral region. Orthop Clin North Am 6/1:163

Donisch EW, Basmajian JV (1971) Electromyography of deep back muscles in man. Am J Anat 113:25

Donisch EW, Trapp W (1971) The cartilage endplates of the human vertebral column (some considerations of postnatal development). Anat Rec 169/4:705

Dubuisson D, Melzack R (1976) Classification and clinical pain descriptions by multiple group discriminant analysis. Exp Neurol 51:480

Duhamel B (1966) Morphogénèse pathologique. Masson, Paris

Eckenhoff JE (1970) The physiological significance of the vertebral venous plexus. Surg Gynecol Obstet 131:72

Edgar MA, Ghadially JA (1976) Innervation of the lumbar spine. Clin Orthop 115:35

Edgar MA, Nundy S (1966) Innervation of the spinal dura mater. J Neurol Neurosurg Psychiatry 29:530

Eger W, Gerner HJ, Ammerer H (1967) Structure and density of the human spongy bone of the ribs, vertebrae and pelvis in relation to the static function. Arch Orthop Unfallchir 62/2:97

Ehrenhaft JL (1943) Development of the vertebral column as related to certain congenital and pathological changes. Surg Gynecol Obstet 76:282

Eie N (1966) Load capacity of the low back. J Oslo City Hosp 16:73–98

Eisenstein S (1976) Measurements of the lumbar spinal canal in 2 racial groups. Clin Orthop 115:42

Eisenstein S (1977) Morphometry and pathological anatomy of the lumbar spine in South African negroes and caucasoids with specific reference to spinal stenosis. J Bone Joint Surg [Br] 59:173

Elsberg CA (1916) Diagnosis and treatment of surgical diseases of the spinal cord and its membranes. Saunders, Philadelphia

Elward JF (1939) Motion in the vertebral column. AJR 42/91

Emminger E (1972) Les articulations interapophysaires et leurs structures méniscoides vues sous l'angle de la pathologie. Ann Med Phys 15:219

Ennabli E (1966) L'artère intercostale supérieure. Arch Anat Cytol Pathol 14:98

Ennabli E (1967) Différents types d'anastomoses entre les artères intercostales dans la région postérieure du thorax. CR Assoc Anat 138:479

Enslin TB (1977) Combined anterior and posterior instrumentation and fusion in scoliosis. J Bone Joint Surg [Br] 59/2:225

Epstein BS (1962) The spine. A radiological text and atlas, 2nd edn Lea & Febiger, Philadelphia

Epstein BS (1976) The spine. A radiological text and atlas, 4th edn. Lea & Febiger, Philadelphia

Epstein BS (1976) The spine. A radiological text and atlas, 4th edn. Lea & Febiger, Philadelphia

Ericksen MF (1978) Aging in the lumbar spine. II. L1 and L2. am J Phys Anthropol 48/2:241

Etemadi AA (1973) Cervical thoracic and lumbar posterior primary rami in man. Pahlavi Med J 4/2:239

Evans FG, Lissner HR (1959) Biomechanical studies on the lumbar spine and pelvis. J Bone Joint Surg [Am] 41:273

Fairbank JCT, O'Brian JP, Davis PR (1980) Intraabdominal pressure rise during weight lifting as an objective measure of low-back pain. Spine 5/2:179–184

Fang HSY, Ong GB (1962) Direct anterior approach to the upper cervical spine. J Bone Joint Surg [Am] 44:1588

Farabeuf LH (1894) Sur l'anatomie et la physiologie des articulations sacroiliaques avant et après la symphyséotomie. Ann Gynecd Obstet 41:407

Farfan HF (1973) Mechanical disorders of the low back. Lea & Febiger, Philadelphia

Farfan HF, Lamy C (1975) The human spine in the performance of the dead lift. St. Mary's Hospital Internal Report, Montreal

Farfan HF, Sullivan JD (1967) The relation of facet orientation to intervertebral disc failure. Can J Surg 10:179

Farfan HF, Cossette JW, Wells RV, Robertson GH, Kraus H (1970) The effects of torsion on the lumbar intervertebral joints: The role of torsion in the production of disc degeneration. J Bone Joint Surg [Am] 52:468

Ferguson WP (1950) Some observations on the circulation in fetal and infant spines. J Bone Joint Surg 31:640

Ferlic D (1962) The range of motion of the «normal» cervical spine. Bull Johns Hopkins Hosp 110/59

Ferlic DC (1963) The nerve supply of the cervical intervetebral disc in man. Bull Johns Hopkins Hosp 113:347

Ferraz de Carvalho CA (1970) Further observations on the functional anatomy of the human fetus spine. Rev Bras Pesqui Med Biol 3/3.4:59

Fick R (1904) Handbuch der Anatomie und Mechanik der Gelenke unter Berücksichtigung der bewegenden Muskeln, T 3. Fischer, Jena

Fielding JW (1957) Cineroentgenography of the normal cervical spine. J Bone Joint Surg [Am] 39:1280

Fielding W (1964) Normal and selected abnormal motion of the cervical spine from the second cervical vertebra to the seventh cervical vertebra based on cine-roentgenography. J Bone Joint Surg [Am] 46/8:1779

Fielding JW, Griffin PP (1974) Os odontoideum: An acquired lesion. J Bone Joint Surg elding[Am] 56:187

Fi JW, Hensinger RN, Hawkins RJ (1980) Os odontoideum. J Bone Joint Surg 62/3:376

Fielding JW, Burstein AA, Frantzel VH (1976) The nuchal ligament Spine I:3

Finneson BE (1973) Low back pain, Lippincott, Philadelphia, p 358

Fischer F, Giere W (1970) Changes in the size of the skeletal sectors of the vertebral column and the lower extremities in adult men and women. Part 1. Changes in the breadth of the vertebral bodies of the normal thoracic and lumbar vertebral column. Z Orthop 107/4:620

Fischer LP, Dimnet H, Gonon GP, Carret JP (1976a) Méthode d'exploitation des radiographies pour une étude cinématique articulaire. Acta Orthop Belg [Suppl 1] 42:125

Fischer LP, Gonon JP, Carret JP et al. (1976b) Vascularisation artérielle des vertèbres lombaires. Bull Assoc Anat (Nancy) 60/169:347

Fishgold H, Adam I, Escoiffier J, Piecquet I (1952) Opacification des plexus rachidiens et des veines azygos par voie osseuse. Presse Med 60:144

Flausen K (1965) The form and function of the loaded human spine. Acta Physiol Scand 65:175

Florent J, Gillot C (1966) Eléments d'anatomie fonctionelle du rachis cervical. Ann Med Phys 9:206

Floyd WF, Silver PHS (1950) Electromyographic study of patterns of activity of the anterior abdominal wall muscles in man. J Anat 84:132

Floyd WF, Silver PHS (1951) Function of erectores spinae in flexion of the trunk. Lancet 260:133

Floyd WF, Silver PHS (1955) The function of the erector spinae muscles in certain movements and postures in man. J Physiol London 129:184

Fountain SS (1979) A single-stage combined surgical approach for vertebral resections. J Bone Joint Surg 61/7:1011

Fox JL, Rizzoli HV (1973) Identification of radiological coordinates for the posterior articular nerve of Luschka in the lumbar spine. Surg Neurol 1:343

Francis CP (1955a) Variations in the articular facets of the cervical vertebrae. Anat Rec 122:589

Francis CP 1955b) Dimensions of the cervical vertebrae. Anat Rec 122:603

Francis CC (1956) Certain changes in the aged male white cervical spine. Anat Rec 125:783

Francois RJ (1975) Ligament insertions into the human lumbar vertebral body. Acta Anat (Basel) 91:467

Frankel VH, Burnstein AH (1970) Orthopaedic biomechanics. Lea & Febiger, Philadelphia

Frazer JE (1965) Anatomy of the human skeleton, 6th edu. Churchill, London

Freeman MAR (1974) Adult articular cartilage. Grune & Stratton, New York

Freund E, Schumacher GH, Fanghanel J (1972) Quantitative studies on morphologic changes in the vertebral column in autopsy material. Folia Morphol Praha 31/4:495

Frigerio NA, Stowe RR, Howe JW (1974) Movement of the sacroiliac joint. Clin Orthop 100:370

Frymoyer JW, Frymoyer WW, Wilder DG, Pope MH (1979) The mechanical and kinematic analysis of the lumbar spine in normal living Human subjects in vivo. J Biomech 12/2:165

Fujiwara M, Hasue M, Numasaki K, Miura H (1978) Relationship between the strength of abdominal and back muscles and the value of integrated electromyogram. Presented at the annual meeting of the Japanese Association of Electroencephalography and Electromyography, Meeting in Kanazawa, October 25, 1978

Fung YC, Perrone N, Anliker M (1972) Biomechanics. Its foundations and objectives. Prentice-Hall, Englewood Cliffs

Gadow HF (1933) The evolution of the vertebral column. Gaskell JF, Green HLHH (eds) Cambridge University Press, Cambridge, p 2/231, 3/156

Galante JO (1967) Tensile properties of the human lumbar annulus fibrosus. Acta Orthop Scand [Suppl 100] 1

Ganguly DN, Roy KK (1964) A study on the cranio-vertebral joint in the man. Anat Anz 4/68:433

Garber JN (1964) Abnormalities of the atlas and axis vertebrae, congenital and traumatic. J Bone Joint Surg [Am] 46:1782

Gardner WJ (1966) Embryologic origin of spinal malformation. Acta Radiol [Diagn] (Stockh) 5:1012

Gargano FP, Jacobson R (1974) Transverse axial tomography of the spine. Neuroradiology 6:254

Geipel P (1955) Zur Kenntnis der Spaltbildung des Atlas and Epistropheus, IV. Zentralbl Allg Pathol 94:19

Ghadially FN (1978) The joint and synovial fluid. I. Edited by L Sokoloff. Academic Press, New York, pp 155

Ghormley RK (1933) Low back pain with special reference to the articular facets, with presentation of an operative procedure. JAMA 101:1773

Gillilan LA (1958) The arterial blood supply of the human spinal cord. J Comp Neurol 110:75

Gillilan LA (1970) Veins of the spinal cord. Anatomic détails suggested clinical applications. Neurology 20:860

Gillot C (1978) La veine rénale gauche. Anat clin 1/2:139–155

Gjorup PA, Gjorup L (1964) Congenital synostosis in the cervical spine. Acta Orthop Scand 34:33

Glenn WV Jr, Rhodes ML, Altshuler EM, Wiltse LL, Kostanek C, Ming Kuo Y (1979) Multiplanar display computerized body tomography applications in the lumbar spine. Spine 4/4:282–352

Goldthwaite JE (1920) Variations in anatomical structure of the lumbar spine. Am J Orthop Surg 2/146:1920

Golub BS, Silverman B (1969) Transforaminal ligaments of the lumbar spine. J Bone Joint Surg [Am] 51:947

Gonon GP (1975) Etude biomécanique de la colonne dorsolombaire de D10 à S1. Thèse Médecine, Lyon.

Gonon GP, Rousson B, Fischer LP (1974a) Données métriques concernant l'arc postérieur au niveau du rachis dorsolombaire de D8 L5. CR Assoc Anat 58/163:867

Gonon GP, Rousson B, Fischer LP, de Mourgues G (1974) Intérêt chirurgical de la connaissance anatomique des directions pédiculaires au niveau du rachis dorsolombaire. Lyon Chir 70/6:408–410

Gonon GP, Dimmet J, Carret JP, Courcelles P, Fischer LP, de Mourgues G (1978) Etude cinématique de la colonne lombaire en inflexion latérale chez le sujet normal et pathologique. Rev Chir Orthop [Suppl II] 64:101

Gouazé A, Castaing J, Rouzaud M (1964) Etude expérimentale de la vascularisation fonctionnelle de la moelle et du cerveau par les fluorescents biologiques. Rev Neurol (Paris) 111:227

Go'zdziewski S (1979) Correlative relations of spondylometric features and the height of the body in Lower Silesian children and adolescent's process of growth (author's transl). Anat Anz 146/3:277

Go'zdziewski S, Mi'skow M (1979) Correlative relations of spondilo metric features in human feti. Anat Anz 146/1:69

Gracovetsky S, Farfan HF, Lamy C (1977) A mathematical model of the lumbar spine using an optimized system to control muscles and ligaments. Orthop Clin North Am 8/1:135

Grant JCB (1944) A method of anatomy. Williams & Wilkins, Baltimore

Gray H (1973a) Gray's anatomy, 35th edn. Edited by R Warwick and PL Williams. Longmans, London

Gray H (1973b) Anatomy of the human body. Edited by SM Goss. Lea & Febiger, Philadelphia

Gray SW, Romaine CBL, Skandalakis JE (1964) Congenital fusion of the cervical vertebrae. Surg Gynecol Obstet 118:373

Greenberg AD, Scoville WB, Davey LM (1968) Transoral decompression of atlantoaxial dislocation due to odontoid hypoplasia: Report of 2 cases. J Neurosurg 28:266

Gregersen GG, Lucas DB (1967) An in vivo study of the axial rotation of the human thoracolumbar spine. J Bone Joint Surg [Am] 49:247

Guerinel G, Artignan P, Richelme H (1966) A propos des veines lombaires. CR Assoc Anat 132:513

Guida G, Cigala F, Riccio V (1969) The vascularization of the vertebral body in the human fetus at term. Clin Orthop 65:229

Guilleminet M, Stagnara P (1952) Rôle de l'entorse vertébrale dans les rachialgies. Presse Med 60:1274

Gunderson CH, Greenspan RH, Glasser GH, Lubs HA (1967) The Klippel-Feil syndrome: Genetic and clinical reevaluation of cervical fusion. Medicine 46:491

Gunn DR, Tupper JW (1976) The combined anterior and posterior approach to the spine in trauma. Presented at the Annual Meeting of the Scoliosis Research Society, Ottawa, Canada, September 1976

Hadley LA (1961) Anatomico-roentgenographic studies of the posterior spinal articulations. AJR 86:270

Hadley LA (1976) Anatomico-roentgenographic studies of the spine. Thomas, Springfield

Hakuba A (1976) Trans-unco-discal approach. A combined anterior and lateral approach to cervical discs. J Neurosurg 45/3:284

Hall MC (1965) Luschka's joint. Thomas, Springfield

Hallock H (1948) Low back lesions – Anatomical considerations. In: Edwards JW (ed) American academy of orthopaedic surgeons instructional course lectures, rd IV. pp 87 Ann Arbor

Hamilton WJ, Boyd JD, Mossman HW (1962) Human embryology Heffer, Cambridge

Hanley EN, Matteri RE, Frymoyer JW (1976) Accurate roentgenographic determination of lumbar flexion extension. Clin Orthop 115:145

Hansson T, Roos, B (1980) The influence of age, height, and weight on the bone mineral content in lumbar vertebrae. Spine 5:545

Hansson T, Roos B, Nachemson A The bone mineral content and ultimate compressive strength in lumbar vertebrae. Spine 5:46

Happey F (1976) A biological study of the human intervertebral disc. In: Jayson MIV (ed) The lumbar spine and back pain. Sector Publishing, London, 293

Hartman WF (1974) Deformation and failure of spinal materials. Exp Mech 3:98

Harris RS, Jones DM (1956) The arterial supply to the adult cervical vertebral bodies. J Bone Joint Surg [Br] 38:922

Hassler O (1966) Blood supply to human spinal cord. A microangiographic study. Arch Neurol 15/3:302–307

Hassler O (1970) The human intervertebral disc: A microangiographical study on its vascular supply at various ages. Acta Orthop Scand 40:765

Hasue M (1972) Evaluation of circulatory dynamics with radioisotopic methods spine and joint diseases. J Jpn Orthop Assoc 46:761

Hasue M, Fujiwara M, Takemura K, Kikuta K, Sato M (1977) Measurement of the strength of abdominal and back muscles with a cybex machine. A preliminary report. Proceedings of the Second Meeting of the Japanese Society for the Study of Muscle Exercise, pp 50

Hasue M, Fujiwara M, Kikuchi S (1980) A new method of quantitative measurement of abdominal and back muscle strength. Spine 5/2:143–200

Haughton VM, Syvertsen A, Williams AL (1980) Soft tissue anatomy within the spinal canal as seen on computed tomography. Radiology 134/3:649

Hayashi K, Yabuki T, Kurokawa T, Seki H, Hogaki M, Minoura S (1977) The anterior and the posterior longitudinal ligaments of the lower cervical spine. J Anat 124/3:633

Henriques CA (1962) The veins of the vertebral column and their role in the spread of cancer. Ann R Coll Surg Engl 31:1

Hensinger RN, Lang JE, MacEwen GD (1974) Klippel-Fiel syndrome. A constellation of associated anomallies. J Bone Joint Surg [Am] 56:1246

Herlihy WF (1947) Revision of the venous system: The role of the vertebral veins. Med J Aust 34:661

Heylings UJ (1978) Supraspinous and interspinous ligaments of the human lumbar spine. J Anat 125/1:127

Hirsch C, Galante J (1967) Laboratory conditions for tensile tests in annulus fibrosus from human intervertebral discs. Acta Orthop Scand 38:148

Hirsch C, Lewin T (1968) Lumbosacral synovial joints in flexion-extension. Acta Orthop Scand 39:303

Hirsch C, Nachemson A (1954) New observations on the mechanical behavior of lumbar disc. Acta Orthop Scand 23:254

Hirsch C, Schajowicz F (1953) Studies on the structural changes in the lumbar annulus fibrosus. Acta Orthop Scand 22:184

Hirsch C, Inglemark BE, Miller M (1963/1964) The anatomical basis for low back pain. Studies on the presence of sensory nerve endings in ligamentous, capsular and intervertebral disc structures in the human lumbar spine. Acta Orthop Scand 33:1–17

Hohl M, Baker HR (1964) The atlantoaxial joint. Bone Joint Surg [Am] 46/1739

Hollinshead WH (1965) Anatomy of the spine; points of interest to orthopaedic surgeons. J Bone Joint Surg [Am] 47:209

Hollinshead WH (1969) The back and limbs. In: Anatomy for surgeons, 2nd. vol 3. Harper & Row, New York

Honnart F (1978) Voies d'abord en chirurgie orthopédique et traumatologique. Masson, Paris

Horton JM (1977) Anesthesia for surgery of the spine and spinal cord. Clin Anesth 15/3:253

Horton WG (1958) Further observations on the elastic mechanism of the intervertebral disc. J Bone Joint Surg [Br] 40:552

Houdart R, Djindjian R, Jullian H, Hurth M (1965) Données nouvelles sur la vascularisation de la moelle dorsolombaire. Rev Neurol (Paris) 112/5:472

Hovelacque A (1925) Le nerf sinu-vertebral. Ann Anat Pathol Anat Norm Med Chir 11:5

Hovelacque A (1927) Anatomie des nerfs crâniens et rachidiens et du système grand sympathique chez l'homme. Doin, Paris 7/938; 8/147

Hsu A (1977) Intra-active three-dimensional display of computerized tomography scanned images. Master's thesis, Los Angeles (UCLA Computer Science)

Huizinga J, Heiden JA, Vinken PJG (1952) The human vertebral canal. A biometric study. Proc R Neth Acad Sci C 55:22

Hukuda S, Ota H, Okabe N, Tazima K (1980) Traumatic atlantoaxial dislocation causing os odontoideum in infants. Spine 5/3:207–210

Huson A, Verbout A (1969) La relation entre la chorde et le tube neural au cours du dévelopement de la colonne vértébrale (note préliminaire). CR Assoc Anat 142:1029

Hutton WC, Stott JRR, Cyron BM (1977) Is spondylolysis a fatigue fracture? Spine 2:202

Hutton WC, Cyron BM, Stott JRR (1979) The compressive strength of lumbar vertebrae. J Anat 129:753

Inoue H (1973) Three-dimensional observation of collagen framework of intervertebral discs in rats, dogs and humans. Arch Histol Jpn 36:39

Inoue H (1981) Three-dimensial architecture of lumbar intervertebral discs. Spine 6/2:139–146

Inoue H, Takeda T (1975) Three-dimensional observation of collagen framework of lumbar intervertebral discs. Acta Orthop Scand 46:949

Isherwood I (1962) Spinal intraosseous venography. J Fac Radiol 13:73

Isherwood I, Fawcitt RA, Nettle JRL, Spencer JW, Pullan BR (1977) Computed tomography of the spine: A preliminary report. In: du Boulay GH, Moseley IF (eds) The first European seminar on computerized axial tomography in clinical practice. Springer Berlin Heidelberg New York pp 322–335

Itoh M, Sihma K, Ishikawa S. Ono Y (1978) A case of cervical canal stenosis accompanied with congenital cervical fusion and extracranial occlusion of vertebrae artery. A clinical and embryological study. No Shinkei Geka 6:591

Jackson HC, Winkelmann RK, Brickel WH (1966) Nerve endings in the human lumbar spinal column and related structures. J Bone Joint Surg [Am] 48/7:1272

Jamiokowska K (1979) Arterial vascularization of the arches of lumbar vertebrae in man. Folia Morphol (Warsz) 38/1:65

Jayson MIV, Barks JS (1973) Structural changes in the intervertebral disc. Ann Rheum Dis 32:10

Johnson PH (1979) The lumbar disc. J Arkansas Med Soc 75/8:297

Johnson RM, Southwick WO (1975) Surgical approaches to the spine. In: (eds) The spine. Rothman, RH, Simeons FF, Saunders, Philadelphia, pp 103

Johnson RM, Crelin ES, White AA, Panjabi MM, Southwick WO (1975) Some new observations on the functional anatomy of the lower cervical spine. Clin Orthop 111:192

Johnson C, Penry JB, Barwood RJ (1972) An unusual presentation of cervical block vertebrae. Australas Radiol 16:63

Johnston HM (1908) The cutaneous branches of the posterior primary divisions of the spinal nerves and their distribution in the skin. J Anat 43:80

Jones MD (1908) The cutaneous branches of the posterior primary divisions of the spinal nerves and their distribution in the skin. J Anat 43:80

Jones MD (1960) Cineradiographic studies of the normal cervical spine. Calcif Med 93:293

Jones RA. Thomson J (1968) The narrow lumbar canal. J Bone Joint Surg [Br] 50:595

Jonsson B (1969) Morphology, innervation, and electromyographic study of the erector spinae. Arch Phys Med Rehabil 50/11:638

Judet R (1969) Inegalités des membres inférieurs – chirurgie du rachis. Masson, Paris

Jung A (1963) Résection de l'articulation uncovertébrale et ouverture du trou de conjugatison par voie antérieure dans le traitement de la névralgie cervico-brachiale. Technique opératoire. Mém Acad Chir 89:361

Jung A, Brunschwig A (1932) Recherches histologiques sur l'innervation des articulations des corps vértébraux. Presse Med 40:316

Junghanns H (1929) Der Lumbosacralwinkel. Dtsch Z Chir 213:332

Juskiewinski S (1963) Branche postérieure des nerfs rachidiens et articulation interapophysaire vertébrale. Thèse Med., Toulouse

Kadyi H (1886) Über die Blutgefäße des menschlichen Rückenmarkes. Anat Anz 1:304

Kapandji JA (1969) The functional anatomy of the lumbosacral spine. Acta Orthop Belg 35/3–4:543

Kapandji IA (1972) Physiologie articulaire. In: Tronc et rachis, fasc III. Maloine, Paris, 1–255

Kapandji IA (1974) The physiology of the joints part III. Churchill-Livingstone, New York

Kazarian L (1972) Dynamic response characteristic of the human vertebral column. An experimental study on human autopsy specimens. Acta Orthop Scand [Suppl] 146:186

Kazarian L, Graves GA (1977) Compressive strength characteristics of the human vertebral centrum. Spine 1:1–14

Keele KD, Stern PRS (1973) Serum lipid changes in relation to pain. J R Coll Physicians Lond 7:319

Keene CW (1906/1907) Some experiments on the mechanical rotation of the normal spine. Am J Orthop Surg 4:69

Keim HA (1976) The adolescent spine. Grune & Straton, New York San Francisco London

Keith A (1933) Human embryology and morphology, 5thedn. Arnold, London, pp 77

Kellgren JG, Lawrence JS (1958) Osteoarthrosis and disc degeneration in an urban population. Ann Rheum Dis 17:338

Keyes DC, Compere EL (1932) The normal and pathological physiology of the nucleus pulposus of the intervertebral disc. J Bone Joint Surg 14:897

King AI, Vulcan AP (1971) Elastic deformation characteristics of the spine. J Biomech 4/5:413

Kinzel GL, Hall AS, Hillberry BM (1972) Measurement of the total motion between two body segments. I. Analytical development J Biomech 5:93

Kippel M, Feil A (1975) A case of absence of cervical vertebrae with the thoracic cage rising to the base of the cranium (cervical thoracic cage). Translated by EM Bick. Clin Orthop 109:3

Klein G (1891) Zur Mechanik des Ileosacralgelenkes. Z Geburtshilfe Gynaekol 21:74

Klinger A, Rhodes ML, Glenn WV (1978) General view imagery from parallel image planes. Proceedings of the San Diego Biomedical Symposium, February 1–3, 1978, 387

Koreska J, Robertson D, Mills RH, Gibson DA, Albisser AM (1977) Biomechanics of the lumbar spine and its clinical significance. Orthop Clin North Am 8/1:121

Kos J, Wolf J (1972) Les ménisques intervertébraux et leur rôle possible dans les blocages vertébraux. Ann Med Phys 15:203

Kottle FJ, Mundale MO (1959) Range of mobility on the cervical spine. Arch Phys Med 40:379

Kovbasenko LA (1978) Surgical anatomical characteristics of the operative approaches to the posterior portion of the sacrum. Ortop Travmatol Protez 7:71

Kovbasenko LA (1979) Surgical anatomical basis for extra-articular resections of the sacrum. Klin Khir 12:19

Kubik S (1966) Topography of spinal nerve roots. I. Changes in the course of stimuli through cervithoracic nerve roots during prenatal and postnatal development and their behaviour in adult. Acta Anat (Basel) 63/3:324

Kulak RF, Schultz AB, Belytschko T, Galante J (1975) Biomechanical characteristics of vertebral motion segments and intervertebral discs. Orthop Clin North Am 1:121

Kumar S, Davis PR (1973) Lumbar vertebral innervation and intra-abdominal pressure. J Anat 114:47

Kwoh YS, Reed IS, Truong TK (1977) A generalized w-filter for 3-D reconstruction. IEEE Trans Nucl Sci 24:1990

Kwoh YS, Reed IS, Truong TK (1977b) Back projection speed improvement for 3-D reconstruction. IEEE Trans Nucl Sci 24:1999

Lacapere J, Drieux H, Kriegel A (1952) La vascularisation du corps vertébral. Rev Rhum 447:82

Lainée J, Bolgert F, Vallot JP, Zhepova F, Derome P (1979) Double malformation discovered during investigations for hypertension single pelvic kidney and occipitovertebral joint malformation. Ann Med Interne (Paris) 130/6–7:377

Lamberty BGH, Zivanovic S (1973) The retro articular vertebral artery ring of the atlas and its significance. Acta Anat (Basel) 85/1:113

Lancourt JE, Glenn WV, Wiltse LL (1979) Multiplanar computerized tomography in the normal spine and in the diagnosis of spinal stenosis: A gross anatomic-computerized tomographic correlation. Spine 4:379

Larsen GN, Glenn WV, Kishore PRS, Davis K, McFarland W, Dwyer SJ (1977) Computer processing of CT images: Advances and prospects. Neurosurgery 1

Lazorthes G (1962) La vascularisation de la moelle épinière. Rev Neurol (Paris), 106:535

Lazorthes G (1972) Les branches posterieures des nerfs rachidiens et le plan articulaire vertébral postérieur. Ann Med Phys 15:192

Lazorthes G, Gaubert J (1966) La branche postérieure des nerfs rachidiens. L'innervation des articulations interapophysaires vertébrales. R Assoc Annat 43:488

Lazorthes G, Gouazé A (1968) Les voies anatomotiques de suppléance (ou système de sécurité) de la vascularisation artérielle de l'axe cérébromédullaire. C R Assoc Anat 140:1–223

Lazorthes G, Juskiewinski S (1964) Etude comparative des branches postérieures des nerfs dorsaux et lombaires et de leurs rapports avec les articulations interapophysaires vertébrales. Bull Assoc Anat (Nancy) 49:1025

Lazorthes G, Poulhes J, Bastide G, Roulleau J, Chancholle AR (1957) Recherches sur la vascularisation artérielle de la moelle. Applications à la pathologie médullaire. Bull Acad Nat Med (Paris) 41:464

Lazorthes G, Poulhes HJ, Bastide G, Roulleau J, Chancholle AR (1958a) Les artères de la moelle. C R Assoc Anat 99:410

Lazorthes G, Poules J, Bastide G, Roulleau J, Chancholle AR (1958b) La vascularisation artérielle de la moelle. Neurochirurgie 4:3–19

Lazorthes G, Gaubert J, Chancholle AR, Lazorthes Y (1962) Les rapports de la branche posterieure des nerfs cervicaux avec les articulations interapophysaires vertebrales. Bull Assoc Anat (Nancy) 48:887

Lazorthes G, Bastide G, Chancholle AR, Zadeth O (1964) Etude anatomique sur l'artère du renflement lombaire. C R Assoc Anat 120:883

Lazorthes G, Gouazé A, Bastide G, Santini JJ, Zadeth H, Burdin P (1966a) La vascularisation artérielle de la moelle cervicale. Etude des suppléances. Rev Neurol (Neurol) 115:1055

Lazorthes G, Gouazé A, Bastide G, Soutoul JH, Zadeth O, Santini JJ (1966b) La participation des artères radiculaires lombosacrées à la vascularisation fonctionnelle du renflement lombaire. C R Assoc Anat 135:580

Lazorthes Y, Zadeb JO, Lagarrigue J (1972) Chirurgie du rachis cervical par voie d'abord antérolatérale. Technique. Rev Med Toulouse 8:741

Le Double AF (1977) Traité des variations de la colonne vertébrale de l'homme, 4th edn. Excerpta Medica Amsterdam (Nomina Antomica)

Le Guyader A, Boucher J, Delteil C (1965) Note sur la collatéralité de l'aorte abdominale chez le nouveau-né. C R Assoc Anat 127:1080

Lethe P (1975) Quelques particularités anatomo-fonctionnelles de l'axe vertébral. C R Assoc Anat 59/164:207

Lewin T, Reichmann S (1968) Bony contacts between the tips of the articular processes and adjacent parts of the vertebral arch in the lumbar spine in young individuals. Acta Morphol Neerl Scand 7/2:185

Lewin T, Moffett B, Vidiik A (1962) The morphology of the lumbar synovial joints. Acta Morphol Neerl Scand 4:299

Ley F (1974) Contribution à l'étude des cavités articulaires interapophysaires vertébrales thoraciques. Arch Anat Histol Embryol 57:61–114

Lin HS, Liu YK, Adams KH (1978) Mechanical response of the lumbar intervertebral joint under physiological (complex) loading. J Bone Joint Surg [Am] 60/1:41

Liu YK, Ray G, Hirsch C (1975) The resistance of the lumbar spine to direct shear. Orthop Clin North Am 6:33

Liu YK, Wickstrom JK (1973) Estimation of the inertial property distribution of the human torso from segmented cadaveric data. In: Kenedi RM (ed) Perspectives in biomedical engineering. Macmillan, London pp 203–213

Lora J, Long D (1976) So-called facet denervation in the management of intractable back pain. Spine 1:121

Louis R (1961) Contribution à l'étude topographique des racines rachidiennes et de la moelle avec les lames et les disques intervertébraux.
Thèse, Marseille

Louis R (1969) Topographie vertébromédullaire. Bull Assoc Anat (Nancy), 54:272

Louis R (1970) Technique de l'ostéotomie cervicale par double abord
pour les lésions traumatiques anciennes. Rev Med Orthop 56:325

Louis R (1973) Chirurgie de la charnière dorsolombaire. In: SOFCOT,
Orthopédie et traumatologie. Conf. d'Enseignement L'Expansion
Scientifique, Paris pp 95–128

Louis R (1978a) Topographic relationships of the vertebral column, spinal cord and nerve roots. Anat Clin 1/1:3–12

Louis R (1978b) Bases anatomiques pour la chirurgie vertébrale de la
jonction thoracolombaire. Anat Clin 1/1:73

Louis R (1978c) Topographie vertébromédullaire et vertébroradiculaire.
Anat Clin 1/1:73

Louis R (1980) Dynamique radiculomédullaire. Anat Clin 3/1:3–12

Louis R, Argenson C (1962–63) Les veines vertébrales. Trav Inst Anat
Marseille 21:21–25

Louis R, Baille Y (1964) La mobilité des racines lombosacrées. Bull Assoc Anat (Nancy) 127:1117–1134

Louis R, Sylla S (1973) Poids des vertèbres chez l'Africain. Bull Assoc
Anat (Nancy) 57/158:549

Louis R, Guérinel G, Mambrini A (1964) Modifications évolutives de
l'isthme vertébral lombosacré. Bull Assoc Anat (Nancy) 49:1135–1152

Louis R, Salamon G, Guérinel G (1962–1963) Le fourreau dural lombo-
sacré. Etude radio-anatomique. Trav Inst Anat Marseille 21/53–60
Acta Radiol 5:1107–1966

Louis R, Laffont J, Conty CR, Argème M (1967a) Mobilité de la moelle
épinière. Bull Assoc Anat (Nancy) 139

Louis R, Laffont J, Obounou-Akong D (1967b) Charnière lombosacrée
de l'Africain. Bull Assoc Anat (Nancy) 139:828–837

Louis R, Ouiminga RM, Conty CR, Obounou E, N'Doye (1971a) Circulation veineuse vertébrale. Livre du IXe Congrès Int Anat Léningrad.
1970. Bull Soc Med. Afr Noire Lang Fr 16/3:383

Louis R, Obounou-Akong D, Ouiminga RM (1971b) Les voies d'accès
antérieur de la région termino-aortique. Bull Soc Med Afr Noire Lang
Fr 16/3:313

Louis R, Obounou-Akong D, Ouiminga RM (1971e) Le mode d'émer-
gence des artères pariétales aortiques chez l'Africain. Bull Soc Med
Afr Noire Lang Fr 16:2–257

Louis R, Obounou-Akong D, Ouiminga RM (1974) Etude topographique de la région termino-aortique. Bull Assoc Anat (Nancy) 154:1089

Louis R, Ouiminga RM, Obounou-Akong D (1971g) Etude topographique de la veine cave inférieure chez l'Africain. Bull Soc Med Afr Noire
Lang Fr 16/1:90

Louis R, Obounou – Akong D, Ouiminga RM (1975) Topographie vascu-
laire de la charnière dorsolombaire chez le Noir Africain (105 cas).
Bull Assoc Anat (Nancy) 59/166:657

Louis R, Sorbier J, Bonnoit J (1977) Instabilité expérimentale. Expé-
riences anatomiques. Rev Chir Orthop 63:428

Louis R, Ouiminga RM, Obounou-Akong D (1978) Le système azygos ou
système veineux anastomotique vertébropariétal. Bull Assoc Anat
(Nancy) 60/169:381

Lovett RW (1902) A contribution to the study on the mechanics of the
spine. Am J Anat 2:457

Lowrance EW, Latimer HB (1967) Weights and variability of components of the human vertebral column. Anat Rec 159/1:83

Lucas DB (1970) Mechanics of the spine. Bull Hosp It Dis 31/2:115

Lucas DB, Bresler B (1961) Stability of the ligamentous spine. Biomechanics Laboratory, University of California

Luschka H (1850) Die Nerven des menschlichen Wirbelkanales. Lapp

Lysell E (1969) Motion in the cervical spine. Acta Orthop Scand 123:7

Maciver DA, Letts RM (1968) Intraosseous vertebral venography as a
diagnostic aid in intervertebral disc disease. Can J Surg 11/16

Macnab I, Dall D (1971) The blood supply of the lumbar spine and its application to the technique of intertransverse lumbar fusion. J Bone
Joint Surg [Br] 53:628

Macrae IF, Wright V (1969) Measurement of back movement. Ann
Rheum Dis 28:584

Madley LA (1961) Anatomico-roentgenographic studies of the posterior
spinal articulations. AJR 86:270

Maigne R (1968) Douleurs d'origine vertébrale et traitements par manipulations. Expansion Scientifique, Paris

Maigne R (1974) Origine dorsolombaire de certaines lombalgies basses.
Rôle des articulations interapophysaires et des branches postérieures
des nerfs rachidiens. Rev Rhum 12:781

Malinsky J (1959) The ontogenetic development of nerve terminations in
the intervertebral discs of man. Acta Anat (Basel) 38:96

Malinsky J, Malinska J (1970) Developmental stages of the prenatal spinal cord in man. Folia Morphol Praha 18/3:228

Malinska J, Malinsky J Zrzavy J (1970) An anatomical study of the spinal
cord in man during the first half of prenatal development. Folia Morphol 18/4:400

Marcozzi G, Messinetti S, Columbati M, De Sanctis M (1960) I plessi venosi rachidei. Ann Ital Chir 37:161

Maresca C, Ghafar W (1979) Le nerf présacré. Plexus hypogastricus superior. Anat Clin 2/1:5–12

Markhashov AM (1970) The functional anatomy of the collateral communications between the vertebral veins and those of adjacent organs.
Arkh Anat Gistol Embriol 59/9:104

Markoff KL (1972) Deformation of the thoracolumbar intervertebral
joints in response to external loads. J Bone Joint Surg [Am] 54:511

Markoff KL, Morris JM (1974) The structural components of the intervertebral disc. J Bone Joint Surg [Am] 56/4:675

Maslow GS (1975) The facet joints another book. Bull NY Acad Med
51/11:1294

Massare C, Bard M, Busson J (1979) Tomodensitometry and spinal pathology. Rev Rhum Mal Osteoartic 46/5:327

Maupoux F, Fuentes JM (1980) L'arthrographie postérieure. La
sciatique et le nerf sciatique sous la direction de L Simon. Masson,
Paris

Meachim G, Cornalh MS (1970) Fine structure of juvenile human nucleus pulposus. J Anat 107/2:337

Meijenhorst GC (1979) Final word on «Epidural double catheter venography in intervertebral disk prolapse; an unknown vein in the vertebral canal». Roefo 131/1:101

Mendes JC (1963) Contribuicão para o estudo das relações entre o terri-
tório da veia cava inferior e as veias do raquis. Theses, universidale de
Lisboa

Mercer W (1950) Orthopedic surgery, 4th edn, Williams & Willkins, Baltimore

Mercier R, Vanneuville G (1968) Anatomie radiologique de l'aorte abdominale et de ses branches collatérales et terminales. Expansion Scientifique, Paris

Mestdagh H (1969) Anatomie fonctionnelle du rachis cervical (C3 à C7).
Thèse Med, Lille

Mestdagh H (1976) Morphological aspects and biochemical properties
of the vertebroaxial joint. Acta Morphol Neerl Scand 14:19

Meyer GH (1873) Die Statik und Mechanik des menschlichen Knochen-
gerüstes. Engelmann, Leipzig

Michaels L, Prevost MJ, Crang DF (1969) Pathological changes in a case
of os odontoideum (separate odontoid process). J Bone Joint Surg
[Am] 51:965

Michie MI, Clark M (1968) Neurological syndromes associated with cervical and craniocervical anomalies. Arch Neurol 18:241

Miles M, Sullivan WE (1961) Lateral bending at the lumbar and lumbosacral joint. Anat Rec 139:387

Mineiro JD (1965) Columna vertebral humana. Socieda de Industrial
Grafica, Rua de Campolide 133B–C Lisboa

Minne J, Depreux R, Francke JP (1970) The peri-odontoid arteries in the
second cervical vertebra. C R Assoc Anat 149:914

Mitchell F (1970) Roentgenographic measurement of sacroiliac respiratory movement. JAOA 69:81

Mitchell GAG (1936) The significance of lumbosacral transitional vertebrae. Br J Surg 24:147

Miyasaka K, Takei H, Ito T, Taschiro K, Abe H, Tsuru M (1979) Catheter
cervical vertebral venography. Neuroradiology 16:413

Moret J (1979) Indications and technique of cervical phlebography.
Diagn Imaging 48/4:253

Morris JM (1973) Biomechanics of the spine. Arch Surg 107:418

Morris JM, Lucas DB, Bresler B (1961) Role of trunc in stability of the spine. J Bone Joint Surg [Am] 42:327

Morris JM, Benner G, Lucas DB (1962) An electromyographic study of intrinsic muscles of the back in man. J Anat 96 /4:509

Morscher E, Dick W (1978) Operations on vertebral bodies by anterior approach. Zentralbl Chir 103/17:1105

Mosberg WH, Lippman EM (1960) Anterior approach to the cervical vertebral bodies. Bull Univ Md Sch Med 45:10–17

Motvkin PA, Belikoula AS (1969) Proper spinal nerves in man. Arkh Anat Gistol Embriol 57/12:66

Nachemson A (1960) Lumbar intradiscal pressure. Experimental studies on post-mortem material. Acta Orthop Scand [Suppl] 43/4/61:1

Nachemson A (1962) Some mechanical properties of the lumbar inter-vertebral discs. Bull Hosp Joint Dis 23:130

Nachemson A (1966 a) The load on the lumbar disc in different positions of the body. Clin Orthop 45:107

Nachemson A (1966 b) Electromyographic studies on the vertebral portion of the psoas muscle. Acta Orthop Scand 37:177

Nachemson A (1975) Towards a better understanding of low-back pain: A review of the mechanics of the lumbar disc. Rheumatol Rehabil 14:129

Nachemson A (1976 a) The lumbar spine an orthopaedic challenge. Spine 1:59

Nachemson A (1976 b) Lumbar intra-discal pressure. In: Jayson MIV (ed). Lumbar spine and back pain. Pitman, Tunbridge Wells

Nachemson A, Elfstrom G (1970) Intravital dynamic pressure measurements in lumbar discs. A study of common movements, manoeuvers and exercises. Almqvist & Wiksell, Stockholm

Nachemson A, Evans J (1968) Some mechanical properties of the third human lumbar interlaminar ligament. J Biomech 1:211

Nachemson A, Lindh M (1969) Measurement of abdominal and back muscle strength with and without low back pain. Scand J Rehabil Med 1:60

Nachemson A, Morris JM (1963) Lumbar discometry. Lumbar intradiscal pressure measurements in vivo. Lancet I:1140

Nachemson A, Morris JM (1964) In vivo measurements of intradiscal pressure. J Bone Joint Surg [Am] 46:1077

Nachemson A, Lewis T, Maroudas A, Freeman MAR (1970) In vitro diffusion of dye through the endplates and the annulus fibrosus of human intervertebral discs. Acta Orthop Scand 41:589

Nachemson A, Schultz AB, Berkson MH (1979) Mechanical properties of human lumbar spine motion segments. Influence of age, sex, disc level, and degeneration. Spine 4/1:1

Nash CL, Moe JH (1969) A study of vertebral rotation. J Bone Joint Surg [Am] 51:223

Nathan MH, Blum L (1960) Evaluation of vertebral venography. AJR 83:1027

Noback CR, Robertson GC (1951) Sequence of appearance of ossification centers in the human skeleton during the first five prenatal months. Am J Anat 89:1

Nomina Anatomica (1966) Excerpta Medica, Amsterdam

Obounou-Akong D (1969) Contribution à l'étude topographique des artères rachidiennes et médullaires. (110 pièces anatomiques). Theses, Dakar

Okada M, Kogi K, Ishii M (1970) Endurance capacity of the erectores spinae muscles in static work. J Anthropol Soc Nippon (Zinruigaku Zasshi) 78/2:99

Ooi Y, Kaminuma S, Mikanagi K, Tsukamoto S, Ijichi M (1976) Theory of isokinetic muscle contraction and its application to the field of orthopaedic surgery. J Jpn Orthop Assoc 50:1011

O' Rahilly R, Meyer DB (1979) The timing and sequence of events in the development of the human vertebral column during the embryonic period proper. Anat Embryol (Berl) 157/2:167

Orofino C, Scherman MS, Schechter D (1969) Luschka's joint – a degenerative phenomenon. J Bone Joint Surg [Am] 42:853

Ouiminga RM (1969) Contribution à l'étude topographique des veines rachidiennes et médullaires. (100 pièces anatomiques.) Thèse Dakar

Overton LM, Grossmann JW (1952) Anatomical variations in the articulation between the 2nd and 3rd vertebrae. J Bone Joint Surg [Am] 34:158

Panjabi MM, White AA, Johnson RM (1975) Cervical spine mechanics as a function of transection of components. J Biomech 8/4:327

Panjabi MM, Brand RA, White AA (1976) Mechanical properties of the human thoracic spine: As shown by three-dimensional load-displacement curves. J Bone Joint Surg [Am] 58/5:642

Panjabi MM, Kras MH, White AA, Southwick WO (1977) Effects of pre-load on load displacement curves of the lumbar spine. Orthop Clin North Am 8/8:181

Panjabi MM (1973) Three dimensional mathematical model of the human spine structure. J Biomech 6:761

Panjabi MM, White AA, Keller D, Southwick WO, Friedlaender G (1978) Stability of the cervical spine under tension. J Biomech 1/4:189–197

Parke WW, Valsamis MP (1967) The ampulloglomerular organ: An unusual neurovascular complex in the suboccipital region. Anat Rec 159:193

Parke WW (1978) The vascular relations of the upper cervical vertebrae. Orthop Clin North Am 9/4:879

Patterson RH Jr, Arbit E (1978) A surgical approach through the pedicle to protruded thoracic discs. J Neurosurg 48/5:768

Paturet G (1958) Traité d'anatomie humaine (appareil circulatoire), vol 3. Masson, Paris

Pauly JE (1967) An electromyographic analysis of certain movements and exercises. Anat Rec 155:223

Peacock A (1951) Observations on the prenatal development of the inter-vertebral disc in man. J Anat 85:260

Pedersen HE, Blunck CFJ, Gardner E (1956) The anatomy of the lumbo-sacral posterior rami and meningeal branches of spinal nerves (sinu-vertebral nerves). J Bone Joint Surg [Am] 38:377

Penning L (1978) Normal movements of the cervical spine. AJR 130/2:317

Perey O (1957) Fracture of the vertebral end-plate in the lumbar spine. An experimental biomechanical investigation. Acta Orthop Scand [Suppl] 26:1

Pernkopf E (1963) Atlas of topographical and applied human anatomy, vol 1–2. Saunders, Philadelphia London

Perpetuo FO, Machado RE (1979) Surgical treatment of atlanto-axial subluxation by transoropharyngeal approach. Report of a case Arq Neuropsiquiatr 37/2:192

Petter CK (1933) Methods of measuring the pressure of the intervertebral disc. J Bone Joint Surg 15:365

Piersol GA (1916) Human anatomy, 5th edn, vol 1. Lippincott, Philadelphia

Pizon P (1972) La colonne lombosacrée, vol 1. Doin, Paris

Pope MH (1975) Biplanar x-ray of the spine. Report of engineering round table. Orthop Clin North Am 6:48

Pope MH, Wilder DG, Matteri RE, et al (1975) Experimental measurements of vertebral motion under load. Presented at the Second Annual Meeting of the International Society for the Study of the Lumbar Spine. London, July 4. 1975

Pope MH, Hanley EN, Matteri RE, Wilder DG, Frymoyer JW (1977 a) Measurement of intervertebral disc space height. Spine 2:282

Pope MH, Wilder DG, Matteri RE, et al (1977 b) Experimental measurements of vertebral motion under load. Orthop Clin North Am 8:155

Pope MH, Wilder DG, Frymoyer JW, et al (1977 c) In vivo load-deflection studies of the lumbar spine. Presented at the Fourth Annual Meeting of the International Society for the Study of the Lumbar Spine. Utrecht, May 5, 1977. Proceedings of the Oxford Orthopaedic Engineering Centre Symposium. New York, Pergamon Press, 1979

Pope MH, Wilder DG, Moreland MS, et al (1978) Moire fringe topography of the scoliotic back. J Bone Joint Surg 2:175

Pope MH, Wilder DG, Stokes IAF, Frymoyer JW (1979) Biomechanical testing as an aid to decision making in low-back pain patients. Spine 4:135

Porter RW, Wicks M, Ottewell D (1978) Measurement of the spinal canal by diagnostic ultrasound. J Bone Joint Surg [Br] 60:481

Portnoy H, Morin F (1956) Electromyographic study of postural muscles in various positions and movements. Am J Physiol 86:122

Pritzer KPH (1977) Aging and degeneration in the lumbar intervertebral disc. Orthop Clin North Am 8:65

Putti V, Logroscino D (1937/1938) Anatomia dell'artritismo vertebrale apofisario. Chir Organi Mov 23:317

Putz R, Pomaroli A (1972) The form and function of the lateral atlanto-axial joint. Acta Anat (Basel) 83/3:333

Rabischong P, Louis R, Vignaud J (1978) Le disque intervertébral. Anat Clin 1:55

Rainer F, Cotaescu I (1946) Contribution à l'étude de l'appareil fibreux de la colonne vertébrale. L'oeuvre scientifique. Acad. Române, Bucuresti

Rakitianskaia AF (1979) Method of mobilizing the diaphragm in the extraperitoneal and extrapleural approach to the thoraco-lumbar spine in disseminated forms of tuberculous spondylitis. Probl Tuberk 3:39

Ramos A, Tavares A (1964) Aspects de l'anatomie du système azygos. C R Assoc Anat 122:322

Ratcliffe JF (1978) Microarteriography of the cadaveric human lumbar spine. Evaluation of a new technique of injection in the anastomotic arterial system. Acta Radiol [Diagn] (Stockh) 19/4:656

Reichmann S, Lewin T (1971) Growth processus in the lumbar neural arch. Z Anat Entwicklungsgesch 133/1:89

Reichmann S, Berglund E, Lundgren K (1972) Motion centre in flexion and extension of the lumbar spine. Z Anat Entwicklungsgesch 138/3:283

Renard M, Larde D, Masson JP, Roland JR (1979) Etude anatomique et radio-anatomique des plexus veineux intrarachidiens lombosacrés. Anat Clin 2/1:21

Rickenbacher J (1969) The ontogenesis of the vertebral column. Praxis 58/6:179

Rigaud A, Cabanie M, Mathé (1959) Note sur le mode d'origine des veines azygos. C R Assoc Anat 46:712

Rizzi MA (1976) Biomechanics of the spine with special reference to its shape. Z Unfallmed Berufskr 69/1:3

Roaf R (1958) Rotation movements of the spine with special reference to scoliosis. J Bone Joint Surg [Br] 40:312

Roaf R (1960) A study of the mechanics of spinal injuries. J Bone Joint Surg [Br] 4:810

Roberts SB, Chen PH (1970) Elastostatic analysis of the human thoracic skeleton: J Biomech 3:527

Rockwell SB, Evans FG, Pheasant HC (1938) The comparative morphology of the vertebral spinal column. Its form as related to function. J Morphol 63:87

Rolander SD (1966) Motion of the lumbar spine with special reference to the stabilising effect of posterior fusion. Acta Orthop Scand [Suppl] 90

Rolander SD, Blair WE (1975) Deformation and fracture of the lumbar vertebral endplate. Orthop Clin North Am 6:75

Romanes GJ (1965) The arterial blood supply of the human spinal cord. Paraplegia 2:199

Roofe PG (1940) Innervation of anulus fibrosus and posterior longitudinal ligament. Arch Neurol Psychiatry 44:100

Rosemeyer B (1974) Standing and sitting posture. Z Orthop 112/1:151

Rothman RH, Simeone FA (1975) The spine, vol 1–2, Saunders, Philadelphia London Toronto

Rouviere H (1962) Anatomie humaine, descriptive et topographique, vol 1–2. Masson, Paris

Rowe GG, Roche MB (1950) The lumbar neural arch. J Bone Joint Surg [Am] 32:554

Roy-Camille R (1979) Rachis cervical traumatique non neurologique. Masson, Paris

Ruge D, Wiltse LL (1977) Spinal disorders. Lea & Febiger, Philadelphia

Saillant G (1976) Anatomical study of the vertebral pedicles. Surgical application. Rev Chir Orthop 62/2:151

Salcman M, Jamaris J, Leveque H, Ducker TB (1979) Transoral cervical corpectomy with the aid of the microscope. Spine 4/3:209

Salmon M (1933) Artères des muscles de la tête et du cou. Masson, Paris

Sand PG (1970) The human lumbo-sacral vertebral column. An osteometric study. Universitets Forlaget Trynkningssentral, Oslo

Santini JJ (1966) Etude anatomique et expérimentale de la vascularisation artérielle fonctionnelle de la moelle épinière. Applications cliniques. Thèse Médecine, Tours

Sarpyener MA (1945) Congenital structure of the spinal canal. J Bone Joint Surg 27:70

Schiff DDM, Parke WW (1972) The arterial supply of the odontoid process. Anat Rec 172:399

Schmorl G, Junghans H (1968) Die gesunde und die kranke Wirbelsäule in Röntgenbild und Klinik. Thieme, Stuttgart

Schmorl G, Junghans H (1971) The human spine in health and disease, 2nd ed. Grund & Stratton, New York.

Schoening HA, Hannan V (1964) Factors related to cervical spine mobility. Arch Phys Med 45:602

Scholder P (1971) Functional anatomy of the cervical spine. Z Unfallmed Berufskr 64/4:233

Schultz AB, Galante JO (1970) A mathematical model for the study of the mechanics of the human vertebral column. J Biomech 3:405

Schultz AB, Belytschko TB, Andriacchi TP, Galante JO (1973) Analog studies of forces in the human spine. Mechanical properties and motion segment behaviour. J Biomech 6:373

Schuwytzer FX (1977) Study of the growth of the vertebral bodies in adolescents. Acta Anat (Basel) 98/1:52

Seib GA (1934) Azygos system of veins in american whites and american negroes, including observations in inferior caval venous system. Am J Phys Anthropd 19:36

Seireg A, Arvikar RJ (1973) A mathematical model for the evaluation of forces in the lower extremities of the musculoskeletal system. J Biomech 6:313

Seireg A, Arvikar RJ (1975) A comprehensive musculoskeletal model for the human vertebral column, Advances in bioengineering. Proceedings of the Winter Annual Meeting of the Bioengineering Division of American Society of Mechanical Engineers Houston, Texas, November 1975, pp 74

Selecki BR (1969) The effects of rotation of the atlas on the axis: Experimental work. Med J Aust 1:1012

Sensening EC (1949) The early development of the human vertebral column. Contrib Embryol Carnegie Inst 33:21

Shah JS, Hampson WG, Jayson MI (1978) The distribution of surface strain in the cadaveric lumbar spine. J Bone Joint Surg [Br] 60/2:246

Shapiro R (1968) Myelography, 2nd ed. Year Book Medical Publishers, Chicago

Shealy CN (1974 The role of the spinal facets in back and sciatic pain. Headache 14:101

Sheldon JJ, Sersland T, Leborgne J (1977) Computed tomography of the lower lumbar vertebral column. Normal anatomy and the stenotic canal. Radiology 124:113

Shinohara H (1970) A study on lumbar disc lesions. J Jpn Orthop Assoc 44:553

Siberstein CE (1965) The evolution of degenerative changes in the cervical spine and an investigation into the «joints of Luschka». Clin Orthop 40:184

Sicard A (1959) Chirurgie du rachis. Masson, Paris

Silver PHS (1954) Direct observations of changes in tension in the supraspinous and interspinous ligaments during flexion and extension of vertebral column in man. J Anat 88:550

Simmons EH, Mouradian WH (1977) Unusual malunion of odontoid process. J Bone Joint Surg [Am] 59:552

Singh S (1965) Variations of the superior articular facets of atlas vertebrae. J Anat 99/3:565

Slabaugh PB, Winter RB, Lonstein JE, Moe JH (1980) Lumbosacral hemivertebrae: A review of twentyfour patients, with excision in eight. Spine 5/3:234–244

Sobotta J, Figg'e FHJ (1963) Atlas of human anatomy. Hafner, New York

Solonen KA (1957) The sacroiliac joint in the light of anatomical, roentgenological and clinical studies. Acta Orthop Scand [Suppl] 27

Somogyi B (1964) The blood supply of the foetal spine. Acta Morphol Acad Sci Hung 12:261

Southworth JD, Bersack SR (1950) Anomalies of the lumbosacral vertebrae in five hundred and fifty individuals without symptoms referable to the low back. AJR 64:624

Spencer DL, Dewald RL (1979) Simultaneous anterior and posterior surgical approach to the thoracic and lumbar spine. Spine 4/1:29

Spencer DL, Ray RD, Spigos DG, Kanakis C (1981) Intraosseous pressure in the lumbar spine. Spine 6/2:159–161

Stanczyk JL (1979) Canal of vertebral artery of atlas. Folia Morphol Praha 38/2:353

Stanley JK, Owen R, Koff S (1979) Congenital sacral anomalies. J Bone Joint Surg [Br] 61/4:401

Steindler A (1955) Kinesiology of the human body. Thomas, Springfield

Stilwell DL Jr (1956) The nerve supply of the vertebral column and the associated structures in the monkey. Anat Rec 125:139

Stilwell DL (1959) The vascular supply of vertebral structures (gross anatomy: Rabbit and monkey). Anat Rec 135:169

Stoff E (1973) Morphology of the suspensory apparatus of the spinal cord in the region of the cervical spine. Radiology 13/12:531

Stoff E, Wiebecke K. Muller G (1969) Flaval ligaments of the human spine. Verh Anat Ges 63:363

Sundaram SH, Feng CC (1977) Finite element analysis of the human thorax. J Biomech 10:505

Suth TH, Alexander J (1939) Vascular system of the human spinal cord. Arch Neurol Psychiatry 41:659

Suzuki N, Ooe K, Inoue H (1977) The strength of abdominal and back muscles in low back pain patients. Centr Jpn Orthop Traum Surg 20:332

Swatko A, Matusewicz M (1979) Variation of the place of origin and course of posterior and anterior spinal arteries in men. Folia Morphol (Warsz) 38/1:77

Szostakiewicz Sawicka H, Narkiewicz O, Reicher M (1972) Body posture and dorsal muscles in phylogenesis. Folia Morphol Praha 31/4:459

Takeda T (1975) Three-dimensional observation of collagen framework of human lumbar discs. J Jpn Orthop Assoc 49:45

Tanz SS (1953) Motion of the lumbar spine. AJR 69:399

Taylor JR (1972) Persistence of the notochondal canal in vertebrae. J Anat 111/2:211

Taylor JR (1975) Growth of human intervertebral discs and vertebral bodies. J Anat 120/1:49

Taylor TK, Ryan MD (1979) A simplified surgical approach for lumbar disc excision. Aust NZ J Surg 49/1:122

Theron J, Houtteville JP, Ammerich H, Alves de Sonsa A, Adam H, Thurel C, Rey A, Houdard R (1976) Lumbar phlebography by catheterization of the lateral sacral and ascending lumbar veins with abdominal compression. Neuroradiology 11:175

Theron J, Houtteville JP, Ammerich M, Alves de Souza A, Adam M, Thurel CL, Rey A, Loyau G (1977) La phlébographie lombaire. Rev Rhum 44:165

Thistle HG, Hislop HJ, Moffroid M, Lowman EW (1967) Isokinetic contraction: A new concept of resistive exercise. Arch Phys Med Rehabil 48:279

Tillmann B (1975) Functional morphology of the human atlanto-occipital joint. Proceedings of the 10th international congress of anatomy. Tokyo.

Tkaczuk H (1968) Tensile properties of human lumbar longitudinal ligaments. Acta Orthop Scand [Suppl] 115:602

Tondury G (1959) La colonne cervicale, son développement et ses modifications durant la vie. Acta Orthop Belg 25:602

Tondury G (1972) Anatomie fonctionelle des petites articulations du rachis. Ann Med Phys 15:173

Tombol T (1964) Über die Ontogenese der vertebralen Blutzirkulation. Verh Anat Ges 7:85

Torr JBD (1957a) The arterial supply of the foetal spine cord. J Anat 91:576

Torr JBD (1957b) The blood supply of the human cord. MD Thesis, University of Manchester

Torr JBD (1958) Division of intercostal arteries. Br Med J 7:1106

Townsend EH, Rowe ML (1952) Mobility of the upper cervical spine in health and disease. Pediatrics 10:567

Trotter M (1964) Accessory sacroiliac articulations in East African skeletons. Am J Phys Antropol 22:137

Troup Hood, Chapmann (1967) Measurement of the sagittal mobility of the lumbar spine and hips. Ann Phys Med 9:308

Truex RC Jr, Johnson CH (1978) Congenital anomalies of the upper cervical spine. Orthop Clin North Am 9/4:891

Tsukada K (1939) Histologische Studien über die Zwischenwirbelscheibe des Menschen. Altersveränderungen. Akad Kioto 25:1–29, 207

Tulsi RS (1971) Growth of the human vertebral column. An osteological study. Acta Anat (Basel) 79/4:570

Tureen LL (1938) Circulation of the spinal cord and the effect of vascular occlusion. Res Publ Assoc Res Nerv Ment Dis 18:394

Turnbull IM, Brieg A, Hassler O (1966) Blood supply of cervical spinal cord in man. J Neurosurg 24:951

Tveten L (1976a) Spinal cord vascularity. I. Extraspinal sources of spinal cord arteries in man. Acta Radiol [Diagn] (Stockh) 17/1:1

Tveten L (1976b) Spinal cord vascularity. III. The spinal cord arteries in man. Acta Radiol [Diagn] (Stockh) 17/3:257

Ullrich C (1980) Quantitative assessment of the lumbar spinal canal by computed tomography. Radiology 134:137

Van Buskirk C (1941) Nerves in the vertebral canal. Their relation to the sympathetic innervation of the upper extremities. Arch Surg 43:427

Vare AM (1965) The development of spinal meninges in human embryos and fetuses. J Anat Soc India 14/2:70

Veleanu C (1971) Vertebral structural peculiarities with a role in the cervical spine mechanics. Folia Morphol (Praha) 19/4:388

Veleanu C (1975) Contributions of the anatomy of the cervical spine. Functional and pathogenetic significance of certain structures of the cervical vertebrae. Acta Anat (Basel) 92/3:467

Veleanu C, Diaconescu N (1975) Contribution to the clinical anatomy of the vertebral column. Considerations on the stability and the instability at the height of the «vertebral units». Anat Anz 137/3:287

Veleanu C, Grun V, Diaconescu M, Cocota E (1972) Structural peculiarities of the thoracic spine: their functional significance. Acta Anat (Basel) 82/1:97

Verbiest H (1949) Sur certaines formes rares de compression de la queue de cheval. I. Les sténoses osseuses du canal vértébral. In: Hommage à Clovis Vincent. Paris, Maloine, pp 161

Verbiest H (1955) Further experiences on the pathological influence of a developmental narrowness of the bony lumbar vertebral canal. J Bone Joint Surg [Br] 37:576

Verbiest H (1968) A lateral approach of the cervical spine. Technique and indications. J Neurosurg 28:191

Verbiest H (1970) La chirurgie antérieure et latérale du rachis cervical. Neurochirurgie [Suppl 2] 16:212

Verbiest H (1976a) Fallacies of the present definition, nomenclature and classification of the stenoses of the lumbar vertebral canal. Spine 1/4:217

Verbiest H (1976b) L'abord antérolatéral dans le traitement des fractures et luxations de la colonne cervicale. Louvain Med 95:435

Vessilopoulos D (1977) Fetal development of the human cervical spine and cord. Acta Anat (Basel) 98/1:116

Virgin WJ (1951) Experimental investigations into the physical properties of the intervertebral disc. J Bone Joint Surg [Br] 33:607

Vlach O (1978) An anterior approach to the thoracolumbar junction by a transthoracoretroperitoneal route. Acta Chir Orthop Traumatol Cech 45/1:15

Voena G (1956) Ricerche anatomiche sulla configurazione e sulla architecttura del legamenti interspinosi del segmento lombare del rachide dell'uomo. Boll Soc Ital Biol Sper 32:130

Vogelsang H (1970) Intraosseous spinal venography. Excerpta Medica, Amsterdam

von Ludinghausen MH (1968) The veins of the human vertebral canal and their function. MMW 110/1:20

von Luschka H (1850) Die Nerven des menschlichen Wirbelkanales. Laupp & Siebeck, Tübingen von Luschka H (1858) Die Halbgelenke des menschlichen Körpers. Karpess, Berlin

von Sudinghansen M, Dziallas P (1972a) The venous system of the human vertebral column. Folia Angiol 20/3:100

von Sudinghansen M, Dziallas P (1972b) The development of the human epidural space. Anat Anz 130/5:571

Wagoner G, Pendergrass EP (1932) Intrinsic circulation of the vertebral body with roentgenologic considerations. AJR 27:818

Walter (1885) Veines du rachis. Thèse Médecine, Paris

Walmsley R (1953) The development and growth of the intervertebral disc. Edinburgh Med J 60. 4/56:341

Warwick R, Williams PL (1973) Gray's anatomy, 35th edn. Longman, Edinburgh

Watkins MB (1953) Posteriolateral fusion of the lumbar and lumbosacral spine. J Bone Joint Surg 35 A: 1014–1018

Weisl H (1954) The ligaments of the sacroiliac joint examined with particular reference to the function. Acta Anat (Basel) 20:201

Weisl H (1955) The articular surfaces of the sacroiliac joint and their relation to the movements of the sacrum. Acta Anat (Basel) 22:1

Weisl H (1955) The movements of the sacroiliac joint. Acta Anat (Basel) 23:80

Werner S (1957) Studies in spontaneous atlas dislocation. Acta Orthop Scand 23 (Suppl)

White AA (1969) Analysis of the mechanics of the thoracic spine in man. An experimental study of autopsy specimens. Acta Orthop Scand [Suppl] 127:8–88

White AA, Hirsch C (1971) The significance of the vertebral posterior elements in the mechanics of the thoracic spine. Clin Orthop 81:2

White AA, Johnson RM, Panjabi MM, Southwick WO (1975) Biomechanical analysis of clinical stability in the cervical spine. Clin Orthop 109:185

White AA (1971) Kinematics of the normal spine as related to scoliosis. J Biomech. 4:405

White AA, Panjabi MM (1978a) The basic kinematics of the human spine. A review of past and current knowledge. Spine 3/1:12

White AA, Panjabi MM (1978b) Clinical biomechanics of the spine. Lippincott, Philadelphia 1–534

Whitesides TF Jr Bhazanfar ASS (1976) On the management of unstable fractures of the thoracolumbar spine. Spine 1:99

Whitesides TE Jr, McDonald AP (1978) Lateral retropharyngeal approach to the upper cervical spine. Orthop Clin North Am 9/4:1115

Wiberg G (1949) Black pain in relation to nerve supply of intervertebral disc. Acta Orthop Scand 19:211–221

Wigh RE (1980) The thoracolumbar and lumbosacral transitional junctions. Spine 5/3:215–222

Wilder DG, Pope MH, Frymoyer JW (1980) The functional topography of the sacroiliac joint. Spine 5/6:575–579

Wilkie R, Beetham R (1980) Trans-femoral lumbar epidural venography. Spine 5/3:424–431

Willis TA (1923/1924) The lumbosacral vertebral column in man, its stability of form and function. Am J Anat 32:95

Willis TA (1929) An analysis of vertebral anomalies. Am J Surg 6:163

Willis TA (1949) Nutrient arteries of the vertebral bodies. J Bone Joint Surg [Am] 31:538

Willis TA (1959) Lumbosacral anomalies. J Bone Joint Surg [Am] 41:935

Wiltse LL, Bateman JG, Hutchinson RH, Nelson WE (1968) The paraspinal sacrospinalis-splitting approach to the lumbar spine. J Bone Joint Surg 50 A: 919

Winckler G (1964) Manuel d'anatomie topographique et fonctionnelle. Masson, Paris

Wollin DG (1963) The os odontoideum. Separate odontoid process. J Bone Joint Surg [Am] 45:1459

Wood PM (1979) Applied anatomy and physiology of the vertebral column. Physiotherapy 10/65/8:248

Woolam DHM, Millen JW (1955) The arterial supply of the spinal cord and its significance. J Neurol Neurosurg Psychiatry 18:97

Yettram AL, Jackman MJ (1980) Equilibrium analysis for the forces in the human spinal column and its musculature. Spine 5/3:402–411

Yinchuan (1978) Anatomical observations on lumbar nerve posterior rami. Chin Med J 4/6:492

Yune SH, Lee HK (1972) A study of motion and height of the lumbar discs by lumbar dynamogram. Korea Univ Med J 9/2:273

Zaborowski Z (1978) Extrafetal development of the axis on the basis of roentgenoanthropometric measurements. Folia Morphol Praha 37/2:167

Zaki W (1973) Aspects morphologiques et fonctionnels de l'annulus fibrosus du disque intervertébral de la colonne dorsale. Arch Anat Pathol 21/4:401

Zolima EJ (1966) Epidural veins of the vertebral canal and their role in collateral circulation in men and animals (in Russian). Mat 2. Itogov Nanch Konf Prob Kompensat Krokoobrashch Innervat Organov (Ryazan) 408

Zuckschwerdt L, Emminger E, Bidermann F, Zettel H (1955) Wirbelgelenk und Bandscheibe. Hippocrates, Stuttgart

Zyablov VI (1965) The development and age related features of the nervous elements of the spinal meninges in man (in Russian). Trudy 6 Nanchnoi. Konferentsi Povozrastnoi Morphologü Fiziologü I Bioklimii. 422

Subject Index

W. Seeger

Microsurgery of the Spinal Cord and Surrounding Structures

Anatomical and Technical Principles

1982. 201 figures. VII, 410 pages. ISBN 3-211-81648-8

Contents: Introduction. – Operations on the Craniovertebral Junction. – Operations on the Cervical Spine. – Operations on the Thoracic Spine. – Operations in the Lumbar and Lumbosacral Regions. – Appendix. – References. – Subject Index.

H. A. Keim

The Adolescent Spine

With contributions by J. R. Denton, H. M. Dick, J. G. McMurtry, III., D. P. Roye Jr.

2nd edition. 1982. 366 figures. XV, 254 pages. ISBN 3-540-90612-6

Contents: Embryology and Anatomy of the Human Spine. – Neurology of the Spine. – Biomechanics of the Adolescent Spine. – Congenital Problems in the Adolescent Spine. – Tumors in the Adolescent Spine. – Trauma and the Adolescent Spine. – The Cervical Adolescent Spine. – Infections and Inflammatory Lesions of the Adolescent Spine. – Scoliosis. – Clinical and Roentgenographic Evaluation of the Scoliosis Patient. – Nonoperative Treatment for Scoliosis. – The Operative Management of Scoliosis. – Kyphosis and Lordosis. – Index.

H. Pettersson, D. C. F. Harwood-Nash

CT and Myelography of the Spine and Cord

Techniques, Anatomy and Pathology in Children

1982. 93 figures. XIV, 122 pages. ISBN 3-540-11322-3

Contents: Introduction. – Technique. – The Normal Spine and Spinal Cord. – Spinal Dysraphism. – Neoplasms. – Trauma, Infection, and Inflammation. – Musculoskeletal Disorders and Dysplasias Involving the Spinal Column and Canal. – Scoliosis. – The Diagnostic Accuracy of CTMM. – Adverse Effects of the Examination. – Diagnostic Protocols. – Reference List. – Subject Index.

G. M. Bedbrook

The Care and Management of Spinal Cord Injuries

Foreword by R. W. Jackson

1981. 147 figures. XVI, 351 pages. ISBN 3-540-90494-8

Contents: Prevention of Spinal Paralysis: Emergency Management. – Examination. – Diagnosis. – Nontraumatic Causes of Spinal Paralysis. – Early Management of Spinal Injuries. – Surgical Procedures for Associated Injuries. – Rehabilitation. – Nursing Management. – Medical Management. – Physical and Occupational Therapy. – Orthotics. – Follow-up Service. – General Medical Care of Spinal Paralytic Patients. – Decubitus Ulcers (Pressure Sores). – Contractures and Spasm. – Pain and Phantom Sensation. – Pott's Paraplegia. – Traumatic Paraplegia in Children. – Care of Children with Spinal Bifida. – Physiologic Studies. – Pathologic Considerations of Spinal Paralysis. – Recent Research in Spinal Cord Injuries. – Design, Organization, and Staffing of a Spinal Paralysis Unit. – Home Nursing Care and Volunteer Organizations. – Paraplegia in Developing Countries. – The Future. – Index.

Springer-Verlag
Berlin
Heidelberg
New York

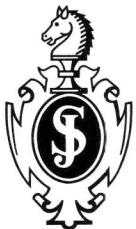

R. Bombelli
Osteoarthritis of the Hip
Classification and Pathogenesis
The Role of Osteotomy an a Consequent Therapy

With a Foreword by M. E. Müller
2nd, revised and enlarged edition. 1982. 374 figures
(128 figures in color), 6 tables. Approx. 392 pages.
ISBN 3-540-11422-X

Bone and Joint Disease
With contributions by numerous experts
Editor: C. L. Berry
1982. 110 figures. IX, 307 pages (Current Topics in
Pathology, Volume 71)
ISBN 3-540-11235-9

C. F. Brunner, B. G. Weber
Special Techniques in Internal Fixation
Translated from the German by T. C. Telger
1982. 91 figures. X, 198 pages
ISBN 3-540-11056-9

Current Concepts of External Fixation of Fractures
Editor: H. K. Uhthoff
Associate Editor: E. Stahl
1982. 227 figures. X, 442 pages
ISBN 3-540-11314-2

J. Guyot
Atlas of Human Limb Joints
Illustrations by J. L. Vannson
Translated from the French by R. A. Elson
1981. 133 figures. X, 252 pages
ISBN 3-540-10380-5

U. Heim, K. M. Pfeiffer
Small Fragment Set Manual
Technique Recommended by the ASIF Group
ASIF: Swiss Association for the Study of Internal Fixation
Translated from the German by R. L. Batten, K. M. Pfeiffer
2nd edition. 1982. 215 figures in more than 500 separate illustrations. IX, 396 pages
ISBN 3-540-11143-3

F. Horan, P. Beighton
Orthopaedic Problems in Inherited Skeletal Disorders
Foreword by W. J. W. Sharrard
1982. 98 figures. XVI, 142 pages
ISBN 3-540-11311-8

E. Letournel, R. Judet
Fractures of the Acetabulum
Translated from the French and Edited by R. A. Elson
1981. 289 figures in 980 separate illustrations. XXI, 428 pages
ISBN 3-540-09875-5

A. Sarmiento, L. L. Latta
Closed Functional Treatment of Fractures
1981. 545 figures, 85 tables. XII, 608 pages
ISBN 3-540-10384-8

F. Schajowicz
Tumors and Tumorlike Lesions of Bone and Joints
1981. 948 figures, 2 color inserts. XIV, 581 pages
ISBN 3-540-90492-1

F. Séquin, R. Texhammar
AO/ASIF Instrumentation
Manual of Use and Care
Introduction and Scientific Aspects by H. Willenegger
Translated from the German by T. C. Telger
1981. Approx. 1300 figures. 17 separate Checklists.
XVI, 306 pages
ISBN 3-540-10337-6

Shoulder Surgery
Editors: I. Bayley, L. Kessel
Foreword by H. Osmond-Clarke
1982. 199 figures. XVI, 221 pages
ISBN 3-540-11040-2

E. W. Sommerville
Displacement of the Hip in Childhood
Aetiology, Management and Sequelae
1982. 262 figures. XIII, 200 pages
ISBN 3-540-10936-6

Springer-Verlag
Berlin Heidelberg New York

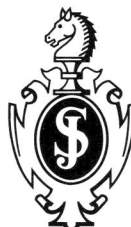